3rd Edition

Nursing Health Assessment

THE FOUNDATION OF CLINICAL PRACTICE

3rd Edition

Nursing Health Assessment

THE FOUNDATION OF CLINICAL PRACTICE

PATRICIA M. DILLON, PhD, RN

Associate Professor
La Salle University
School of Nursing and Health Sciences
Philadelphia, Pennsylvania

F.A. Davis Company • Philadelphia

F. A. Davis Company
1915 Arch Street
Philadelphia, PA 19103
www.fadavis.com

Printed in the United States of America

Last digit indicates print number: 10 9 8 7 6 5 4 3 2 1

Publisher: Lisa Houck
Senior Content Project Manager: Elizabeth Hart
Electronic Product Manager: Sandra Glennie
Design and Illustration Manager: Carolyn O'Brien

As new scientific information becomes available through basic and clinical research, recommended treatments and drug therapies undergo changes. The author(s) and publisher have done everything possible to make this book accurate, up to date, and in accord with accepted standards at the time of publication. The author(s), editors, and publisher are not responsible for errors or omissions or for consequences from application of the book, and make no warranty, expressed or implied, in regard to the contents of the book. Any practice described in this book should be applied by the reader in accordance with professional standards of care used in regard to the unique circumstances that may apply in each situation. The reader is advised always to check product information (package inserts) for changes and new information regarding dose and contraindications before administering any drug. Caution is especially urged when using new or infrequently ordered drugs.

Library of Congress Cataloging-in-Publication Data

Dillon, Patricia M., author.
Nursing health assessment. The foundation of clinical practice / Patricia M. Dillon. — Edition 3.
p. ; cm.
Foundation of clinical practice
Preceded by: Nursing health assessment. Clinical pocket guide / Patricia M. Dillon. 2nd ed. c2007.
Includes bibliographical references and index.
ISBN 978-0-8036-4400-7
I. Title. II. Title: Foundation of clinical practice.
[DNLM: 1. Nursing Assessment—Case Reports. 2. Nursing Assessment—Handbooks. 3. Medical History Taking—methods—Case Reports. 4. Medical History Taking—methods—Handbooks. 5. Physical Examination—methods—Case Reports. 6. Physical Examination—methods—Handbooks. WY 49]
RT48
616.07'5—dc23

2015036276

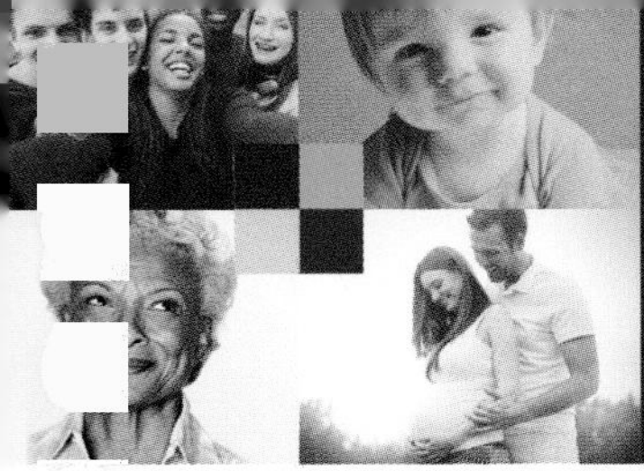

DEDICATION

To my patients and students

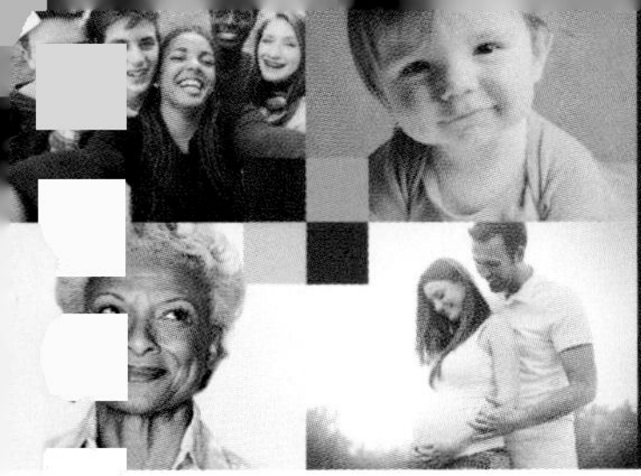

ACKNOWLEDGMENTS

I would like to acknowledge the staff of F.A. Davis, especially Lisa Houck, Elizabeth Hart, and Teresa Wilson, for their support and expertise throughout this project.

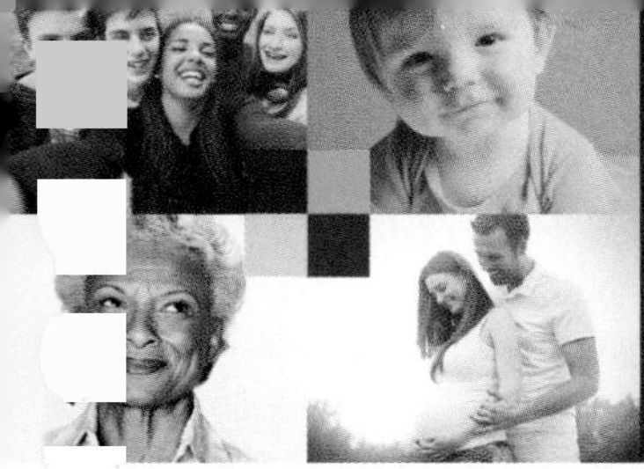

PREFACE

Welcome to F. A. Davis's *Nursing Health Assessment: The Foundation of Clinical Practice 3rd Edition.* Assessment is the first step in the nursing process and is the most important. Assessment directs the rest of the nursing process. It does not matter what your outcomes and goals are if you "missed it on assessment."

Assessment is a thinking, doing, and feeling process. You need to think as you interact with your patients. Think critically as you proceed through the assessment process and make clinical decisions. To do assessment well, you need to develop trusting relationships with your patients. Assessment is a skill, and as with any skill, the more you practice, the better you become. This book will walk you through the assessment process, but it is up to you to develop the skill. As a beginning practitioner, focus on learning the normal. Once you are able to identify normal, if something abnormal occurs, you will know! Initially, you may not be able to identify the abnormal, but you will know that it doesn't belong. Don't worry; with practice, soon you will not only know normal, but will be able to identify the abnormal.

Nursing Health Assessment: The Foundation for Clinical Practice contains:

- Primary function of every system
- Developmental and cultural considerations
- Key history questions with specific symptoms
- Integration with other systems
- The physical assessment, which includes:
  - Anatomical landmarks
  - Approach
  - Position for exam
  - Tools needed for exam
  - Assessment procedure and normal and abnormal findings with helpful hints identified by this symbol and alerts identified by this symbol

This edition provides you with the essentials to perform a thorough assessment. Take this with you wherever you are practicing nursing: the hospital, the home, the community, schools, and long-term care facilities. As a valuable resource, use it to:

- Perfect your assessment skills
- Differentiate normal from abnormal findings
- Validate your assessment findings

Never forget that you learn much from your patients, so view your encounters with them as a means to learn assessment and develop your skills. And practice, practice, practice!

Patricia M. Dillon, PhD, RN

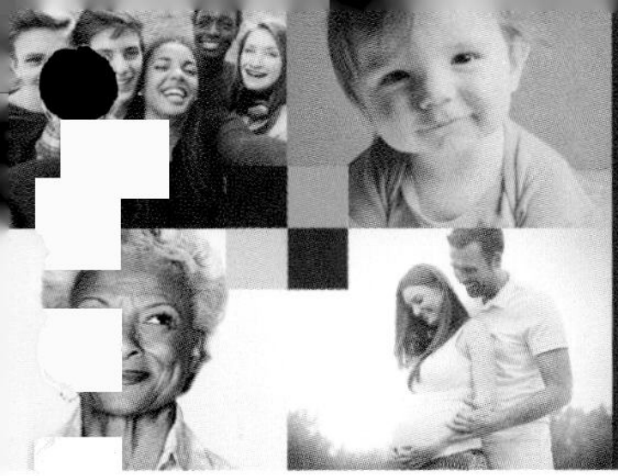

CONTENTS

CHAPTER 1
Introduction to Assessment 1

CHAPTER 2
Assessing the Integumentary System 29

CHAPTER 3
Assessing the Head, Face, and Neck 73

CHAPTER 4
Assessing the Eyes and the Ears 107

CHAPTER 5
Assessing the Respiratory System 152

CHAPTER 6
Assessing the Cardiovascular System 172

CHAPTER 7
Assessing the Peripheral-Vascular and Lymphatic Systems 204

CHAPTER 8
Assessing the Breasts 226

CHAPTER 9
Assessing the Abdomen 245

CHAPTER 10
Assessing the Female Genitourinary System 275

CHAPTER 11
Assessing the Male Genitourinary System 297

CHAPTER 12
Assessing the Motor-Musculoskeletal System 314

CHAPTER 13
Assessing the Sensory-Neurologic System 345

CHAPTER 14
Assessing the Mother-to-Be 375

CHAPTER 15
Assessing the Newborn and Infant 401

CHAPTER 16
Assessing the Toddler and Preschooler 438

CHAPTER 17
Assessing the School-Age Child and Adolescent 448

CHAPTER 18
Assessing the Older Adult 472

CHAPTER 19
Assessing the Homeless Person 502

CHAPTER 20
Assessing Pain 509

CHAPTER 21
Approach to the Mental Health Assessment 529

CHAPTER 22
Assessing Nutrition 562

CHAPTER 23
Assessing Spirituality 569

CHAPTER 24
Assessing Culture 573

CHAPTER 25
Assessing the Patient's Environment 580

CHAPTER 26
Assessing Abuse 591

CHAPTER 27
Assessing the Dying Patient 599

Index 610

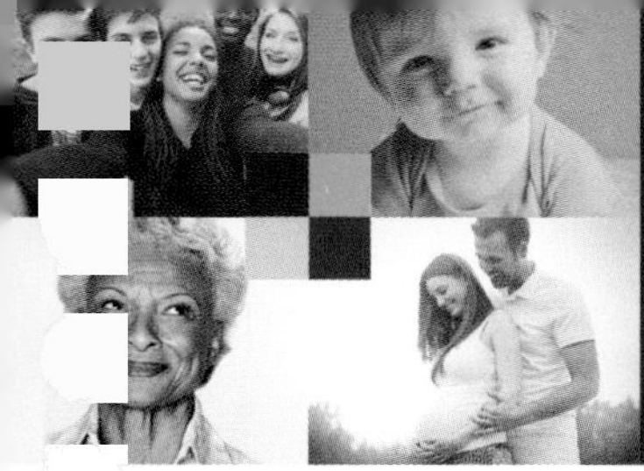

Introduction to Assessment

Assessment: An Overview

Assessment

- The first step in the nursing process
- A data collection process
- A continuous process
- A thinking, doing, feeling process

Thinking Process

Essentials of Critical Thinking

- Intellectual integrity
  - High standards
  - Hold yourself to same standards
- Intellectual perseverance
  - Persist to find answer, to understand
- Faith in reason
  - Look out for best interest of all
  - Consider consequences
- Intellectual justice
  - Open to all viewpoints, impartiality and fairness

Critical Thinking Skills

- Divergent thinking: analyzing different point of view
- Reasoning: differentiating fact (truth) from assumptions (beliefs)
- Reflection: step back and consider "if. . . then" possibilities
- Creativity: think outside of the box
- Clarification: addressing assumptions, comparing, contrasting. Ask, "What is similar, what is different?"
- Basic support: evidence-based practice

Doing Process

Psychomotor skills are needed to perform the four techniques of physical assessment

- Inspection
- Palpation
- Percussion
- Auscultation

Feeling Process

- Interpersonal/affective skills needed to develop caring, therapeutic nurse-client relationships

Ethical Skills

- Responsible and accountable for practice
- Patient advocate
- Respect clients' rights
- Assure confidentiality
- Health Insurance Portability and Accountability Act (HIPAA)

The nurse's goal is to diagnose and treat human responses to actual or potential health problems. Clinical decisions are made through critical thinking, evidence-based practice, and experience.

Levels of Preventative Health Care

- Primary: focus on health promotion and prevention (e.g., health fairs)
- Secondary: focus on early detection, prompt intervention and health maintenance (e.g., acute care)
- Tertiary: focus on rehabilitative, extended, or end-of-life care (e.g., home care)

Data

Types

- Subjective: what the patient tells you or is feeling, symptoms, (e.g., the history)
- Objective: measurable, observable, signs, (e.g., physical findings, diagnostic test results)

Sources

- Primary: the patient
- Secondary: family members, healthcare providers, friends

Prioritizing Data

- Primary: life threatening problems (e.g., airway obstruction)
- Secondary: require prompt attention to prevent further progression or deterioration (e.g., pain)
- Tertiary: important, but doesn't require immediate attention (e.g., Patient teaching)

Communication Tips

- Introduce yourself.
- Don't rush.
- Avoid interruptions.
- Establish eye contact.
- Explain what you are doing.
- Work at same level as patient.
- Consider personal space.
- Begin with the patient's problem.
- Leave sensitive topics until the end.
- Consider patient's cultural background.
- Consider developmental level of patient.
- Be nonjudgmental.
- Avoid "why" questions.
- Nonverbal communication more valid than verbal.
- Be honest.
- Present reality.
- Look for teachable moments.
- Provide reassurance.
- Be respectful.
- Avoid medical jargon.
- Avoid leading the patient.
- Ask one question at a time.
- Listen!

SBAR

- S = situation
- B = background
- A = assessment
- R = recommendation

Documentation

Electronic Health Records are being used more and more as the preferred method for documentation.

- Source-oriented: discipline/department specific
- Problem-oriented:

SOAPIE

S = subjective data
O = objective data
A = assessment
P = plan
I = intervention
E = evaluation

DAR

D = data
A = action
R = response

PIE

P = problem
I = interventions
E = evaluation

Physical Assessment

When performing the skills of physical assessment, you are using your senses to collect data.

Inspection

- Types: direct, indirect
  - Direct: direct visualization
  - Indirect: using a light source and/or magnifier for visualization (e.g., otoscope)
- Senses: sight, smell

- Data: surface characteristics, symmetry, gross abnormalities, signs of distress, unusual odors

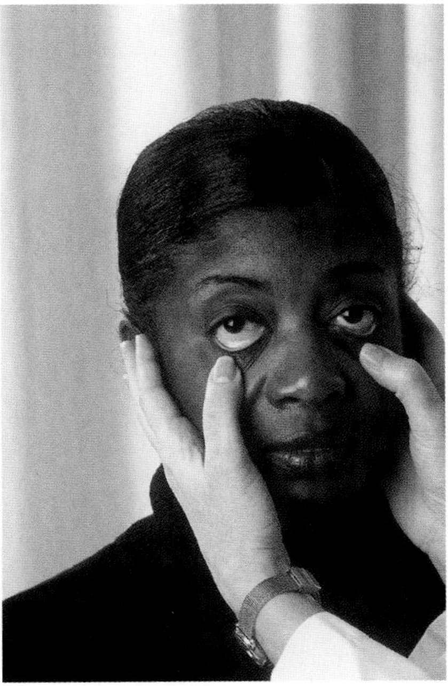

Inspection

Palpation

- Types: single handed or bimanual
  - Light: indenting the skin no more than ½ inch

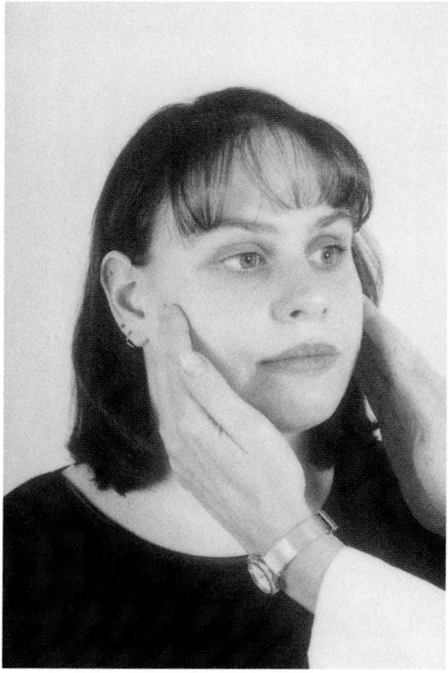

Light palpation

  - Deep: indenting the skin more than ½ inch

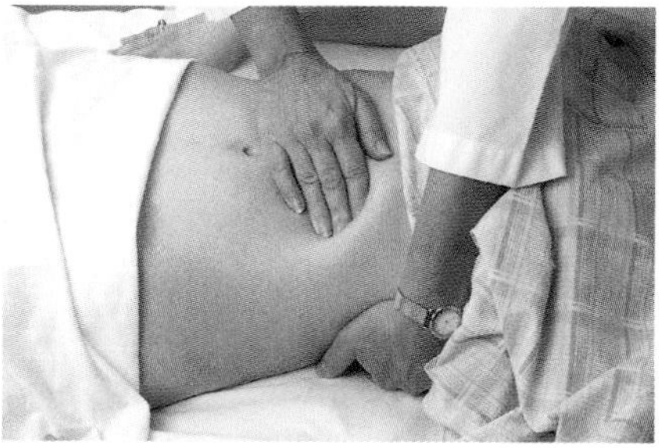

Deep palpation, bimanual

- Ballottement: assess partially free floating objects

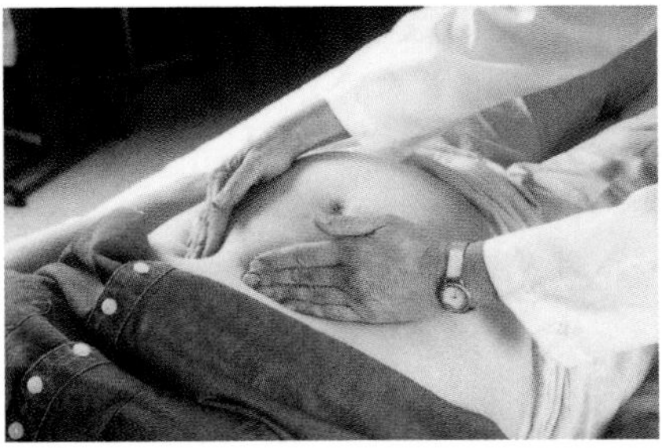

Ballottement

- Different parts of the hand are best for assessment data.
  - Dorsal aspect of hand: best to assess temperature changes

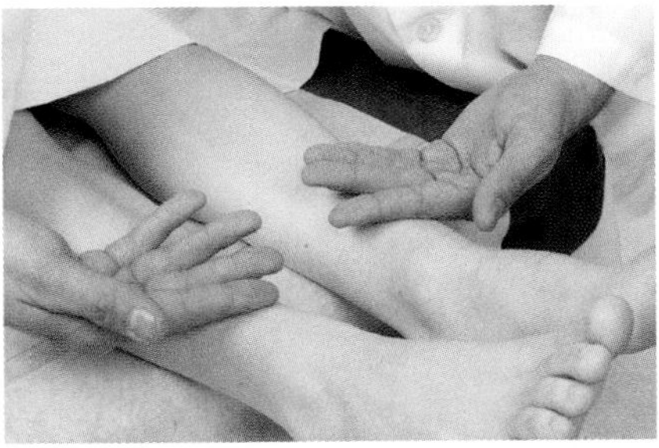

Palpating temperature changes with dorsal part of hand

  - Balls and ulnar surface of hands (bones): best to assess vibrations
  - Finger pads/tips: best to assess fine sensations
- Sense: touch
- Data:
  - Light palpation: surface characteristics (e.g., temperature, texture)
  - Deep palpation: organs, masses, tenderness
  - Ballottement: size, shape of partially free floating objects (e.g., fetal position)

Percussion

- Types: direct, indirect
  - Direct (immediate): directly tapping over body surface to elicit a sound or area of tenderness

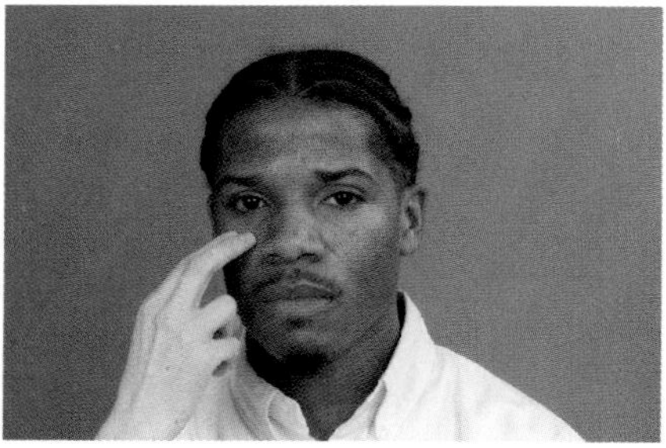

Direct percussion

  - Indirect (mediate): placing nondominant hand over body surface, striking to elicit a sound or area of tenderness

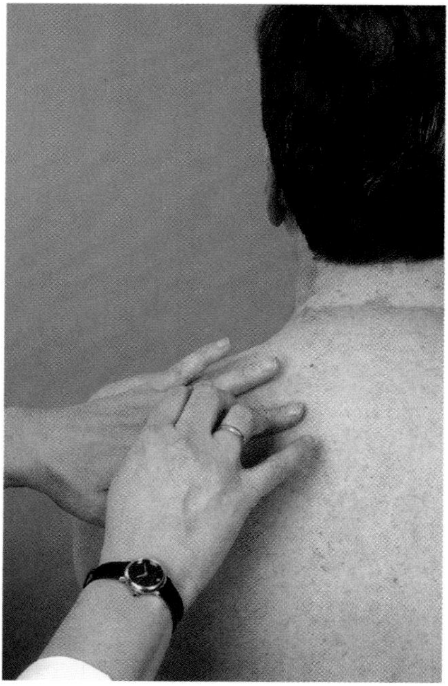

Indirect percussion

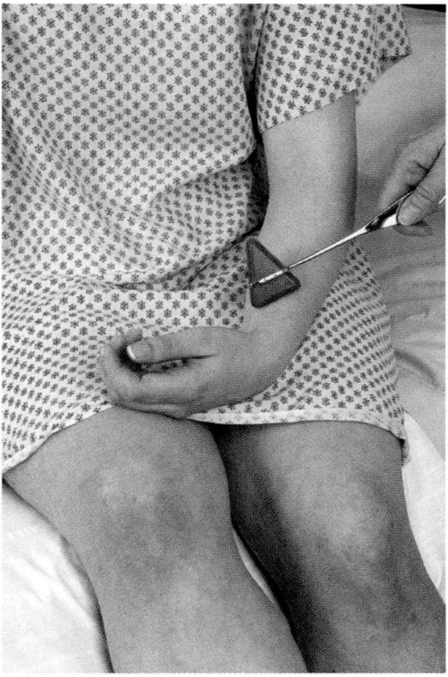

Using a percussion hammer

- Fist or blunt: directly or indirectly striking a body surface to note area of tenderness

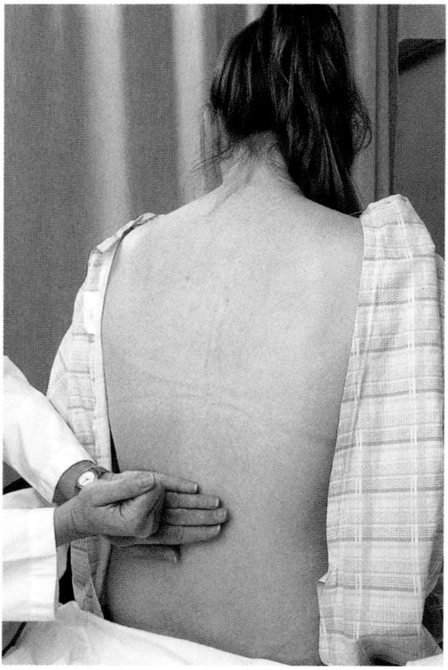

Percussing for costovertebral angle tenderness

- Senses: touch and hearing
- Data: direct or indirect:
  - Density (air, fluid, solid)
  - Size and shape
  - Tenderness
  - Deep tendon reflexes
- Percussion sounds
  - Resonance: low, loud, long (e.g., lung)
  - Hyperresonance: very low, very loud, very long (e.g., emphysema)
  - Dull: high, soft, short (e.g., liver)
  - Flat: very high, very soft, very short (e.g., soft tissue)
  - Tympany: medium, medium, medium, musical, drumlike (e.g., stomach)
- Fist/Blunt:
  - Tenderness

Auscultation

- Types: direct, indirect
  - Direct: directly listening for sounds
  - Indirectly: using a stethoscope to hear sounds
- Stethoscope types:
  - Single head: pressure-sensitive to detect high- and low-pitch sounds; apply heavy pressure for high-pitch sounds and light pressure for low-pitch sounds
  - Combination head with bell and diaphragm: diaphragm (flat side) best for high-pitch sounds; use heavy pressure. Bell (cone shaped) best for low-pitch sounds; use light pressure.

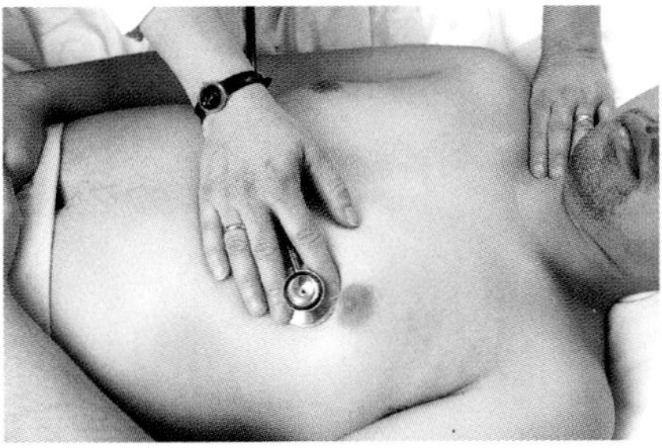

Listening with diaphragm of stethoscope

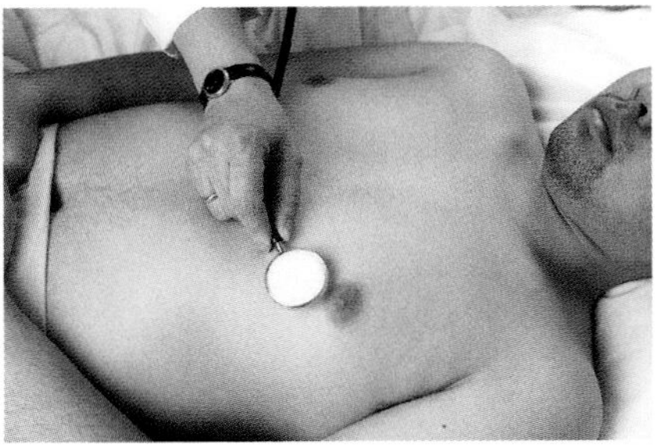

Listening with bell of stethoscope

- Senses: hearing
- Data:
  - Heart sounds (high, medium and low pitch)
  - Lung sounds (high)
  - Bowel sounds (high)
  - Vascular sounds (low)

Tools of Assessment

EQUIPMENT	PURPOSE	TYPES
Thermometer	Body temperature	Oral (glass thermometers are becoming obsolete due to mercury). Electronic for oral, rectal, axillary. Tympanic uses infrared sensors to measure tympanic membrane temperature. Temporal scanners: use infrared sensors to measure temporal artery temperature. Disposable paper strips with temperature sensitive dots for oral/skin surface.
Stethoscope	Heart sounds Lung sounds Bowel sounds Vascular sounds	Single pressure sensitive: heavy pressure for high-pitch sound; light for low-pitch sounds. Combination with bell (best for low pitch, light pressure) and diaphragm (best for high pitch, heavy pressure). Electronic: detects high and low best for hearing impaired. Fetoscope: best for fetal heart sounds. Doppler: uses ultrasound to detect fetal heart sounds and vascular sounds. **When using stethoscope, ear pieces should always be pointing forward.**
Sphygmomanometer	Blood pressure	Mercury (becoming obsolete due to toxicity of mercury). Aneroid.

EQUIPMENT	PURPOSE	TYPES
		Electronic. **Incorrect cuff size can lead to inaccurate readings.**
Visual acuity charts	Visual acuity Far vision Color vision	Snellen eye chart (letters or "E"). Stycar: used for children over 2½ years or illiterate adults Allen cards: used for children as young as 24 months). Pocket vision screener (scaled Snellen chart. **Test each eye separately, with and without glasses. No more than 2 mistakes with Snellen.**
Pen light	Pupils, hard to see places, such as mouth, nose	
Opthalmoscope	Funduscopic examination of the eyes Red light reflex Optic disk and physiologic cup Retinal blood vessels Retina Macula and fovea centralis	**Perform in darkened room. Use same eye as that being examined; your right eye to patient's right eye, your left eye to patient's left eye.**
Otoscope	External ear canal Tympanic membrane	**Always palpate the tragus and mastoid and pull the helix forward to check for tenderness prior to insertion of otoscope.** **Pull earlobe up and back and insert ½ inch for adult.** **Pull earlobe down and back and insert ¼ inch for child.**
Tuning fork	Hearing tests: Weber, Rinne	Low frequency (256-Hz) best for

(continued)

Tools of Assessment (continued)

EQUIPMENT	PURPOSE	TYPES
	Neurological exam: vibratory sensation	neurological vibratory examination. High frequency (52-Hz) best for assessing hearing. **Do not hold tuning fork by tines—will dampen sound.**
Nasoscope	Nostrils Nasal mucosa Turbinates Septum	
Transilluminator	Sinuses Scrotum Fontanels	**Perform in darkened room.**
Tape measure Ruler	Lengths Circumferences (e.g., legs, arms, head) Liver size Jugular venous pressure Lesions	**Centimeters are used more often than inches.**
Goniometer	Range of motion of a joint	
Triceps skinfold calipers	Body fat	
Marking pen	Marking measurements such as liver, diaphragmatic excursion, pulse sites	Markers should be washable.
Scales	Weight	Platform Bed scales Floor scales **Scales need to be calibrated.**
Tongue depressor	Mouth, gag reflex and strength of masseter muscles	**Break and discard after use.**
Cotton balls	Neurological examination: sensory	
Test tubes	Neurological examination: temperature	

EQUIPMENT	PURPOSE	TYPES
Scent Sugar, salt, lemon	Neurological examination: sensory Smell, taste	
Cup of water	Thyroid Swallowing	
Paper clip, coins	Neurological examination Stereognosis	
Gloves	Wear gloves when at risk for exposure to blood or body fluids	**Wear non-latex gloves**
Cytology brush Scraper Pap test slides Fixative Potassium hydroxide Lubricant (water soluble) Speculum Hemoccult test	Pelvic examination Rectal examination	

Approach to Assessment

- Determine system or region.
- Be systematic.
- Minimize position change.
- Expose only the area being assessed.
- Explain as you go.
- Share findings with client and teach.
- Ensure privacy and confidentiality.
- Consider developmental level of client.
- Consider cultural background of client.

Before You Begin and Before You Leave!

- Wash hands! When in doubt, wear gloves.
- General survey
- Patient safety
- Bed low position
- Side rails
- Call bell
- Personal items

- Lighting
- Tubes (oxygen, IVs, catheters)
- Wash hands!

General Survey

- Age: actual and apparent
- Gender
- Race
- Affect
- Level of consciousness
- Dress
- Posture
- Speech
- Obvious abnormalities or signs of distress

Vital Signs and Anthropometric Measurements

- Temperature
- Pulse
- Respirations
- Pulse oximetry
- Blood pressure
- Height
- Weight
- Body mass index

Head-to-Toe Approach

- Integumentary
- Head, eyes, ears, nose, and throat
- Breast
- Respiratory
- Cardiovascular
- Gastrointestinal
- Musculoskeletal
- Neurological
- Genitourinary/reproductive

Documentation

- Accurate
- Concise
- Objective
- Record by systems
- Chart pertinent negatives

Initially, as you begin to develop your assessment and clinical decision-making skills, your focus is limited. You have difficulty looking at your patient as a whole; instead you tend to focus on the parts while you strive to develop skills. But remember, no single finding stands alone. All of the systems are related, so a problem in one system will eventually affect every other system. With experience, as you develop your assessment and clinical decision-making skills, you will begin to recognize patterns and to see the entire picture while zooming in on the acute problem.

With practice, you will develop competence in your skills and confidence in your findings. So, practice and learn from your patients—they can teach you so much!

THE COMPLETE HEALTH ASSESSMENT

A complete health assessment includes a comprehensive history and a complete physical assessment.

Complete Health History

Biographical Data

Includes name, address, phone number, contact person, age, birth date, place of birth, gender, race/ethnicity/nationality, religion, marital status, number of dependents, educational level, occupation, social security number/health insurance, source of history/reliability, referral, advance directive.

Current Health Status

Includes symptom analysis for chief complaint and current medications (prescribed, over the counter, and/or herbal supplements), and allergies with reaction (food, drug, and environmental). (At primary level of health care when the patient does not have an acute problem, current health status should include: usual state of health, any major health problems, usual patterns of health care and any health concerns.)

Past Health History

Includes childhood illnesses, surgeries, hospitalizations, serious injuries, medical problems, immunizations, and recent travel or military service.

Family History

Includes patient, spouse, children, siblings, parents, aunts, uncles, and grandparents' health status, or, if deceased, age and cause of death.

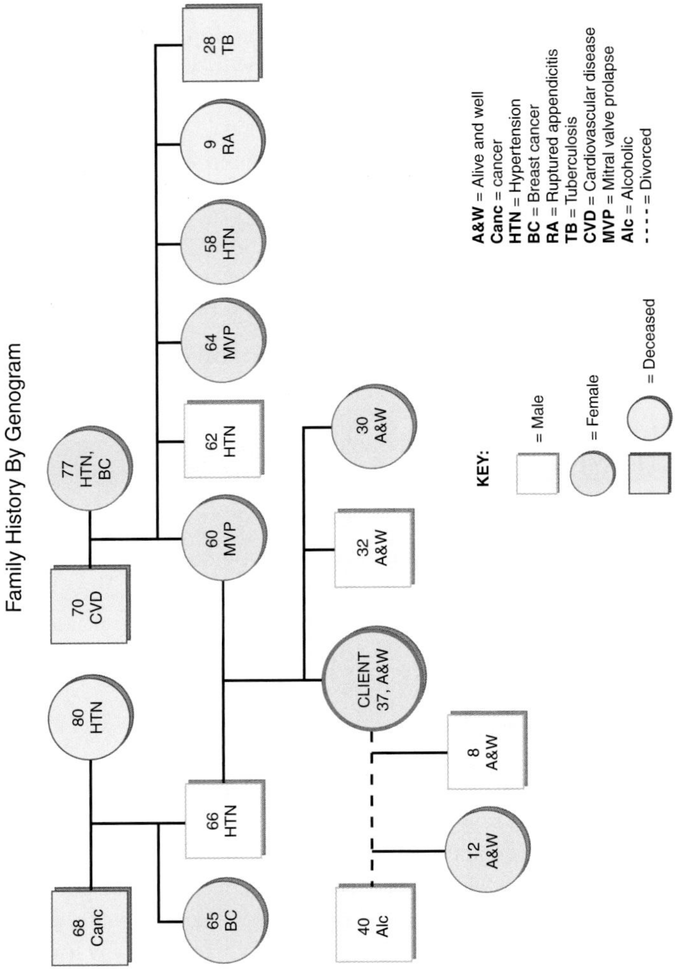

Family history by genogram.

Review of Systems

Includes questions specific to each body system and analysis of any positive symptoms.

- General: usual state of health, fatigue, weakness, changes in weight, difficulty performing activities of daily living (ADLs) Integumentrary: skin disorders, rashes, itching, scars, sores, moles, changes in skin lesions, changes in hair or nails.
  - Helpful Hint: Recommend annual skin examination.
- Head and neck: headaches, lumps, trauma, concussions, loss of consciousness, surgery, dizzy spells, fainting, stiff neck, pain with movement of head and neck, swollen glands, nodes or masses.
- Eyes: wear glasses/contacts, visual deficit, last eye examination, last glaucoma check, eye injury, tearing, pain, discharge, floaters, halos, loss of vision, double vision (diplopia), colored lights, flashes, light sensitivity, twitching, cataracts, glaucoma, eye surgery, retinal detachment, strabismus, astigmatism, amblyopia
  - Recommend routine eye examination and glaucoma check for adults every 2 years.
- Ears: last hearing test, difficulty hearing, sensitivity to sounds, ear pain, drainage, vertigo, ear infections, ringing (tinnitus), fullness, ear wax problems, hearing aids, ear care.
  - Recommend annual hearing test with physical examinations and screening for hearing deficits in elderly patients.
- Nose and sinuses: nosebleeds, broken nose, deviated septum, snoring, post-nasal drip, runny nose, sneezing, allergies, use of recreational drugs, difficulty breathing through nose, problems with sense of smell, pain over sinuses, sinus infections.
- Mouth and throat: sore throats, streptococcal infections, mouth sores, herpes, bleeding or receding gums, hoarseness, changes in quality of voice, difficulty chewing or swallowing, changes in sense of taste, dentures or bridges, last dental examination, dental surgery, dental hygiene.
  - Recommend annual dental examination.
- Respiratory: breathing problems, cough, sputum, shortness of breath (SOB) at rest or with activity, wheezing/congestion, pneumonia, asthma, bronchitis, tuberculosis (TB), last chest x-ray and results, TB testing and results, history of smoking.
- Cardiovascular: chest pain, palpitations, murmurs, skipped beats, hypertension, wakening at night SOB, dizzy spells, coldness, numbness, tingling, color changes, edema in hands and

feet, pain in legs when walking, hair loss on legs, nonhealing wounds, abnormal electrocardiogram results.
  - Recommend BP check every 1 to 2 years.
- Breasts: breast masses, lumps, pain, discharge, swelling, changes in breasts or nipples, cystic breast disease, breast cancer, breast surgery (reduction/enhancement), breast self-examination (BSE), last clinical breast examination, last mammogram.
  - Recommend BSE monthly, clinical breast examination annually, mammogram annually for patients age 40 years and older unless indicated earlier.
- Gastrointestinal: changes in appetite, indigestion, heartburn, gastroesophageal reflux (GERD), nausea, vomiting, vomiting blood, liver/gall bladder disease, jaundice, abdominal swelling, bowel pattern, changes in bowel pattern, color of stool, constipation, diarrhea, hemorrhoid, weight changes, use of laxatives and antacids, last Hematest.
  - Recommend annual fecal occult blood test and sigmoidoscopy/colonoscopy every 5–10 years for patients over age 50.
- Genitourinary: pain during urination, burning, frequency, urgency, dribbling, incontinence, hesitancy, changes in urinary stream, color of urine, history of urinary tract infections, kidney infections, kidney disease, kidney stones, nighttime urination.
- Female reproductive: menarche, description of cycle, last menstrual period, painful menstruation, excessive bleeding, irregular menses, bleeding between periods, use of contraceptives, history of sexually transmitted diseases (STDs), knowledge of STD prevention, including HIV, infertility problems, obstetrical history (pregnancies, live births, miscarriages, and abortions).
  - Recommend annual pelvic examination with Pap test for sexually active women.
- Male reproductive: lesions, discharge, painful urination, painful intercourse, prostate or scrotal problems, history of STDs, infertility problems, impotence or sterility, satisfaction with sexual performance, knowledge of STD prevention including HIV, use of contraceptives, testicular self-examination (TSE), prostate examination.
  - Recommend monthly TSE.
  - Annual digital rectal prostate examination for men age 50 or older.
- Musculoskeletal: fractures, sprains, muscle cramps, pain, weakness, joint swelling, redness, limited range of motion, joint

deformity, noise with movement, spinal deformities, low back pain, loss of height, osteoporosis, DJD, rheumatoid arthritis, difficulty with ADLs, use of calcium supplements.
  - Recommend dexascan for bone density for postmenopausal women.
- Neurological: loss of consciousness, fainting, seizures, head injury, changes in cognition or memory, hallucinations, speech problems, sensory disturbances (numbness, tingling, loss of sensation), motor problems with gait, balance, coordination, inability to perform ADLs.
- Endocrine: thyroid disease, diabetes, unexplained changes in weight or height, increased thirst, increased hunger, increased urination, heat and cold intolerance, goiter, weakness, hormone therapy, changes in skin and hair.

Psychosocial Profile

Includes health practices and beliefs, typical day, nutritional patterns, activity/exercise patterns, recreation, pets/hobbies, sleep/rest patterns, personal habits, occupational health patterns, socioeconomic status, environmental health patterns, roles/relationships, sexuality patterns, social supports, and stress/coping patterns.

Complete Physical Assessment

Approach

Two methods are used for completing a total physical assessment: a systems approach and a head-to-toe approach.

- A systems approach allows for a thorough assessment of each system, doing all assessments related to one system before moving on to the next. Better for a focused assessment.
- A head-to-toe assessment includes the same examinations as a systems assessment, but you assess each region of the body before moving on to the next. Better for a complete assessment.

No matter which approach you use, be systematic and consistent.

All four assessment techniques—inspection, percussion, palpation, and auscultation—are used to perform a complete assessment. Remember:

- Inspect for abnormalities and normal variations of visible body parts.
- Palpate to identify surface characteristics, areas of pain or tenderness, organs, and abnormalities, including masses and fremitus.

- Percuss to determine the density of underlying tissues and to detect abnormalities in underlying organs.
- Auscultate for sounds made by body organs, including the heart, lungs, intestines, and vascular structures.

Assessment data are usually charted by systems (e.g., respiratory or neurological) and by regions to a limited extent (e.g., head/neck). Your documentation can focus only on positive findings or on both positive and negative findings. No matter which format you use, always be brief and to the point and avoid generalizations.

Toolbox

You will need all of the tools of assessment identified in the other chapters of this book.

Performing a Head-to-Toe Physical Assessment

Here are some helpful hints to keep in mind as you conduct the assessment:

- Wash your hands before you begin.
- Listen to your patient.
- Provide a warm environment.
- If your patient has a problem, start at that point.
- Work from head to toe.
- Compare side to side.
- Let your patient know your findings.
- Use your time not only to assess but also to teach your patient.
- Leave sensitive or painful areas until the end of the examination.

General Survey

Get anthropometric data and vital signs, and evaluate patient's clothing, hygiene, state of well-being, nutritional status, emotional status, speech patterns, level of consciousness, affect, posture, gait, coordination and balance, and gross deformities.

Skin/Hair/Nails

- Inspect and palpate patient's visible skin for color, lesions, texture, turgor, and warmth. Continue observation throughout the examination.
- Note hair color, texture, and distribution over body.
- Observe hands and nails for clubbing or other abnormalities.

Head/Face

- Note head size, shape, and position.
- Note scalp tenderness, lesions, or masses.

PERCUSSION SOUNDS

Percussion produces sounds that vary according to the tissue being percussed. This chart shows important percussion sounds along with their characteristics and typical locations.

SOUND	INTENSITY	PITCH	DURATION	QUALITY	SOURCE
Resonance	Loud	Low	Long	Hollow	Normal lung
Tympany	Moderate to loud	Medium	Moderate	Drumlike	Gastric air bubble; intestinal air
Dullness	Soft to moderate	High	Moderate	Thudlike	Liver; full bladder; pregnant uterus
Hyperresonance	Very loud	Very low	Long	Booming	Hyperinflated lung (as in emphysema)
Flatness	Soft	Very high	Short	Flat	Muscle

THE EFFECT OF AGE ON VITAL SIGNS

Normal vital sign ranges vary with age, as this chart shows.

AGE	TEMPERATURE		PULSE RATE	RESPIRATORY RATE	BLOOD PRESSURE
	°Fahrenheit	°Celsius			
Newborn	98.6–99.8	37–37.7	120–160	30–80	Systolic: 50–52; diastolic: 25–30; mean: 35–40
3 Yr	98.5–99.5	36.9–37.5	80–125	20–30	Systolic: 78–114; diastolic: 46–78
10 Yr	97.5–98.6	36.3–37	70–110	16–22	Systolic: 90–132; diastolic: 56–86
16 Yr	97.6–98.8	36.4–37.1	55–100	15–20	Systolic: 104–108; diastolic: 60–92
Adult	96.8–99.5	36–37.5	60–100	15–20	Systolic: <120; diastolic: <80
Older Adult	96.5–97.5	35.9–36.3	60–100	15–25	Systolic: <120; diastolic: <80

- Observe for facial symmetry and note facial expressions (cranial nerve [CN] VII).
- Test sensation on face (CN V).
- Palpate temporomandibular joint for popping or tenderness.

Eyes

- Test visual acuity (CN II) with Snellen test or pocket vision screener.
- Perform test of extraocular movements (CNs III, IV, VI).
- Perform cover test and corneal light reflex test.
- Test visual fields by confrontation.
- Inspect general appearance and eyelids.
- Inspect cornea, iris, and lens with oblique lighting.
- Observe sclera and conjunctivae.
- Perform pupillary reaction to light and accommodation.
- Perform fundoscopic examination to test for red reflex and to observe disks and retinal vessels.

Ears

- Inspect external ear and canal.
- Inspect position and angle of attachment.
- Palpate tragus, mastoid, and helix for tenderness.
- Perform Weber test for lateralization, Rinne test for bone and air conduction, and whisper test for low-pitched or low-tone hearing loss (CN VIII).
- Perform otoscopic examination of canal and tympanic membrane.

Nose

- Test for patency of each nostril.
- Test sense of smell (CN I).
- Palpate for sinus tenderness.
- Observe nasal mucosa, septum, and turbinates with speculum.

Mouth/Pharynx

- Inspect and palpate lips and oral mucosa.
- Inspect teeth, gingiva, and palate.
- Inspect pharynx and tonsils.
- Test gag and swallow reflexes, and have patient say "ah" (CNs IX, X).
- Test taste on anterior and posterior tongue (CNs VII, IX).
- Inspect tongue for abnormalities, and check ROM of tongue by having patient say "d, l, n, t" (CN XII).

Neck

- Inspect and palpate thyroid gland.
- Inspect for masses, abnormal pulsations, or tracheal deviation.
- Palpate carotid pulse and listen for bruits.
- Inspect jugular veins.
- Measure jugular venous pressure.
- Palpate lymph nodes in head, neck, and clavicular areas.
- Test ROM of neck.
- Test muscle strength of neck and shoulder muscles (CN XI).

Upper Extremities

- Test for ROM and muscle strength.
- Inspect joints for swelling, redness, and deformities.
- Test hand grip.
- Test superficial and deep sensations.
- Palpate radial, ulnar, and brachial pulses.
- Test for deep tendon reflexes of biceps, triceps, and brachioradialis.
- Test coordination, rapid alternating movements, and finger-thumb opposition.
- Inspect and palpate nails, checking capillary refill and angle of attachment.
- Test for pronator drift.
- Test for accuracy of movements with point-to-point movements.

Posterior Thorax/Back

- Palpate thyroid from behind (if not done previously).
- Inspect spine and palpate muscles along spine.
- Percuss and auscultate lung fields.
- Fist/blunt percuss costovertebral angle tenderness.
- Palpate and percuss chest excursion.
- Palpate tactile fremitus.
- Note normal curvatures of spine.
- Test for kyphosis, scoliosis, and lordosis.
- Check ROM of spine.

Anterior Thorax

- Inspect, palpate, percuss, and auscultate lungs.
- Inspect and palpate precordium for pulsations, point of maximal impulse, and thrills.

- Auscultate heart.
- Inspect and palpate breasts.
- Palpate axillary and epitrochlear lymph nodes.

Abdomen

- Inspect for shape, scars, movements, and abnormalities.
- Auscultate for bowel sounds and vascular sounds.
- Percuss abdomen and organs for size.
- Obtain a liver measurement.
- Palpate lightly for tenderness.
- Palpate deeply for masses and enlarged liver, spleen, kidneys, and aorta.
- Palpate femoral arteries and inguinal lymph nodes.
- If ascites suspected, percuss for shifting dullness.

Lower Extremities

- Inspect for skin color, hair distribution, temperature, edema, and varicose veins.
- Test for ROM, muscle strength, and superficial and deep sensations.
- Palpate pulses.
- Test deep tendon reflexes (patellar and achilles) and plantar reflex.
- Observe gait, toe walk, heel walk, heel-to-toe walk, and deep knee bend.
- Perform Romberg's test and proprioception test.
- Test coordination with toe tapping and heel down shin.
- If indicated, test knees for fluid with bulge sign or patellar tap.
- If indicated, test for torn meniscus with Apley's or McMurray's test.
- Observe ROM of lower extremities.
- Test muscle strength of lower extremities.

Female Genitalia/Rectum

- Inspect and palpate external genitalia and inguinal lymph nodes.
- Perform internal examination: Inspect vagina and cervix, collect Pap smear and cultures.
- Palpate uterus and adnexa, assess cervical mobility.
- Inspect perianal area and palpate anal canal and rectum.
- Test stool for occult blood.

Male Genitalia/Rectum

- Inspect and palpate external genitalia.
- Palpate for hernias.
- Inspect perianal area for hemorrhoids or abnormalities.
- Palpate anal canal, rectum, and prostate.
- Test stool on glove for occult blood.

Documenting Physical Assessment Findings

Document physical assessment findings by system, using the following sequence:

- General survey, including anthropometric measurements and vital signs
- Integumentary
- Head, face, and neck
- Eyes
- Ears, nose, and throat
- Respiratory
- Cardiovascular
- Breasts
- Abdomen
- Male/female genitourinary
- Musculoskeletal
- Neurologic

Focused Physical Assessments

- Focused assessments are only partial ones, dealing only with systems that relate to the patient's problem, so less data are collected.
- Focused assessments are used when the patient's condition or time restraints preclude a comprehensive assessment.
- A focused physical assessment should include:
  - A general survey with vital signs and weight.
  - Assessment of level of consciousness.
  - Assessment of skin color, temperature, and texture.
  - Testing of gross motor balance and coordination.
  - Testing of extraocular movements.
  - Testing of pupillary reaction.
  - Testing of gross vision and hearing.
  - Inspection of oral mucosa as patient says "ah."
  - Auscultation of anterior and posterior breath sounds.

- Palpation of apical impulse, point of maximal impulse.
- Auscultation of heart sounds.
- Inspect abdomen.
- Auscultation of abdomen.
- Percussion of abdomen.
- Palpation of abdomen.
- Palpation of peripheral pulses.
- Testing sensation to touch on extremities.
- Palpation of muscle strength of upper and lower extremities.

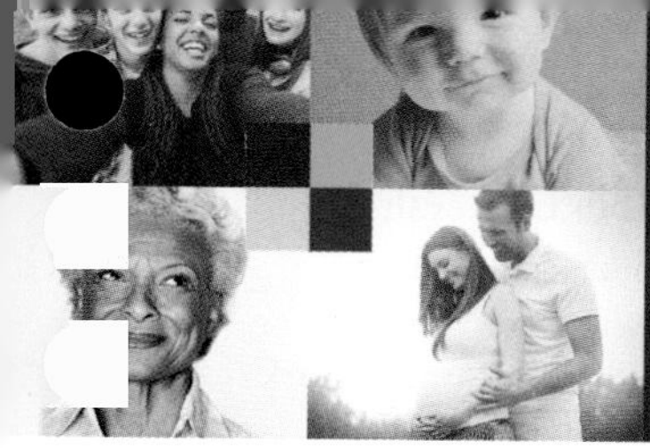

CHAPTER 2

Assessing the Integumentary System

Primary Functions

- Body's first line of defense
- Protects against trauma
- Protects against ultraviolet radiation
- Supports nerve tissue, blood vessels, sweat and sebum glands, and hair follicles
- Helps maintain body temperature
- Helps maintain fluid balance
- Provides sensation with external environment
- Involved in absorption and excretion
- Involved with immunity
- Synthesizes vitamin D

Developmental Considerations

Infants

- Skin is smooth, with little subcutaneous tissue.
- Color changes can be seen readily. Newborns often appear pinker/redder because of the lack of subcutaneous tissue.
- Physiological jaundice may occur 2 to 3 days after birth.
- Newborns have little or no coarse terminal hair; hair is shed at approximately 3 months and then is soon replaced.
- Eccrine sweat glands begin to function within a month after birth.
- Immature sweat glands lead to poor thermoregulation.
- Because there are no functioning apocrine sweat glands, babies' skin is less oily than adults' and lacks offensive odor.

- Secretion of sebum by the sebaceous glands can result in cradle cap.
- Numerous skin lesions, such as mongolian spots , nevus flammeus (port-wine stains), capillary hemangiomas (stork bites), hemangioma simplex (strawberry marks), milia, and erythema toxicum neonatorum, may be seen on the newborn.

Adolescents

- Apocrine glands begin to enlarge and function.
- Axillary sweating increases, with the potential for a more pronounced body odor.
- Sebum production increases and the skin becomes more oily, leading to acne.
- Pubic and axillary hair appear, and male and female body hair patterns become apparent.

Pregnant Clients

- Increased blood flow to the skin, particularly to the hands and feet, occurs as vessels dilate and the number of capillaries increases to dissipate heat.
- Sweating and sebaceous activity increase.
- Skin thickens and separates with stretching, with the appearance of striae.
- Hormonal changes result in hyperpigmentation. Pigmentary changes occur on the face (resulting in chloasma); on abdominal midline (the linea alba becomes the linea nigra); and on the nipples, areolae, axillae, and vulva.

Menopausal Women

- Hormonal fluctuations result in hot flashes, often accompanied by flushing of the skin and increased pigmentation.
- Facial hair increases, and there is some degree of scalp hair loss.
- Incidence of skin tags increases at menopause.

Older Adults

- Skin atrophies.
- Sebum and sweat production decreases.
- Skin becomes drier and flattens, often becoming paper-like.

- Elasticity decreases and wrinkles develop.
- Decreased melanocyte function causes gray hair and pale skin. Target areas of increased melanocyte function result in "age spots."
- Decrease in axillary, pubic, and scalp hair. Women may have increased facial hair as estrogen function is lost; men have increased nasal and ear hair growth.
- Nails grow more slowly and become thicker and more brittle.
- Specific skin lesions, including actinic keratoses, basal cell carcinomas, seborrheic keratoses, stasis ulcers, senile pruritus , and keratotic horns, are more common in elderly persons.

Age-Related Skin Disorders

AGE	DISORDER
Children	Impetigo Atopic dermatitis or eczema Pityriasis rosea Juvenile plantar dermatosis Rashes secondary to bacterial or viral infections Pediculosis capitis Varicella
Adolescents/ Young Adults	Acne Pityriasis rosea Tinea versicolor Psoriasis
Adults	Seborrheic dermatitis Malignant melanoma Herpes simplex virus type 2 Tinea cruris Seborrheic intertrigo Rosacea
Older Adults	Actinic keratosis Seborrheic keratosis Basal cell carcinoma Squamous cell carcinoma Xerosis Herpes zoster
Children and Adults	Nummular eczema/dermatitis Scabies Insect bites, poisonous plants Contact dermatitis Herpes zoster Tinea pedis

Cultural Considerations

- The oral mucosa is best for assessing color changes in dark-skinned persons.
- Assessing the sclera, rather than the skin, for jaundice is more accurate in Asians.
- Fair-skinned persons of Irish, German, or Polish descent have an increased risk for skin cancer with prolonged sun exposure.
- African Americans have a higher incidence of keloids, pseudofolliculitis, and mongolian spots.
- Asians often have black, straight, silky hair, and Chinese men have very little facial hair.
- Hair texture of African Americans is often thick and kinky.
- Asians produce less sweat and so have less body odor.

Assessment

History

Symptoms ("PQRST" Any + Symptom)

- Change in mole or lesion
  - When did you first notice a change in the mole or lesion?
  - What changes did you notice?
  - Have you ever had any severe sunburns?
  - Do you use sun block? If yes, what type?
  - Do you have a family history of skin cancer?
- Pruritus
  - Do you have any allergies?
  - Have you noticed any rashes?
  - Do you have any medical problems?
  - Are you on any medications, prescribed or over-the-counter (OTC)?
  - Do you typically have any sinus congestion, runny nose, or watery eyes?
  - Have you noticed any change in your overall skin coloring?
  - Have you had any loss of appetite or nausea?
  - Have you recently experienced any abdominal pain?
  - Have you had a change in your energy level?
- Nonhealing lesion or ulceration
  - How long have you had the sore/ulcer?
  - Do you remember bumping or hurting the area?
  - What have you used to treat the sore?
  - Does the sore hurt?

- Is there drainage? If yes, does it have an odor?
- Do you have any history of vascular disease or diabetes?

■ Rashes
- Do you have any allergies?
- Do you have any medical problems?
- Are you taking any medications, prescribed or OTC?
- Have you been exposed to anything different or new, such as soaps or detergents?
- Have you experienced any fevers?
- Have you noticed any swollen lymph nodes?
- Have you had any associated symptoms such as runny nose, sore throat, or headache?
- Have you had any pain in your joints or muscles?

■ Changes in hair
- Can you describe the changes in your hair?
- Do you have any medical problems?
- Are you taking any medications, either prescribed or OTC?
- What are your usual patterns of hair care—washing, perms, curling, and so forth?

■ Changes in nails
- Have you noticed any changes in color of your nails?
- Are your nails brittle?
- What are your usual patterns of nail care?
- Do you smoke?
- Do you bite your nails?

Focused Integumentary History

- Do you have changes in your skin, hair, or nails?
- Do you have any food, drug, or environmental allergies?
- Do you have any medical problems? Endocrine problems, diabetes, peripheral vascular disease, or cardiovascular disease?
- Are you taking any medications, either prescribed or OTC (Table 2.1)?

Seasonal Skin Disorders

SEASON	SKIN DISORDERS
Spring	Pityriasis rosea Chickenpox Acne flare-ups
Summer	Contact dermatitis Tinea Candida

(continued)

Seasonal Skin Disorders (continued)

SEASON	SKIN DISORDERS
	Impetigo Insect bites
Fall	Senile pruritus/winter itch Pityriasis rosea Urticaria Acne flare-ups
Winter	Contact dermatitis of hands Senile pruritus/winter itch Psoriasis Eczema

TABLE 2.1 Drugs That Adversely Affect the Integumentary System

DRUG CLASS	DRUG	POSSIBLE ADVERSE REACTIONS
Anticonvulsants	Carbamazepine	Pruritic rash, toxic epidermal necrolysis, Stevens-Johnson syndrome
	Lamotrigine	Same as carbamazepine
	Valproic acid	Alopecia
	Phenytoin	Morbilliform (measles-like) rash, hirsutism
	Ethosuximide	Urticaria, pruritic (itchy) and erythematous (reddened) rashes
Antimalarial	Chloroquine	Pruritus; pigmentary skin changes, eruptions resembling lichen planus (with prolonged therapy)
Antineoplastic agents	Bleomycin	Skin toxicity may be accompanied by hypoesthesia that may progress to hyperesthesia, urticaria, erythematous swelling, hyperpigmentation, patchy hyperkeratosis, alopecia
	Busulfan	Cheilosis, hyperpigmentation, urticaria, dry skin, alopecia, anhidrosis (absent or deficient sweating)
	Cyclophosphamide	Skin and fingernail pigmentation, alopecia
Barbiturates	Pentobarbital, phenobarbital	Urticaria; maculopapular, morbilliform, or scarlatiniform rash
Cephalosporins	Cefazolin, cefoxitin, cefuroxime, ceftriaxone, cefotaxime, and others in this class	Rash, pruritus, urticaria, erythema multiforme

DRUG CLASS	DRUG	POSSIBLE ADVERSE REACTIONS
Corticosteroids	Methylprednisolone, prednisone, dexamethasone	Urticaria, skin atrophy and thinning, acne, facial erythema, striae, allergic dermatitis, petechiae, ecchymoses
	Corticotropin (ACTH)	Urticaria, pruritus, scarlatiniform exanthema, skin atrophy and thinning, acne, facial erythema, hyperpigmentation
Gold salts	Auranofin, gold sodium thiomalate	Rash, pruritus, alopecia, photosensitivity, urticaria
Nonsteroidal anti-inflammatory agents	Diflunisal	Rash, pruritus, erythema multiforme, Stevens-Johnson syndrome
	Ibuprofen	Rash, erythema multiforme, Stevens-Johnson syndrome
	Sulindac	Rash, pruritus, photosensitivity, erythema multiforme, Stevens-Johnson syndrome
Oral antidiabetic agents	All types	Photosensitivity, various skin eruptions
Penicillins	Amoxicillin, ampicillin, dicloxacillin, penicillin G potassium, penicillin V potassium, piperacillin, ticarcillin, nafcillin	Urticaria, erythema, maculopapular rash, pruritus
Phenothiazines	Chlorpromazine, thioridazine, trifluoperazine, and others in this class	Dermatoses, pruritus, marked photosensitivity, urticaria, erythema, eczema, exfoliative dermatitis
Sulfonamides	Sulfamethoxazole, sulfasalazine, sulfisoxazole	Rash, pruritus, erythema nodosum, erythema multiforme, Stevens-Johnson syndrome, exfoliative dermatitis, photosensitivity
Tetracyclines	Demeclocycline, doxycycline, minocycline, tetracycline	Photosensitivity
Miscellaneous agents	Allopurinol	Pruritic maculopapular rash, exfoliative dermatitis, urticaria, erythematous dermatitis
	Captopril	Maculopapular rash, pruritus, erythema

(continued)

TABLE 2.1 Drugs That Adversely Affect the Integumentary System (continued)

DRUG CLASS	DRUG	POSSIBLE ADVERSE REACTIONS
	Griseofulvin	Rash, urticaria, photosensitivity, erythema multiforme or lupus-like syndrome
	Isotretinoin	Alopecia, photosensitivity, hirsutism, pruritus, urticaria
	Oral contraceptives (estrogen)	Chloasma or melasma, rash, urticaria, erythema
	Thiazide and loop diuretics	Photosensitivity
	Lithium	Acne, alopecia
	Warfarin	Skin necrosis

Assessment of the Integumentary System's Relationship to Other Systems

Remember, all systems are related. As you assess the integumentary system, look at the relationship between it and all other systems.

(text continues on page 42)

Assessment of the Integumentary System's Relationship to Other Systems

SUBJECTIVE DATA/RATIONALE	OBJECTIVE DATA/ RATIONALE
Area/System: General	
Ask about:	*Inspect for:*
Changes in energy level	*Confusion and irritability:* May indicate hypoxia resulting from cyanosis.
Weight changes	*Inability to recall information/provide history:* May indicate neurologic disorders that cause impaired judgment and altered sensation, placing skin at risk for injury. *Lethargy/somnolence:* May indicate a variety of disorders including disease of thyroid, liver, kidney, or cardiovascular or neurologic systems, which may be reflected in skin.
Fevers	*Measure:* Vital signs. Height and weight.
Level of consciousness	
Assessing for changes in energy level and weight changes, fevers, and level of	

SUBJECTIVE DATA/RATIONALE	OBJECTIVE DATA/ RATIONALE
consciousness helps identify problems that are relatively nonspecific to any one system. Many endocrine and immune diseases present with this type of complaint.	
Area/System: HEENT	
Head and neck	
Ask about:	*Inspect for:*
Lumps or swelling in neck: Swollen glands or nodes may be associated with infectious or malignant cause of skin problems.	*Facial expression and movements:* Facial expressions and movements often reflect neurologic or psychological diseases. For example, pruritus may be associated with depression and neurotic excoriations. Depression may also show in the client's facial expression.
Difficulty swallowing: Congestion and sore throat are common symptoms of several viral illnesses that typically cause skin changes.	*Neck vein distension:* Altered cardiac function that could be reflected with cyanosis of skin.
History of endocrine problems	*Enlarged accessory muscles:* Normal in a person who lifts weights. Otherwise, suggests chronic pulmonary disease, with potential for cyanosis or ruddy skin. *Palpate for:* *Lymph node enlargement:* May indicate infectious process or malignancy that could cause skin rashes, pruritus. *Thyroid gland enlargement:* Hyper- or hypothyroidism, both of which cause integumentary changes.
Eyes	
Ask about:	*Inspect for:*
Watery eyes and allergies: Congestion with watery/itchy eyes is common in atopic disorders that may be associated with urticaria, eczema, and other skin problems.	*Red eyes:* Allergies.
Changes in eye color.	*Sclera icterus (yellow sclera):* Jaundice. *Exophthalmos:* Hyperthyroidism with associated skin changes.

(continued)

Assessment of the Integumentary System's Relationship to Other Systems (continued)

SUBJECTIVE DATA/RATIONALE	OBJECTIVE DATA/ RATIONALE
Area/System: HEENT *(cont'd)* **Ears, nose, and throat**	
Ask about:	*Inspect for:*
Ear, throat, or sinus infections	*Red, swollen nasal and oral mucous membranes:* Allergy or infection. Infections such as streptococcal infection or mononucleosis can cause a macular rash.
Sore throat	
Nasal discharge	
Area/System: Respiratory	
Ask about:	*Inspect for:*
	Tachypnea: Respiratory distress.
Cough, breathing difficulty	Signs of hypoxia.
History of respiratory disease: Chronic lung disorders such as emphysema and bronchitis may limit oxygenation to the point of cyanosis. Reactive airway disease (asthma) may be associated with atopic disorders of the skin.	*Asymmetrical chest movement:* Pneumothorax or chronic restrictive lung diseases.
	Auscultate for:
	Abnormal/adventitious breath sounds (crackles, wheezes, rhonchi, or bronchial breath sounds): Altered pulmonary function.
	Percuss for:
	Dull percussion tones/increased fremitus: Consolidation within pulmonary tissue.
	Hyperresonant percussion tones and decreased/absent fremitus: Emphysemic changes.
	All of these respiratory alterations have the potential to impair oxygenation and cause cyanosis. Chronic cardiopulmonary disease with hypoxia can result in clubbing.
Area/System: Cardiovascular	
Ask about:	*Inspect for:*
History of cardiovascular disease: Dyspnea, palpitations, and chest pain are seen with cardiac disease and result in poor output, which contributes to cyanosis.	Signs of impaired circulation.

SUBJECTIVE DATA/RATIONALE	OBJECTIVE DATA/ RATIONALE
Leg pain: Claudication is common in vascular disorders and results in discoloration, hair loss, and ulceration of skin over lower extremities.	*Skin changes in extremities (thin, shiny, hairless, cool skin with decreased pulses):* Arterial insufficiency.
	Palpate for:
	Pedal pulses.
	Edema (peripheral edema, leathery skin with cyanosis and brownish discoloration): Venous insufficiency.
	Auscultate for:
	Irregular heart rate/extra heart sounds: Cardiovascular disease impairs cardiac output and/or peripheral oxygenation, causing altered skin appearance and integrity, such as diaphoresis and cyanosis.
Area/System: Gastrointestinal	
Ask about:	*Inspect for:*
History of liver disease: Liver disease can result in jaundice and pruritus.	Ascites.
Nausea/vomiting, loss of appetite.	*Palpate for:*
	Liver enlargement, tenderness (hepatomegaly): May cause jaundice and pruritus.
	Percuss for:
Change in stool to clay color.	Liver size.
Abdominal pain, anorexia, nausea, changes in bowel habits and clay-colored stools occur with liver diseases.	
Area/System: Genitourinary/ Reproductive	
Ask about:	*Inspect for:*
Changes in urine color: Dark orange urine is often seen with obstructive jaundice.	*Lesions on external genitalia skin (Genital warts, condyloma acuminata):* Human papillomavirus.
Urinary tract infections (UTIs): UTIs are frequently seen in type 2 diabetes, which can lead to skin changes.	*Burning, itching, vesicles:* Herpes simplex type 2.

(continued)

Assessment of the Integumentary System's Relationship to Other Systems (continued)

SUBJECTIVE DATA/RATIONALE	OBJECTIVE DATA/ RATIONALE
Area/System: Genitourinary/ Reproductive *(cont'd)*	
Incontinence: Can cause dermatitis.	
Menstrual irregularities, last menstrual period, pregnant: Menstrual irregularities are often found in endocrine disorders, including hypothyroidism and glucose intolerance. Pregnancy may explain localized changes in skin pigmentation.	
History of sexually transmitted diseases (STDs) and safe-sex practices: Unprotected sex increases the risk for STDs. Discharge may be associated with STD and may also cause skin lesions of genitalia or other skin.	
Area/System: Musculoskeletal	
Ask about:	*Inspect for:*
History of joint disease, rheumatoid arthritis, gout: Common in some autoimmune disorders, such as lupus, and in infectious syndromes, such as Reiter's syndrome, that affect the skin. Gout is associated with development of tophi, uric acid deposits beneath the skin.	Joint deformity.
	Decreased ROM. Skin changes over joints.
Area/System: Neurologic	
Ask about:	*Test for:*
Loss of sensation: The altered sensation found in neuropathic disorders can predispose to skin injuries. Altered sensation is also found in some	Sensory perception changes, both superficial and deep sensations.

SUBJECTIVE DATA/RATIONALE	OBJECTIVE DATA/ RATIONALE
neurologic disorders that result in skin dryness.	
	Percuss for:
	Deep tendon reflexes (decreased sensation/DTRs): Associated with neuropathy, which increases risk for injury to skin.
Area/System: Endocrine	
Ask about:	
History of thyroid disease, diabetes: Polyuria, polydipsia, polyphagia, fatigue, and weight loss are common symptoms in diabetes, which alters the healing ability of the skin and promotes other changes through alterations in circulation and sensation. Fatigue and weight gain are commonly found in hypothyroid disorders, which result in dry skin and pruritus.	
Area/System: Immunological/ Hematological	
Ask about:	*Inspect for:*
Immune disorders: Immune diseases such as lupus or human immuno deficiency virus (HIV) often have skin manifestations, such as Kaposi's sarcoma.	Ecchymoses or petechiae.
Use of immunosuppressive drugs: Can cause skin changes. For example, steroids can cause acne, decreased wound healing, ecchymosis, thinning of skin, hirsutism, and petechiae.	
Bleeding disorders or use of aspirin or anticoagulants: Bleeding disorders or use of anticoagulants may result in vascular lesions such as petechiae, purpura, and ecchymosis.	

HEENT = Head, eyes, ears, nose, and throat; ROM = range of motion.

Physical Assessment

APPROACH: Inspection, palpation

Assessment can be approached in any of three ways:

- Using a head-to-toe approach.
- Observing all skin on the anterior, posterior, and lateral surfaces of the body.
- Inspecting the skin by regions, as you assess the other body systems.

POSITION: Dependent on approach used

TOOLBOX: Gloves; flexible, transparent ruler; marker; penlight; glass slide; magnifier

Physical Assessment

AREA/PA SKILL	NORMAL FINDINGS	ABNORMAL FINDINGS
Inspection		
Skin		
Note color, odor, and integrity.	Uniform skin color with slightly darker exposed areas. No jaundice, cyanosis, pallor, erythema, or hyper/hypopigmentation. No unusual odors.	Color changes may be benign or may indicate underlying pathology. (See Table 2.2.) *Unusual body odor:* Poor hygiene or underlying disease. If from poor hygiene, may be related to self-care deficit that warrants nursing intervention. *Odors from excessive sweating (hyperhidrosis):* Possible thyrotoxicosis. *Odors from night sweats:* Possible tuberculosis. *Urine odor:* Incontinence problem. Stale urine odor may be associated with uremia. *Mousy odor:* Liver disease.
Cold or hot weather can affect surface characteristics of skin and nails.	Ethnic/racial differences account for many variations in color. Mucous membranes and conjunctiva pink.	

AREA/PA SKILL	NORMAL FINDINGS	ABNORMAL FINDINGS
Differentiate central (mouth and conjunctiva) vs. peripheral cyanosis (extremities).		

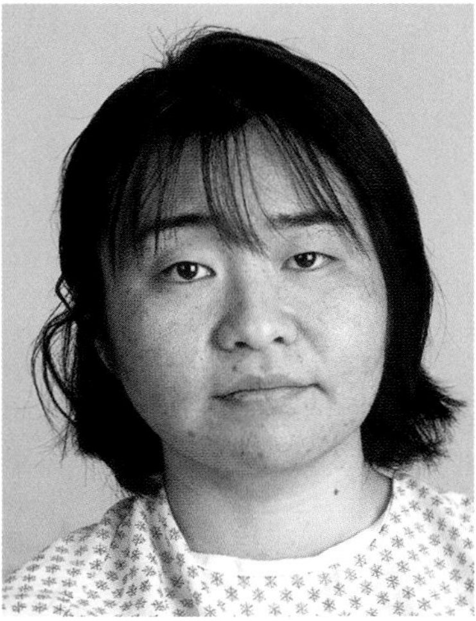

Inspect both exposed and unexposed areas

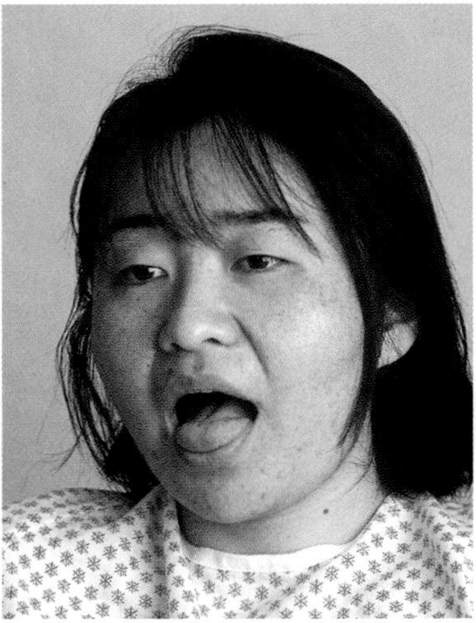

Inspect oral mucosa and conjunctiva

(box continued on page 44)

Physical Assessment (continued)

AREA/PA SKILL	NORMAL FINDINGS	ABNORMAL FINDINGS

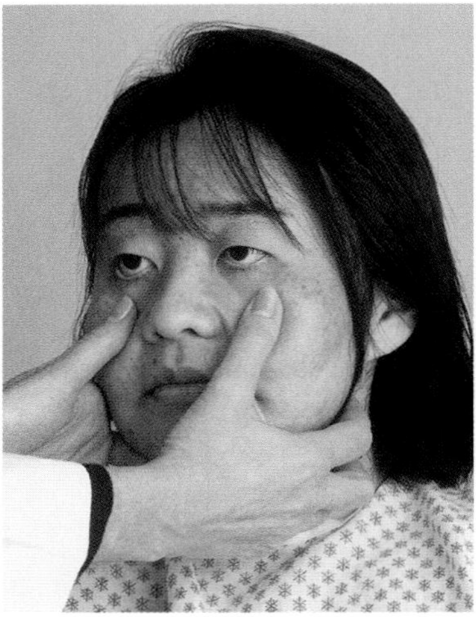

Gently pull lover eyelids down

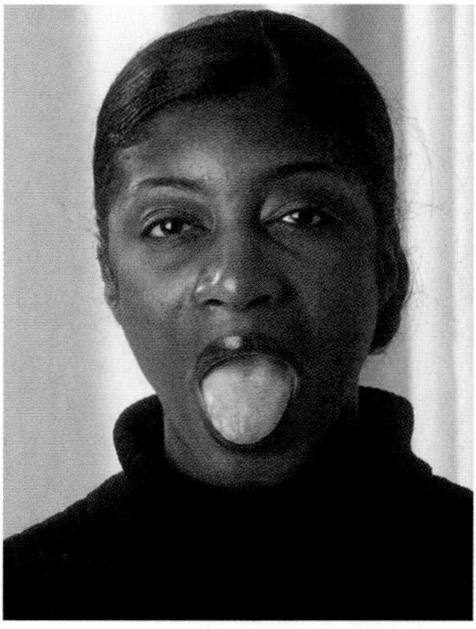

Oral mucous membranes pink

When assessing for color changes in dark-skinned patients, check oral mucous membranes.

AREA/PA SKILL	NORMAL FINDINGS	ABNORMAL FINDINGS

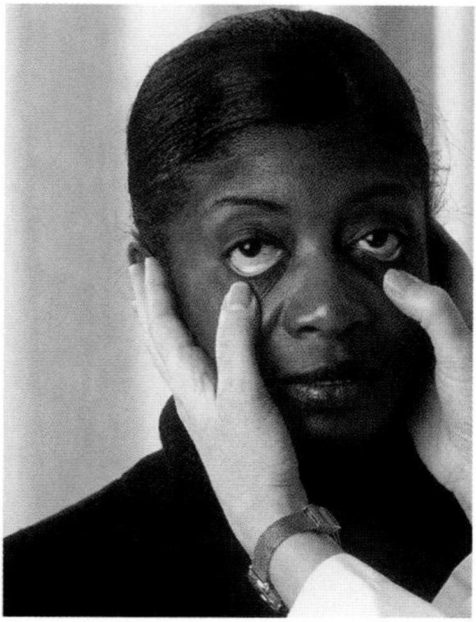

Conjunctiva pink

AREA/PA SKILL	NORMAL FINDINGS	ABNORMAL FINDINGS
Identify any lesions: Primary, secondary, or vascular. (See Tables 2.3 through 2.5.)	Skin intact, no suspicious lesions.	*Primary lesions:* See Table 2.3. *Secondary lesions:* See Table 2.4. *Vascular lesions:* See Table 2.5.
Assess for pressure ulcers. (See Table 2.6.) **Pressure ulcers often develop over bony prominences, such as the sacrum and heels, so inspect these areas carefully.**		*Pressure ulcers:* See Table 2.6.

(box continued on page 46)

Physical Assessment (continued)

AREA/PA SKILL	NORMAL FINDINGS	ABNORMAL FINDINGS
Inspection: *Skin (cont'd)* **With pressure ulcers, extensive undermining often occurs, extending through the dermal layer to the bone. The visible pressure ulcer may be only the "tip of the iceberg."** *Risk factors for pressure ulcers:* Impaired mental status, impaired nutritional status, sensory deficits, immobility, mechanical forces, shearing and friction, and excessive exposure to moisture from bodily secretions. Describe morphology, distribution, pattern, and location of lesions. (See Tables 2.7 through 2.9.) Assess for malignant lesions. A = Asymmetry. B = Border irregularity. C = Color variation. D = Diameter > 0.5 cm. E = Evolution/ enlarging 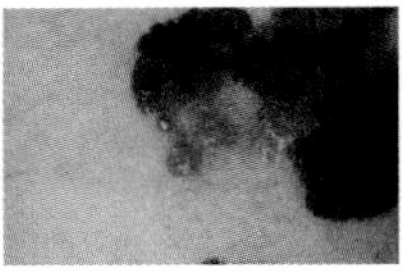 *Skin*		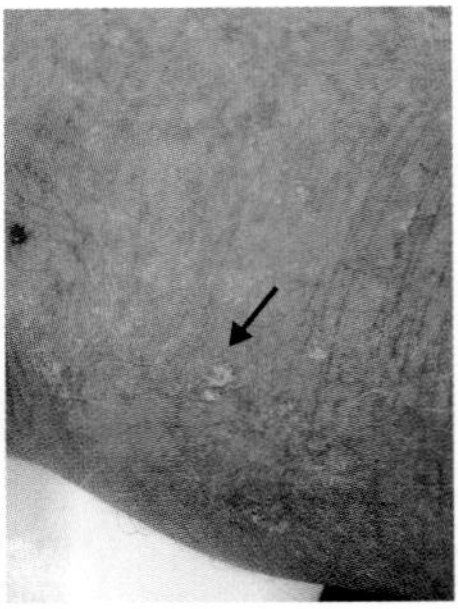 *Actinic keratosis* 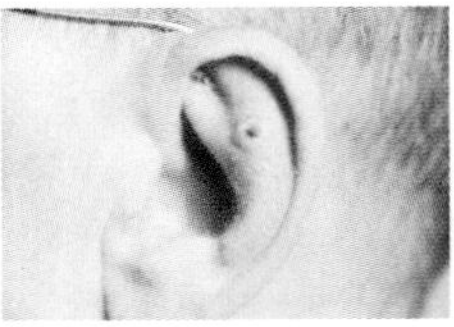 *Basal cell carcinoma* 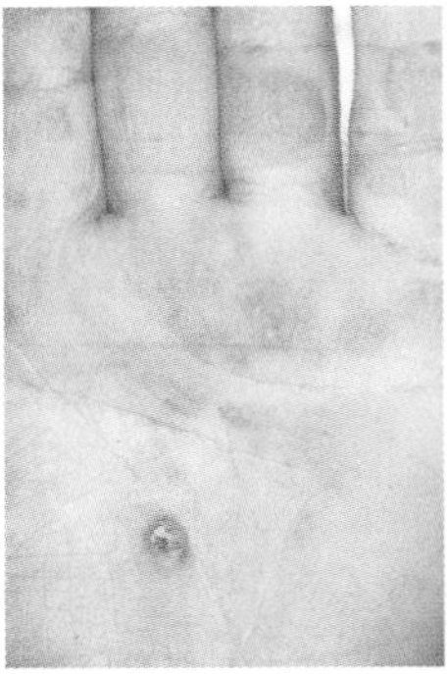 *Kaposi's sarcoma* 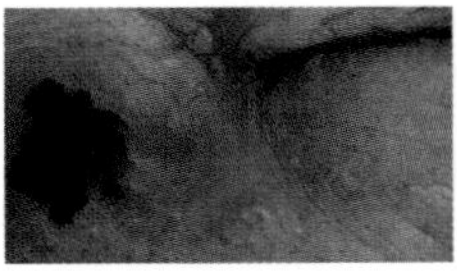 *Malignant melanoma*

AREA/PA SKILL	NORMAL FINDINGS	ABNORMAL FINDINGS
Palpation Maintain standard pre-cautions. Wear gloves if assessing an open area.		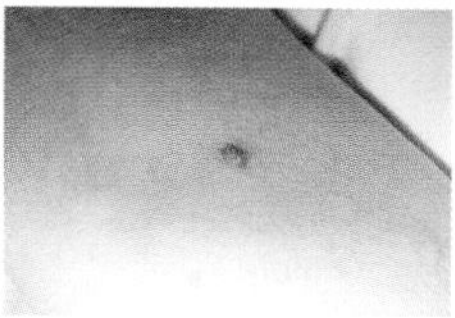 *Squamous cell carcinoma.*
Temperature **(Use dorsal part of hand.)**	Skin warm.	*Local area with increased temperature:* Inflammatory process, infection, or burn; caused by increased circulation to area.

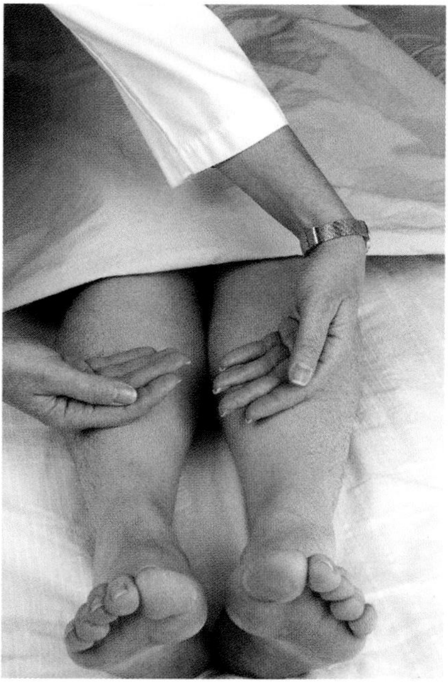

Palpating skin temperature with the dorsal aspect of hands

	Temperature varies depending on area being assessed; for example, exposed areas may be cooler than unexposed areas.	*Generalized decrease in skin temperature:* Exposure or shock. *Generalized increase in temperature:* Fever. *Local area with decreased temperature:* Decreased circulation to area, arterial occlusion.

(box continued on page 48)

Physical Assessment (continued)

AREA/PA SKILL	NORMAL FINDINGS	ABNORMAL FINDINGS
Palpate for tenderness and surface characteristics of any lesions. Check for pulsations and blanching of vascular lesions.	Nontender	Tenderness may indicate underlying problem, such as inflamation
Moisture	Skin warm and dry. Moisture dependent upon body area. Exposed areas tend to be drier.	*Increased moisture:* Fever or thyrotoxicosis.
		Decreased moisture: Dehydration, myxedema, chronic nephritis.
Texture	Texture varies from soft/fine to coarse/thick depending upon area and age of client. Skin coarser on extensor surfaces.	*Coarse, thick, dry skin:* Hypothyroidism.
		Skin more fine-textured: Hyperthyroidism. *Smooth, thin, shiny skin:* Arterial insufficiency. *Thick, rough skin:* Venous insufficiency.
Turgor	Good skin turgor, no tenting.	*Decreased turgor or tenting:* Dehydration or normal aging.

AREA/PA SKILL	NORMAL FINDINGS	ABNORMAL FINDINGS
(Test unexposed area such as below clavicle.)		*Increased turgor and tension:* Scleroderma and edema.

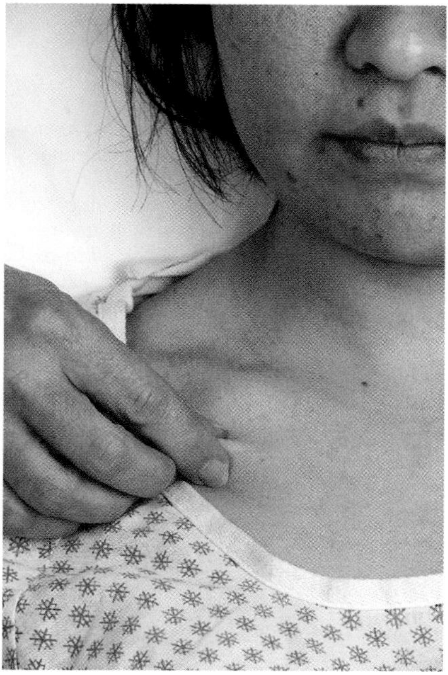

Turgor

AREA/PA SKILL	NORMAL FINDINGS	ABNORMAL FINDINGS
Inspection		
Nails		
Note color, condition, angle of attachment, and presence of focal or generalized abnormalities, for example, ridges, clubbing.	Color varies from pink to light brown in darker-skinned individuals.	*Color changes in nails:* Local or systemic problem.

(box continued on page 50)

Physical Assessment (continued)

AREA/PA SKILL	NORMAL FINDINGS	ABNORMAL FINDINGS
Inspection *Nails (cont'd)*		*Yellow nails:* Cigarette smoking, fungal infections, psoriasis. 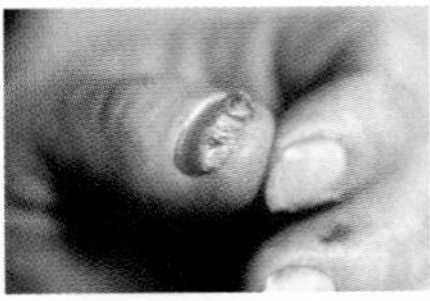 *Fungal infection* *Very distal band of reddish-pink or brown covering < 20% of nail (Terry's nails):* Cirrhosis, disorders causing hypoalbuminemia. *Distal band of reddish-pink or brown covering 20% to 60% of nails (Lindsay's nails or half-and-half nails):* Renal disease, hypoalbuminemia. 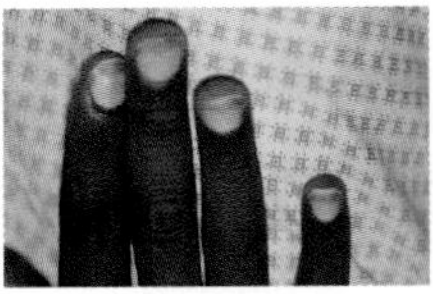 *Half-and-half nails* *Blue (cyanotic) nails:* Peripheral disease or hypoxia. 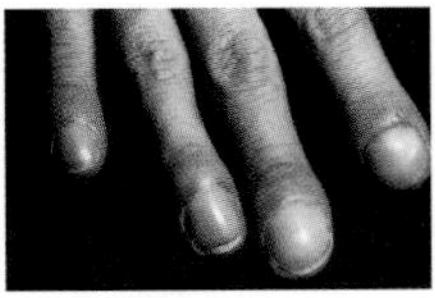 *Blue nails*

AREA/PA SKILL	NORMAL FINDINGS	ABNORMAL FINDINGS
		Green nails: *Pseudomonas* infections. *White nails (leukonychia):* Trauma, cardiovascular, liver, or renal disease. 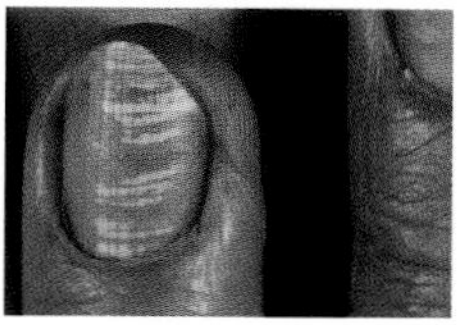 *Leukonychia* *Black nails:* Trauma. *Splinter hemorrhages:* Bacterial endocarditis or trauma. 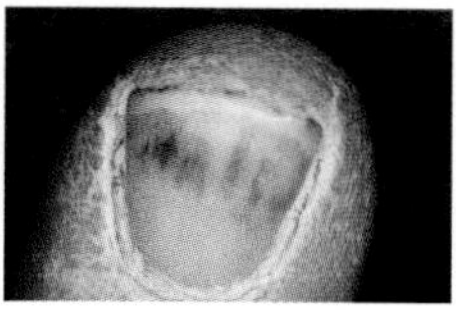 *Splinter hemorrhages* 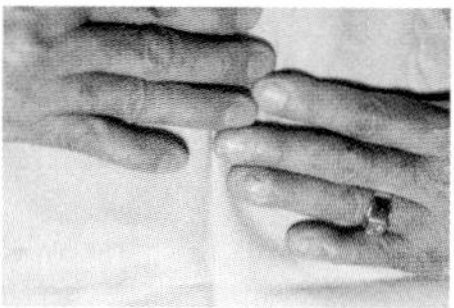 *Onycholysis* 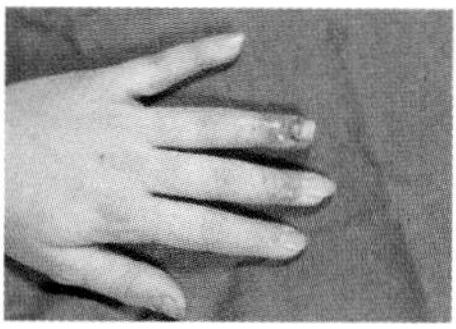 *Paronychia* *(box continued on page 52)*

Physical Assessment (continued)

AREA/PA SKILL	NORMAL FINDINGS	ABNORMAL FINDINGS
Inspection *Nails (cont'd)*		
Shape	Angle of attachment 160 degrees. Nails convex.	*Angle of nail attachment 180 degrees or more (clubbing):* Congenital heart disorders, cystic fibrosis, and chronic pulmonary diseases.

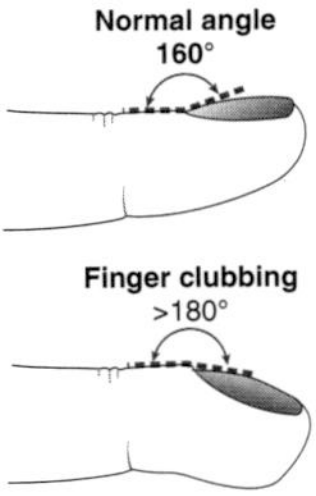

Nail clubbing

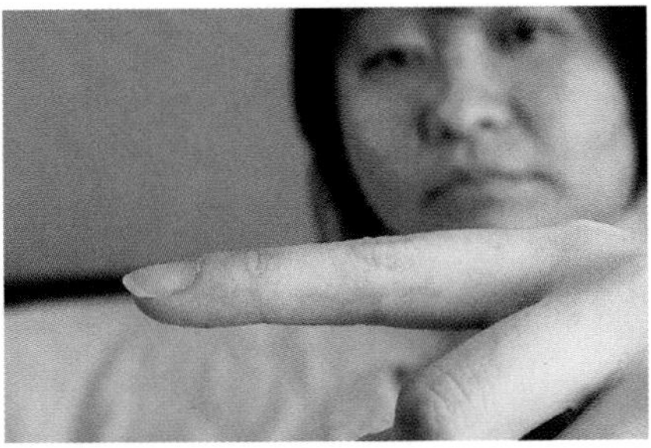

Inspect nail shape

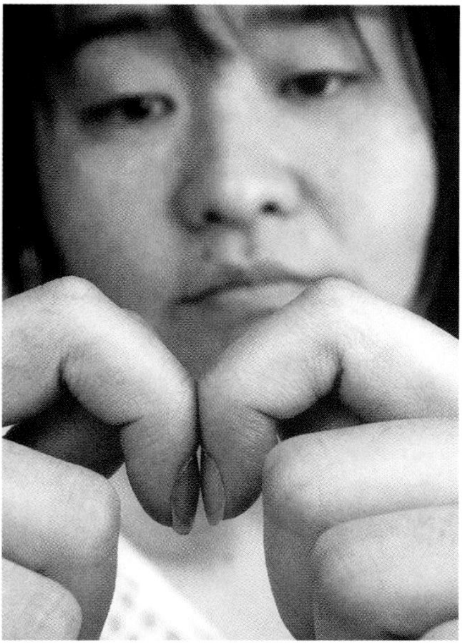

Note space between nails

AREA/PA SKILL	NORMAL FINDINGS	ABNORMAL FINDINGS
		Spooning or concave nail (koilonychia): Severe iron deficiency anemia, hemochromatosis, thyroid and circulatory diseases, in response to some skin diseases and local trauma.
Nail and cuticle	Nails well groomed. Cuticle pink and intact.	*Onycholysis, separation of the nail from nail bed:* Fungal infections, psoriasis, thyrotoxicosis, eczema, systemic diseases, following trauma, or as allergic response to nail products/ contactants. *Pitting:* Psoriasis. *Red and inflamed perionychium (paronychia):* Infection or ingrown nail.
Palpation		
Texture	Nails smooth and firm, no ridges, adhere well to nailbed.	*Soft, boggy nails:* Clubbing resulting from poor oxygenation.

(box continued on page 54)

Physical Assessment (continued)

AREA/PA SKILL	NORMAL FINDINGS	ABNORMAL FINDINGS
		Brittle nails: Hyperthyroidism, malnutrition, calcium and iron deficiency, repeated use of harsh nail contactants or products. *Pitted nails:* Psoriasis. 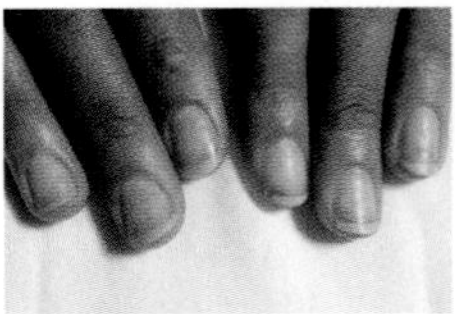 *Pitted nails* *Beau's lines (transverse ridges):* Serious illness that causes nail growth to slow or halt. 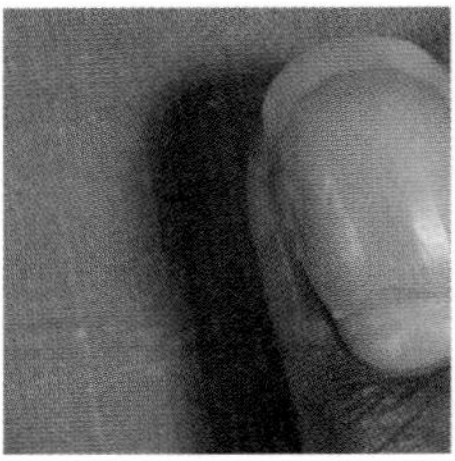 *Beau's lines* *Thick, brittle nails:* Arterial insufficiency. 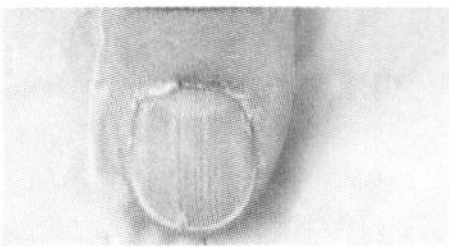 *Longitudinal ridges (usually benign)*
Capillary refill	Brisk capillary refill < 3 sec.	*Poor capillary refill:* Cardiopulmonary problems or anemia.
Inspection *Hair and Scalp* Note quantity and distribution of hair, condition of scalp, presence of lesions or pediculosis.	Hair evenly distributed over scalp, no alopecia.	*Generalized hair loss:* Nutritional deficiencies, hypothyroidism, lupus erythematosus, thyroid disease, serious illnesses, or side effects of medications.

AREA/PA SKILL	NORMAL FINDINGS	ABNORMAL FINDINGS
Gender, genetics, and age affect hair distribution.	Normal balding patterns common to men and elderly persons. No lesions or pediculosis.	
Note actual hair loss, with smooth skin beneath, or whether hair has been broken off near the scalp, with palpable stubble over the skin.		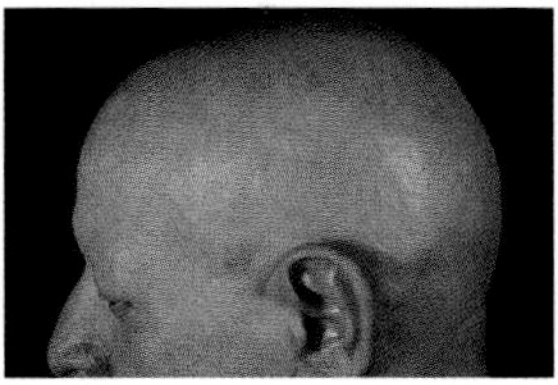 *Alopecia* *Patchy alopecia:* Alopecia areata, trichotillomania, and fungal infections such as tinea capitis. *Scaling of scalp:* Dandruff, seborrhea, psoriasis, certain tineas, and eczema (atopic dermatitis). 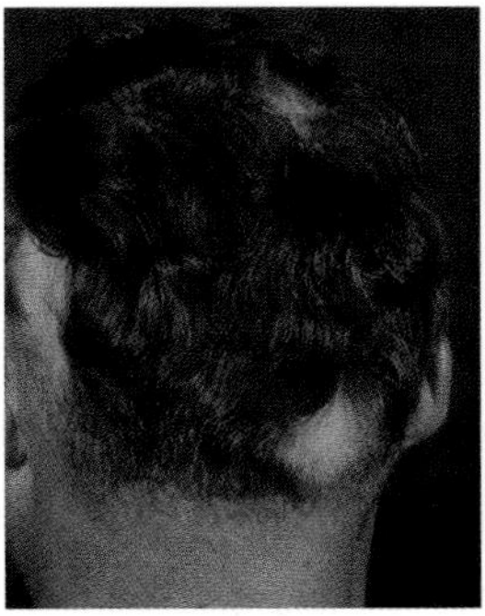 *Alopecia areata* 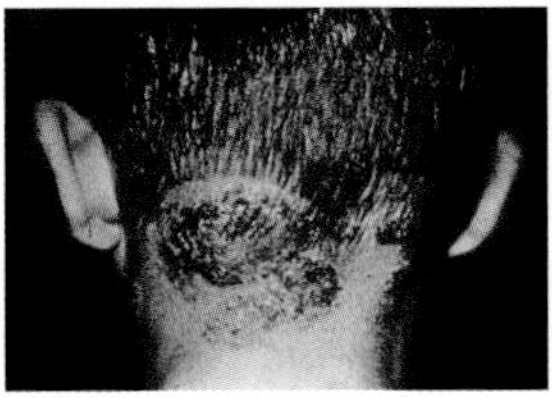 *Tinea capitis*

(box continued on page 56)

Physical Assessment (continued)

AREA/PA SKILL	NORMAL FINDINGS	ABNORMAL FINDINGS
Inspection *Hair and Scalp (cont'd)*		
Assess the body for normal distribution of hair.	Fine body hair (vellus) noted over most of body.	*Hirsutism, hair in male patterns in a woman (e.g., excess facial or trunk hair):* Endocrine disorders or medications such as steroids. 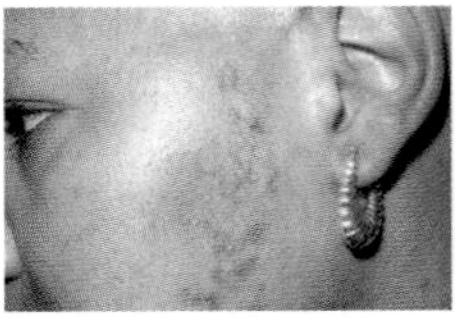 *Hirsutism*
Note color of hair.	Hair color appropriate, thins and grays with age.	*Localized areas of white or gray hair:* Recovering from alopecia areata, or having vitiligo and piebaldism. *Diffuse white hair:* Albinism. *Green hair:* Copper exposure and pernicious anemia.
Palpation Palpate scalp for tenderness, masses, and mobility.	Scalp mobile, nontender.	*Dry, coarse hair:* Hypothyroidism.
Note texture of hair.	Hair texture varies (fine, medium, coarse) depending on genetics and treatments, (e.g., perms).	*Fine, silky hair:* Hyperthyroidism.

PA = Physical assessment.

TABLE 2.2 Skin Color Variations

COLOR	CAUSE/DESCRIPTION
Bronzing/ tanning	*Addison's disease/adrenal insufficiency:* Generalized, most evident over exposed areas. 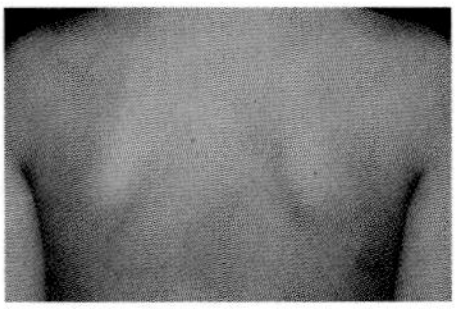 *Addison's disease*

COLOR	CAUSE/DESCRIPTION
	Hemochromatosis: Generalized, may be gray-brown coloring.
Tan	*Ichthyosis:* With coarse scaliness. *Sprue:* Tan/brown patches of any area. *Scleroderma:* Generalized tanning/yellowing of skin, associated with loss of elasticity. *Chloasma:* "Mask of pregnancy" (on face). 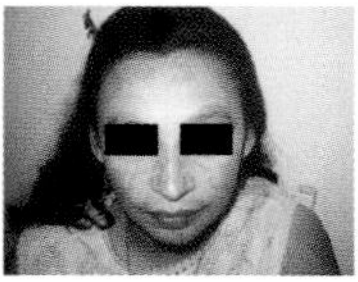 *Chloasma* *Lupus:* Butterfly rash on face. *Tinea versicolor:* Fawn color or yellow patchy.
Yellow	*Uremia:* Generalized. *Liver disease, such as hepatitis, cirrhosis, liver cancer, or gallbladder disease with obstructive jaundice. Generalized carotenemia:* not found in conjunctiva or sclera. 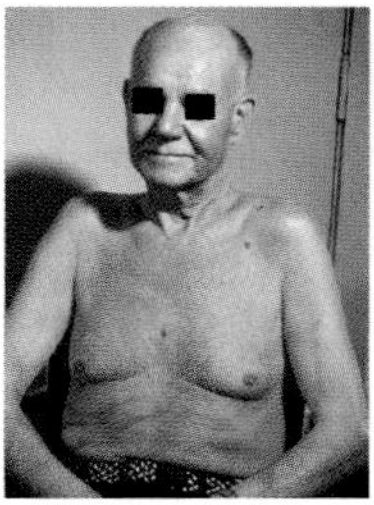 *Jaundice* 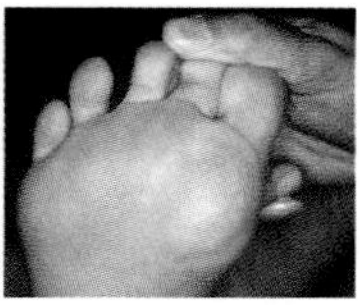 *Carotenemia* **Jaundice from liver disease is seen in the sclera and conjunctiva. Pseudojaundice—yellow color variations associated with carotenemia—is seen on the skin but not in the eyes.**

(continued)

TABLE 2.2 Skin Color Variations (continued)

COLOR	CAUSE/DESCRIPTION
Dusky blue	*Arsenic poisoning:* Paler spots on trunk and extremities. *Central cyanosis with hypoxia; peripheral cyanosis from vasoconstriction:* Caused by cold exposure or vascular disease. 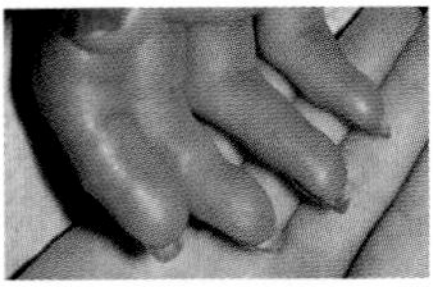 *Cyanosis* **To differentiate peripheral cyanosis (caused by vasoconstriction or decreased circulation) from central cyanosis (caused by hypoxia), check the oral mucous membranes and conjunctiva. Cyanotic mucous membranes and conjunctiva indicate a central process.**
Pallor	*Anemia:* Also on conjunctiva and mucous membranes. *Vitiligo:* Patchy. 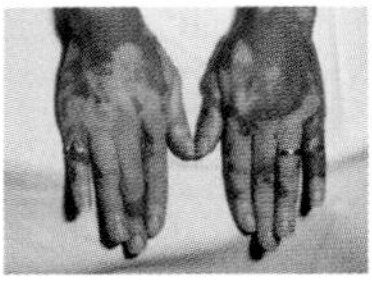 *Vitiligo* *Albinism:* Generalized. 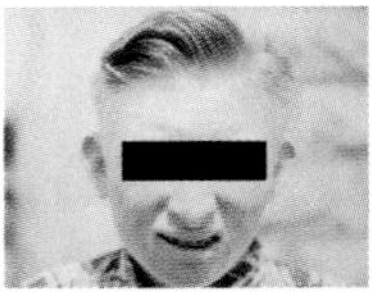 *Albinism*
Red	Polycythemia. *Erythema:* Dilated superficial capillaries, such as in rosacea. 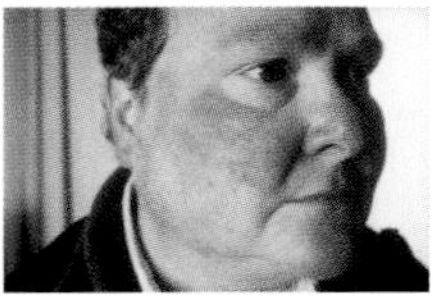 *Erythema of rosacea* *Cherry red:* Carbon monoxide poisoning.

TABLE 2.3 Primary Lesions

SURFACE CHARACTERISTICS	LESION	EXAMPLES
Flat, nonpalpable 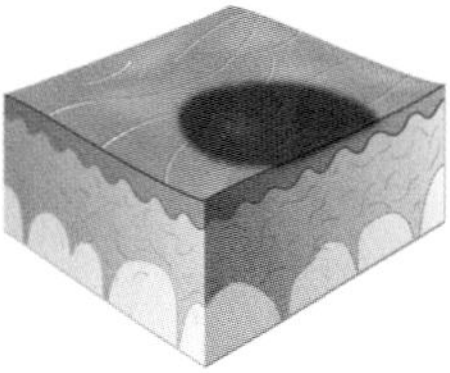 *Macule*	**Macule** < 1 cm	Cherry angioma, freckle, flat mole, measles, melanoma 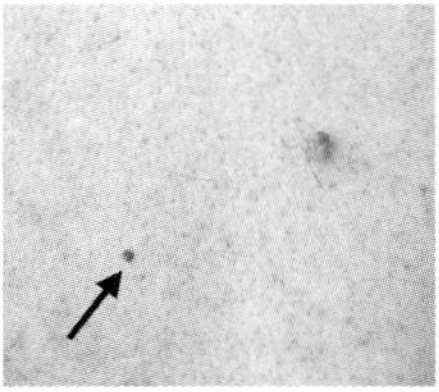 *Cherry angioma*
	Patch > 1 cm	Vitiligo, tinea versicolor, mongolian spot 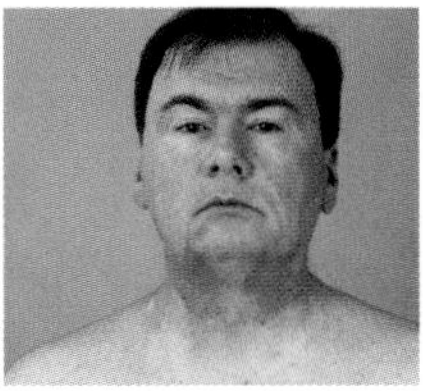 *Vitiligo*
Palpable, raised, but superficial 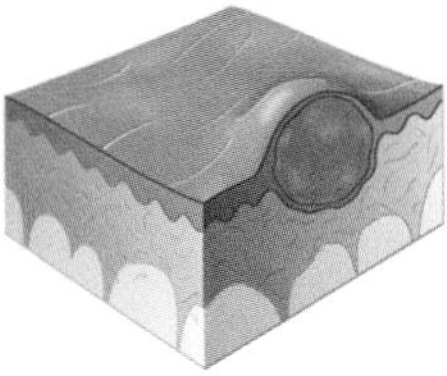 *Papule*	**Papule** < 1 cm	Raised mole, wart, lichen planus 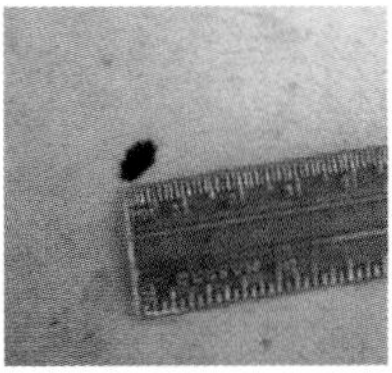 *Mole*
	Plaque > 1 cm	Seborrheic keratosis, psoriasis 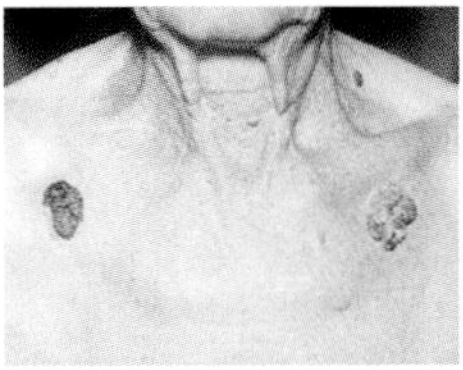 *Seborrheic keratosis*

(continued)

TABLE 2.3 Primary Lesions (continued)

SURFACE CHARACTERISTICS	LESION	EXAMPLES
Raised, superficial 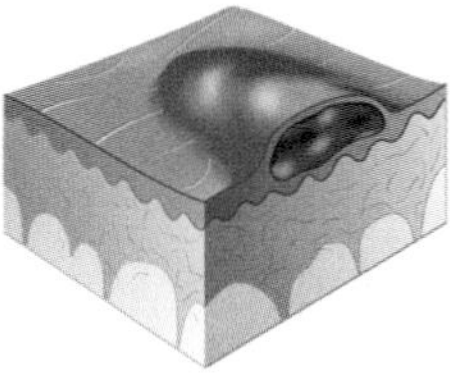 *Wheal/hive*	**Wheal/hive** Hives (urticaria) are groups of wheals	Transient lesion 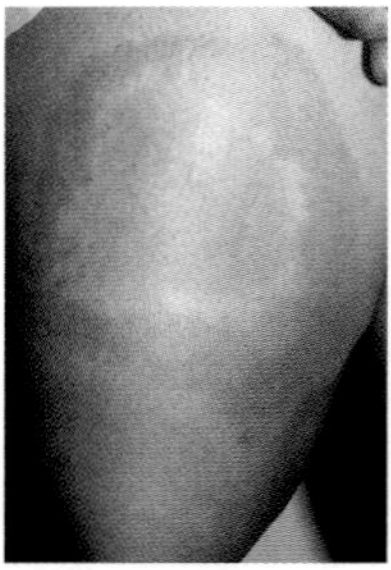 *Transient lesion (hive)*
Palpable, solid with depth into dermis 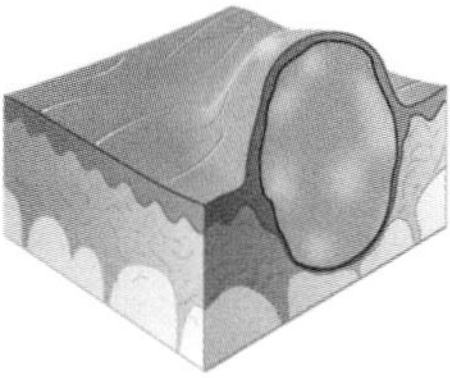 *Cyst*	Nodule < 2 cm If fluid filled and encapsulated, called a *cyst*	Erythema nodosum, fibroma, xanthoma, keratogenous cyst 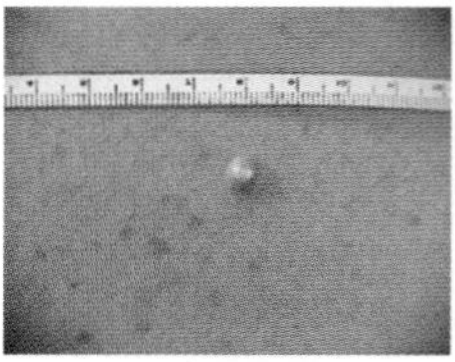 *Keratogenous cyst* 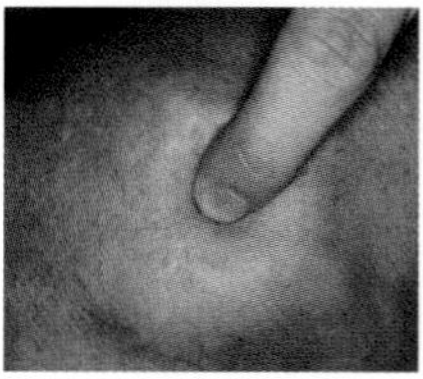 *Neoplasm (lipoma)*
Palpable, fluid filled 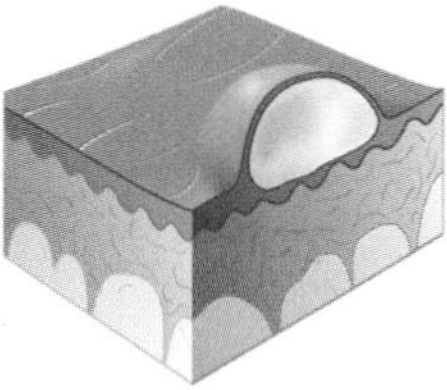 *Vesicle (serous)*	**Tumor** > 2 cm **Vesicle (serous)** < 1 cm	Blister, herpes simplex, contact dermatitis 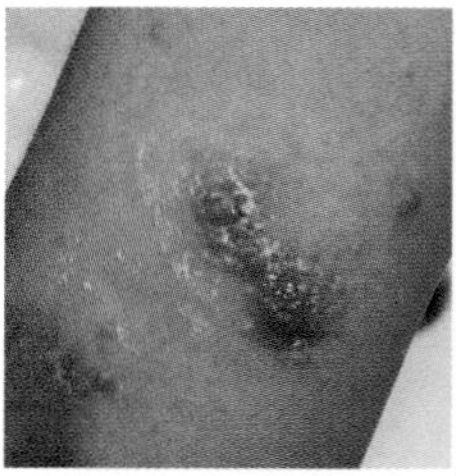 *Vesicles from poison ivy*

SURFACE CHARACTERISTICS	LESION	EXAMPLES
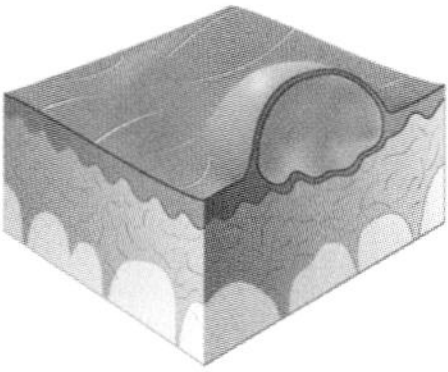 *Pustule (pus filled)*	**Bulla (serous) > 1 cm**	Blister, contact dermatitis, burns 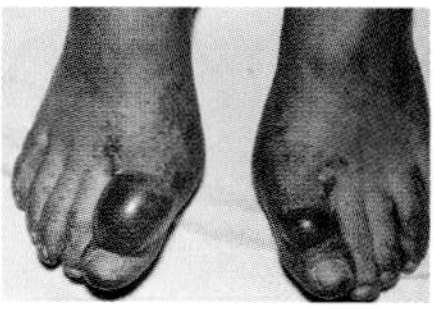 *Blister*
	Pustule (pus filled)	Acne, impetigo 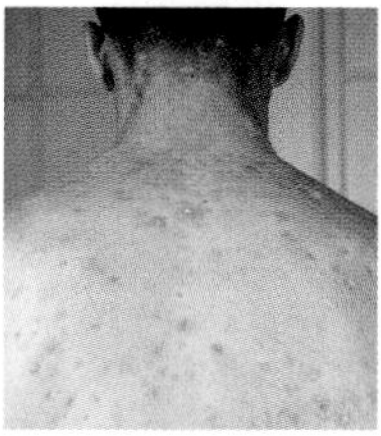 *Acne vulgaris*

TABLE 2.4 Secondary Lesions

SURFACE CHARACTERISTICS	LESION	EXAMPLES
Secondary Lesions That Add To: Thickening and scaling with increased skin markings	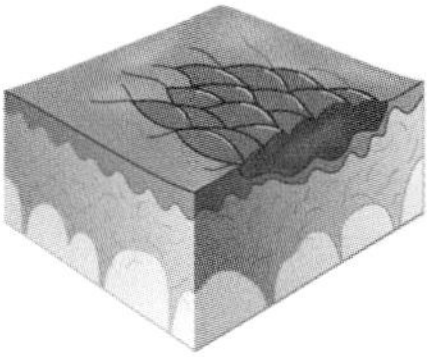 *Lichenification*	Eczema, contact dermatitis 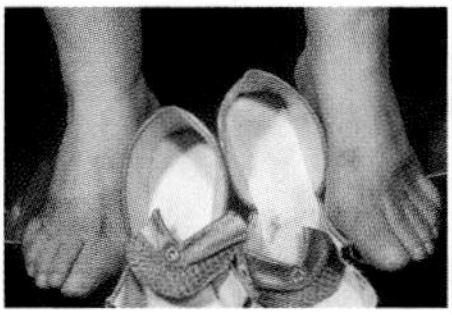 *Contact dermatitis*
Shedding, dead skin cells; scales can be either dry or oily, adherent or loose, variable in color	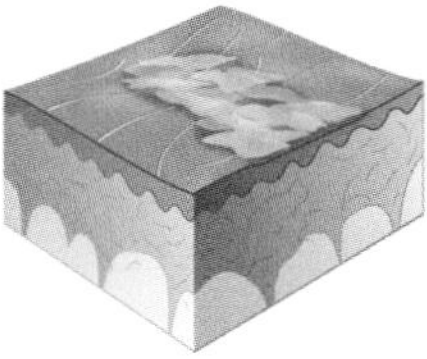 *Scales*	Dandruff, psoriasis 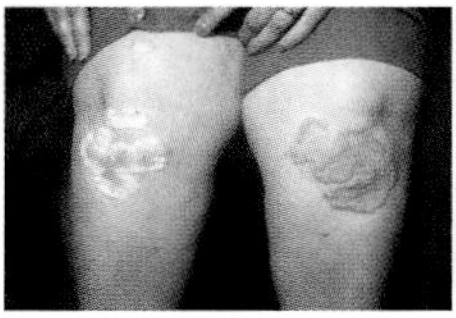 *Psoriasis*

(continued)

TABLE 2.4 Secondary Lesions (continued)

SURFACE CHARACTERISTICS	LESION	EXAMPLES
Dried exudates	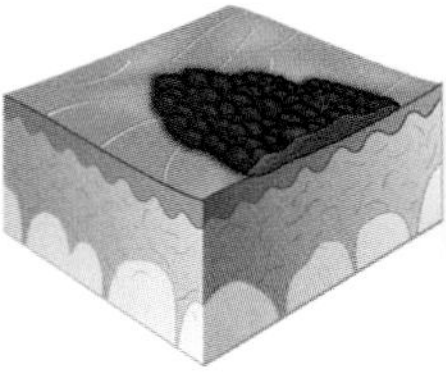 *Crust*	Impetigo, dried herpes simplex 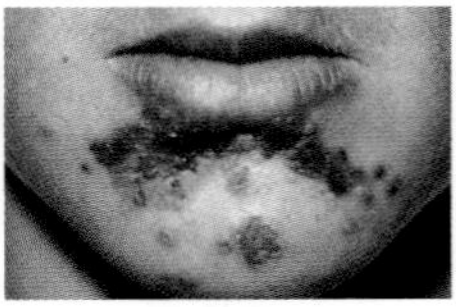 *Dried herpes simplex*
Replacement connective tissue formations	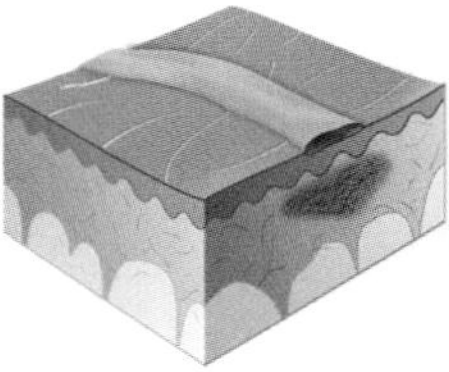 *Scar*	Surgical site, trauma sites 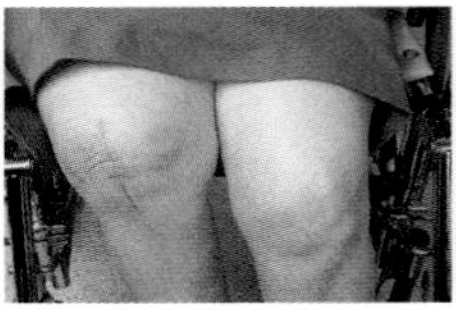 *Surgical site*
Hypertrophic scarring caused by excess collagen formation; raised and irregular	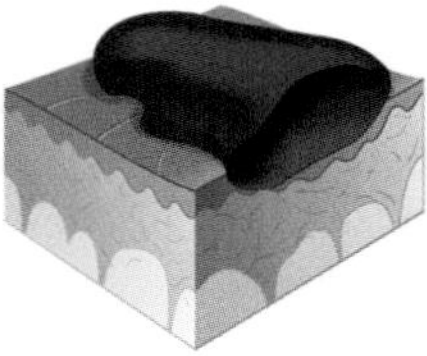 *Keloid*	Surgical site, tattoo, ear-piercing site 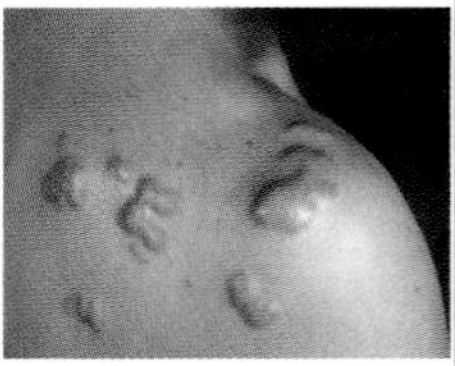 *Keloids*
Secondary Lesions That Take Away From: Abrasions or other loss that does not extend beyond the superficial epidermis	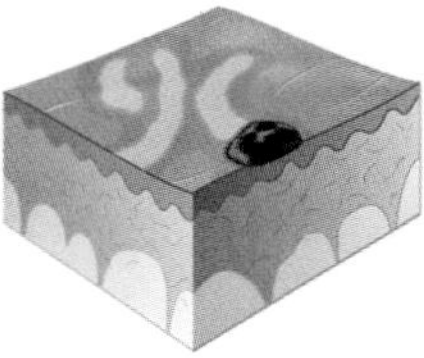 *Excoriation*	Scratch marks, scabies, vascular rupture sites 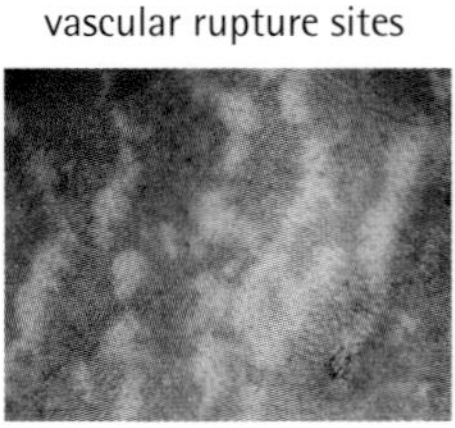 *Excoriation from uremic pruritus*

SURFACE CHARACTERISTICS	LESION	EXAMPLES
Loss of superficial epidermis	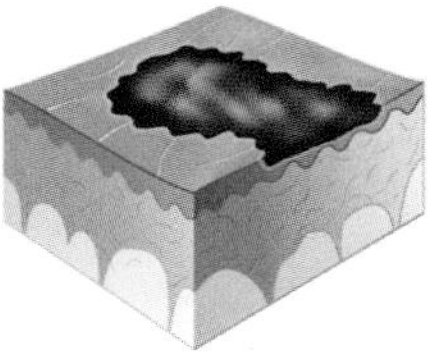 *Erosion*	Abrasion; some fungal infections such as candidiasis can cause erosion 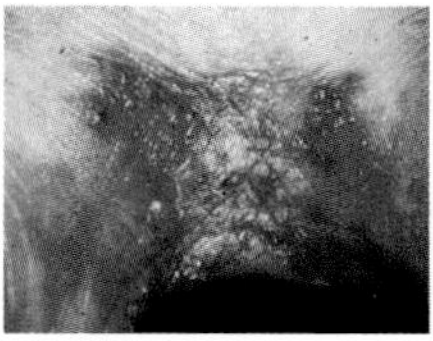 *Candidiasis*
Linear breaks in the skin with well-defined borders, may extend to the dermis	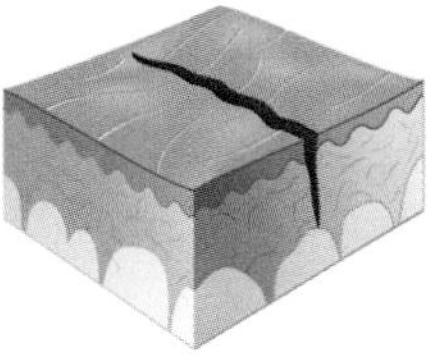 *Fissure*	Athlete's foot, syphilis, cheilitis 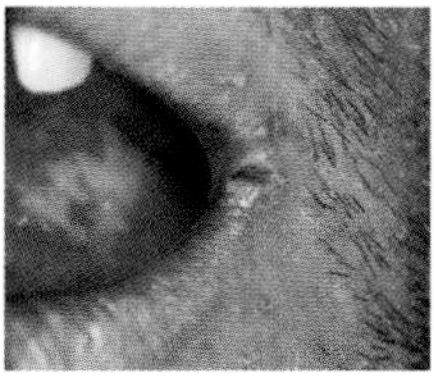 *Cheilitis*
Irregularly shaped loss extending to or through the dermis; may be necrotic	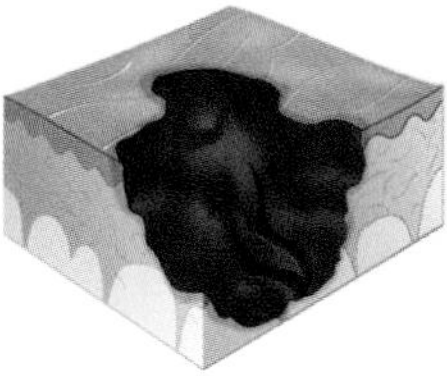 *Ulcer*	Stasis ulcer, pressure ulcer 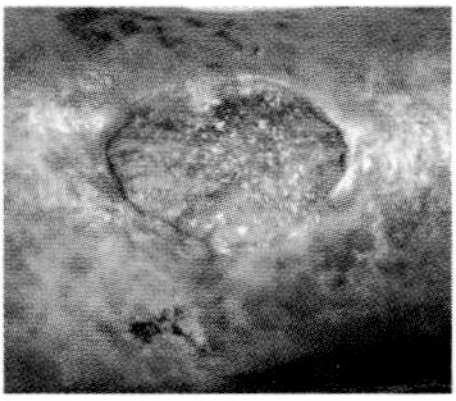 *Stasis ulcer*
Thinning of skin with transparent appearance and loss of markings	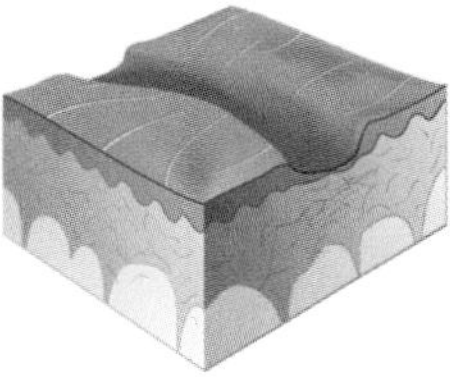 *Atrophy*	Arterial insufficiency, aging 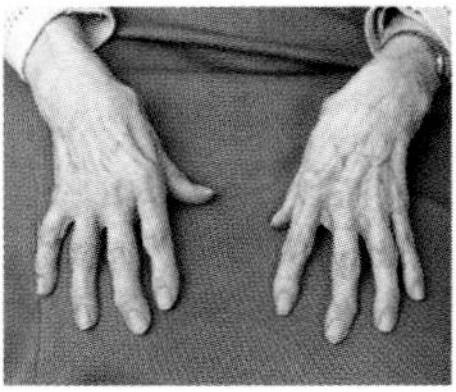 *Aging*

TABLE 2.5 Vascular Lesions

LESION	EXAMPLE	CHARACTERISTICS
Ecchymosis	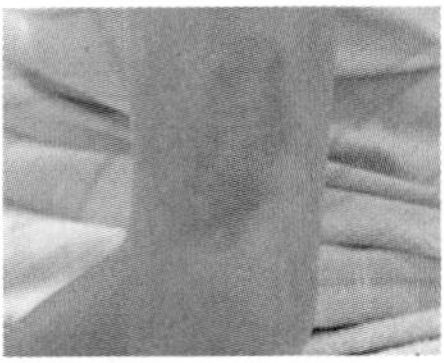 *Ecchymosis*	Extravasation of blood into skin layer Caused by trauma/injury Does not blanch
Petechiae or purpura	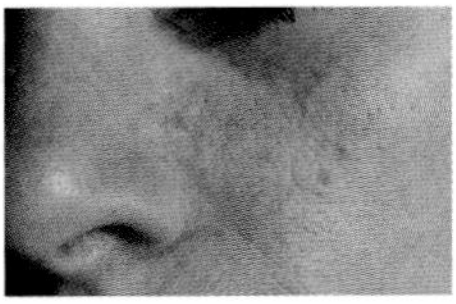 *Petechiae*	Extravasations of blood into skin Caused by steroids, vasculitis, systemic diseases Does not blanch
Venous star	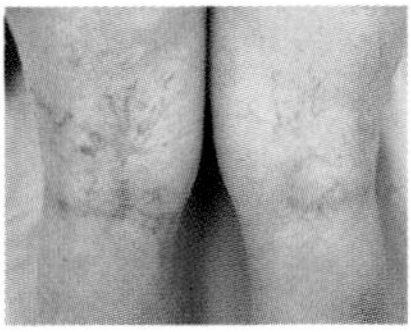 *Venous star*	Blue color Irregularly shaped, linear, spider Does not blanch Caused by increased pressure on superficial veins
Telangiectasia	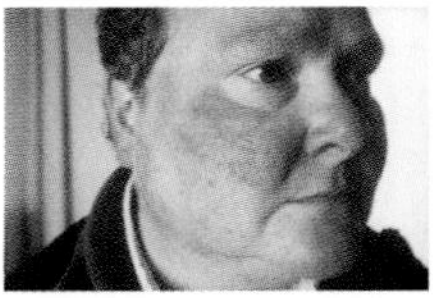 *Telangiectasia*	Red color Very fine and irregular vessels Blanches Seen with dilation of capillaries
Spider angioma	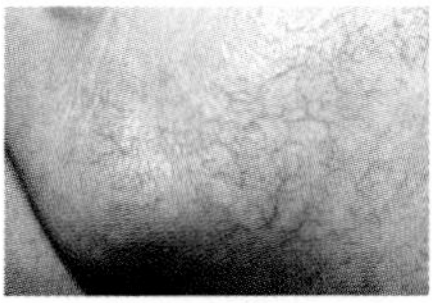 *Spider angioma*	Red color, type of telangiectasia Looks like a spider, with central body and fine radiating legs Blanches Seen in liver disease, vitamin B deficiencies, idiopathic origin
Capillary hemangioma	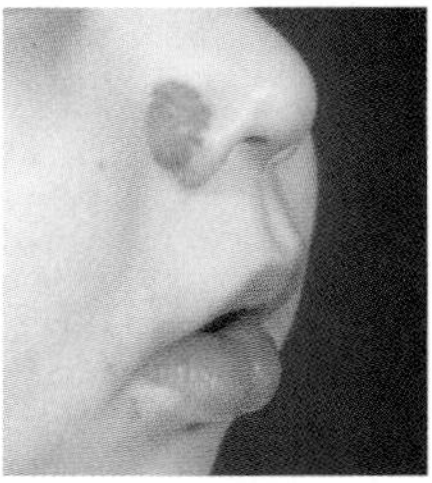 *Capillary hemangioma*	Red color Irregularly shaped macular patch

LESION	EXAMPLE	CHARACTERISTICS
Port-wine stain	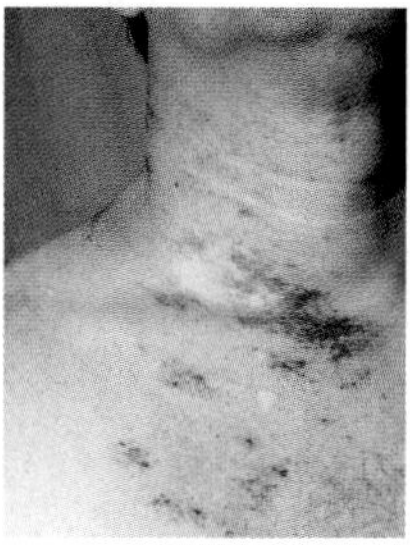 *Port-wine stain*	Red color Does not blanch Seen with dilation of dermal capillaries

TABLE 2.6 Staging Criteria for Pressure Ulcers

STAGE	APPEARANCE	CHARACTERISTICS
I	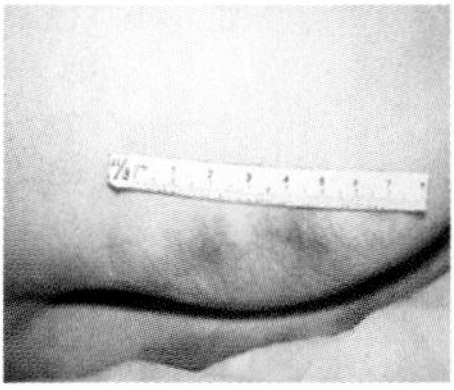	Nonblanchable erythema of intact skin; indicates potential for ulceration.
II	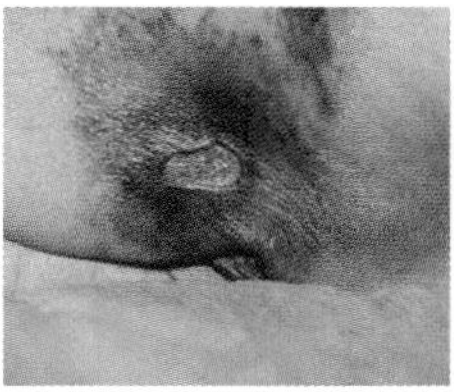	Partial-thickness loss involving both epidermis and dermis. Ulcer is still superficial and appears as a blister, abrasion, or very shallow crater
III	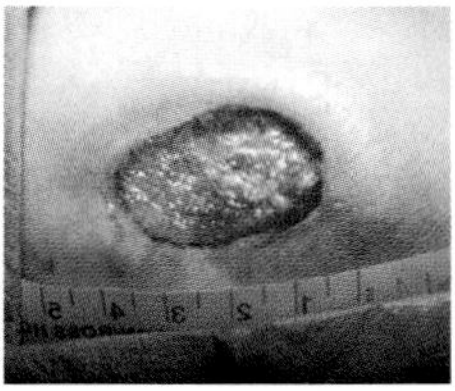	Full-thickness loss involving subcutaneous tissue. Ulcer may extend to but not through fascia. A deep crater that may undermine adjacent tissues.

(continued)

TABLE 2.6 Staging Criteria for Pressure Ulcers (continued)

STAGE	APPEARANCE	CHARACTERISTICS
IV	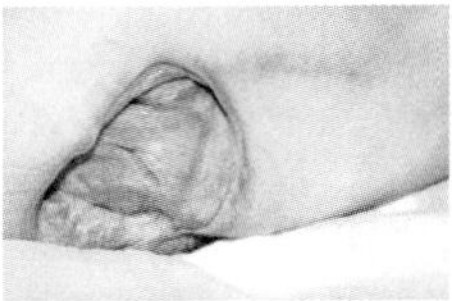	Full-thickness loss with extensive involvement of muscle, bone, or supporting structures. This deep ulcer may involve undermining and sinus tracts of adjacent tissues.
	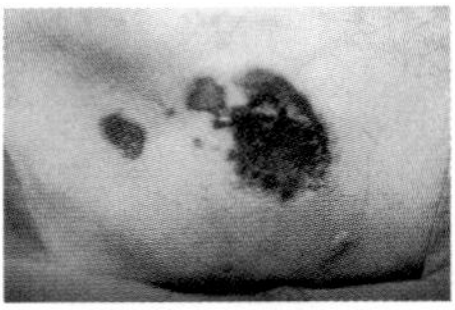	Ulcers that are covered with eschar cannot be staged without débridement.
	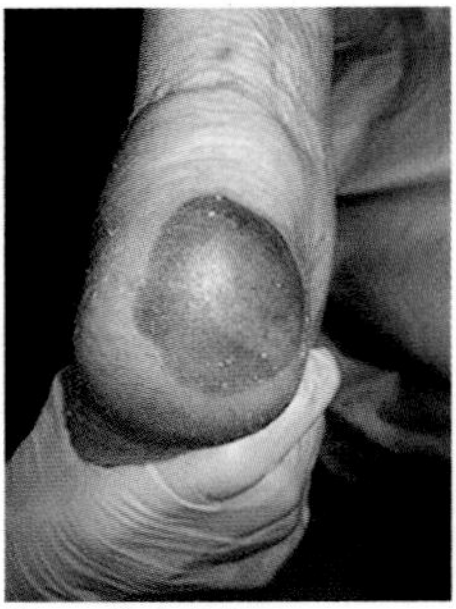 *Deep tissue injury*	Deep tissue injury is a pressure-related injury that appears as a deep bruise with intact skin.

TABLE 2.7 Clinical Description of Lesions

CHARACTERISTICS	SIGNIFICANCE
Size	Major determinant of correct category for primary lesions. Pigmented lesions are typically < 0.5 cm. If larger, consider potential for malignancy. Depth of pressure ulcers is major determinant of assigned grade. (See Table 2.6.)
Shape	Macules, wheals, and vesicles are circumscribed. Fissures are linear. Irregular borders associated with melanoma.
Color	Varies widely, and many changes are diagnostic of specific skin diseases. Variegated-colored lesions may signal melanoma.

CHARACTERISTICS	SIGNIFICANCE
	Pustules are usually yellow-white. New scars are red and raised; old scars, white or silver. Petechiae are red. Purpura are red to purplish. Vitiligo is white.
Texture	Macules are smooth. Warts are rough. Psoriasis is scaly.
Surface Relationship	Surface characteristics help differentiate between potential causes of a change and between various primary and secondary lesions. *Flat (nonpalpable):* Macules, patches, purpura, ecchymoses, spider angioma, venous spider. *Raised (palpable) solid:* Papules, plaques, nodules, tumors, wheals, scale, crust. *Raised (palpable) cystic:* Vesicles, pustules, bullae, cysts. *Depressed:* Atrophy, erosion, ulcer, fissures. *Pedunculated:* Skin tags, cutaneous horns.
Exudate	*Clear or pale, straw-yellow exudate:* Serous oozing/weeping from noninfected lesion. *Thicker, purulent discharge:* Infected lesion. *Clear serous exudates:* Vesicles, as seen with herpes simplex; or bullae, larger than vesicles, as seen with second-degree burns. *Yellow pus exudates:* Pustules, as seen with impetigo or acne
Tenderness/Pain	Tenderness or pain associated with a lesion depends on the underlying cause. May be associated with bullae from a burn or ecchymosis (bruise).

TABLE 2.8 Pattern and Configuration of Lesions

PATTERN	EXAMPLE
Round/Oval 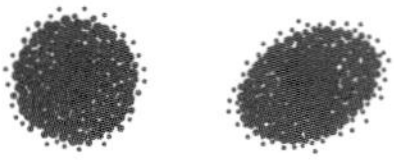 Coin- or oval-shaped, such as in nummular eczema.	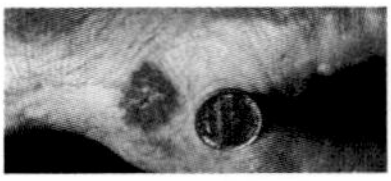
Discrete 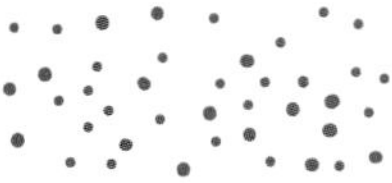 Lesions that remain separate and apart are common to many skin disorders. Moles (nevi) are an example.	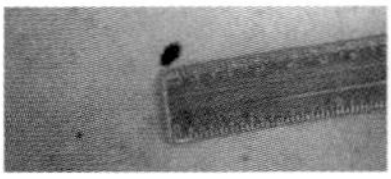
Grouped 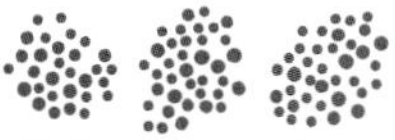 Lesions that are grouped, or clustered, such as herpes simplex.	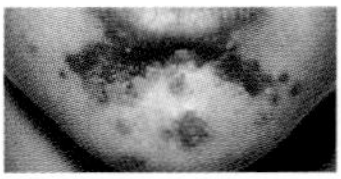
Confluent 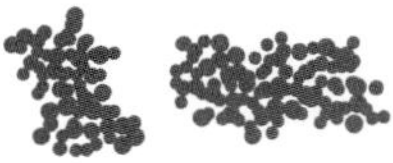 Lesions that run together or are confluent are common in childhood diseases such as rubella.	
Linear 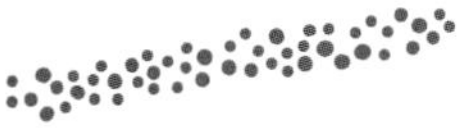 Lesions arranged in lines are common with contact dermatitis resulting from poison ivy or herpes zoster.	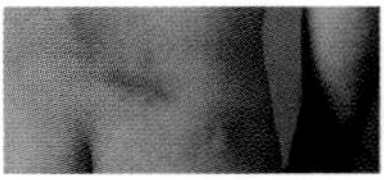
Annular/Circular 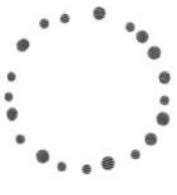 Ring-shaped lesions may be ringworm.	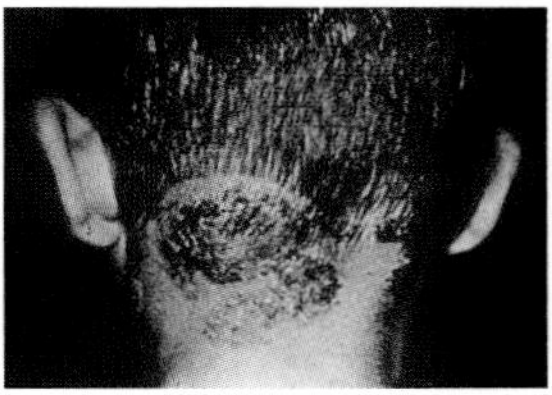

PATTERN	EXAMPLE
Arciform 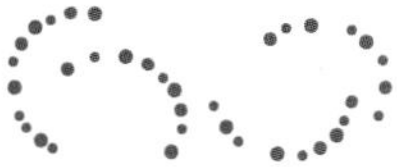 Lesions arranged in partial rings, or arcs, occur in syphilis.	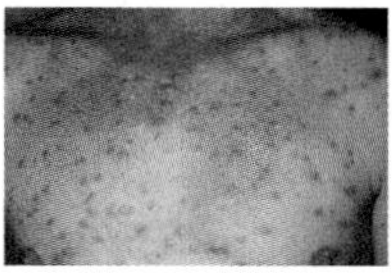
Iris 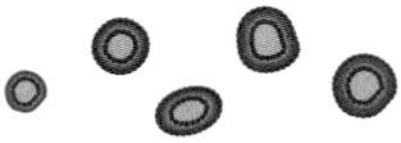 A bull's-eye lesion, or round lesion with central clearing, is typical of erythema multiforme and Lyme disease.	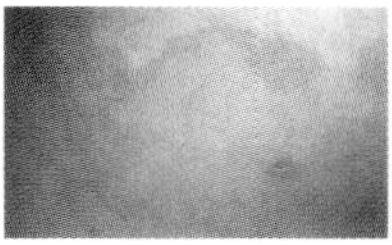
Reticular 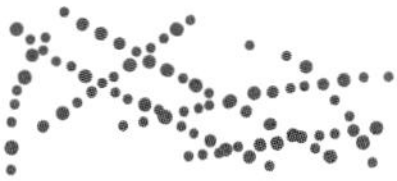 Meshlike pattern as in lichen planus.	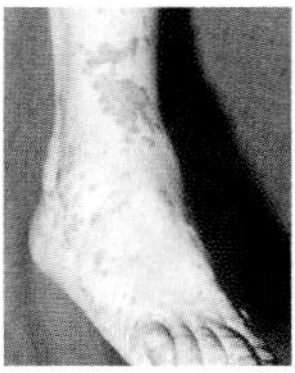
Gyrate 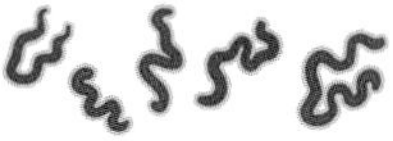 Lesions have serpentine configuration, as in gyrate erythema.	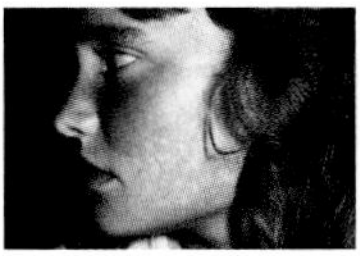
Polycyclic 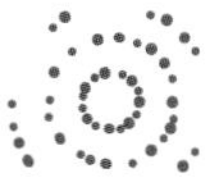 Coalesced, concentric circles, such as in urticaria.	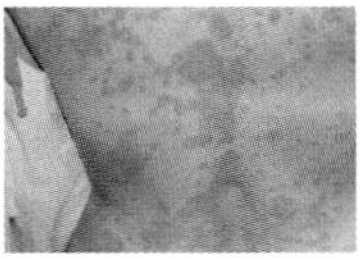

TABLE 2.9 Distribution of Skin Lesions

AREA	EXAMPLE
Diffuse/Generalized 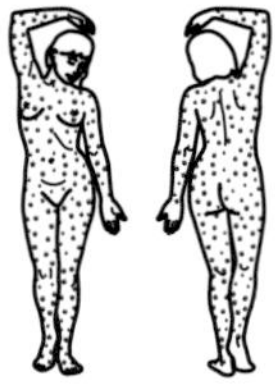 Lesions distributed over entire body, such as urticaria from allergic reactions.	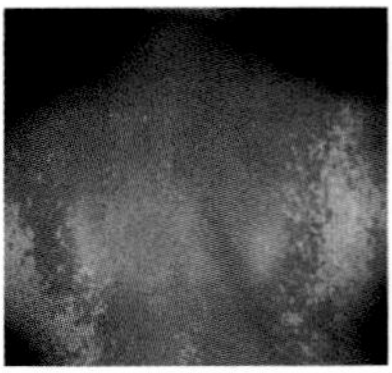
Scattered 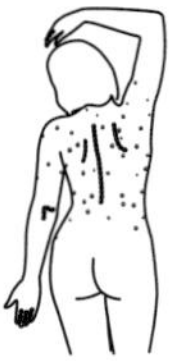 Lesions that are sparsely distributed, as in seborrheic keratosis.	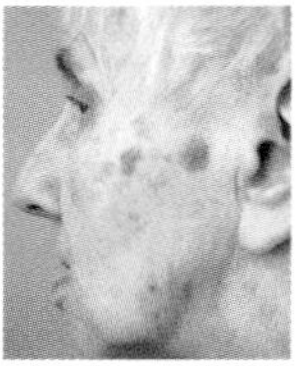
Localized 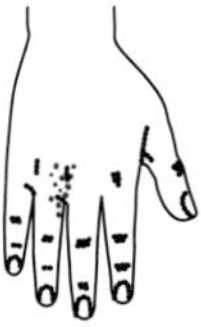 Lesions in a very limited, discrete area. Location may indicate contact with an allergen or a wheal from insect bite.	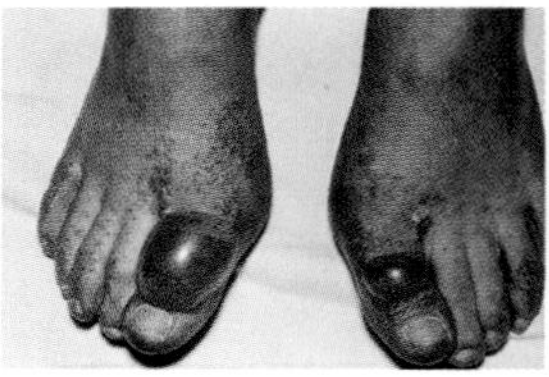
Regional **Head** 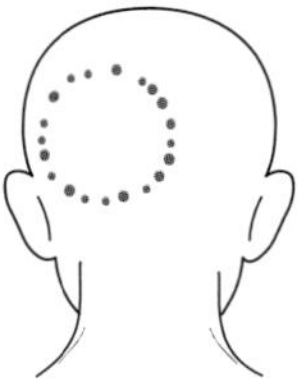 Confined to a specific body area, Tinea capitis.	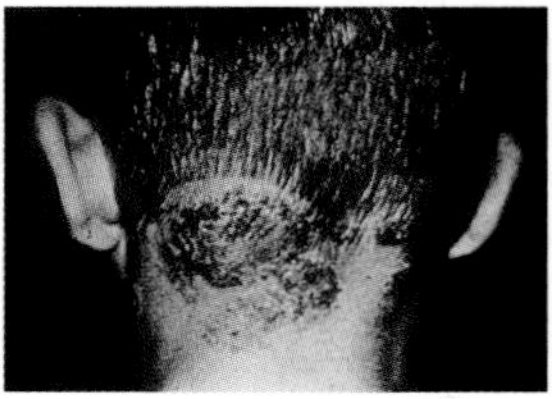

AREA	EXAMPLE
Regional *(cont'd)* **Torso** 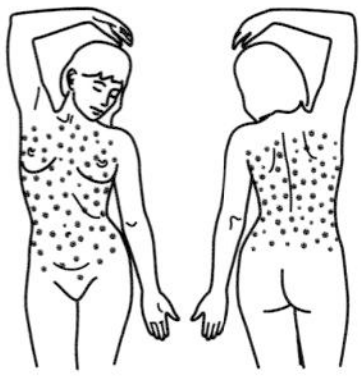 Pityriasis rosea.	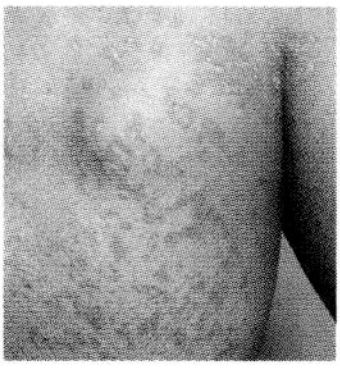
Extensor surfaces 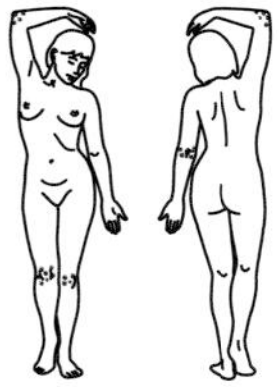 Psoriasis.	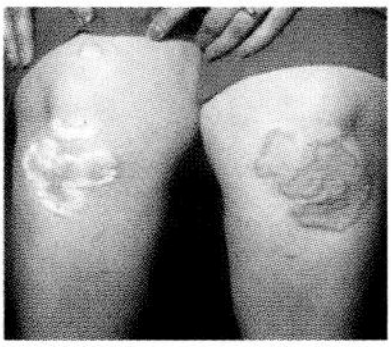
Flexor surfaces 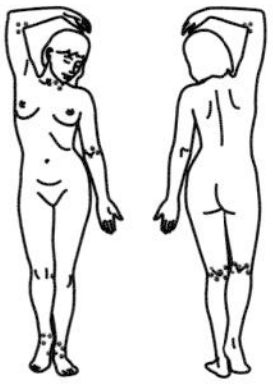 Intertrigo.	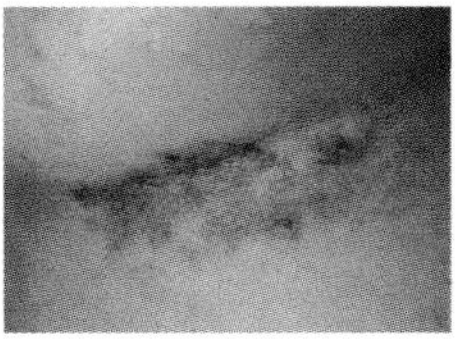
Dermatome 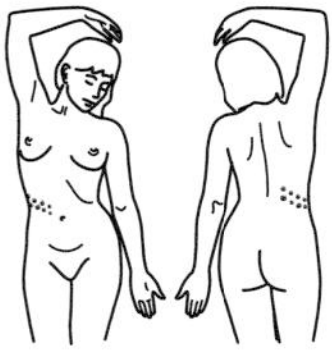 Herpes zoster.	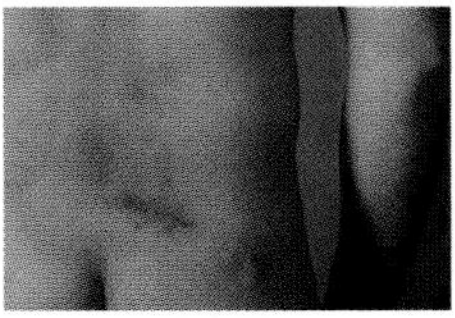

(continued)

TABLE 2.9 Distribution of Skin Lesions (continued)

AREA	EXAMPLE
Hairy areas 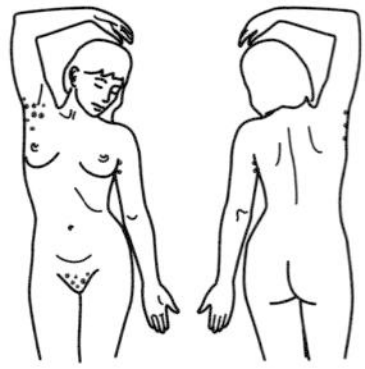 Herpes simplex virus type 2, pediculosis pubis.	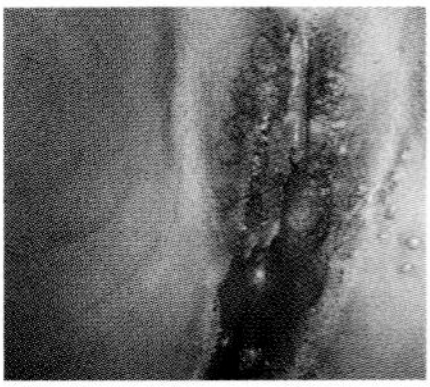
Intertriginous areas (folds of skin) 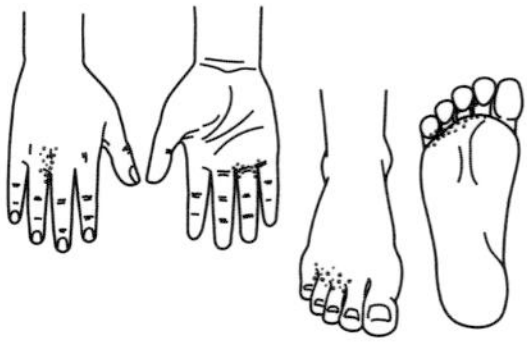 Contact dermatitis, diaper rash, intertrigo (erythema and scaling of body folds).	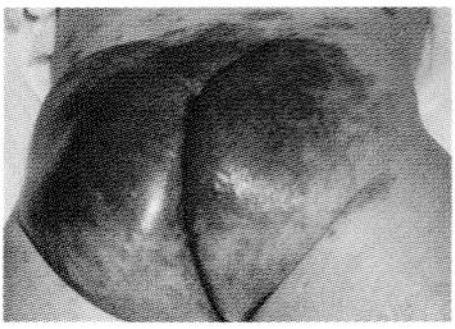
Sun-exposed areas 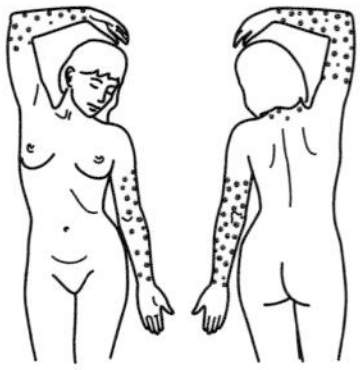 Actinic keratosis.	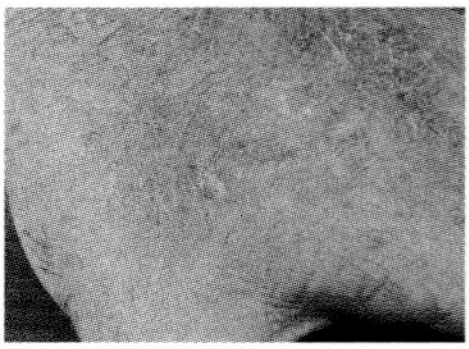

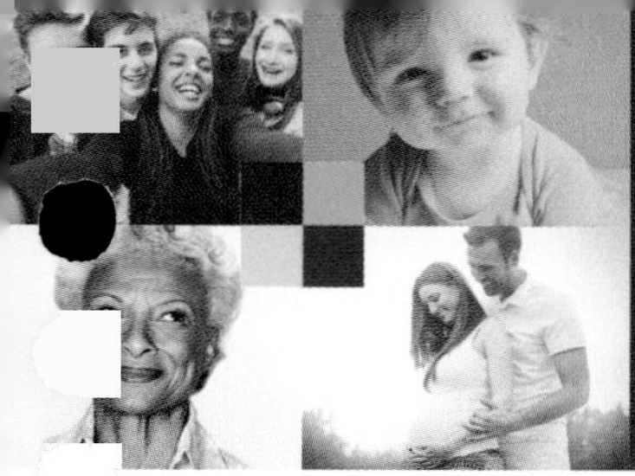

CHAPTER 3

Assessing the Head, Face, and Neck

Primary Functions

The head, face, and neck are not systems but regions of the body in which most of the systems are included.

- Integumentary system: Covers and protects the head, face, and neck.
- Respiratory system: Begins at the nose.
- Cardiovascular (CV) system: Major CV vessels (carotids and jugulars) provide blood supply to the brain.
- Gastrointestinal (GI) system: Begins at the mouth.
- Musculoskeletal system: Facial, mouth, and neck muscles allow for movement, eating, and communication; the skull protects the brain.
- Neurologic system: Skull houses brain; cranial nerves innervate head, face, and neck.
- Endocrine system: The thyroid, the largest endocrine gland, is located in the neck.
- Lymphatic system: The cervical lymph nodes are located in the neck.

Developmental Considerations

Infants and Children

- Molding of the head occurs during vaginal delivery, yet the head assumes a symmetrical, rounded shape within several days of birth.
- Fontanels ("soft spots") allow for growth.
- Sinuses are not fully developed until age 7.

- Children have 20 deciduous teeth.
- Lymphatic tissue (nodes and tonsils) is larger in children than in adults.

Pregnant Clients

- The thyroid is more active during pregnancy and is often palpable.
- Chloasma occurs on face.
- Gums may hypertrophy.

Older Adults

- Gum disease and tooth loss are often problems.
- Salivation decreases.
- Senses of taste and smell diminished.

Cultural Considerations

- African Americans may develop pseudofolliculitis.
- Chinese Americans have very little facial hair.
- Irish Americans are at increased risk for skin cancer on sun-exposed areas.
- Filipino Americans have almond-shaped eyes, mildly flared nostrils, and a low, flat nose bridge.

Assessment

History

Symptoms ("PQRST" Any + Symptom)

- Head pain
  - How long have you had this pain?
  - Have you had any recent head trauma or other injury/accident?
  - What have you done to treat the pain?
- Jaw tightness/pain
  - How long have you had this tightness or pain?
  - When does it usually occur?
  - Do you have a personal or family history of heart disease?
  - Please describe the discomfort, using your own words.
- Neck pain/stiffness
  - How would you describe the stiffness or pain?
  - How has the pain or stiffness affected your usual activities?

- What do you believe may have caused the pain/stiffness?
- Have you recently had any injury or done any unusual activity?
- Have you had similar symptoms before?
- Have you been sick—upper respiratory infection (URI), sore throat?

■ Neck mass
- When did you first notice the mass?
- Have you had any recent illness, sore throat, rashes, or other symptoms?
- Do you have a personal or family history of malignancies?

■ Nasal congestion
- Have you ever had similar congestion before?
- What other symptoms have you recently noticed?
- When is the congestion at its worst?

■ Nosebleeds (epistaxis)
- When did you first have a nosebleed?
- Describe the typical episode.
- Are there any particular settings or situations in which the bleeding is most likely to occur?
- Do you have a personal or family history of a bleeding disorder or high blood pressure?
- Have you had any recent trauma, injury, or procedure to your nose or sinuses?

■ Mouth lesions
- When did you first notice the sore?
- Does the area hurt or have other related symptoms?
- How has it changed since you first noticed it?
- What do you think caused the sore?
- Do you use tobacco or alcohol?

■ Mouth/dental pain
- Describe the pain you are having in your own terms.
- When did the pain first occur?
- Does the pain occur in certain situations more frequently than in others?
- Do you have any family or personal history of cancer or heart disease?

■ Sore throat
- Please describe the pain or discomfort in your own words.
- Where, exactly, is the pain located?
- How would you describe the onset/frequency of the pain?
- Difficulty swallowing?
- Are there any other symptoms?

- Hoarseness
  - Tell me about the progression of the hoarseness since the time you first noticed it.
  - Do you use tobacco or alcohol?
  - Is there any family or personal history of cancer or throat disease?
  - Have you had any problems with heartburn, wheezing, or indigestion?
  - What, if any, other symptoms have you recently noticed?
  - Have you recently had an injury to the throat area, surgery, or any other procedure?

Focused Head, Neck, and Throat History

- Do you have any problems or complaints related to your head, face, nose, mouth, throat, or neck? Some examples might be head pain, nasal congestion, nosebleeds, nasal discharge, mouth sores or pain, sore throat, postnasal drip, difficulty swallowing, or neck pain.
- Do you have any allergies to any medications, foods, or environmental factors?
- What, if any, health problems do you have?
- What, if any, over-the-counter or prescribed medications do you take (Table 3.1)?

TABLE 3.1 Drugs That Adversely Affect the Head, Face, and Neck

DRUG CLASS	DRUG	POSSIBLE ADVERSE REACTIONS
Anticholinergics	Atropine, scopolamine, glycopyrrolate, propantheline, belladonna alkaloids, dicyclomine, hyoscyamine	Decreased salivation, dry mouth
Anticonvulsants	Phenytoin Valproic acid	Gingival hyperplasia Alopecia
Antidepressants	Tricyclics, including amitriptyline and nortriptyline, paroxetine	Dry mouth
Antihistamines	Diphenhydramine, brompheniramine, chlorpheniramine	Dry mouth

DRUG CLASS	DRUG	POSSIBLE ADVERSE REACTIONS
Antihypertensives	Guanabenz, clonidine, methyldopa	Dry mouth
	(All calcium channel blockers)	Gingival hyperplasia
	Propranolol	Hyperkeratosis and psoriasis of the scalp, alopecia
Antineoplastics	Bleomycin	Ulcerated tongue and lips, alopecia
	Dactinomycin	Mouth lesions, alopecia
	Melphalan	Mouth lesions, alopecia
	Mitomycin	Mouth lesions, alopecia
	Methotrexate	Gingivitis, mouth lesions, alopecia
	Cyclophosphamide	Mouth lesions, alopecia
	Vincristine	Mouth lesions, alopecia
	Chlorambucil	Mouth lesions
	Uracil mustard	Mouth lesions
	Cisplatin	Gingival platinum line, alopecia
	Hydroxyurea	Mouth lesions
	Fluorouracil	Alopecia, epistaxis
	Doxorubicin	Mouth lesions, alopecia
	Cytarabine	Mouth lesions, alopecia
	Daunorubicin	Mouth lesions, alopecia
	Etoposide	Alopecia
Cardiac agents	Disopyramide	Dry mouth
Genitourinary smooth-muscle relaxants	Flavoxate, oxybutynin, propantheline	Dry mouth
Gold salts	Gold sodium thiomalate	Gingivitis, mouth lesions, alopecia
	Auranofin	Mouth lesions, alopecia
Miscellaneous agents	Lithium	Dry mouth, dry hair, alopecia
	Metoclopramide	Dry mouth, glossal or periorbital edema

(continued)

TABLE 3.1 Drugs That Adversely Affect the Head, Face, and Neck (continued)

DRUG CLASS	DRUG	POSSIBLE ADVERSE REACTIONS
	Penicillamine	Mouth lesions
	Isotretinoin	Inflamed and bleeding gums, epistaxis, hirutism
	Edrophonium	Increased salivation
	Pyridostigmine	Increased salivation, increased tracheobronchial secretions
	Fluorides	Staining or mottling of teeth
	Warfarin	Epistaxis
	Amphetamines	Dry mouth, continuous chewing or bruxism (tooth grinding) with prolonged use
	Tetracycline	Enamel hypoplasia and permanent yellow-gray to brown tooth discoloration in children under age 8 and in offspring of pregnant patients
	Cyclosporine	Gingival hyperplasia

- Is there anything specific that you think I should know in relation to your overall health or this specific complaint?

Assessment of the Head, Face, and Neck's Relationship to Other Systems

Remember, all systems are related! As you assess the head, face, and neck, look at the relationship between them and all other systems.

(text continues on page 85)

Assessment of The Head, Face, and Neck's Relationship to Other Systems

SUBJECTIVE DATA/ RATIONALE	OBJECTIVE DATA/ RATIONALE
Area/System: General	
Ask about:	*Inspect:*
Changes in energy level and mental status: Altered mental status may indicate meningeal infection, which could be associated with head or neck pain or stiffness. Forgetfulness or slow mental processes are associated with hypothyroidism; mood lability, personality changes, and restlessness are associated with hyperthyroidism.	Features for symmetry and proportion.
Weight changes.	
Fevers.	*Measure:*
Night sweats.	Vital signs. Height and weight.
Endocrine and lymphatic system disorders often result in nonspecific symptoms, which are best elicited through the general review of systems. Examples include thyroid disorders and allergies, both of which are important to the assessment of the head, face, and neck.	
Area/System: Integumentary	
Ask about:	*Inspect:*
Changes in skin, hair, and nails: Changes in the texture of skin, hair, and nails commonly occur with thyroid disorders. Color changes may be associated with endocrine disorders, such as the bronze color change of Addison's disease. Hirsutism (increase in facial or body hair growth) may be a result of Cushing's disease or a side effect of steroids.	*Skin for color changes (e.g., cyanosis, pallor), lesions, hair distribution:* Color changes can readily be seen in mucous membranes. For example, cyanosis related to hypoxia, jaundice related to liver dysfunction, pallor related to anemia, or bronze/tan discoloration related to Addison's disease. Dry, sparse, coarse hair seen with hypothyroidism; patchy alopecia, and fine, silky hair, with hyperthyroidism. Increased facial hair in women is associated with Cushing's disease or steroid use.

(continued)

Assessment of the Head, Face, and Neck's Relationship to Other Systems (continued)

SUBJECTIVE DATA/ RATIONALE	OBJECTIVE DATA/ RATIONALE
Area/System: Integumentary *(cont'd)*	
Rashes, itching: People with allergic rhinitis often have allergies affecting other systems, including the skin, and could have atopic rashes or pruritus. Sores or lesions might cause enlarged lymph nodes.	*Palpate:* *Skin for temperature, turgor, texture:* Dry, thick, cool skin with poor turgor is associated with hypothyroidism; warm, smooth, moist skin is associated with hyperthyroidism. *Nails and hair texture:* Thick, brittle nails seen with hypothyroidism; thin, brittle nails with hyperthyroidism.
Area/System: HEENT	
Head and neck	
Ask about:	*Inspect:*
Head or neck pain: May indicate a musculoskeletal problem or an infection, such as meningitis.	Size, shape, symmetry of head and facial features.
Masses or swollen nodes: Infection may cause enlarged lymph nodes. Thyroid disease may cause enlarged thyroid gland.	Facial expression.
	Palpate: Thyroid. Lymph nodes.
Eyes	
Ask about:	*Inspect:*
Vision changes.	*Conjunctiva:* Conjunctival redness and drainage suggest infection or allergy, both of which may involve the nose and sinuses.
Drainage, itching, pain.	*Palpebral fissures:* Lid lag from exopthalmos associated with hyperthyroidism.
	Test: Visual acuity.
Ears, nose, and throat	
Ask about:	*Inspect:*
Changes in hearing.	*Gross hearing:* Hearing changes and altered appearance of tympanic membrane and landmarks associated with fluid accumulations behind the tympanic membrane (serous otitis) or infection (otitis media), both of which may affect the nose or throat.

SUBJECTIVE DATA/ RATIONALE	OBJECTIVE DATA/ RATIONALE
Ear drainage, itching, pain.	Structures of the mouth and throat.
Nasal congestion, drainage, sinus pain.	External ear and tympanic membrane.
	Bleeding from the ear and nose signals possible skull fracture.
Nosebleeds. Mouth sores or dental pain. Jaw pain.	
Because of their proximity, disorders that affect the eyes and ears may also affect other organs of the head, face, and neck. The ears communicate with the rest of the upper airways, so infections involving one structure may move to the other. Allergic disorders causing rhinitis often involve the ears and/or eyes as well.	
Area/System: Respiratory *Ask about:*	*Measure:*
Cough, congestion, wheezing, mucus production: The upper and lower respiratory tracks are closely related, so infections in one often influence the other. People with asthma have a high incidence of allergic rhinitis.	Respiratory rate.
	Auscultate: *Breath sounds:* Tachypnea, cough, and wheezing may indicate asthma, which is highly related to other atopic diseases, such as allergic rhinitis or a respiratory infection that may also involve the upper respiratory tract. Masses or lesions in the nose, mouth, or throat can influence respiratory status.

(continued)

Assessment of the Head, Face, and Neck's Relationship to Other Systems (continued)

SUBJECTIVE DATA/ RATIONALE	OBJECTIVE DATA/ RATIONALE
Area/System: Cardiovascular *Ask about:*	*Measure/Palpate:*
History of cardiovascular disease (e.g., coronary artery disease, hypertension).	Heart rate, pulse. *Pulse amplitude:* Bounding temporal arteries paired with temporal pain suggests temporal arteritis, an explanation for head pain.
Chest pain, palpitations.	*Auscultate:*
CV disorders can result in fluid imbalances that cause facial edema. Veins may become distended and arterial pulses may be bounding. Extreme elevations in blood pressure can cause nose-bleeds. Other symptoms of cardiac ischemia may help to explain jaw, tooth, or neck discomfort. Thyroid disorders have profound CV effects, including tachycardia and/or arrhythmias.	*Heart sounds, bruits:* Bruits of the carotid arteries are detected during the examination of the neck and may indicate carotid stenosis. Proper examination should differentiate between bruits of the carotids and vascular sounds over the thyroid.
Area/System: Gastrointestinal *Ask about:*	*Inspect:*
Changes in appetite.	*Abdomen for size, shape, and symmetry:* The mouth is the beginning of the GI tract, so oral problems may affect the GI system. Jaundice can be seen on the palate.
Bowel changes, nausea, and vomiting: Thyroid disorders can alter bowel habits. Infections that involve the upper respiratory tract, particularly viral ones, are often associated with nausea, abdominal discomfort, vomiting, and/or diarrhea.	*Palpate:* For organomegaly. *Auscultate:* Bowel sounds.
Area/System: Genitourinary/ Reproductive *Ask about:*	*Inspect:*
History of renal disease: Chronic renal failure may cause periorbital edema. Uremic frost may be seen on the face in end-stage renal disease.	

SUBJECTIVE DATA/ RATIONALE	OBJECTIVE DATA/ RATIONALE
History of STDs.	*External genitals for lesions or discharge:* Oral lesions may be caused by STDs.
Changes in libido: Decreased libido is associated with both hypothyroid and hyperthyroid disease. *For women:* *Last menstrual period and menstrual changes:* Thyroid disorders frequently alter the menstrual pattern. *Vaginal discharge or sores:* Oral lesions and pharyngitis may be found in people with STDs. **Pregnancy may cause nasal congestion.** **For men:** *Penile discharge or sores:* Oral lesions and pharyngitis may be found in people with STDs.	
Area/System: Musculoskeletal *Ask about:*	*Inspect:*
Joint pain: Joint and muscle symptoms suggest arthritic or neuromuscular disorders that would cause head, face, and neck discomfort or limit motion. Infectious diseases affecting the head, face, and neck may also cause generalized aches and pains.	*ROM of head and neck:* Muscle weakness and limitations of motion, pain, and/or joint deformities are found with various forms of arthritis and may affect the TMJ and cervical joints. Weakness can be a sign of thyroid disorder, as well as of various neuromuscular disorders that may affect expression, speech, and eating. Limited ROM of the neck and nuchal rigidity (resistance to neck flexion) are associated with meningitis.
Limited movement: Hypothyroidism can result in an overall sense of fatigue or weakness; hyperthy-roidism causes weakness of the proximal muscle groups of the extremities.	*Palpate:* For muscle strength, joint deformities.

(continued)

Assessment of the Head, Face, and Neck's Relationship to Other Systems (continued)

SUBJECTIVE DATA/ RATIONALE	OBJECTIVE DATA/ RATIONALE
Area/System: Neurologic	
Ask about:	*Test:*
Nervousness: Nervousness, fine tremors, restlessness, and labile moods are associated with hyperthyroidism.	Level of orientation.
	Thought process and memory.
Apathy, lethargy, difficulty staying focused, forgetfulness, slowed speech, and slowed mental processes: Associated with hypothy-roidism.	*Cranial nerves:* Cranial nerves innervate most structures of the head, face, and neck and affect their function. Changes in sensation and coordination indicate neurologic disorders that influence function of the nose (olfaction) and muscles of facial expression, eating, and speech.
Changes in level of consciousness.	
Numbness and tingling.	*Inspect:*
Headaches, head injury: Neurologic disorders can cause head pain and neck pain/stiffness.	For abnormal movements.
Paresthesias, paralysis, or weakness from neurologic disorders may have a profound influence on facial expressions and ability to swallow.	
Thyroid disease may manifest as neurologic symptoms. A history of head trauma or headaches may also explain physical findings.	
Area/System: Endocrine	
Ask about:	*Inspect:*
Changes in shoe size or ring size.	For masses, goiters.
Changes in facial features: Acromegaly, a pituitary hypersecretory disorder, causes enlargement and hypertrophy of bone and connective tissues, with profound alterations in facial structures and headaches.	*Palpate:* For thyroid enlargement and nodules.

SUBJECTIVE DATA/ RATIONALE	OBJECTIVE DATA/ RATIONALE
Changes in energy level: Associated with thyroid disorders.	*Auscultate:*
Weight changes: Associated with thyroid disorders.	Thyroid, if palpable.
Sleep problems: Associated with thyroid disorders.	
Area/System: Immunological/ Hematological	
Ask about:	*Inspect:*
Unusual bleeding, bruising.	For ecchymoses, petechiae.
Current/recent infection.	*Palpate:*
History of cancer.	For lymph node enlargement.
Disorders of the hematological system may become evident through bleeding of other structures and help to explain nasal or oral bleeding.	

HEENT = Head, eye, ear, nose, and throat.

Physical Assessment

ANATOMICAL LANDMARKS: Palpebral fissures (opening between the eyelids) and nasolabial (corner of the nose to edge of the lip) folds; anterior and posterior triangles

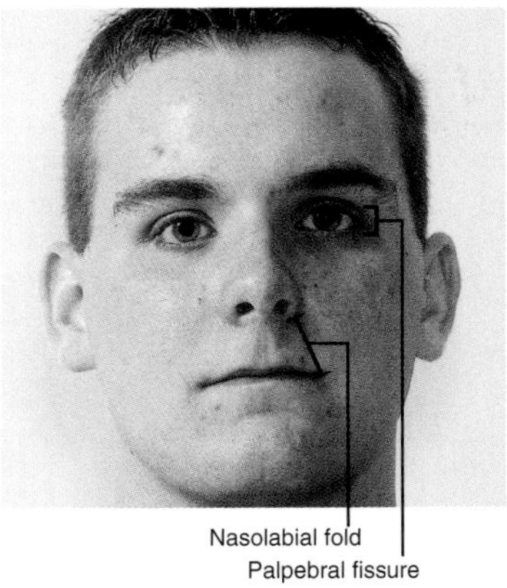

Palpebral fissures and nasolabial folds

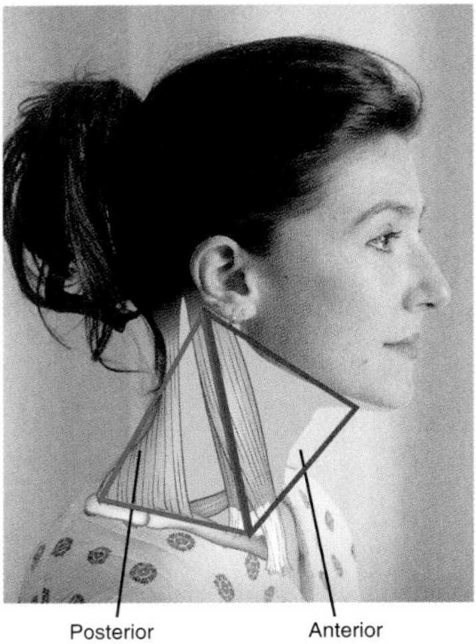

Anterior and posterior triangles

APPROACH (ANTERIOR AND POSTERIOR): Inspection, palpation, percussion, auscultation

POSITION: Sitting

TOOLBOX: Penlight or otoscope for focused light, tongue blades, gauze, stethoscope, transilluminator, cup of water, gloves, nasal speculum

Physical Assessment

AREA/PA SKILL	NORMAL FINDINGS	ABNORMAL FINDINGS
Inspection *Head*		
Note size, shape, symmetry, and position.	Normocephalic, erect, midline.	*Increasing head circumference in children:* Hydrocephalus.
Assess fontanels and head circumference in infants.		*Increasing head size in adolescents or adults:* Acromegaly. 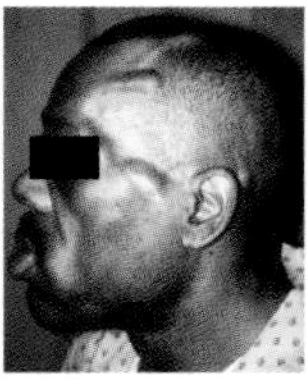 *Acromegaly* *Asymmetry:* Trauma or congenital deformity.

AREA/PA SKILL	NORMAL FINDINGS	ABNORMAL FINDINGS
Face		
Assess facial expression.	Facial expression appropriate.	*Facial appearance inconsistent with gender, age, or racial/ethnic group:* Inherited or chronic disorder with typical facies (e.g., Graves' disease, hypothyroidism with myxedema, Cushing's syndrome, or acromegaly). 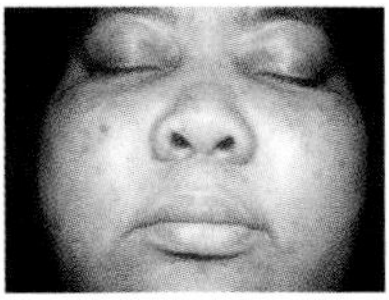 *Cushing's syndrome*
Check for symmetry of facial features.	Nasolabial folds and palpebral fissures symmetrical.	*Asymmetry of features:* Previous trauma, surgical alterations, congenital deformity, paralysis, or edema. Also seen with Bell's palsy and stroke. 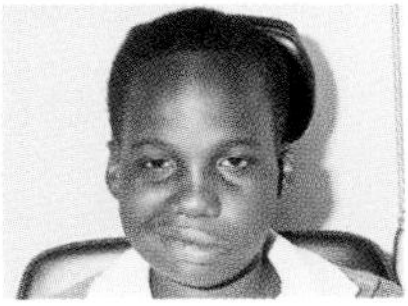 *Bell's Palsy*
Nasolabial folds and palpebral fissures are good places to check for symmetry.		
		Asymmetry of movement: Neuromuscular disorder or paralysis. Tics usually occur in the head and face.
Inspect for abnormal movements, lesions, and hair distribution.	Hair distribution appropriate for client's age, sex, and ethnicity. No lesions or abnormal movements.	*Hirsutism in women:* Steroid use or Cushing's syndrome. 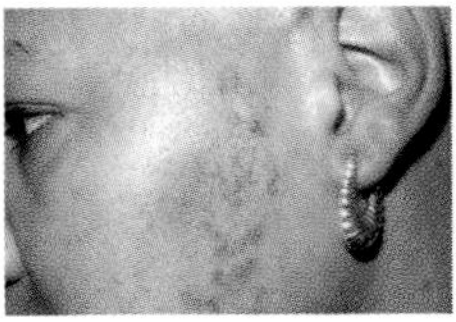 *Hirsutism*

(box continued on page 88)

Physical Assessment (continued)

AREA/PA SKILL	NORMAL FINDINGS	ABNORMAL FINDINGS
Inspection *(cont'd)* *Nose* Note position, deformities, septal deviation, discharge, flaring.	Nose midline, symmetrical, no deviation, no flaring.	*Misalignment of nose, or shape inconsistent with client's history:* Previous trauma, congenital deformity, surgical alteration, or mass; also associated with typical facies, including acromegaly or Down syndrome. **Nasal flaring: Suggests respiratory distress, especially in infants, who are obligatory nose breathers.**
Assess for color, intactness, lesions, edema, and discharge (types of discharge: clear, bloody, purulent).	Nasal mucosa pink, moist; no lesions, edema, or discharge.	*Drainage:* Clear, bilateral: Allergic rhinitis. **Clear, unilateral: May be spinal fluid as a result of head trauma or fracture.** *Clear, mucoid:* Viral rhinitis. *Yellow or green:* Upper respiratory infection. *Bloody:* Trauma, hypertension, or bleeding disorders.
Inspect for color and edema of turbinates.	Septum intact and midline turbinates pink.	*Bright red nasal mucosa:* Inflammation from rhinitis or sinusitis; also suggests cocaine abuse. *Pale/gray mucosa:* Allergic rhinitis. *Copious or colored discharge:* Allergic or infectious disorder, epistaxis, head or nose trauma. *Clustered vesicles:* Herpes infection. *Ulcers or perforations:* Chronic infection, trauma, or cocaine use. *Dried, crusted blood:* Previous nosebleed. *Polyps (elongated, rounded projections):* Allergies. 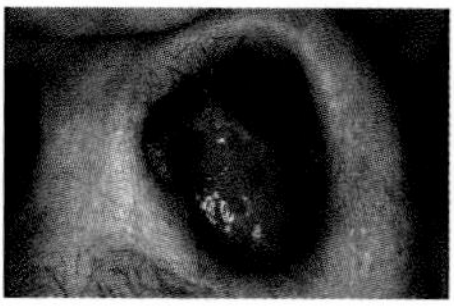 *Polyps*

AREA/PA SKILL	NORMAL FINDINGS	ABNORMAL FINDINGS
		Deviated septum: Normal variant or following trauma. 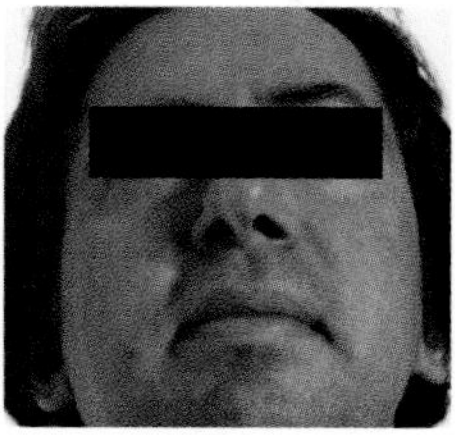 *Deviated septum* *Enlarged, boggy turbinates:* Allergic disorder. *Pale or gray mucosa overlying turbinates:* Allergic disorder.
Frontal and Maxillary Sinuses **Frontal sinuses above eyes; maxillary below eyes.**		
Assess for periorbital edema, dark circles under eyes.	No periorbital edema.	*Periorbital edema and dark under-eye circles:* Sinusitis.
Transilluminate sinuses if indicated.	Sinuses clear, presence of transillumination.	*Absence of transillumination over one sinus when opposite structure transilluminates:* Mucosal thickening or sinus fullness with sinusitis. Absence of transillumination must be considered with other findings.

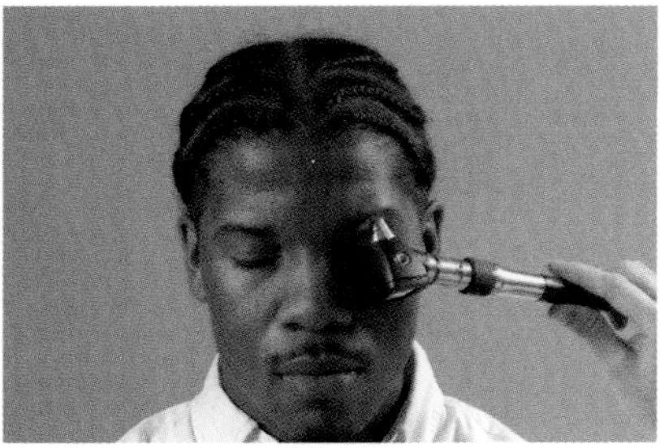

Transilluminating frontal sinuses

(box continued on page 90)

Physical Assessment (continued)

AREA/PA SKILL	NORMAL FINDINGS	ABNORMAL FINDINGS
Inspection *Nose (cont'd)*		

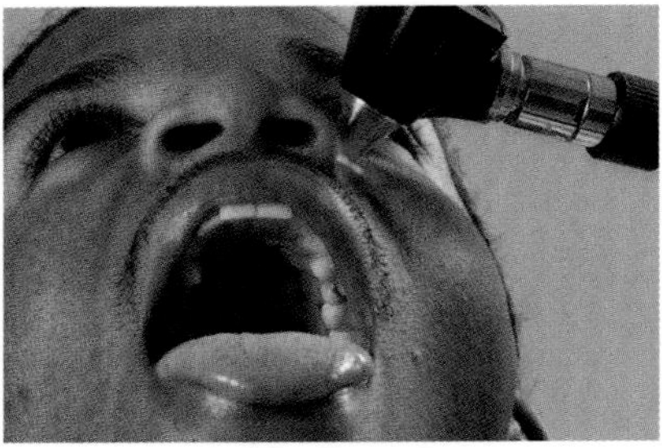

Transilluminating maxillary sinuses

AREA/PA SKILL	NORMAL FINDINGS	ABNORMAL FINDINGS
Parotid and Submandibular Glands **Parotid glands in front of ears; submandibular under mandible.**		
Assess for edema, redness.	No edema or redness over glands.	*Fullness or inflammatory changes of glands:* Blockage of duct by calculi, infection, malignancy.
Lips Note color, condition, lesions.	Lips pink (or consistent with ethnic group/race), moist, intact, no lesions.	*Asymmetry of placement:* Congenital deformity, such as cleft lip, trauma, paralysis, or surgical alteration. *Pallor:* Anemia. *Redness:* Inflammatory or infectious disorder. *Cyanosis:* Vasoconstriction or hypoxia. *Lesions:* Infectious or inflammatory disorder. *Cheilitis, drying, and cracking:* Dehydration, allergy, lip licking. *Cheilosis:* Deficiency of B vitamins or maceration related to overclosure.

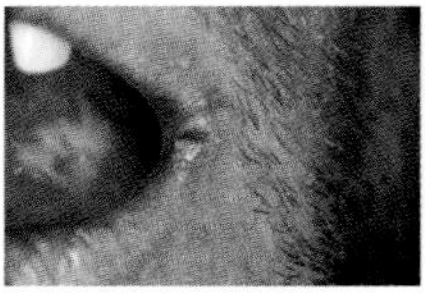

Cheilitis and cheilosis

AREA/PA SKILL	NORMAL FINDINGS	ABNORMAL FINDINGS
		Chancre: Single, painless ulcer of primary syphilis. 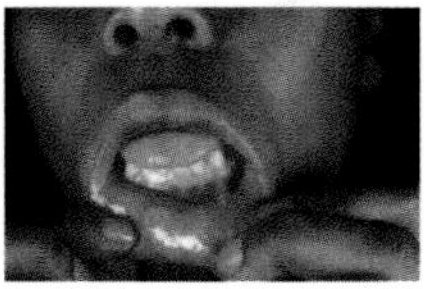 *Chancre*
		Angioedema: Allergic response 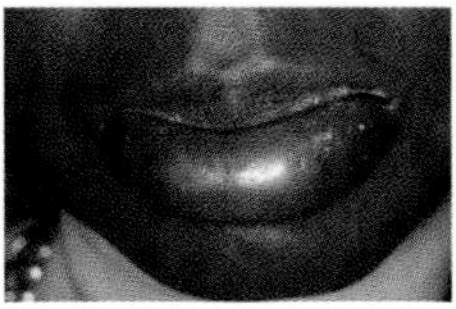 *Angioedema*
		Clustered area of fullness/nodularity that forms vesicles, then ulceration: Herpes simplex viral infection. 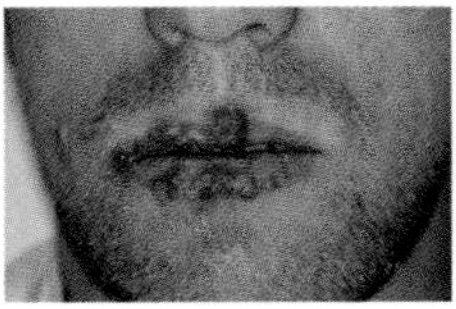 *Herpes viral infection*
Assess for breath odor and pursed-lip breathing.	No unusual odors (halitosis). No pursed-lip breathing.	*Halitosis:* Infections or GI problems. 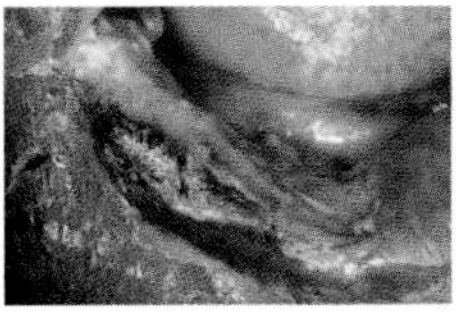 *Cancer on lip*
Oral Mucosa Note color, condition, lesions.	Oral mucosa pink (or consistent with ethnic group/race), moist, intact, no lesions.	*Abrasions, erosion of underlying mucosa:* In denture wearers, poorly fitted dentures. *Painful, reddened mucosa, often with mildly adherent white patches: Candida albicans.*

(box continued on page 92)

Physical Assessment (continued)

AREA/PA SKILL	NORMAL FINDINGS	ABNORMAL FINDINGS
Inspection *Oral Mucosa (cont'd)*		*Reddened, inflamed oral mucosa, sometimes with ulcerations:* Allergic stomatitis. *Small, painful vesicles, often with reddened periphery and a white or pale yellowish base:* Aphthous ulcer caused by viral infection, stress, or trauma. 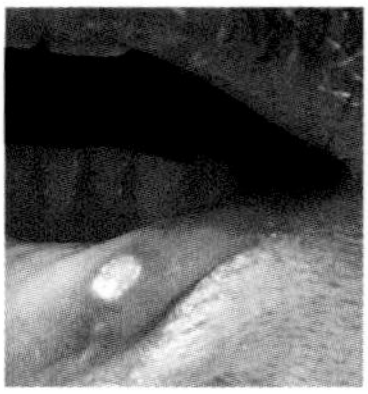 *Aphthous ulcer* *Nodular, macular, or papular lesions widely involving the integument and oral mucosa:* Kaposi's sarcoma. *Inflammatory changes of the integument, often found on oral mucosa as chronic gray, lacy patches with or without ulceration:* Lichen planus. May progress to neoplasm. 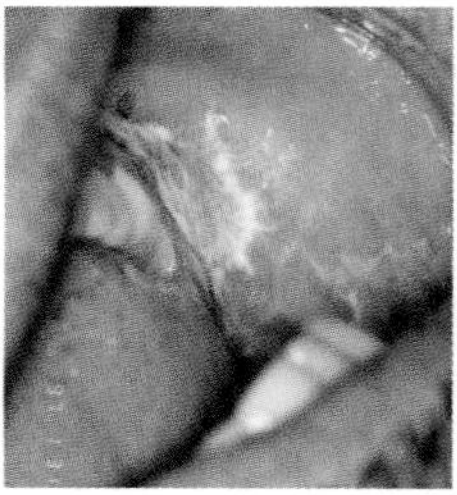 *Lichen planus* *Reddened mucosal change that may progress to form cancer:* Erythroplakia. **White, adherent mucosal thickening: Leukoplakia. Precancerous lesion, warrants follow-up.**

AREA/PA SKILL	NORMAL FINDINGS	ABNORMAL FINDINGS
Assess for inflammation of Stensen's and Wharton's ducts. **(Stensen's ducts opposite second upper molars; Wharton's ducts on floor of mouth under tongue.)**	Stensen's and Wharton's ducts patent, no inflammation.	

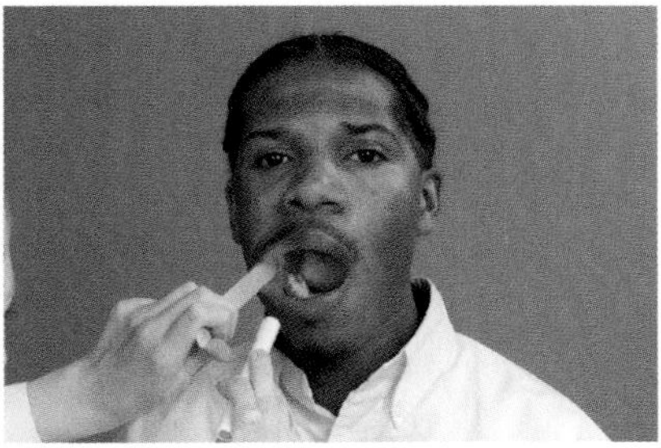
Inspecting the oral mucosa and gums

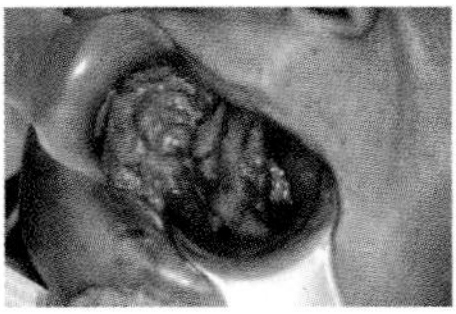
Cancer on oral mucosa

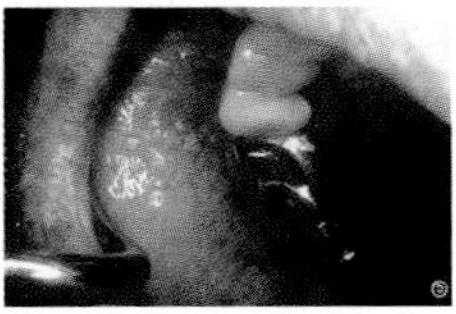
Fordyce granules

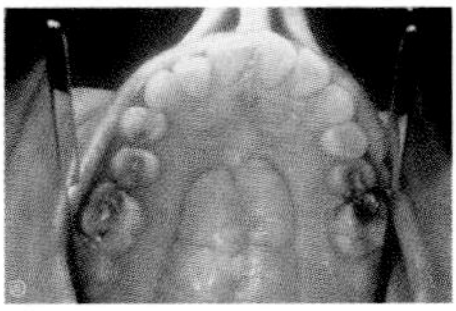
Torus palatinus

(box continued on page 94)

Physical Assessment (continued)

AREA/PA SKILL	NORMAL FINDINGS	ABNORMAL FINDINGS
Inspection *Oral Mucosa (cont'd)*		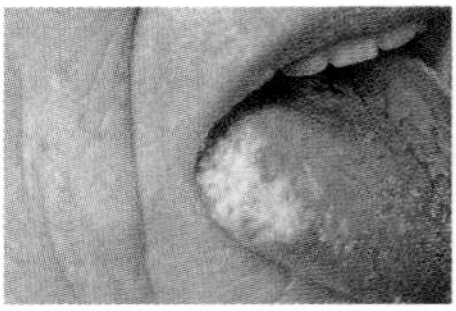 *Leukoplakia* 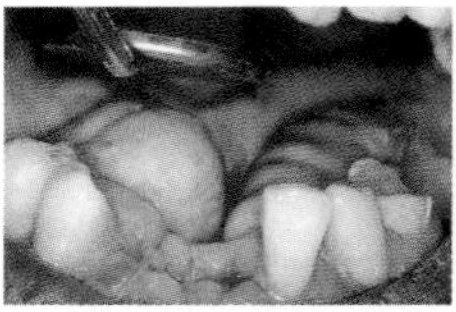 *Torus mandibularis* 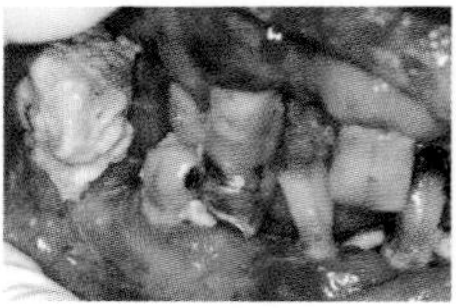 *Parotitis* 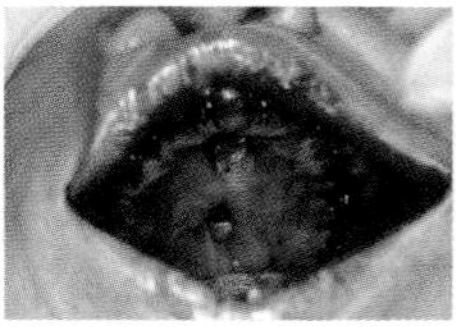 *Cocaine use* 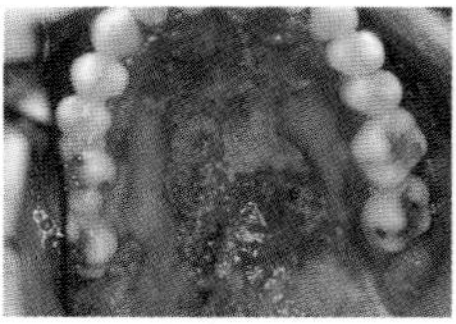 *HIV palatal candidiasis*

AREA/PA SKILL	NORMAL FINDINGS	ABNORMAL FINDINGS
Gingivae Assess for color, condition, retraction, hypertrophy, edema, bleeding, and lesions.	Gingivae pink, moist, intact; no bleeding edema, recession, hypertrophy, or lesions.	*Inflamed, bleeding gingivae:* Leukemia and human immunodeficiency virus (HIV). Also, poorly fitted dentures in denture wearers. 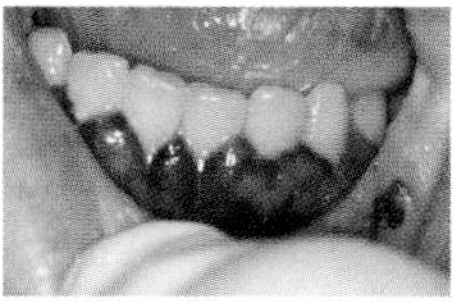 *Leukemia* 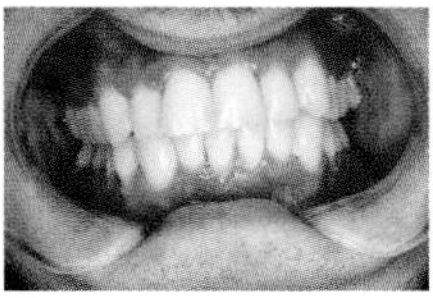 *Early HIV periodontitis* 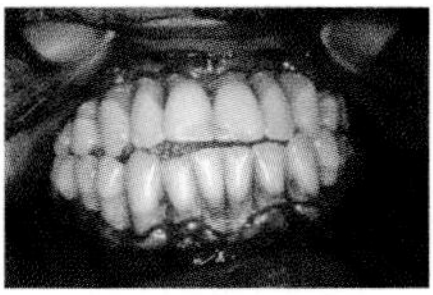 *Advanced HIV periodontitis* *Hyperplasia of gums:* Side effect of medications (e.g., Dilantin or calcium channel blockers). 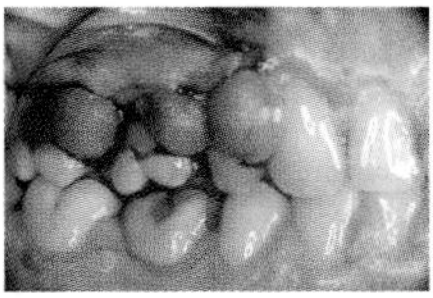 *Gum hyperplasia* *Gum recession or inflammatory gum changes:* Poor dental hygiene or vitamin deficiency. 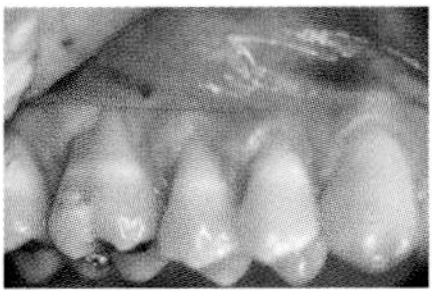 *Gingival recession*

(box continued on page 96)

Physical Assessment (continued)

AREA/PA SKILL	NORMAL FINDINGS	ABNORMAL FINDINGS
Inspection *Gingivae (cont'd)*		*Pale/gray gingivae:* Chronic gingivitis. 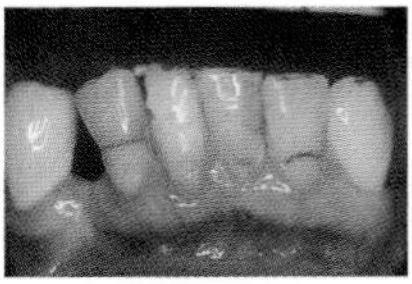 *Chronic gingivitis*
Teeth Assess for number, color, condition. Note any missing or loose teeth.	32 teeth in adults (28 without wisdom teeth), 20 in children; white; edges smooth; in good repair; no caries; no missing or loose teeth.	Various abnormalities include loose, poorly anchored teeth, malalignment, dental caries. 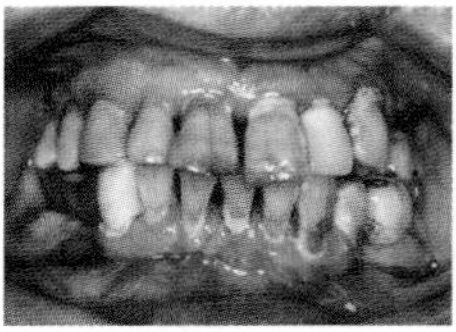 *Dental caries* **A loose tooth poses a threat of airway obstruction.** *Discoloration of teeth:* Chemicals or medications (tetracycline may discolor teeth gray if administered before puberty). 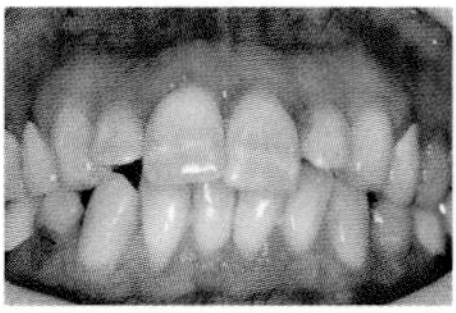 *Tetracycline staining* *Mottled enamel:* Fluorosis. 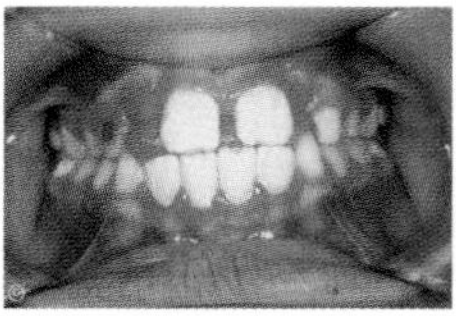 *Fluorosis*

AREA/PA SKILL	NORMAL FINDINGS	ABNORMAL FINDINGS
Check occlusion.	Good occlusion.	Malocclusion. 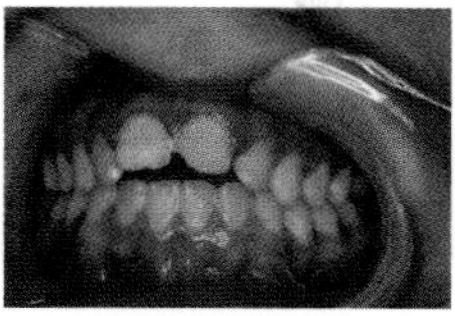 *Malocclusion*
Tongue Assess color, texture, position, and mobility (tests cranial nerve [CN] XII).	Tongue pink, moist, intact; papillae intact; midline with full mobility (CN XII intact).	*Absence of papillae, reddened mucosa, ulcerations:* Allergic, inflammatory, or infectious cause. 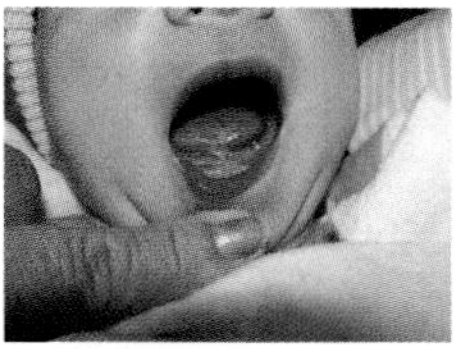 *Tongue tied*
Note any involuntary movements or lesions.	No lesions or involuntary movements.	Color changes may indicate underlying problems (e.g., red "beefy" tongue is seen with pernicious anemia).

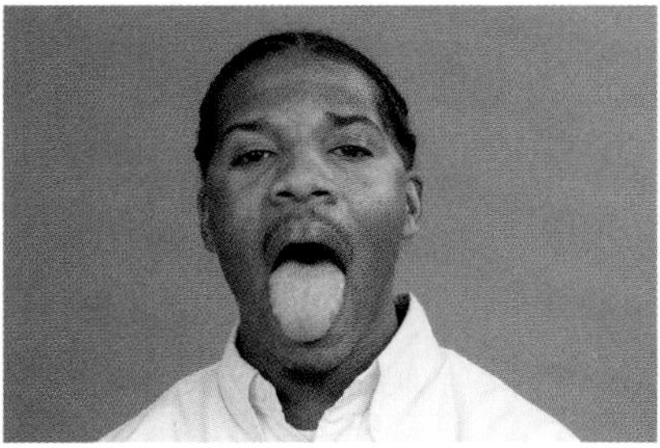

Inspecting the tongue

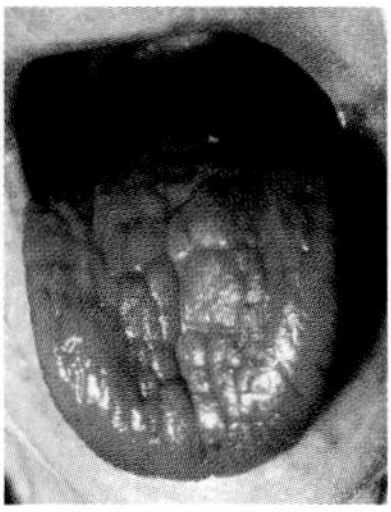

Red "beefy" tongue

(box continued on page 98)

Physical Assessment (continued)

AREA/PA SKILL	NORMAL FINDINGS	ABNORMAL FINDINGS

Inspection
Tongue (cont'd)

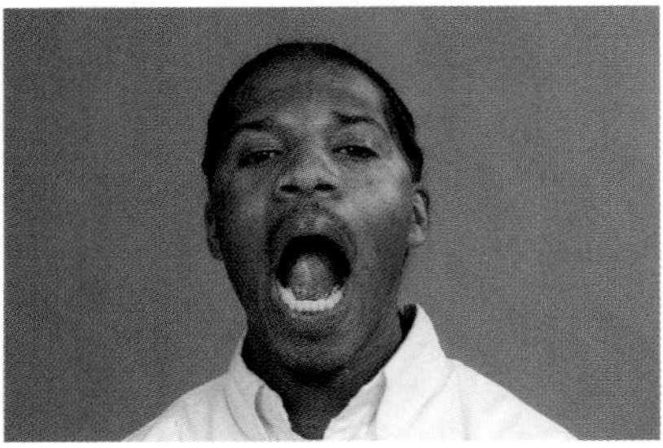

Inspecting the underside of the tongue

Geographic tongue is normal variation.

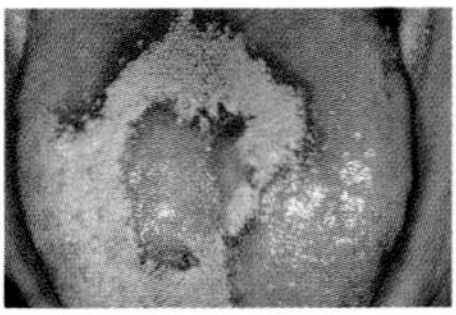

Geographic tongue

Black hairy tongue: Fungal infections.

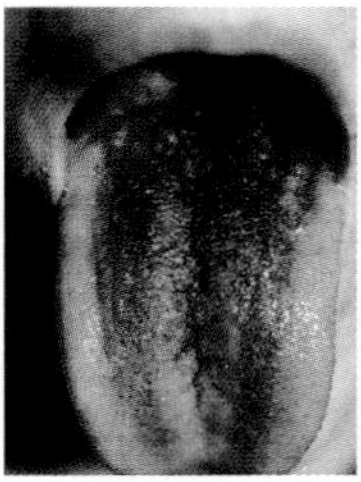

Black, hairy tongue

Hypertrophy and discoloration of the papilla: Antibiotic use.

Reddened, smooth, painful tongue, with or without ulcerations: Anemia, chemical irritants, medications.

AREA/PA SKILL	NORMAL FINDINGS	ABNORMAL FINDINGS
		Cancers may form on the tongue and on other oral mucosa. 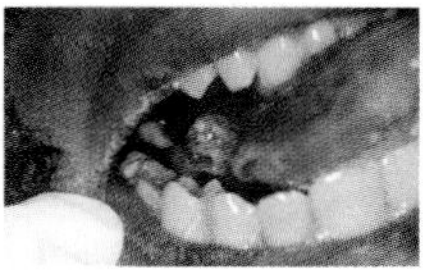 *Cancer of the tongue* 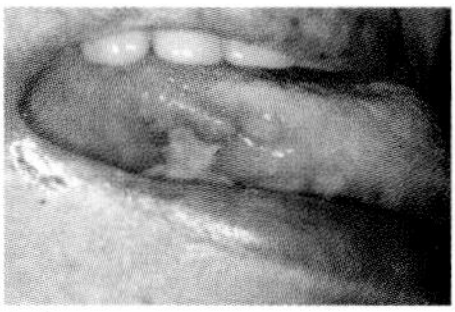 *Glossitis*
Oropharynx, Hard/ Soft Palate, Tonsils, and Uvula		
Assess for color, condition, lesions, drainage, exudates, and edema.	Hard and soft palate pink and intact.	*Reddened, hypertrophic tonsil, with or without exudates:* Acute infection or tonsillitis with lymphoid cobblestoning.
	Tonsils pink, symmetrical, + 1, no exudates.	Enlarged tonsils with exudates.

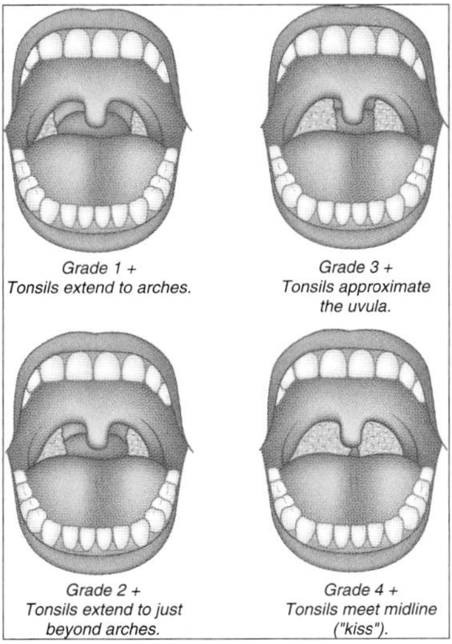

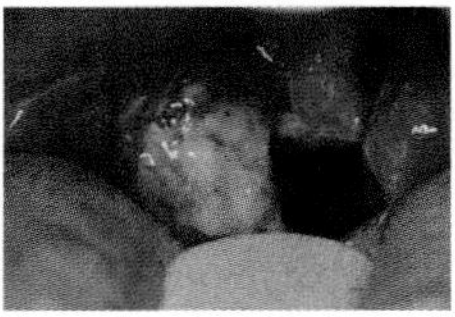

Enlarged tonsils with exudates. See box for specific tonsil grades.

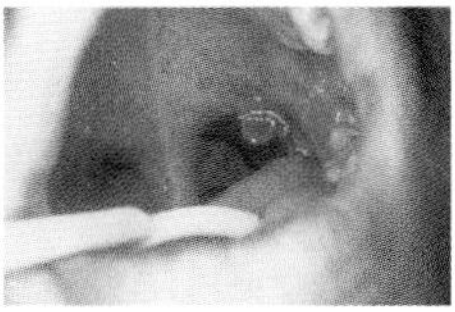

Herpangioma

(box continued on page 100)

Physical Assessment (continued)

AREA/PA SKILL	NORMAL FINDINGS	ABNORMAL FINDINGS
Inspection		
Oropharynx, Hard/ Soft Palate, Tonsils, and Uvula (cont'd)		*Erythema, exudate, lesions:* Infectious process. *Perforation of palate:* Congenital defect, cleft palate, trauma, drug use.
Look for symmetrical rise of the uvula (CN IX, X).	Symmetrical rise of uvula.	*Asymmetrical rise of uvula:* Problem with CNs IX and X.
Test swallow reflex (CNs IX, X).	+ Swallow and gag reflex.	
Neck, Thyroid, Cervical Lymph Nodes		
Inspect neck in neutral position, hyperextended, and as client swallows.	Neck symmetrical, active range of motion (AROM), no masses, skin intact.	*Enlargements:* Lymphadenopathy, lymphoma, or other malignancy.
Assess symmetry, neck ROM, and condition of skin.	Larynx and trachea rise with swallowing.	*Torticollis:* Scars, tonsillitis, adenitis, disease of cervical vertebrae, enlarged cervical glands, cerebellar tumor, rheumatism, retropharyngeal abscess.
Note any thyroid and lymph node enlargement.		*Enlarged, visible thyroid:* Goiter or malignant mass.

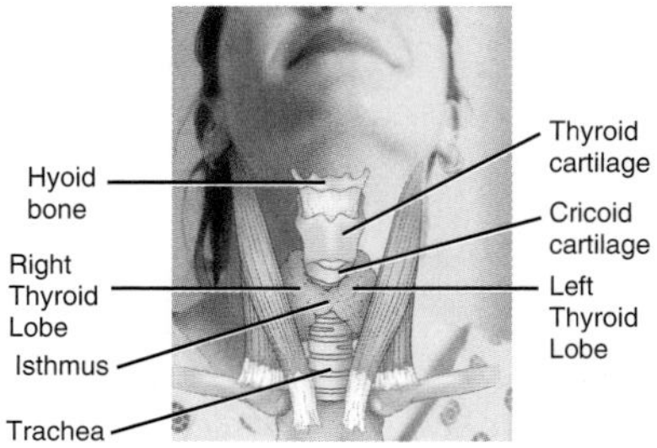

Thyroid gland

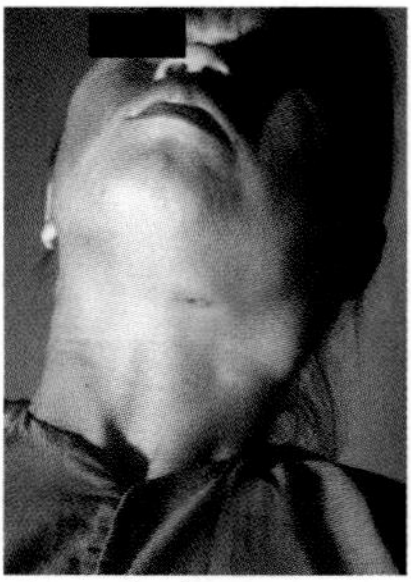

Cervical adenitis

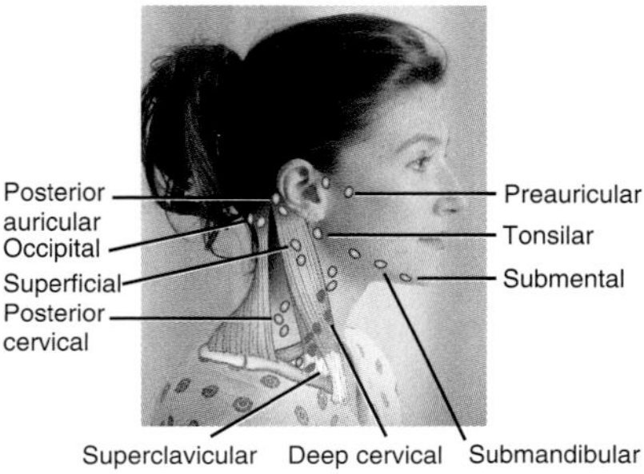

Cervical lymph nodes

Palpation **(Maintain standard precautions—wear gloves when palpating the mouth or if lesion is suspected.)**

AREA/PA SKILL	NORMAL FINDINGS	ABNORMAL FINDINGS
Head		
Assess for masses and tenderness.	Head symmetrical, no masses, nontender; scalp freely movable.	*Bulging fontanels and tight scalp:* Hydrocephalus, increased intracranial pressure (ICP).
Assess scalp mobility.		*Masses, tenderness:* Trauma, cysts.
Palpate fontanels in infants. Anterior fontanel closes between 18 and 24 mo; posterior by 2 mo.		
Face		
Note condition, symmetry, tenderness.	Facial bones smooth, intact, symmetrical, nontender.	*Contour abnormalities, including bulges or projections:* Previous trauma or surgery, or congenital deformity.
Assess muscle tone and temporomandibular joint (TMJ) function.	Facial muscles with good tone.	*Tenderness:* Trauma, TMJ syndrome, temporal arteritis, or inflammatory process.
	TMJ with AROM; no crepitus or tenderness.	

(box continued on page 102)

Physical Assessment (continued)

AREA/PA SKILL	NORMAL FINDINGS	ABNORMAL FINDINGS
Palpation *(cont'd)*		
Nose		
Assess for patency, tenderness, deformity.	Nares patent; no nasal tenderness or deformity.	*Deviations or masses:* Previous trauma or infection.
Frontal and Maxillary Sinuses		
Palpate for tenderness.	Sinuses nontender.	*Tenderness:* May indicate infectious or allergic sinusitis.

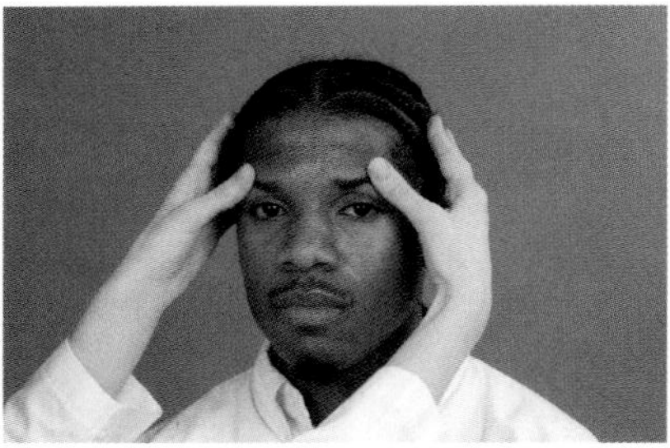

Palpating the frontal sinuses

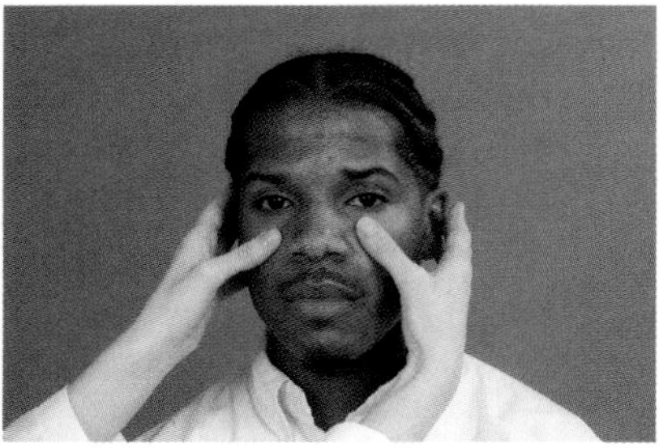

Palpating the maxillary sinuses

AREA/PA SKILL	NORMAL FINDINGS	ABNORMAL FINDINGS
Parotid and Submandibular Glands		
Palpate for tenderness and enlargement.	Parotid and submandibular glands nontender and not enlarged.	*Enlarged, tender parotid glands:* Parotitis, blocked ducts, infection, or malignancy.

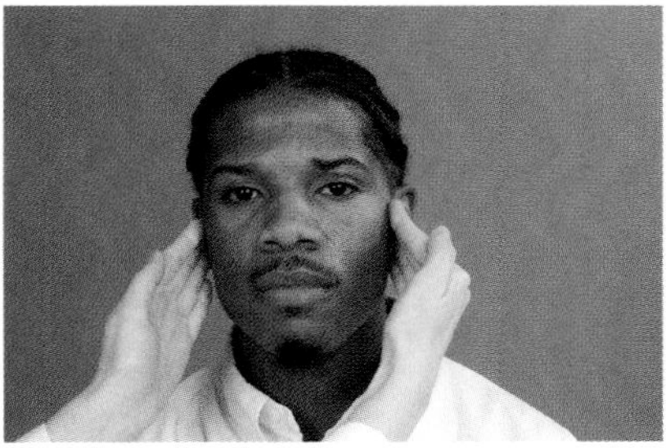

Palpating the parotid gland

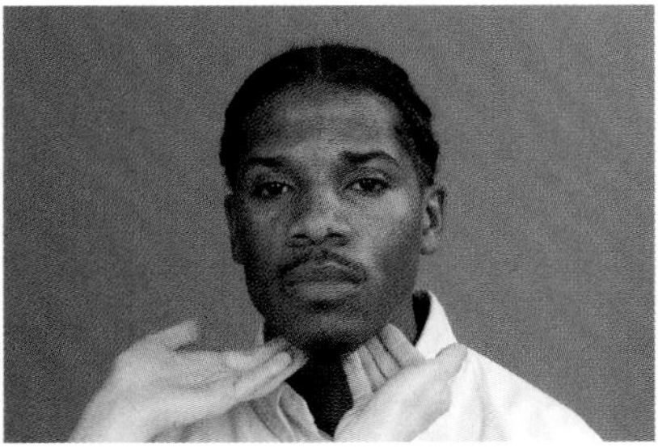

Palpating the sublingual gland

AREA/PA SKILL	NORMAL FINDINGS	ABNORMAL FINDINGS
Lips and Tongue		
Assess for tenderness, muscle tone, and lesions.	Soft, nontender, with good muscle tone.	*Areas of induration, thickening, nodularity, or masses:* Neoplasm, potential malignancy.
	No lesions.	*Tender induration that soon develops vesicles:* Herpes simplex.
		Areas of induration, thickening, nodularity: Potential malignancy.
Oropharynx		
Test gag reflex.	Presence of gag reflex.	**Absent gag reflex: Damage to CNs IX, X; stroke poses risk for aspiration.**

(box continued on page 104)

Physical Assessment (continued)

AREA/PA SKILL	NORMAL FINDINGS	ABNORMAL FINDINGS
Palpation *(cont'd)* *Thyroid Gland* Locate thyroid isthmus below cricoid cartilage.	Thyroid nonpalpable, nontender, or small; smooth edge of thyroid palpable.	*Enlarged thyroid:* Tumor, goiter. Nodular thyroid tissue.

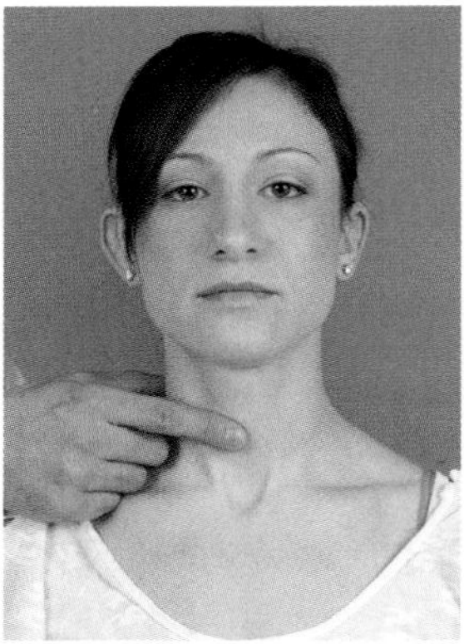

Landmarking the thyroid

AREA/PA SKILL	NORMAL FINDINGS	ABNORMAL FINDINGS
Palpate for size, shape, symmetry, consistency, tenderness, and nodules.		*Tender thyroid:* Inflammatory process such as acute thyroiditis.

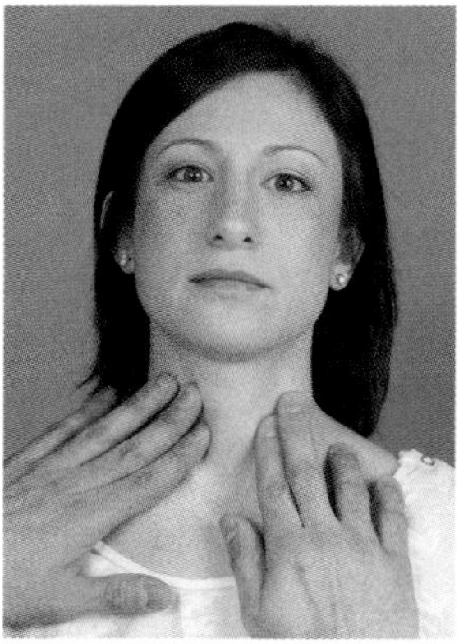

Palpating the thyroid: Anterior approach

AREA/PA SKILL	NORMAL FINDINGS	ABNORMAL FINDINGS

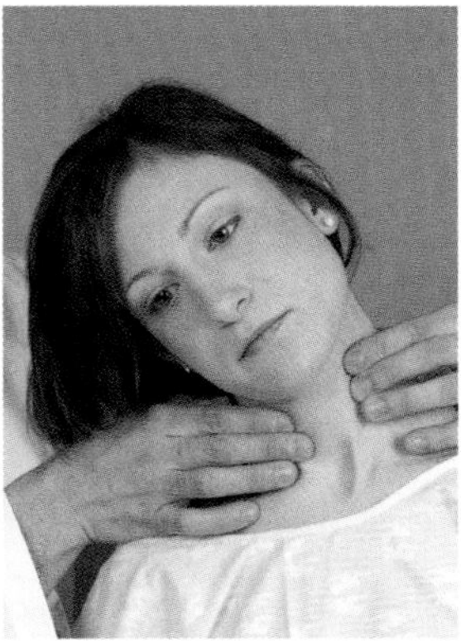

Palpating the thyroid: Right posterior approach

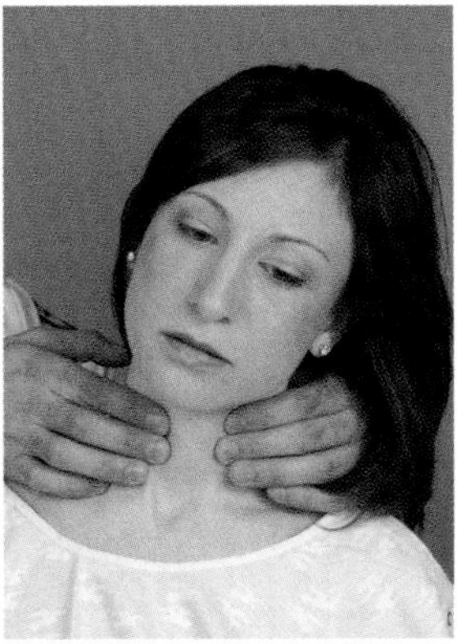

Palpating the thyroid: Left posterior approach

An enlarged thyroid gland may occur with either hypo- or hyperthyroidism. If enlarged, further assessment of signs and symptoms and thyroid function studies are warranted to determine cause.

(box continued on page 106)

Physical Assessment (continued)

AREA/PA SKILL	NORMAL FINDINGS	ABNORMAL FINDINGS
Palpation *(cont'd)* *Cervical Lymph Nodes*		
Use light palpation with your finger pads in a circular movement.	Cervical nodes nonpalpable, nontender; or superficial or shotty node palpable, <1 cm, mobile, soft to firm, nontender.	*Palpable nodes (≥1 cm):* Malignancy, inflammatory or infectious process of glands or area they drain.
Palpate for size, shape, symmetry, consistency, mobility, tenderness, and temperature.		*Significant lymphadenopathy:* Mononucleosis and various forms of lymphoma.
Percussion *Frontal and Maxillary Sinuses*		
(Use direct percussion.)		
Assess for tenderness.	Sinuses nontender, resonant.	*Tenderness:* Sinusitis.
		Dull tone: Thickening or fullness of sinus cavity or cavities, associated with chronic or acute sinusitis.
Auscultation (Use the bell of the stethoscope and have client hold breath.)		
Thyroid		
Listen for bruits.	No bruits over thyroid.	*Bruit:* Increased vascularity of hyperthyroidism.

PA = Physical assessment.

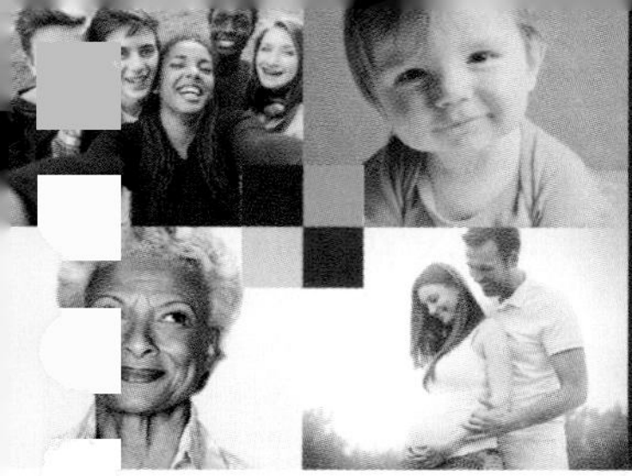

CHAPTER 4

Assessing the Eyes and the Ears

EYES

Primary Function

- Vision

Developmental Considerations

Infants

- Normal spacing measurements are plotted between the 10th and the 90th percentile.
- The color of the iris after birth is normally blue/gray in light-skinned infants and brown in darker-skinned infants. Permanent color is usually established by 9 months of age.
- Brushfield spots can be a normal variant or a sign of Down syndrome.
- Edema of the lids and irritation of the conjunctiva may be caused by birth trauma or silver nitrate prophylaxis.
- The sclera is very thin at birth, so it may have a slightly blue undertone.
- The pupils should normally constrict in response to light. After 3 weeks, if no pupillary light reflex is present, blindness is indicated. However, the presence of pupillary reaction alone does not confirm an infant's ability to see. A blink reflex in response to bright light and observing the infant for ability to follow objects or light with the eyes confirm that some degree of vision is intact.
- By 2 to 4 weeks, an infant should be able to fixate on an object; by 1 month, to fixate on and follow an object.

- An infant's visual acuity is usually about 20/200; 20/20 vision is usually achieved by school age.
- During the first 1 to 2 months, infants' eye movements are often disconjugate, making screening for strabismus difficult. Persistence of disconjugate eye movements after this time may indicate strabismus and warrants referral to a specialist.
- Absence of a red reflex may indicate congenital cataracts or retinal detachment. The general background in infants is typically paler than that in adults. The macula also is not fully developed until about 1 year of age.

Toddlers

- Visual acuity in toddlers is determined by the Allen test.
- Untreated strabismus can lead to permanent visual damage.

Preschoolers

- By age 3 to 5, the Snellen E chart can usually be used to determine visual acuity.
- Normal visual acuity for a 3-year-old is approximately 20/40 or better.
- By the time the child is 4 years old, visual acuity should be about 20/30 or better.

School-Age Children

- By the time the child is about 5 to 6 years old, visual acuity approximates that of the adult—20/20 in both eyes. Use the Snellen E chart until the child has acquired reading skills and can easily verbalize the letters seen on the Snellen chart.
- Screen for color blindness between 4 and 8 years of age.

Older Adults

- Both central and peripheral visual acuity may be diminished with advanced age.
- Changes in near vision occur around the 4th and 5th decades, often resulting in presbyopia.
- Lids lose elasticity and fatty deposits, causing the eyes to appear sunken.
- Ectropion is significant because the punctum is no longer in contact with the globe, resulting in constant tearing.
- Entropion is significant because the punctum may not be able to drain tears and the lashes may rub the conjunctiva and cornea, causing pain and injury to the cornea.

- A decrease in tear production may result in dry eyes.
- Lens becomes more opaque and yellowish, obscuring the transfer of light rays to the retina.
- Arcus senilis may appear.
- Senile cataracts may appear.
- Pupil size at rest is generally smaller than in younger adults.
- Pupillary reaction to light and accommodation slows.
- General fundoscopic background is paler, and the blood vessels of the eye may show signs of the same atherosclerotic processes that are occurring elsewhere throughout the body.
- Visual fields may be less than normal.
- Color vision may be less vivid.
- Night vision may be impaired.
- Macular degeneration and glaucoma are the two leading causes of blindness in older adults.

Cultural Considerations

- Persons of Asian origin typically have an epicanthal fold at the medial canthus.
- In African Americans and others with normally dark skin, muddy sclera is common.
- In dark-skinned people, the color of the optic disc is typically darker orange and the retinal background is darker red than in fair-skinned people.
- An African American person's sclera also may have a blue/gray appearance or a yellowish cast at the peripheral margins.
- Incidence and severity of glaucoma are greater in African Americans than in people of other races.
- Cataracts occur with greater frequency in people living in sunny climates.

Assessment

History

Symptoms ("PQRST" Any + Symptom)

- Vision loss
  - Have you noticed any changes in your vision?
  - Have you experienced any decrease or loss of vision?
  - Was the loss of vision sudden or gradual?
  - Was the loss of vision painful?

- Eye pain
  - Do you have any pain or discomfort in your eyes?
  - Did the pain occur suddenly or gradually?
  - Do you have any other symptoms associated with the eye pain?
  - Does light bother your eyes?
  - Is the pain associated with movement of the eye? With blinking?
  - What makes your eye pain better? What makes it worse?
- Diplopia
  - Does the double vision get worse when you are tired?
  - Did the double vision occur suddenly or gradually?
  - Did the double vision occur after a head injury?
- Eye tearing
  - Have you noticed any tearing of the eyes?
  - Is the tearing associated with pain? With direct contact with chemicals, irritants, or environmental allergens?
- Dry eye
  - Have you noticed any dryness or discomfort of the eye when blinking?
  - Do you wear contact lenses?
  - Do you have a history of corneal abrasion or burns?
  - Are you taking any medications?
- Eye drainage
  - What does the drainage look like?
  - Is the drainage associated with redness? With itching?
- Eye appearance changes
  - Have you noticed any recent changes in the appearance of your eyes?
  - Describe how the appearance of your eyes has changed.
- Blurred vision
  - Do you wear corrective lenses?
  - Is the blurred vision worse for near or for far objects?
  - When was your last eye examination?

Focused Eye History

- Have you noticed any changes in your vision?
- Do you wear glasses or contact lenses?
- Have you ever had an eye injury?
- Have you ever had eye surgery?
- Have you ever had blurred vision?
- Have you ever seen spots or floaters, flashes of light, or halos around lights?

- Do you have a history of frequent or recurring eye infections, styes, tearing, or dryness?
- When was your last eye examination?
- Do you have a history of diabetes or high blood pressure?
- What medications, prescription or over-the-counter (OTC), are you currently taking (Table 4.1)?
- Do you use any prescription or OTC eye drops?

TABLE 4.1 Drugs That Adversely Affect the Eyes

DRUG CLASS	DRUG	POSSIBLE ADVERSE REACTIONS
Antiarrhythmics	Quinidine	Blurred vision, color perception disturbances, night blindness, mydriasis, photophobia, diplopia, reduced visual fields, scotomas, optic neuritis
	Flecainide	Blurred vision, difficulty focusing, spots before eyes, diplopia, photophobia, nystagmus
Anticholinergic agents	All types	Blurred vision, cycloplegia, mydriasis, photophobia
Anti-infectives	Chloramphenicol	Optic neuritis, decreased visual acuity
Antineoplastics	Cisplatin	Optic neuritis, papilledema, cerebral blindness
	Methotrexate	Conjunctivitis
	Tamoxifen	Retinopathy, corneal opacities, decreased visual acuity
Antipsychotics	All phenothiazines	Abnormal corneal lens pigmentation, blurred vision
	Chlorpromazine	Cataracts, retinopathy, visual impairment
	Quetiapine	Lens changes
Antitubercular agents	Isoniazid, pyrazinamide, ethambutol	Optic neuritis, decreased visual acuity, loss of red-green color perception, central and peripheral scotomas (ethambutol only)
Cardiotonic glycosides	Digoxin	Altered color vision, photophobia, diplopia, halos or borders on objects (all are signs of potential toxicity)
Genitourinary smooth muscle relaxants	Flavoxate	Blurred vision, disturbed accommodation

(continued)

TABLE 4.1 Drugs That Adversely Affect the Eyes (continued)

DRUG CLASS	DRUG	POSSIBLE ADVERSE REACTIONS
	Oxybutynin	Transient blurred vision, cycloplegia, mydriasis
Glucocorticoids	Prednisone, methylprednisolone, dexamethasone	Exophthalmos, increased intraocular pressure, cataracts, increased susceptibility to secondary fungal and viral eye infections
Miscellaneous agents	Carbamazepine	Blurred vision, conjunctivitis, transient diplopia, visual hallucinations, lens opacities
	Oral contraceptives (estrogen with progesterone)	Worsening of myopia or astigmatism, intolerance to contact lenses, neuro-ocular lesions
	Isotretinoin	Conjunctivitis, dry eyes, corneal opacities, eye irritation, altered color vision, optic neuritis, photophobia
	Loxapine	Blurred vision
	Pentazocine	Blurred vision, focusing difficulty, nystagmus, diplopia, miosis

Assessment of the Eyes' Relationship to Other Systems

Remember, all systems are related. As you assess the eyes, look at the relationship between them and all other systems.

SUBJECTIVE DATA/ RATIONALE	OBJECTIVE DATA/ RATIONALE
Area/System: General	
Ask about:	*Inspect:*
General state of health: Changes in usual state of health may reflect underlying problems that can affect the eyes.	General appearance.
Recent infections/illnesses.	Level of consciousness. *Changes in mental status:* Head injury or conditions that cause an increase in intracranial pressure.

SUBJECTIVE DATA/ RATIONALE	OBJECTIVE DATA/ RATIONALE
Vision problems.	*Changes in eyes (e.g., in pupils):* Early sign of IICP.
Area/System: Integumentary *Ask about:*	*Inspect for:*
Allergies	*Xanthelasma, chalazion, and other skin lesions on eyelids:* Eyelids are covered by skin, so they are vulnerable to various skin lesions.
Rashes or legions: May be associated with irritation, infection, or allergies that cause eye irritation. May explain physical findings or source of symptoms.	Periorbital edema.
Area/System: HEENT *Ask about:*	*Inspect/Palpate for:*
Headaches/migraines: May be associated with disorders of visual acuity. Visual aura often precedes migraines.	Head, masses.
Head trauma.	Abnormalities in oral, nasal, and ear structures. *Changes in pupil reaction and papilledema:* Head trauma, which can result in IICP and is readily detected in the eye.
Ear infections.	*Watery eyes:* Upper respiratory infection or ear infection.
Runny nose: Associated with environmental allergies or upper respiratory infections.	
Thyroid disease.	Thyroid. *Exophthalmos and eyelid lag:* Hyperthyroid disease.
Area/System: Respiratory *Ask about:*	*Inspect for:*
Breathing problems.	*Cyanotic color changes (pale, cyanotic conjunctiva):* Hypoxia associated with respiratory disease.
Lung disease.	*Auscultate:* Breath sounds.

(box continued on page 114)

SUBJECTIVE DATA/ RATIONALE	OBJECTIVE DATA/ RATIONALE
Area/System: Cardiovascular	
Ask about:	*Measure:*
History of HTN: May be responsible for changes in the blood vessels of the eye and the retinal background.	Blood pressure.
Vascular disease: Linked to deficits in visual fields or damage to the optic track.	*Palpate:*
	Pulses.
	Auscultate:
	Heart sounds.
	Bruits.
	Vascular changes (e.g., cotton, wool, AV nicking, retinal hemorrhages) on funduscopic examination: Cardiovascular disease.
Area/System: Abdomen	
Ask about:	*Palpate:*
History of liver disease: Jaundice may be seen as icteric sclera.	Abdomen.
History of renal disease: Periorbital edema may be seen with renal disease.	Liver. *Yellow sclera:* Jaundice associated with liver disease.
Area/System: Reproductive	
Ask about:	*Inspect:*
History of sexually transmitted disease (STDs), discharge or lesions: Cross-contamination may transmit infections to eyes. Newborns may be exposed to STDs during delivery through the birth canal.	Genitalia. Eye infections can be caused by cross-contamination.
Area/System: Musculoskeletal	
Ask about:	*Inspect:*
Muscle weakness.	Joints for deformities.
Joint swelling, pain, rheumatoid arthritis: Episcleritis and keratoconjunctivitis are associated with rheumatoid arthritis.	ROM.

SUBJECTIVE DATA/ RATIONALE	OBJECTIVE DATA/ RATIONALE
	Palpate: Joints for nodules. Muscle strength. *Ptosis, episcleritis, and keratoconjunctivitis:* Muscle weakness associated with rheumatoid arthritis.
Area/System: Neurologic *Ask about:*	*Test:*
History of multiple sclerosis (MS), myasthenia gravis, or neurologic problems: MS may produce visual disturbances such as partial blindness, diplopia, or nystagmus as a result of demyelinization of nerve fibers. Myasthenia gravis may cause ptosis.	Sensory function.
	CNs II, III, IV, VI. *Ptosis:* Myasthenia gravis and Bell's palsy. *Visual problems and fundoscopic changes:* MS.

Physical Assessment

ANATOMICAL LANDMARKS: Six cardinal fields; fundoscopic structures

APPROACH: Inspection, palpation, ophthalmoscopy, visual acuity, extraocular muscles, external structures, fundoscopy

POSITION: Sitting

TOOLBOX: Visual acuity charts (Snellen and Snellen E charts, Allen cards, Jaeger chart), Ishihara cards, ophthalmoscope, penlight, cotton-tipped swab, cotton ball

(text continues on page 134)

BOX 4.1 Ophthalmoscope Apertures

APERTURE TYPE	PURPOSE
Small white aperture 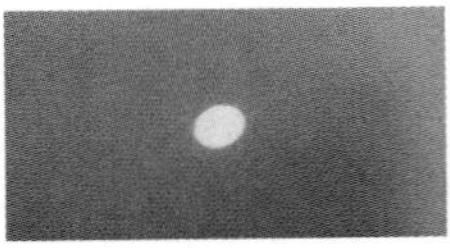	Best for examining the undilated eye. Start the eye exam with this setting.
Large white aperture 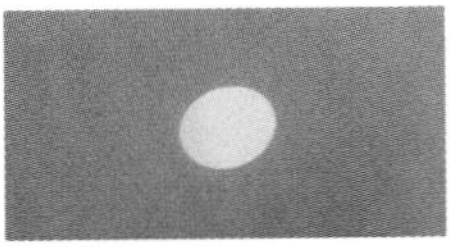	For general examination of the eye and when pupils are dilated.
Red-free filter 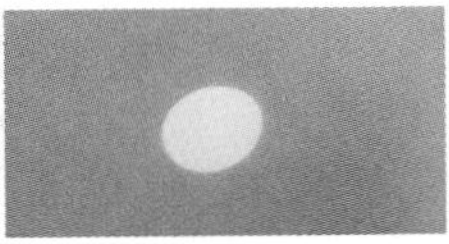	A green light for differentiating hemorrhages, which appear black, from melanin, which looks gray. Also differentiates arteries, which appear black, from veins, which appear blue.
Blue light 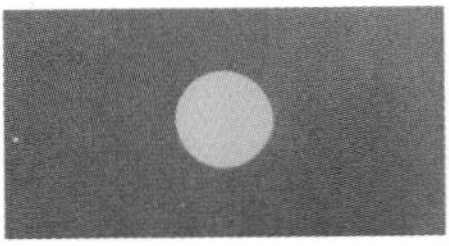	When fluorescein dye is injected into patient intravenously, a blue filter enables examiner to see movement of dye into eye vessels. Useful for detecting hemorrhages, leaking vessels, or vessel abnormalities.
Grid 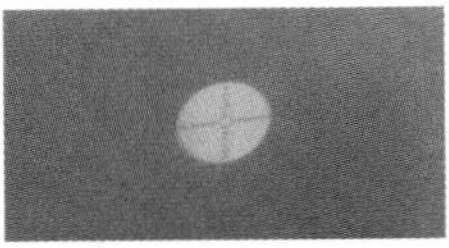	Used to measure size or location of lesions.
Slit or streak 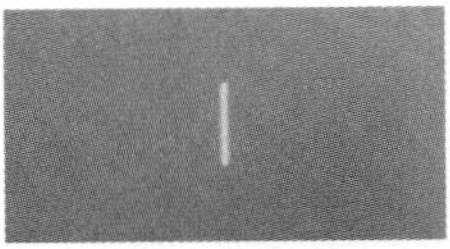	Used to determine levels or depth of lesions.

AREA/PA SKILL	NORMAL FINDINGS	ABNORMAL FINDINGS
Inspection *Visual Acuity* **(Measure each eye separately, then together, with and without corrective lenses. Tests cranial nerve [CN] II.)**		
Far Vision Depending on patient's age and literacy level, use Snellen eye chart, Snellen E chart, or STYCAR chart.	20/20 right eye (OD), left eye (OS), both eyes (OU)	*A smaller fraction (e.g., 20/30, 20/40):* Diminished distant visual acuity. *Myopia:* Impaired far vision. Hypermyopia: Impaired near vision
Numerator = Distance patient stands from chart (20 feet). **Denominator = distance in feet at which person with normal vision could read any given line on chart. No more than two mistakes permitted per line.**		
Near Vision Assess patient's ability to read newsprint held 13 to 15 inches from eyes. Use print-size pictures if patient is unable to read.	Near vision intact.	*A smaller fraction (e.g., 14/18):* Diminished near vision (hyperopia or, if it occurs with aging, presbyopia).
Color Vision Screen for color vision by assessing ability to differentiate patterns of colors on Ishihara cards or identify color bars on Snellen eye chart.	Color vision intact.	*Inability to detect embedded number or letter in Ishihara cards:* Color blindness. Often inherited in an X-linked recessive pattern predominantly affecting males. Can result from macular degeneration or other diseases affecting the cones that mediate color vision.

(box continued on page 118)

AREA/PA SKILL	NORMAL FINDINGS	ABNORMAL FINDINGS
Inspection *(cont'd)*		
Peripheral Vision		
Assess patient's ability to detect movement coming in from the periphery (inferior, superior, temporal, and nasal fields).	Peripheral vision intact OU, all fields.	*Diminished visual fields:* Seen with glaucoma, cataracts and stroke.

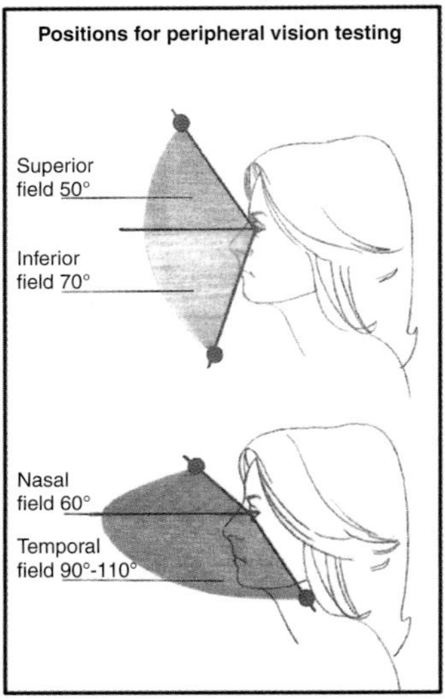

Positions for peripheral vision testing

Sudden loss of peripheral vision needs immediate ophthalmology referral—may be a sign of acute closed-angle glaucoma, a medical emergency.

AREA/PA SKILL	NORMAL FINDINGS	ABNORMAL FINDINGS
Extraocular Muscles		
Inspect eyes for parallel alignment.	Eyes in parallel alignment.	*Asymmetrical corneal light reflex:* Weak extraocular muscles or strabismus.
Perform corneal light reflex test. **(Look for the sparkle in your patient's eyes.)**	Corneal light reflex symmetrical.	
Put eyes through range of motion (ROM), six cardinal fields of vision **(tests CNs III, IV, VI).**	Extraocular motion intact OU, no lid lag or nystagmus.	

AREA/PA SKILL	NORMAL FINDINGS	ABNORMAL FINDINGS
Perform the cover/ uncover test, check for drifting. 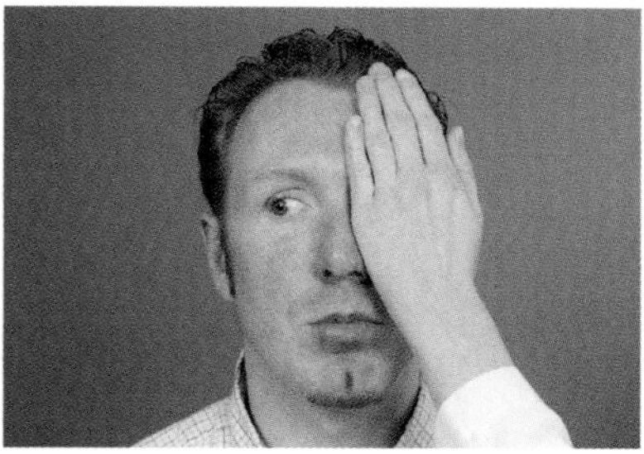 *Cover* 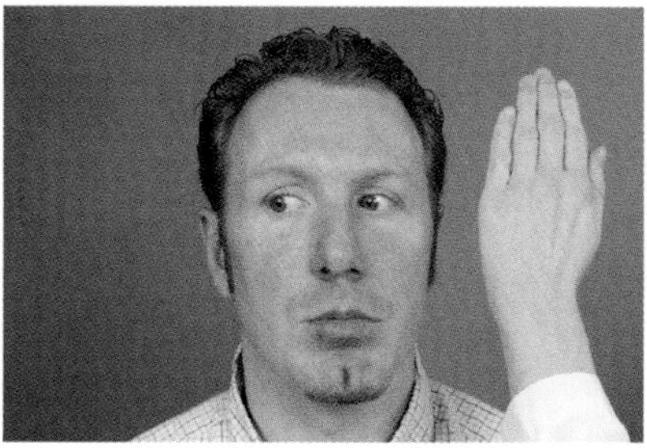 *Uncover*	No wandering with cover/ uncover test.	*Shift in gaze:* One or more eye muscles are weak. When uncovered eye shifts in response to covering opposite eye, covered eye is dominant. When covered eye shifts after being uncovered, it indicates weakness in that eye. *Limited or disconjugate movement in one or more fields of gaze, nystagmus in fields other than extreme lateral, ptosis, and lid lag:* Damage, irritation, or pressure on corresponding extraocular muscle or cranial nerve that innervates the muscle 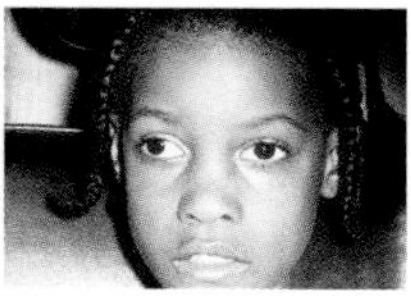 *Exotropia (divergent strabismus)* 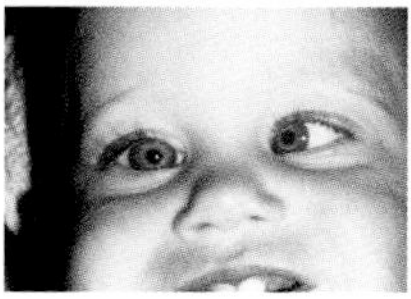 *Congenital exotropia*
External Structures *General Appearance* Appearance and parallel alignment. 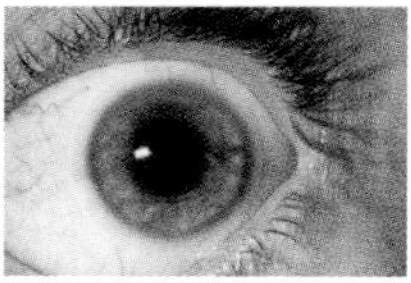 *Soft contact lenses*	Eyes clear and bright, in parallel alignment.	*Glazed eyes:* Febrile state. *Unequal parallel alignment:* Exotropia.

(box continued on page 120)

AREA/PA SKILL	NORMAL FINDINGS	ABNORMAL FINDINGS
Inspection *(cont'd)* 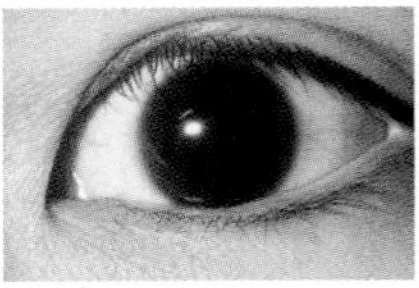 *Hard contact lenses*		
Eyelids Note color, lesions, edema, symmetry of palpebral fissures **(opening of the eyes between upper and lower lids),** and lid lag.	Color consistent with patient's complexion, no lesions or edema, palpebral fissures symmetrical, no lid lag.	*Visible sclera between iris and upper lids (exophthalmos):* Hyperthyroidism or hydrocephalus (setting-sun sign). 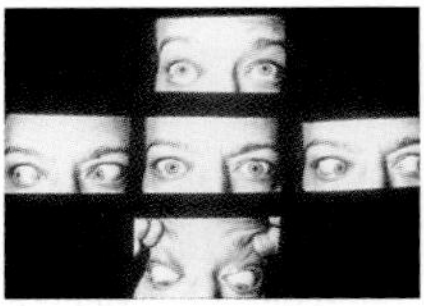 *Exophthalmos* *Asymmetry of lids:* CN III damage, stroke. *Ptosis of both lids:* Myasthenia gravis. Various lesions may be found on lids. 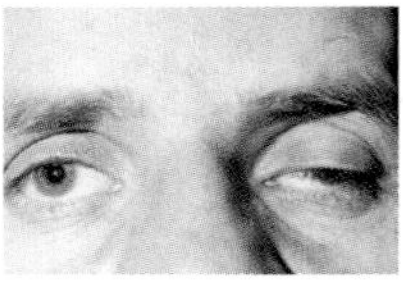 *Ptosis* 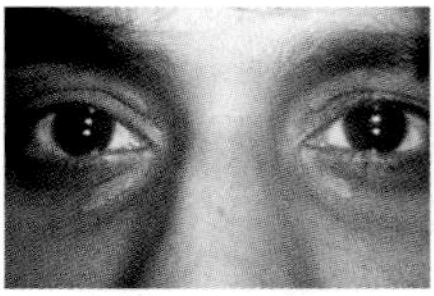 *Xanthelasma* 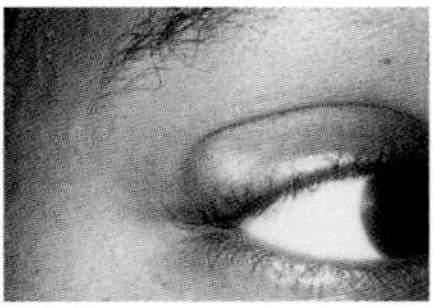 *Chalazion*

AREA/PA SKILL	NORMAL FINDINGS	ABNORMAL FINDINGS
		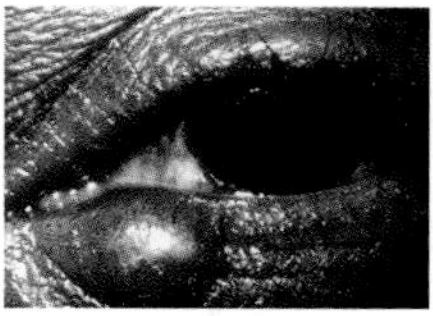 *Hordeolum* 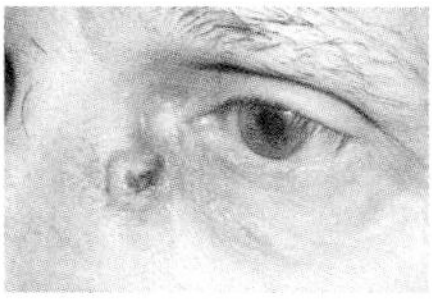 *Basal cell carcinoma* 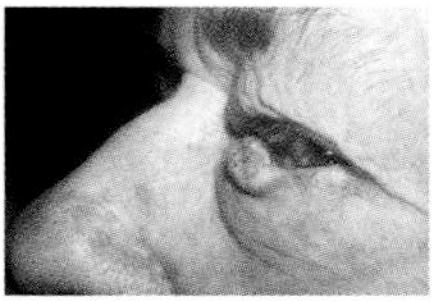 *Squamous cell carcinoma*
Eyelashes Note symmetry and distribution.	Eyelashes evenly distributed, no ectropion or entropion.	*Absence of lashes:* Alopecia universalis. *Lice or ticks at base of lashes:* Infestation. 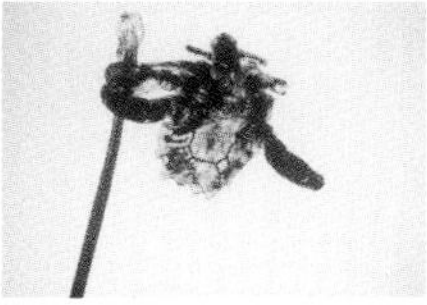 *Lice* Blepharitis (inflammation of lashes and meibomian glands of eyelids). 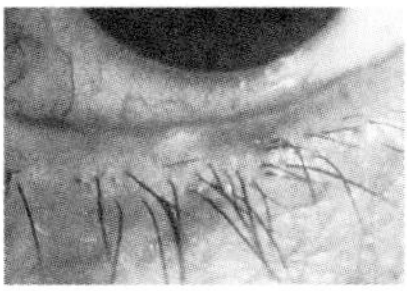 *Blepharoconjunctivitis*

(box continued on page 122)

AREA/PA SKILL	NORMAL FINDINGS	ABNORMAL FINDINGS
Inspection *Eyelashes (cont'd)*		Entropion can scratch the cornea. 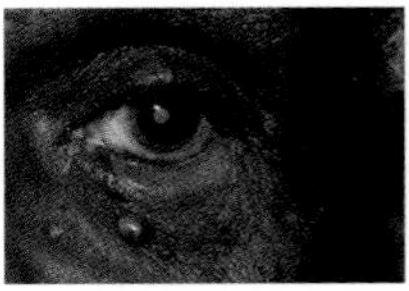 *Entropion* Ectropion can lead to excessive drying of the eyes. 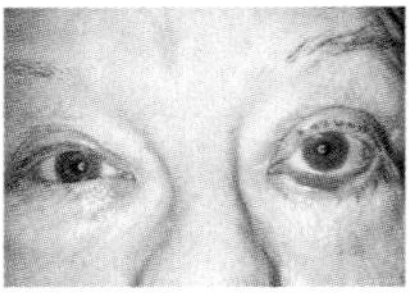 *Ectropion* 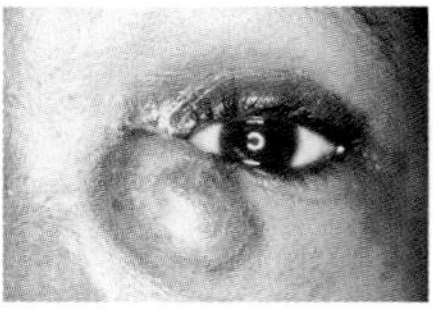 *Dacryocystitis*
Eyeball Inspect for protrusion of eyeball.	No protrusion beyond frontal bone (mild protrusion seen in some African-Americans).	*Protrusion:* Hyperthyroidism or inherited disorders of mucopolysaccharide metabolism.
Lacrimal Ducts, Puncta Note color, edema, excessive tearing or drainage.	Puncta pale pink and patent, no excessive tearing or dryness, drainage, or edema.	*Swelling, redness, drainage, or tenderness:* Obstruction or inflammation.

AREA/PA SKILL	NORMAL FINDINGS	ABNORMAL FINDINGS
Conjunctiva		
Assess color, moisture, lesions, and foreign bodies.	Conjunctiva clear, pink, and moist; no lesions.	*Reddened palpebral and bulbar conjunctiva:* Conjunctivitis.

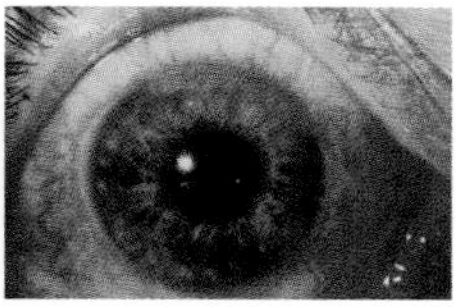

Acute allergic conjunctivitis

Pale pink conjunctiva: Anemia.

Growth and thickening of conjunctiva from inner canthal area toward iris: Pterygium or pinguecula.

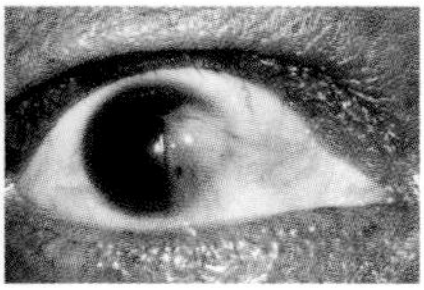

Pterygium

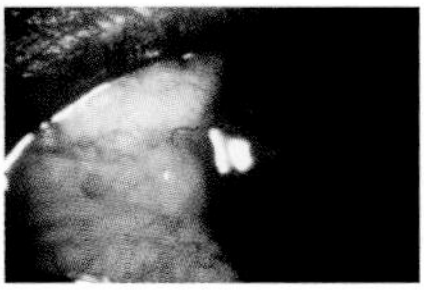

Pinguecula

Subconjunctival hemorrhage: Eye injury.

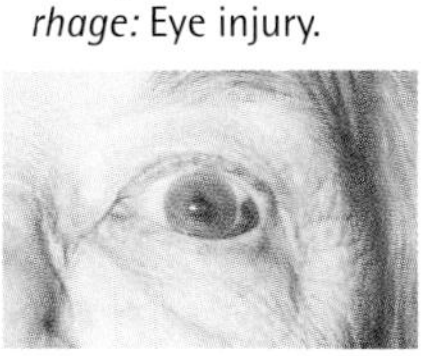

Subconjunctival hemorrhage

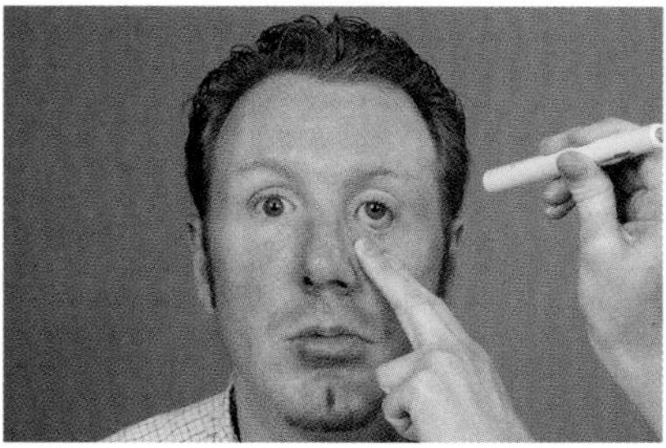

Pulling eyelid down

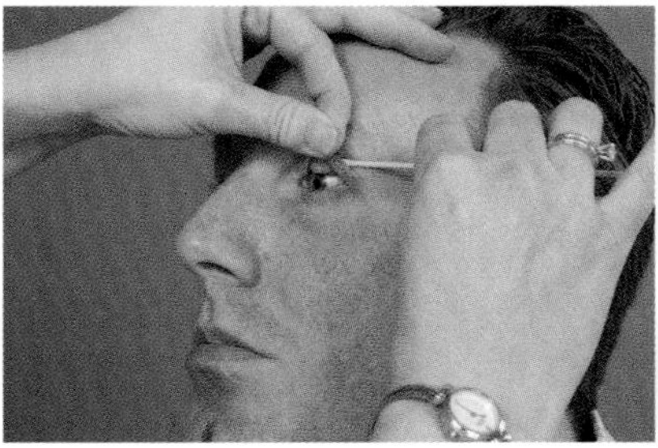

Rolling eyelid up

Palpebral conjunctiva covers the lids; bulbar conjunctiva, the eyeball.

(box continued on page 124)

AREA/PA SKILL	NORMAL FINDINGS	ABNORMAL FINDINGS
Inspection *Conjunctiva (cont'd)*		Conjunctival nevus or papilloma. 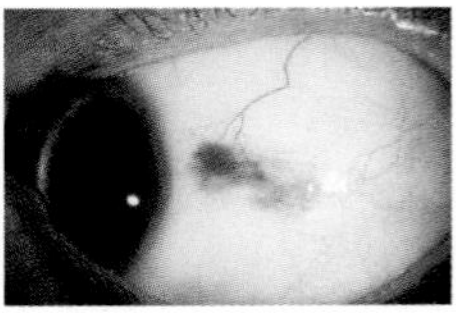 *Nevus* 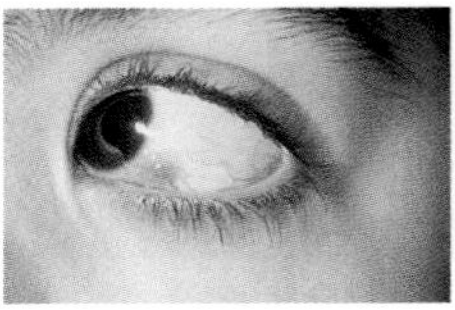 *Papilloma*
Sclera Note color, moisture, and lesions or tears.	Sclera white and intact, no lesions or tears.	*Bluish sclera:* Osteogenesis imperfecta. *Yellow sclera at the limbus:* Jaundice. *Bitot's spots:* Vitamin A deficiency. *Episcleritis:* Inflammation of sclera. 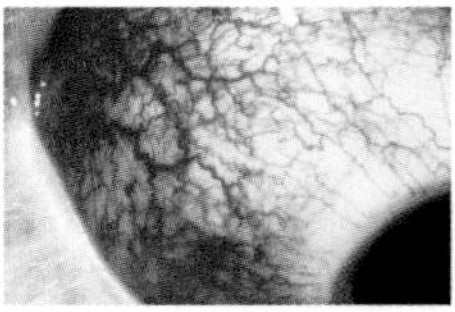 *Diffuse episcleritis*
Cornea Note clarity and lesions or abrasions. **Examine cornea from oblique angle.**	Cornea clear without opacities, lesions, or abrasions. 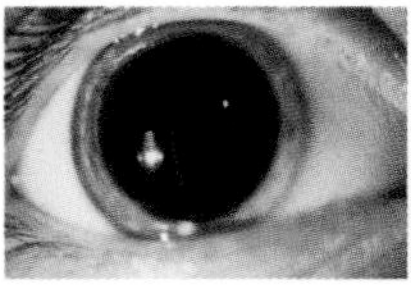 *Normal lens*	*Clouding of cornea:* Infection (hypopyon: Pus in the anterior chamber) or vitamin A deficiency. *Roughness or irregularity of cornea:* Corneal abrasions and ulcers. 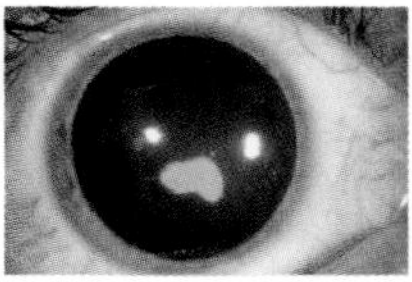 *Corneal abrasion*

AREA/PA SKILL	NORMAL FINDINGS	ABNORMAL FINDINGS
	Arcus senilis: Common finding and normal variant in older adults. 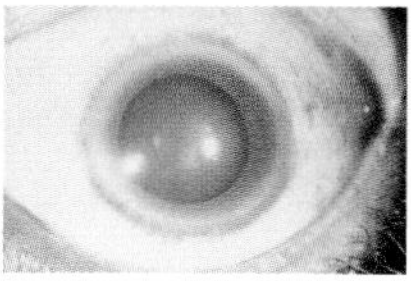 *Arcus senilis*	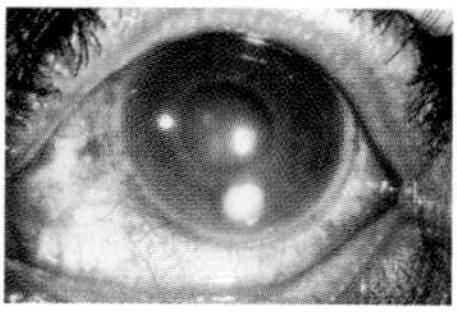 *Healing corneal ulcer*
Test corneal reflex (CNs V and VII) **Instead of touching the cornea with a wisp of cotton, use a needleless syringe and shoot a small amount of air over the cornea, or gently touch lashes and look for blink reflex.**	+ Corneal reflex.	*Kayser-Fleischer ring:* Wilson's disease. Cataracts may also be seen through transparent cornea. 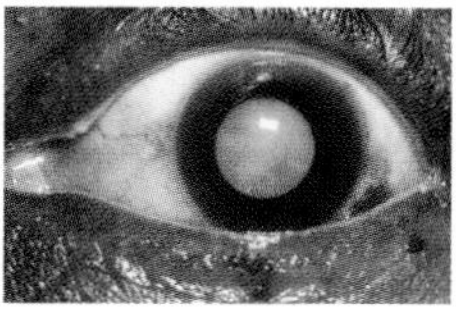 *Mature cataract*
Anterior Chamber Inspect for clarity, bulging of the iris, and blood. **Inspect with patient's eyes looking straight ahead while you look across the eye from the side.**	Anterior chamber clear, no blood or bulging of the iris.	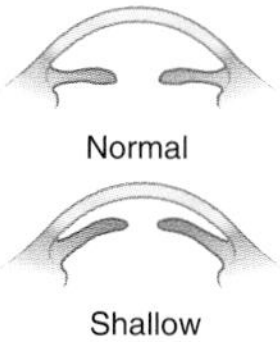 *Hypopyon:* Corneal ulceration or other infection. 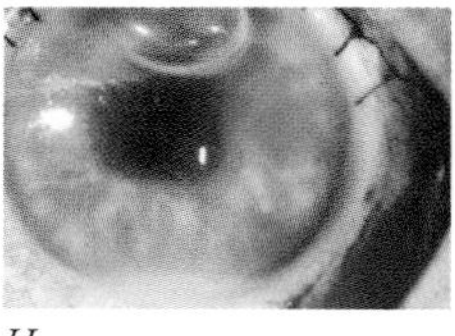 *Hypopyon* *Hyphema:* Trauma or intraocular hemorrhage. 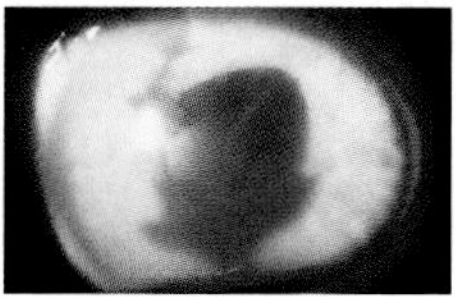 *Hyphema*

(box continued on page 126)

AREA/PA SKILL	NORMAL FINDINGS	ABNORMAL FINDINGS
Inspection *Anterior Chamber (cont'd)*		*Crescent-shaped shadow on nasal side of iris:* Protrusion of iris into anterior chamber from increased intraocular pressure; seen in narrow-angle glaucoma. 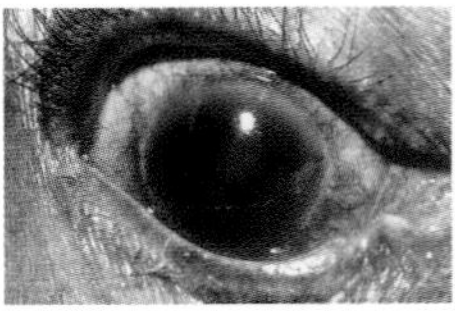 *Acute angle closure*
Iris Note color, size, shape, and symmetry.	Irides round and symmetrical.	*Brushfield spots:* Common in persons with Down syndrome (but sometimes a normal variant). *Red, bloodshot appearance of vessels in iris:* Iritis. *New blood vessel on anterior surface of iris:* Diabetes. *Heterochromia iridis:* Previous damage in lighter colored eye or (rarely) Waardenburg syndrome. *Aniridia:* Congenital absence of part or all of iris. *Keyhole wedges in iris:* Previous eye surgery.
Pupils Note size, shape, reaction to light (direct and consensual); test for accommodation (tests CN III).	Pupil size 3 to 5 mm in adults. (Normal size depends on age: Larger in children, smaller in older adults.) No miosis or mydriasis.	*Miosis:* Brain injury to the pons; use of narcotics, atropine, and other drugs.

AREA/PA SKILL	NORMAL FINDINGS	ABNORMAL FINDINGS
Consensual reaction: The pupil not receiving light stimulus reacts the same as the pupil receiving stimulus.	PERRLA—Pupils equal, round, reactive to light (pupils constrict) and accommodation (pupils converge and constrict) direct and consensual.	*Mydriasis:* Brain herniation, anoxia, use of marijuana or mydriatic eye drops.
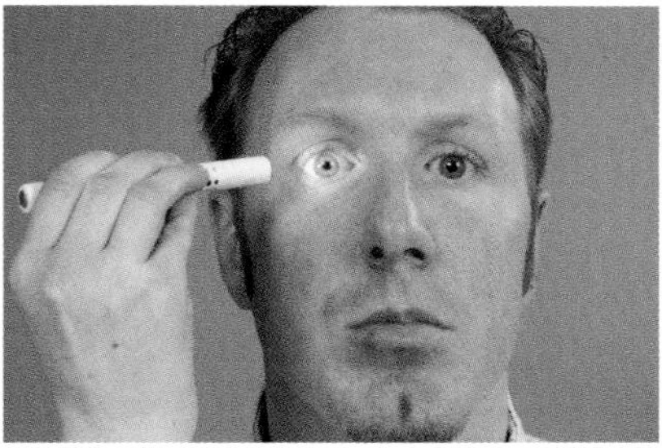 *Testing pupillary reaction to light*		**Changes in pupils, such as unequal or dilated, may be a sign of increased intracranial pressure (IICP).** *Anisocoria:* Unilateral brain herniation; IICP.
	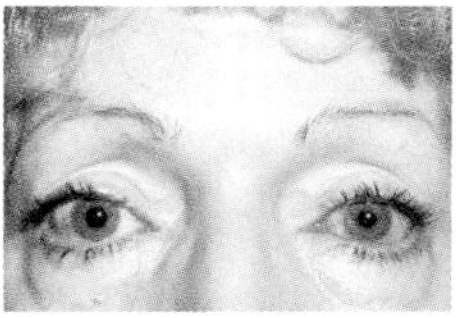 *Anisocoria* Older patient may have decreased accommodation. Anisocoria < 0.5 mm can be normal variation.	*Tonic pupil slow to react to light:* Adie's pupil. 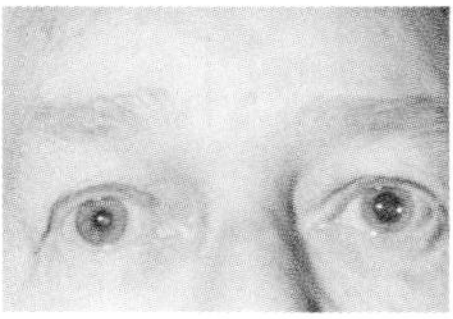 *Adie's pupil* *Pupils unequal, affected pupil small but reacts to light:* Horner's syndrome. 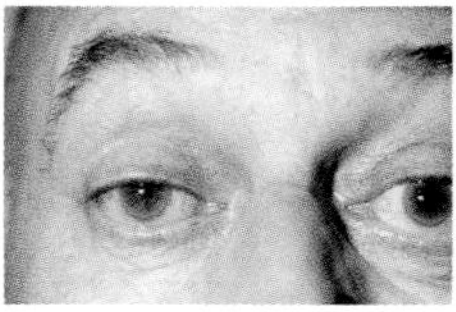 *Horner's syndrome* *Sluggish or fixed pupil reaction to light:* Lack of oxygen to optic nerve or brain, or topical or systemic drug effects.

(box continued on page 128)

AREA/PA SKILL	NORMAL FINDINGS	ABNORMAL FINDINGS
Inspection *Pupils (cont'd)*		*Absence of consensual response:* Conditions that compress or deprive optic nerve and brain of oxygen. One or both pupils fail to dilate or constrict to near or distant objects. Sluggish accommodation in the absence of advanced age may be caused by drugs.
Palpation *External Structures* **(Maintain standard precautions. Wear gloves if there is eye drainage.)**		
Eyeball **Gently palpate globe with fingertips or thumb on upper lids over sclera.**	Eyeball firm and nontender.	*Excessively firm or tender globe:* Glaucoma.
Note consistency and tenderness. **Do not palpate eyeball in patients with eye trauma or known glaucoma.**		
Lacrimal Apparatus (Tear Gland and Ducts)		
Palpate below eyebrow and inner canthus of eye. Note tenderness or excessive tearing or discharge from punctae.	Lacrimal gland nontender, no drainage or excessive tearing.	*Swelling and tenderness:* Inflammation.

AREA/PA SKILL	NORMAL FINDINGS	ABNORMAL FINDINGS
Ophthalmoscopy (Perform in dark room. Examine same eye to same eye, your right to your patient's right. Use small white light aperture for undilated pupil. See Box 4.1.)		

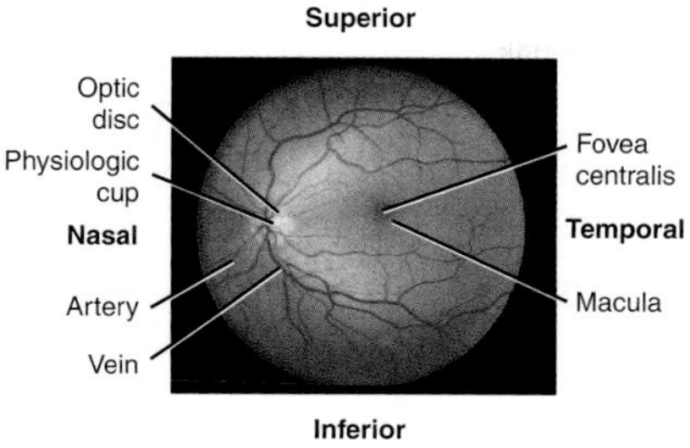

Normal funduscopic structures of the left eye with fields (Courtesy of Wills Eye Hospital, Philadelphia, Pa.)

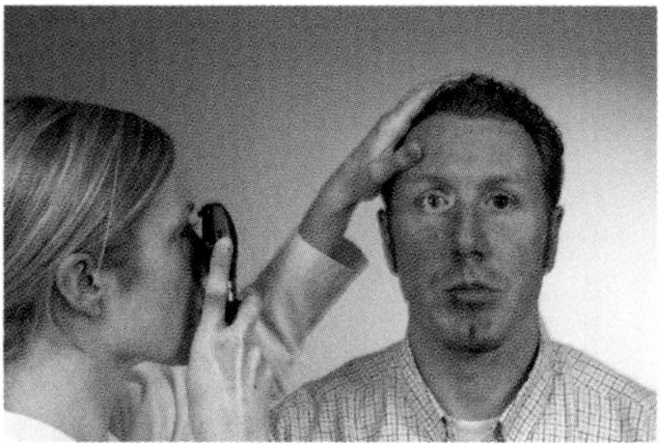

Checking red reflex

AREA/PA SKILL	NORMAL FINDINGS	ABNORMAL FINDINGS
Red Reflex Note presence, opacities.	+ Red reflex, no opacities.	*Opaque/blackened area of red reflex:* Cataracts.
Approach from an oblique angle about 14 inches from patient.		*Dark spots or shadows that interrupt red reflex:* Opacities in lens or vitreous.

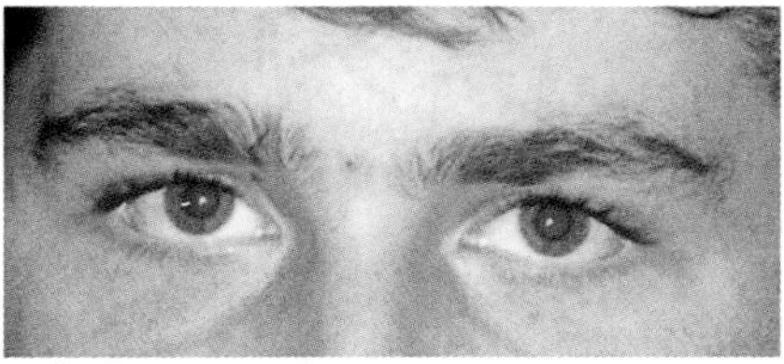

Red reflex over pupil area

Optic Disc and Physiological Cup (Located Nasally)

(box continued on page 130)

AREA/PA SKILL	NORMAL FINDINGS	ABNORMAL FINDINGS
Palpation *Red Reflex (cont'd)* Note size, shape, borders, color, cup-to-disc ratio.	Optic disc round, with sharp margins, cup-to-disc ratio 1:2. Color depends on patient's pigmentation: Yellow to orange with white cup.	*Whitish or gray color of the optic disc:* Partial or complete death of optic nerve- (optic atrophy).

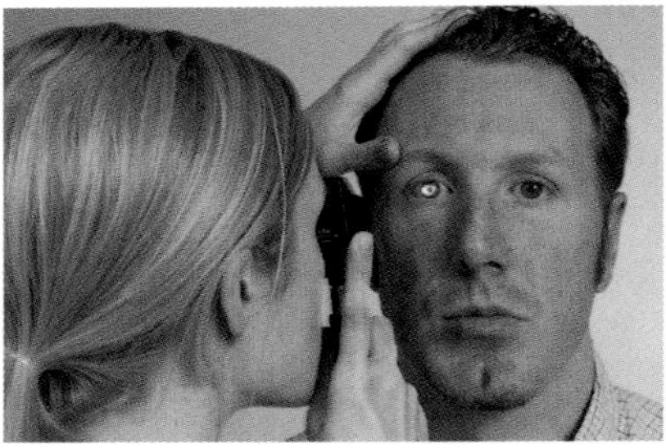

Examining optic disc

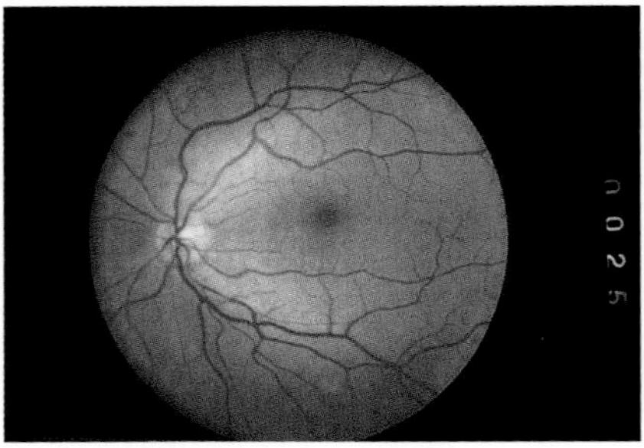

Normal fundus

Blurred margins other than nasally: Hypertension (HTN), glaucoma, or papilledema.

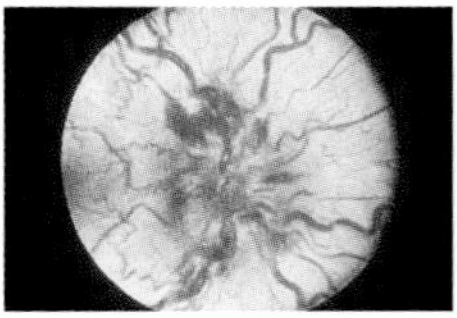

Acute papilledema

AREA/PA SKILL	NORMAL FINDINGS	ABNORMAL FINDINGS
		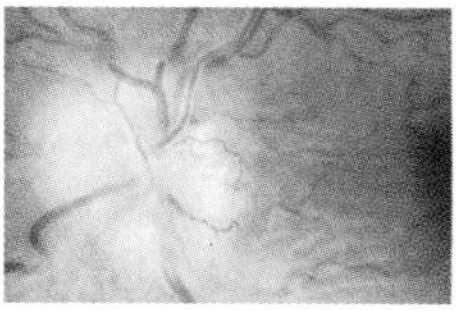 *Chronic papilledema*
		Excessive cup-to-disc ratio greater than 1:2: Open-angle glaucoma.
Retinal Vessels		
Arteries and veins comeout of disc in pairs.		
Assess size ratio of arteries and veins (AV ratio), color, arteriole light reflex, crossings.	Vessels noted. AV ratio 2:3 or 4:5. + Arteriole light reflex. AV crossings smooth, no nicking or narrowing.	*Large AV ratio:* HTN.
Veins normally darker and larger than arteries.		*Narrowed arteries:* Severe HTN, retinitis pigmentosa, and central retinal artery occlusion.
		AV crossings more than 2 disc diameters (DD) from optic disc or nicking or pinching of underlying vessel: HTN.
		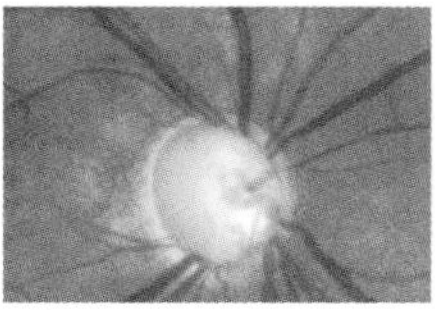 *Glaucomatous optic nerve*
		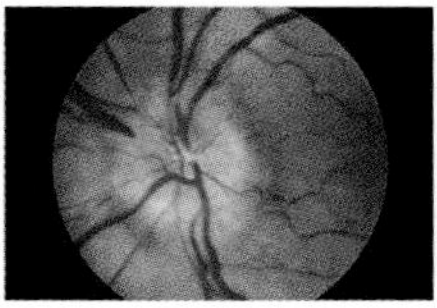 *Optic neuritis*

(box continued on page 132)

AREA/PA SKILL	NORMAL FINDINGS	ABNORMAL FINDINGS
Palpation *Retinal Vessels (cont'd)*		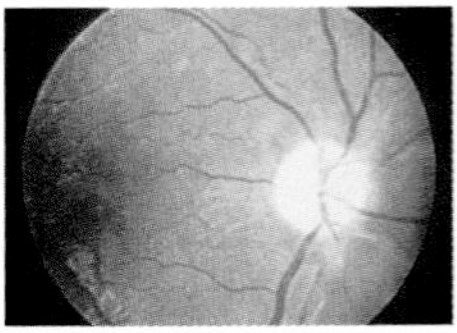 *Optic nerve pallor* 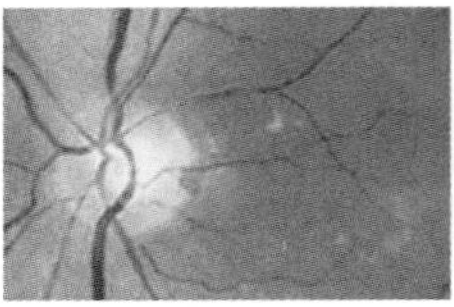 *Hypertensive changes*
Retina Assess color, texture, exudates, lesions, hemorrhages, or aneurysms.	Color varies depending on pigmentation of patient, from pale yellow to orange-red.	*Cotton wool spots:* Microinfarctions that occur with diabetes, HTN, lupus, papilledema. 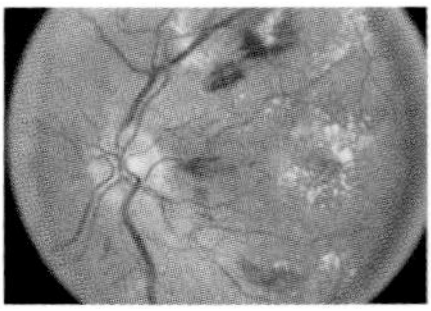 *Diabetic retinopathy*
	The darker the person, the darker the background.	*Dot hemorrhages:* Deep intraretinal hemorrhages seen with diabetes. 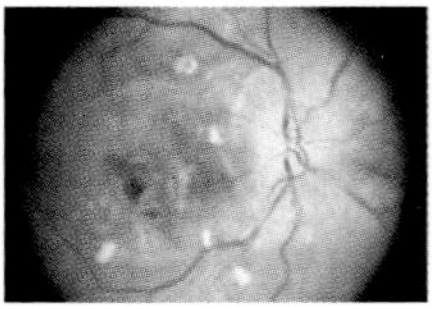 *Malignant HTN*
	Texture finely granular.	*Flame-shaped hemorrhages:* Superficial retinal hemorrhages that occur in HTN.
	No lesions, hemorrhages, exudates, aneurysms.	

AREA/PA SKILL	NORMAL FINDINGS	ABNORMAL FINDINGS
Macula and Fovea Centralis		
Always examine last!		
Note, color, size, location, lesions.	Macula darker area on retina, 2 DD temporal to OD, 1 DD in size, no lesions, + fovea light reflex.	*Excess or clumped pigment:* Trauma or retinal detachment.
Macula is darker area temporal to disc.		*Hemorrhage or exudate in the macula:* Macular degeneration. 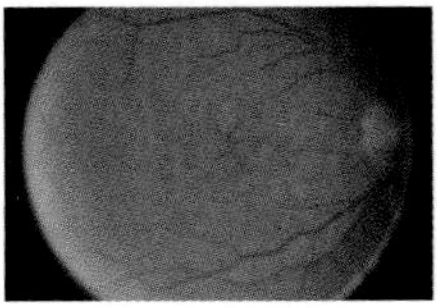 *Age-related macular degeneration ("dry")—vision 20/20* 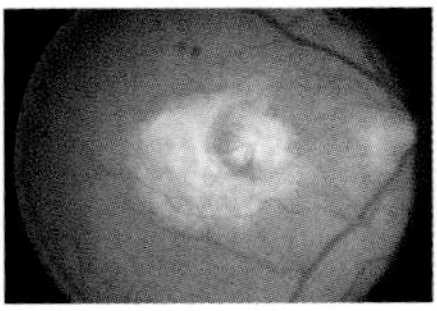 *Advanced macular degeneration ("wet")—vision 20/400*

OD = Right eye; OS = left eye; OU = both eyes; PA = physical assessment.

EARS

Primary Functions

- Hearing
- Balance/equilibrium

Developmental Considerations

Infants and Children

- Abnormalities in the structure and positioning of the ears are more common in infants who have a hearing deficit.
- Low-set ears, ears positioned at greater than a 15-degree angle, or malformed ears are often associated with genetic disorders and developmental delay.
- Infants and children are more prone to inner ear infections than adults because of the shape and position of the external auditory canal and eustachian tube.
- By school age, the external auditory canal has assumed a straighter, adult configuration.

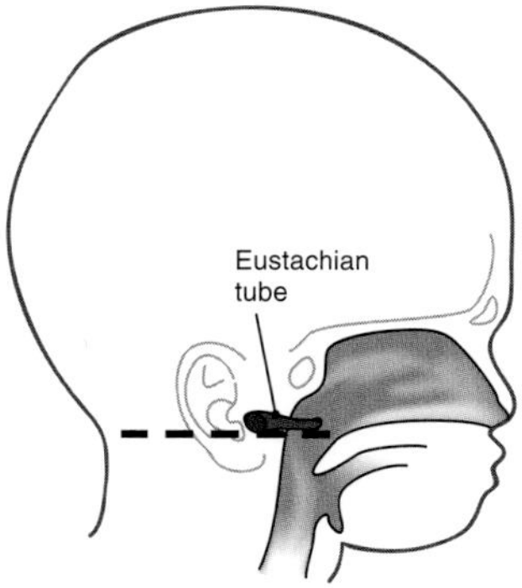

Infant

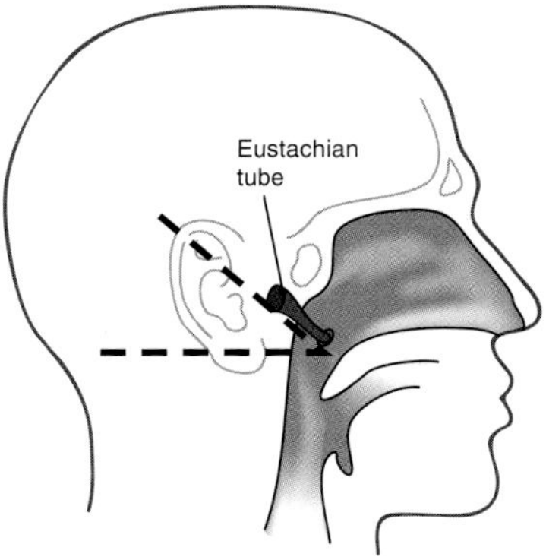

Adult

Young and Middle-Aged Adults

- Noise-induced hearing loss from exposure to loud music or machinery is the most common cause of hearing loss for adults aged 20 to 40 years old.

Older Adults

- Hearing loss in older adults is extremely common and can be associated with sensorineural loss or conductive loss.
- Presbycusis occurs around the 5th decade and gradually progresses. Typically, presbycusis involves hearing loss for high-pitched sounds such as consonants and affects men more often than women.
- Older adults are prone to stiffening of the cilia in the external canal, which impedes the transmission of sound waves and causes cerumen to accumulate more readily and obstruct the membrane. Excess accumulation of cerumen impairs hearing by air conduction and is one of the most common correctable causes of conductive hearing loss in older adults.

Cultural Considerations

- Incidence and severity of otitis media for Native American, Hispanic, and Alaskan infants are even higher than for the general population.
- Cerumen is dry, white, and flaky in the majority of Asians and Native Americans.

- Cerumen is brown, wet, and sticky in the majority of African Americans and whites.
- People living in highly industrialized communities are routinely exposed to sounds above 80 dB, such as traffic and occupational machinery, and are more prone to hearing loss.

Assessment

History

Symptoms ("PQRST" Any + Symptom)

- Hearing loss
  - Was your hearing loss sudden or gradual?
  - Is your hearing loss in one or both ears?
  - Can you hear better when it is noisy?
  - Have you ever been given an antibiotic called gentamicin or streptomycin?
  - Are you, or have you been, exposed repeatedly to continuous or loud noise?
- Vertigo
  - Do you ever feel as though the room is spinning when you are at rest?
  - If so, was the spinning sensation brought on or worsened by a change in position?
  - Does the spinning sensation change if you change position?
  - Is the sensation associated with blurred vision? Nausea? Vomiting? Weakness? Ringing in the ears?
- Tinnitus
  - Is the ringing or buzzing continuous or intermittent?
  - Does anything in particular seem to bring on the ringing or buzzing sound?
  - Does the ringing or buzzing sound pulsate?
- Drainage from ear (otorrhea)
  - Have you had any drainage from the ear?
  - If so, what does it look like (color, clarity)?
  - Does the drainage have an odor?
  - Have you had a recent ear or throat infection?
  - Do you have any dizziness? Ear pain? Change in your hearing?
  - Have you had a recent head or ear injury?

- Ear pain (otalgia)
  - Is the pain associated with decreased hearing?
  - Have you had any recent trauma to the ear?

Focused Ear History

- Do you have any problems with your ears? Ringing? Hearing?
- Do you have any balance problems?
- Do you have any drainage from your ears? If yes, amount, color?
- Have you had recent head trauma?
- Do you have any health problems?
- Are you exposed to noise pollution in your job or environment?
- Are you taking any medications, prescribed or OTC (Table 4.2)?
- Do you have allergies?

TABLE 4.2 Drugs That Adversely Affect the Ear

DRUG CLASS	DRUG	POSSIBLE ADVERSE REACTIONS
Aminoglycosides	All aminoglycosides	Tinnitus, vertigo, hearing loss
Anti-inflammatory agents	All nonsteroidal anti-inflammatory agents (such as diflunisal, ibuprofen, and indomethacin)	Tinnitus, vertigo, hearing loss
Antimalarials	Quinine	Tinnitus, vertigo, hearing loss
Diuretics	Furosemide and bumetanide	Tinnitus, vertigo, hearing loss (with too-rapid intravenous administration)
Nonnarcotic analgesics and antipyretics	All salicylates and all combination products containing salicylates	Tinnitus, dizziness, hearing loss (with high-dose or long-term therapy)
Miscellaneous agents	Capreomycin, cisplatin, erythromycin, ethacrynic acid, quinidine sulfate, and vancomycin	Tinnitus, vertigo, hearing loss

Assessment of the Ears' Relationship to Other Systems

Remember, all systems are related! As you assess the ears, look at the relationship between them and all other systems.

SUBJECTIVE DATA/RATIONALE	OBJECTIVE DATA/RATIONALE
Area/System: General	
Ask about:	*Inspect for:*
General state of health: Change in general health may indicate underlying problem that may affect the ears.	Ear guarding, inattentiveness, inappropriate responses, balance problems.
	Behaviors similar to confusion or disorientation during conversation: Hearing loss.
Recent infections/illnesses.	*Measure:*
Hearing difficulty.	Vital signs.
Area/System: Integumentary	
Ask about:	*Inspect:*
Lesions on ears (sun-exposed area, common site for skin cancer): Six or more brown patches of skin (café-au-lait spots) in the axillary region may signify neurofibromatosis, commonly associated with acoustic neuroma and hearing loss.	Lesion, areas of inflammation. Inflammation may indicate infection. *Axillary freckling, café-au-lait spots, acoustic neuroma, hearing loss:* Neurofibromatosis. *Palpate for:* Tenderness.
Area/System: HEENT	
Head and neck	
Ask about:	*Palpate for:*
Pain.	Lymph node enlargement, sinus swollen nodes, tenderness. *Palpable, tender, warm lymph nodes:* Infection.
Nose and throat	
Ask about:	*Inspect:*
Sore throat	Oral and nasal structures.
Nasal congestion.	*Tearing eyes, ear fullness, and pale, boggy mucosa with watery drainage:* Environmental allergy. *Purulent or mucoid discharge, often with concurrent otitis media:* Upper respiratory infection. *Reddened pharynx, whitish exudate on pharynx or tonsils, or enlarged tonsils:* Upper respiratory infection, often with concurrent otitis.

SUBJECTIVE DATA/RATIONALE	OBJECTIVE DATA/RATIONALE
Area/System: Respiratory	
Ask about:	*Measure:*
Cough, congestion.	Respiratory rate.
Mucus production.	*Auscultate:*
Ear infections often follow upper respiratory infections, especially in children.	Lung sounds.
	Cough with sputum, crackles/wheezes: Upper respiratory infection. (Ear infections often exist concurrently or as a precursor.)
Area/System: Cardiovascular	
Ask about:	*Measure:*
History of cardiovascular disease, HTN, stroke: Tinnitus/vertigo may be a symptom of cardiovascular or cerebrovascular disease.	Heart rate.
	Palpate: Pulses, carotid thrills. *Auscultate:* Heart sounds, bruits. *Tinnitus/vertigo:* Cardiovascular/cerebrovascular disease.
Area/System: Abdomen/Gastrointestinal	
Ask about:	
Change in appetite: Children with ear infections often have a decrease in appetite.	
Area/System: Genitourinary	
Ask about:	
History of kidney disease: The ears and kidneys are formed in utero during similar time periods.	
Area/System: Reproductive	
Ask about:	
For female patients, pregnancy: Increased vascularity may cause fullness and diminished hearing.	

(continued)

SUBJECTIVE DATA/RATIONALE	OBJECTIVE DATA/RATIONALE
Area/System: Musculoskeletal *Ask about:*	*Inspect:*
History of gout: Uric acid deposits can form in ear lobes. *Hearing problems:* Auditory ossicles sclerosis can affect hearing.	Ear lobes for tophi.
	Altered muscle strength, tremors, auditory problems, balance problems: MS.
Area/System: Neurologic *Ask about:*	*Test:*
History of transient ischemic attacks.	Romberg's
Balance problems: Indicates problem with inner ear or cerebellum.	*Tinnitus/balance and gait problems:* MS; balance problems also may indicate problem with inner ear.
Neurologic problem: Tinnitus and balance problems may be associated with MS.	
Area/System: Lymphatic *Ask about:*	
Recent ear infections: May cause lymph node enlargement.	

HEENT = Head, eyes, ears, nose, and throat.

Physical Assessment

ANATOMICAL LANDMARKS: Position of ears; tympanic membrane (TM)

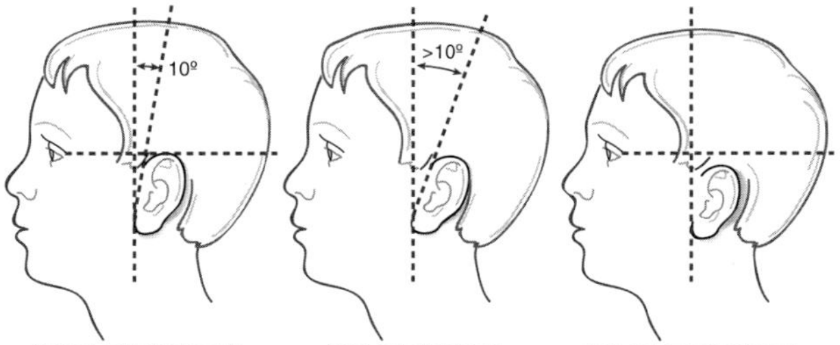

Normal ear attachment Deviated alignment Low-set ear attachment

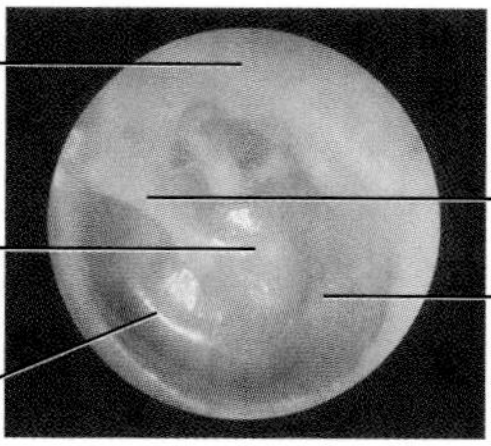

Tympanic membrane, left ear

APPROACH: Inspection and palpation of external structures; otoscopy of external auditory canal and TM; hearing tests

POSITION: Sitting; supine for infants to immobilize head

TOOLBOX: Tuning fork (512 Hz), otoscope with pneumatic attachment, thermometer, watch

AREA/PA SKILL	NORMAL FINDINGS	ABNORMAL FINDINGS
Inspection *External Ear*		
Note position, shape, size, symmetry, angle of attachment, color, lesions, and drainage (clear, bloody, or purulent).	Vertical ear position with < 10-degree lateral posterior slant. Ears aligned with eyes, symmetrical, no redness, lesions, or drainage.	*Microtia:* Small ears < 4 cm vertical height in adults. Seen in some genetic disorders.
		Macrotia: Large ears: 10 cm vertical height in adults.
To assess angle of attachment, draw imaginary line from top of helix to external canthus of eye and then a perpendicular line in front of ear.		*Landmarks missing or malformed:* Associated with hearing deficit. *Creased ear lobe:* Associated with heart conditions. *Ear pits or sinuses usually located anterior to the tragus:* Associated with internal ear anomalies. *Low-set ears or ears rotated posteriorly > 15 degrees:* Associated with mental retardation.

(box continued on page 142)

AREA/PA SKILL	NORMAL FINDINGS	ABNORMAL FINDINGS
Inspection *External Ear (cont'd)*		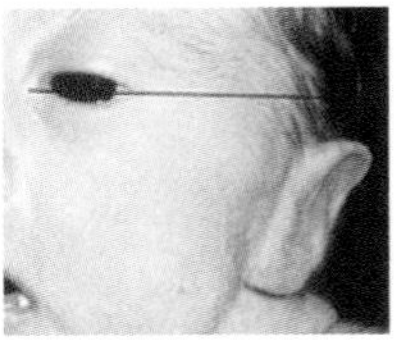 *Low-set ears* 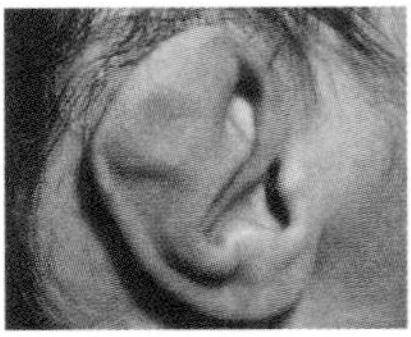 *Congenital ear anomaly* 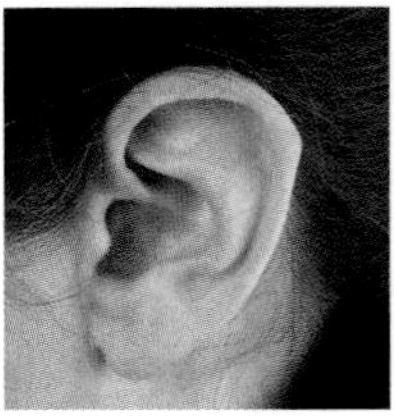 *Darwinian tubercle* If clear drainage noted from nose or ears, secondary to head trauma, suspect cerebrospinal fluid. 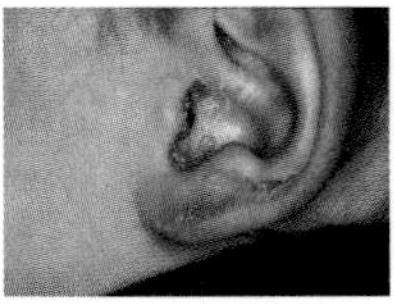 *Impacted cerumen*
Palpation Maintain standard precautions. Wear gloves if drainage is present.		

AREA/PA SKILL	NORMAL FINDINGS	ABNORMAL FINDINGS
External Ear Assess consistency, tenderness, lesions.	Helix soft and pliable, nontender, no nodules or lesions.	*Tenderness of mastoid, helix, tragus, or pinna:* Ear infections or tophi.
Palpate tragus and mastoid process. **Before starting otoscopic exam, palpate tragus and mastoid, pull helix forward.** **If tender, proceed carefully with insertion of otoscope—patient may have ear infection.**		

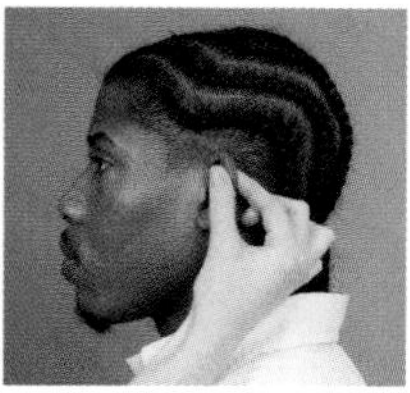

Palpating the ear

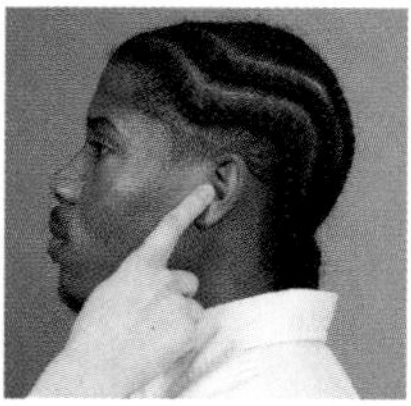

Palpating the tragus

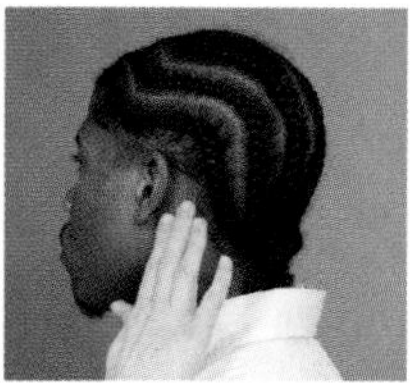

Palpating the mastoid

(box continued on page 142)

AREA/PA SKILL	NORMAL FINDINGS	ABNORMAL FINDINGS

Palpation

External Ear (cont'd)

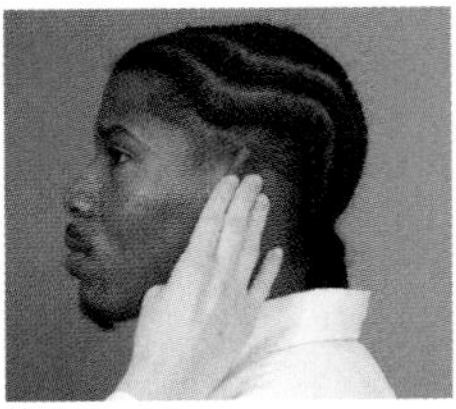

Pulling helix forward

Otoscopic Exam

Use the largest and shortest speculum that the ear canal can accommodate (4, 5, or 6 mm, ½" in length). Have patient tilt head to opposite side to that being examined. Pull helix up and back for an adult and down for a child. Always look into canal before inserting the otoscope.

Insert ½" for adult, ¼" for child

Avoid the inner two-thirds of the canal—it is over the temporal bone and is very sensitive.

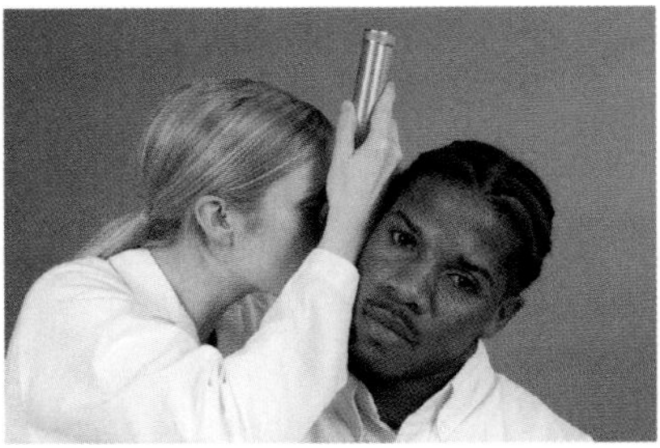

Otoscope insertion with handle up

AREA/PA SKILL	NORMAL FINDINGS	ABNORMAL FINDINGS
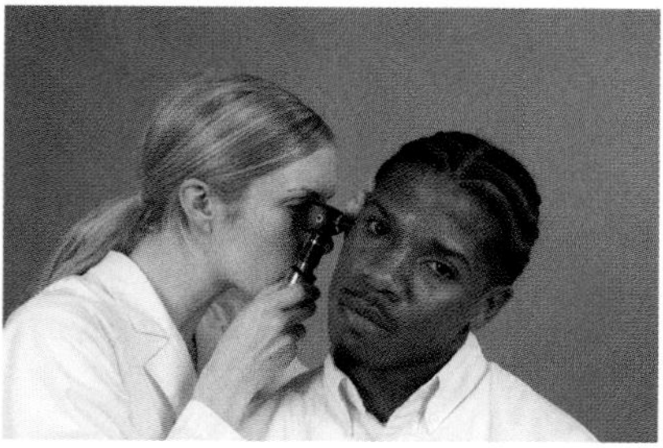 *Otoscope insertion with handle down*		
External Ear Canal Note color, drainage, patency, edema, lesions, or foreign objects.	Ear canal light-colored and patent, small amount of yellow cerumen and hair; no lesions, exudates, or foreign objects.	Ear canal may be blocked by a foreign object or cerumen. *Reddened canal:* Otitis externa.
Cerumen is the only normal drainage in the ear.	*Color and amount of cerumen vary depending on ethnicity.*	Excessive impacted cerumen in older adults can contribute to conductive hearing loss. *Exudate and an edematous canal:* External otitis. 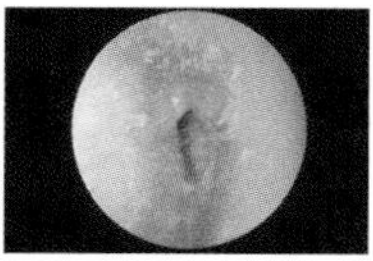 *External otitis* *Drainage:* Bloody drainage can result from trauma; purulent from infection; and clear may be spinal fluid from head injury. Exostosis often results from swimming in cold water. 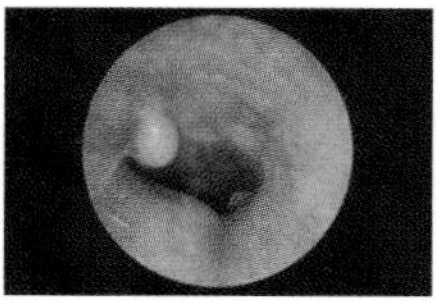 *Exotosis*

(box continued on page 146)

AREA/PA SKILL	NORMAL FINDINGS	ABNORMAL FINDINGS
Inspection *External Ear (cont'd)*		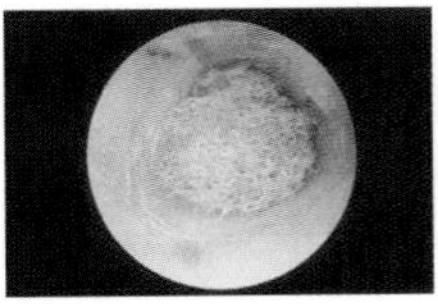 *Foreign body*
Tympanic Membrane Note position of landmarks (cone of light, pars flaccida, pars tensa, malleus, and umbo). **Ears are mirror images, so cone of light is at 7 o'clock in left ear and 5 o'clock in right ear.** Note intactness of TM, color, lesions, and exudates. **Assess mobility of TM in children using pneumatic attachment.** **Never irrigate the ear canal unless you are sure the TM is intact.**	TM shiny, pearly gray, intact, and mobile. No lesions or exudates. Landmarks appropriately noted. No bulging or retraction of the TM.	*Yellowish membrane with fluid and air bubbles visible behind TM:* Serous otitis. 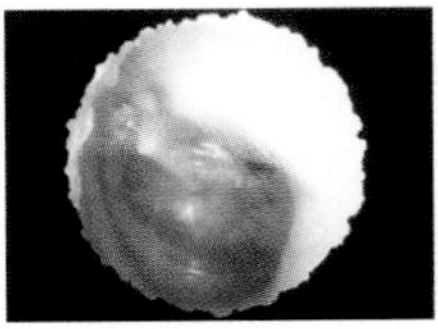 *Serous otitis* *Reddish TM with absent or distorted light reflex:* Otitis media. 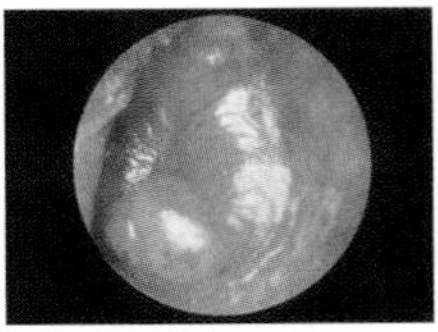 *Otitis media* *Round-/oval-shaped dark area:* Perforated TM. 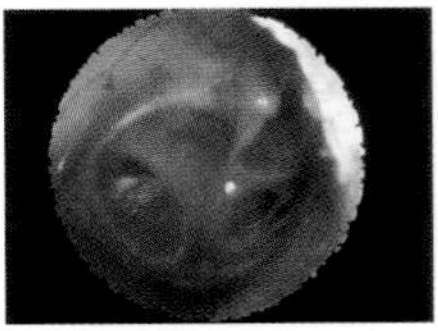 *Perforated TM* *White irregular-shaped area:* Scar tissue.

AREA/PA SKILL	NORMAL FINDINGS	ABNORMAL FINDINGS
		Blue to black TM: Hemotympanum; bleeding usually results from trauma. 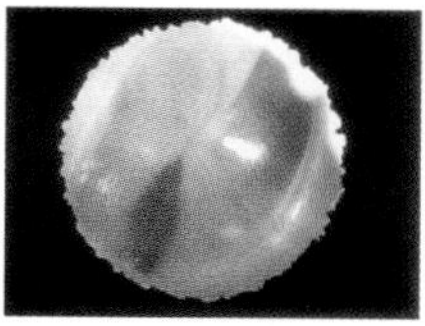 *Hemotympanum* *Golden-brown TM with caramel-color, thick, elastic (like rubber cement) drainage:* Secretory, adhesive otitis media; associated with viral infection. 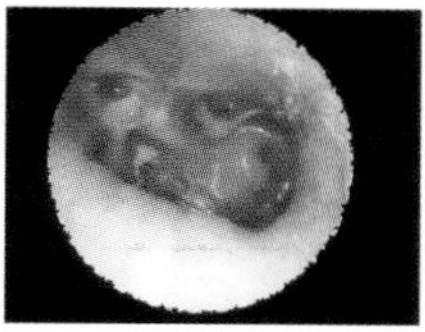 *Adhesive otitis media* *Cystic mass of epithelial cells in middle ear:* Cholesteatoma, a complication of chronic otitis media. 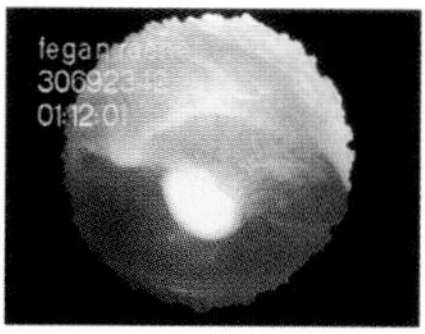 *Cholesteatoma*

(box continued on page 148)

AREA/PA SKILL	NORMAL FINDINGS	ABNORMAL FINDINGS
Inspection *Tympanic Membrane (cont'd)*		Tubes placed in ear to promote drainage and equalize pressure. 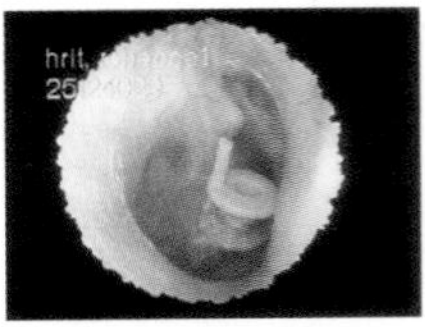 *Pressure equalization tube* 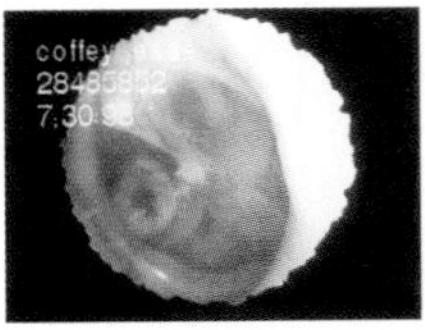 *Tympanotomy* 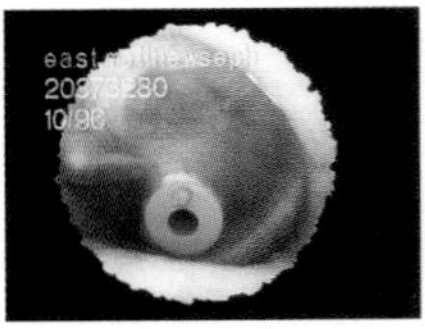 *Intact patient pressure equalization tube* *Change in position or shape of cone of light reflex and absence or exaggeration of bony landmarks:* Imbalance in middle ear pressure. Bony landmarks are more prominent if negative pressure in inner ear, less prominent in infections or conditions in which fluid or pus collects behind membrane. *Limited mobility of drum:* Associated with bulging drum.
Hearing Exam *Gross Hearing* Use whispered voice test to assess for low-pitched deficits (1 to 2 feet from ear).	Gross hearing intact bilaterally.	*Inability to repeat whispered words:* Low-tone frequency loss.

AREA/PA SKILL	NORMAL FINDINGS	ABNORMAL FINDINGS
Use ticking watch to assess for high-pitched deficits **(5 inches from ear).**		*Inability to hear watch ticking:* High-tone frequency loss.
Weber Test		
Place vibrating tuning fork on forehead or top of head to assess bone conduction.	Negative lateralization of sound: Heard equally in both ears.	*Lateralization of sound:* Either conductive or sensorineural loss.
Be careful not to touch the prongs of tuning fork—it will dampen vibration.		

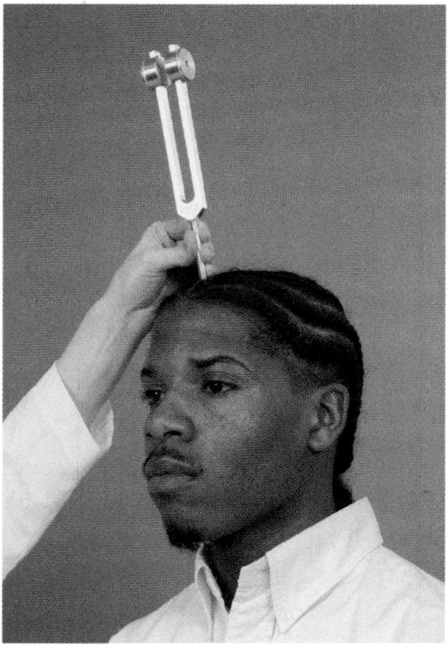

Performing Weber test on head

(box continued on page 150)

AREA/PA SKILL	NORMAL FINDINGS	ABNORMAL FINDINGS
Hearing Exam *Weber Test (cont'd)*		

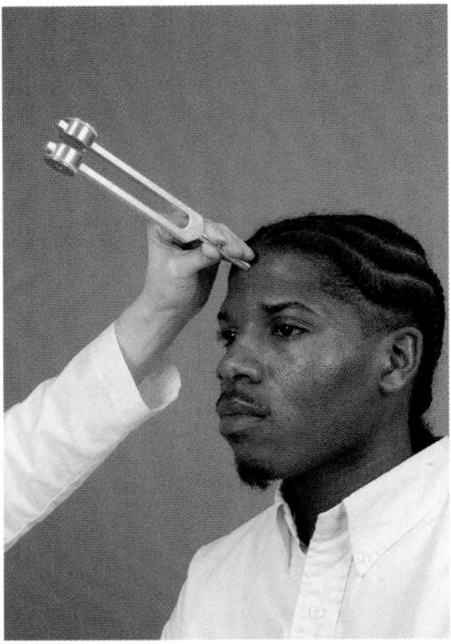

Performing Weber test on forehead

AREA/PA SKILL	NORMAL FINDINGS	ABNORMAL FINDINGS
Rinne Test Compare bone conduction (BC) to air conduction (AC). Place vibrating tuning fork on mastoid (BC) until no longer heard, then move fork to in front of ear (AC). Time how long the sound is heard.	Sound transmission through air is normally twice as long as sound transmission through bone.	*AC-to-BC ratios that differ markedly in each ear:* Unilateral hearing deficit.

AREA/PA SKILL	NORMAL FINDINGS	ABNORMAL FINDINGS
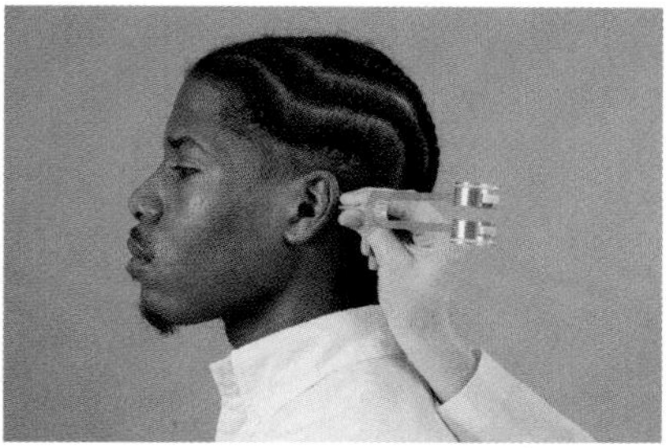 Performing Rinne test on mastoid 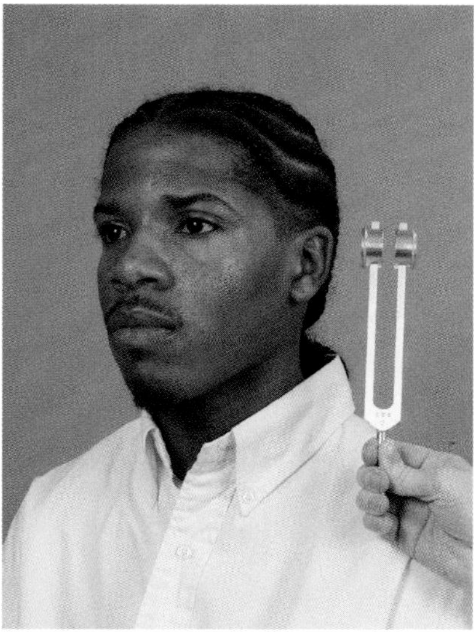 Performing Rinne test in front of ear	AC > BC.	*AC < 2BC:* Hearing loss by AC, possibly caused by ear wax, otitis media, serous otitis, or damage to ossicles of middle ear.
Balance		
Perform Romberg test with patient's eyes open and then closed.	Negative Romberg.	*Positive Romberg test, loss of balance:* Inner ear problem, cerebellar dysfunction, or ingestion of drugs or alcohol.

PA = Physical assessment.

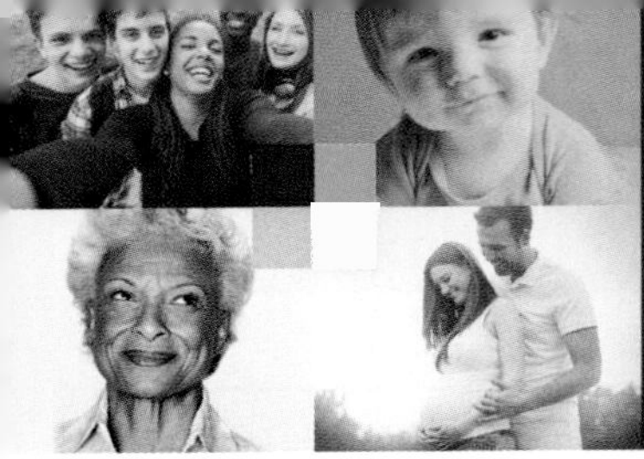

CHAPTER 5

Assessing the Respiratory System

Primary Function

- Exchange of oxygen and carbon dioxide through respirations.
- Plays important role in maintaining acid-base balance.

Developmental Considerations

Infants
- Obligatory nose breathers.
- Irregular respiratory patterns with patterns of apnea.
- Normal breath sounds more bronchial/bronchovesicular.
- Abdominal breathers.
- Anteroposterior (AP): lateral ratio 1:1.

Pregnant Patients
- Increased tidal volume.
- Increased costal angle.
- Diaphragm rises.
- Increased oxygen demands.

Older Adults
- Decreased surface area.
- Decreased breathing and lung capacity.
- Increased dead space.
- Decreased vital capacity.

Cultural Considerations

- Chinese Americans have smaller chests than Caucasians.
- African Americans in urban areas have higher incidence of respiratory disease.
- Appalachians have higher incidence of black lung, tuberculosis (TB), and emphysema.
- Irish have higher incidence of respiratory problems related to coal mining.
- Navajo Native Americans have increased risk for respiratory problems related to close living quarters.

Assessment

History

Symptoms ("PQRST" Any + Symptom)

- Cough
  - How long have you had the cough?
  - When does your cough occur: On awakening, late afternoon, in the evening, after eating, during the night?
  - Do you cough when sitting up, or just when lying down?
  - Do you cough when you exercise?
  - Are you allergic to pollens, animals, or dust?
  - When you cough, what does it sound like? Is it dry or moist sounding? Wheezy?
  - Do you have trouble catching your breath when you start coughing?
  - Do you bring up mucus or sputum when you cough?
  - What color is the sputum? Does it smell or taste bad?
  - Is your sputum thick and hard to get up? Or is it thin? Is it frothy or bubbly?
- Dyspnea
  - Do you ever feel you don't have enough air or you can't catch your breath? If so, please describe what you are doing when this happens, whether it occurs suddenly or over time, and how it affects your activities.
  - How many pillows do you sleep with?

- Do you experience shortness of breath, or breathlessness, with activity or exercise? How much can you do before you become short of breath?
- Can you breathe better after you rest or when you are quiet?
- Do you wake up at night feeling breathless?
- Do you have pain associated with the shortness of breath?
- How long have you noticed this problem of breathlessness?

- Chest pain
  - Do you experience pain in your chest, especially when you take a deep breath?
  - If you have shortness of breath, is it accompanied by pain?
  - Do you have pain when you cough?
  - Where in your chest do you feel the pain?
  - Please describe your pain: Is it aching, sharp, stabbing, gripping? How severe is it on a scale of 1 to 10?
  - Is your chest wall tender or sore when touched?
- Other related symptoms
  - Do you have swelling of your abdomen, legs, ankles, or feet?
  - Do you have enough energy to do your usual daily activities?
  - Do you need to sleep or rest more than usual?

Focused Respiratory History

- Do you have a history of respiratory disease? If yes, are you taking any medications for it? If yes, what are you taking and why?
- Do you have any other medical problems? (Especially note cardiac problems.)
- Do you have allergies? If yes, describe reaction.
- Do you have a cough, shortness of breath, or chest pain?
- Do you smoke? If yes, what do you smoke, how much, and for how long?
- What is your occupation?
- Where do you live?
- When was your last purified protein derivative test, and what were the results?
- Have you ever had a chest x-ray? If yes, what were the results?
- Have you been immunized for influenza or pneumonia?
- Are you taking any medications, prescribed or over-the-counter (OTC) (Table 5.1)?

TABLE 5.1 Drugs That Adversely Affect the Respiratory System

DRUG CLASS	DRUG	POSSIBLE ADVERSE REACTIONS
Adrenergic agents (sympathomimetics)	Epinephrine	Dyspnea, paradoxical bronchospasms
Antineoplastic agents	Bleomycin	Fine crackles, dyspnea (early signs of pulmonary toxicity); interstitial pneumonitis, pulmonary fibrosis
	Busulfan	Irreversible pulmonary fibrosis (busulfan lung)
	Carmustine	Pulmonary fibrosis
	Cyclophosphamide	Pulmonary fibrosis (with high doses)
	Melphalan	Interstitial pneumonitis, pulmonary fibrosis
	Methotrexate	Interstitial pneumonitis
	Mitomycin	Dyspnea, cough, pulmonary infiltrates, interstitial pneumonitis
Antiarrhythmics	Amiodarone	Interstitial pneumonitis, pulmonary fibrosis
Antihypertensives	Enalapril	Cough
	Guanabenz	Nasal congestion, dyspnea
	Reserpine	Nasal congestion
Anti-infectives	Polymyxin B sulfate	Respiratory paralysis
Beta-blockers	All beta-blockers	Bronchospasm, particularly in patients with a history of asthma; dyspnea, wheezing
Cholinergic agents	Bethanecol	Dyspnea, bronchoconstriction (with subcutaneous administration)
	Neostigmine	Increased bronchial secretions, bronchospasm, dyspnea

(continued)

TABLE 5.1 Drugs That Adversely Affect the Respiratory System (continued)

DRUG CLASS	DRUG	POSSIBLE ADVERSE REACTIONS
Gold salts	Aurothioglucose, gold sodium thiomalate	Pulmonary infiltrates, interstitial pneumonitis, interstitial fibrosis, "gold" bronchitis
Narcotic analgesics	All types	Respiratory depression
Nonsteroidal anti-inflammatory agents	Aspirin	Bronchospasm
	Ibuprofen	Bronchospasm, dyspnea
	Indomethacin	Bronchospasm, dyspnea
Penicillins	All types	Anaphylaxis
Sedatives and hypnotics	All types	Respiratory depression, apnea
Urinary tract antiseptics	Nitrofurantoin	Pulmonary sensitivity reactions, such as cough, chest pain, dyspnea, pulmonary infiltrates; interstitial pneumonitis (with prolonged use)
Miscellaneous agents	Cromolyn sodium	Dyspnea, pharyngitis
	Levodopa	Excessive nasal discharge, hoarseness, episodic hyperventilation, bizarre breathing patterns

Assessment of the Respiratory System's Relationship to Other Systems

Remember, all systems are related. As you assess the respiratory system, look at the relationship between it and all other systems.

(text continues on page 163)

Assessment of the Respiratory System's Relationship to Other Systems

SUBJECTIVE DATA/RATIONALE	OBJECTIVE DATA/RATIONALE
Area/System: General	
Ask about:	*Inspect for:*
Fatigue, activity intolerance, changes in energy level: Chronic lung disease often causes fatigue and activity intolerance because so much energy is expended on breathing.	Signs of acute distress, such as shortness of breath, dyspnea on exertion.
Fevers, night sweats: Fevers and night sweats may be associated with a more serious underlying disease such as TB.	*Posture:* Tripod. *Position:* Orthopnea.
Weight changes: Weight gain may correlate with fluid retention associated with right-side congestive heart failure (CHF), a common complication of COPD.	Early signs of hypoxia include confusion, restlessness, irritability, short attention span.
	Short-term memory may also be affected by hypoxia. People with chronic respiratory disease may deny illness, severity of symptoms, or associated risk factors. Anxiety can trigger a respiratory problem, such as hyperventilation, or can result from a respiratory problem such as an acute asthmatic attack or pulmonary emboli. Fatigue is associated with chronic lung disease, lung cancer, and pneumonia because more energy is expended on breathing. *Measure:* Height, weight (check for changes). Temperature, pulse, respirations, blood pressure (check for increases).

(continued)

Assessment of the Respiratory System's Relationship to Other Systems (continued)

SUBJECTIVE DATA/RATIONALE	OBJECTIVE DATA/RATIONALE
Area/System: Integumentary	
Ask about:	*Inspect for:*
Skin color changes.	Skin color changes (e.g., cyanosis, pallor, ruddiness). *Pale, diaphoretic:* Sympathetic response to respiratory distress and hypoxia. *Central cyanosis:* Dusky or blue buccal mucosa and tongue when $Po_2 < 50$. Caused by respiratory failure, shock, pulmonary edema, airway obstruction, ventilation-perfusion problems. May see cyanosis in conjunctiva in end-stage COPD. *Peripheral cyanosis:* Blue, dusky-red, or purple color of lips, nail beds, tips of nose and ears, sometimes face and especially cheeks. Caused by slow or congested blood flow in peripheral vessels or disorders with compensatory polycythemia, such as COPD, CHF. *Ruddy, reddish color:* Associated with polycythemia. *Cyanotic or dusky nails:* Reflect peripheral cyanosis seen in vasoconstriction and slowing of peripheral blood flow. Also associated with central cyanosis. *Yellow-brown stains on nails and fingers:* Nicotine stains from long history of smoking. *Purple/dusky lower extremities:* Venous stasis, especially if Po_2 is low. Central (mucous membranes) vs. peripheral cyanosis.
Cyanosis: Cardiopulmonary disease.	Nail clubbing.
Fluid retention: Right-side cardiac involvement of long-standing respiratory disease.	*Palpate:*
	Skin temperature, turgor, edema. Capillary refill.

SUBJECTIVE DATA/RATIONALE	OBJECTIVE DATA/RATIONALE
	Peripheral edema frequently seen in people with chronic lung disease secondary to right-side CHF. *Clubbing:* Long-standing lung disease.
Area/System: HEENT *Ask about:*	*Inspect for:*
Lumps or swelling in neck: Enlarged thyroid may compromise respiratory function.	Facial expression (e.g., anxious).
Excessive eye tearing: Associated with allergies.	Neck vein distension, hypertrophy, and use of accessory neck muscles.
Ear infections, sore throats, upper respiratory infections (URIs), sinus problems: Postnasal drip, sinus problems may indicate allergies or acute/chronic URI.	Color of conjunctiva.
Difficulty swallowing or breathing.	Ear or nose drainage, nasal flaring.
Enlarged lymph nodes: Infection or malignancy.	Color of mucous membranes, color of tonsils and enlargement. *Palpate:* Sinus tenderness, lymph nodes, tracheal position, thyroid gland, patent nares, tonsillar glands. *Examine:* Fundus, optic disc. External ear and tympanic membrane (TM) (otoscopic exam). Internal nasal mucosa and structures. *Tracheal shifts:* Collapsed lung, tumors, pneumothorax or hemothorax. Pursed-lip breathing, or physiological positive end-expiratory pressure, is a compensatory mechanism used by people with COPD to prolong expiration, help expel trapped air, and keep alveoli open longer for maximum oxygenation of pulmonary blood. Nasal flaring occurs in infants and small children and indicates acute respiratory distress or cyanotic heart disease. *(continued)*

Assessment of the Respiratory System's Relationship to Other Systems (continued)

SUBJECTIVE DATA/RATIONALE	OBJECTIVE DATA/RATIONALE
Area/System: HEENT *(cont'd)*	Neck vein distension is a general sign of respiratory distress or air hunger. When patient sits, elevating head and chest 45 degrees, neck vessels are firm and tortuous. This sign of increased venous pressure is seen in right heart failure and cor pulmonale. People with chronic lung disease may also develop hypertrophied neck muscles from increased efforts to breathe. *Use of scalene, sternocleidomastoideus (SCM), and trapezius accessory muscles:* Sign of respiratory distress or COPD. *Visible/palpable lymph nodes:* Infection or malignancy. Central cyanosis can be seen in the conjunctiva and the oral mucous membranes. *Excessive tearing:* Allergies. *Papilledema:* Hypercapnea or CO_2 narcosis. *Red mucous membranes, red TM, drainage:* URI.
Area/System: Cardiovascular *Ask about:* *Chest pain, palpitations, swelling, tight shoes:* May indicate cardiac involvement.	*Inspect for:* Edema. *Palpate for:* Edema, Homans' sign. *Auscultate:* Right side S_4 and S_3. *Right-sided S_3 and S_4:* Right CHF and pulmonary hypertension (HTN). *Accentuated P_2:* Pulmonary HTN. *Absent/diminished pedal pulses and ankle/pedal edema:* Heart failure and cor pulmonale. Patients with polycythemia are at risk for thrombophlebitis and possibly pulmonary embolism caused by sluggish blood flow. A positive Homans' sign may indicate thrombophlebitis, but it is not conclusive.

SUBJECTIVE DATA/RATIONALE	OBJECTIVE DATA/RATIONALE
Area/System: Gastrointestinal	
Ask about:	*Palpate for:*
Changes in appetite, weight loss, anorexia: Weight loss, anorexia associated with chronic lung disease, TB, or lung malignancy.	Enlarged liver, ascites.
Gastrointestinal (GI) complaints, right upper quadrant (RUQ) pain: GI complaints and RUQ tenderness are associated with right CHF, a common complication of COPD.	*Enlarged liver and ascites:* Right-side CHF, a common complication of chronic lung disease.
Area/System: Genitourinary/ Reproductive	
Ask about:	
Nocturia: Associated with heart failure or diuretic use to treat right-side heart failure.	
Changes in sexual activity: Chronic respiratory disease requires most of the patient's energy for breathing.	
Safe-sex practices: Unprotected sexual activity increases risk for human immunodeficiency virus (HIV).	
Pregnancy: Respiratory changes occur with pregnancy.	
Area/System: Musculoskeletal	
Ask about:	*Inspect for:*
Muscle weakness, wasting: Associated with chronic lung disease.	Hypertrophy and use of accessory muscles, muscle atrophy, spinal deformities.
	Measure:
	Muscle strength, checking for weakness.
	Weakness/muscle wasting: Long-standing respiratory disease.

(continued)

Assessment of the Respiratory System's Relationship to Other Systems (continued)

SUBJECTIVE DATA/RATIONALE	OBJECTIVE DATA/RATIONALE
Area/System: Neurologic *Ask about:*	*Inspect for:*
Memory changes, change in mental status: Early sign of hypoxia.	Impaired mental status, awake, alert, and oriented (AAO) morning headaches x 3.
Tremors: Associated with theophylline toxicity or CO_2 narcosis.	*Asterixis (flapping hand tremors):* CO_2 narcosis.
	Tremors, seizures, decreased deep tendon reflexes (DTRs): Respiratory failure.
Area/System: Endocrine *Ask about:* Thyroid disease. Enlarged thyroid can affect breathing.	
Area/System: Lymphatic/ Hematological *Ask about:* Bleeding, anemia. Allergies. Directly affect respiratory system.	

HEENT = Head, eyes, ears, nose, and throat.

Physical Assessment

Anatomical Landmarks

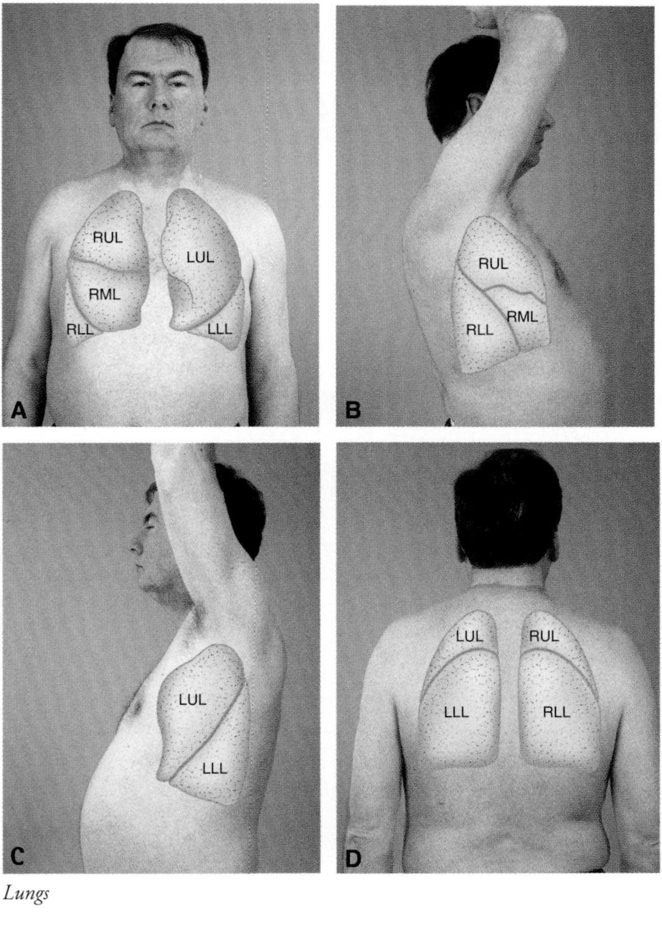

Lungs

APPROACH: Inspection, palpation, percussion, auscultation from anterior, posterior, and lateral approaches. Compare side to side, work apex to base.

POSITION: Sitting.

TOOLBOX: Stethoscope, felt-tipped marker, metric ruler.

Physical Assessment

AREA/PA SKILL	NORMAL FINDINGS	ABNORMAL FINDINGS
Inspection		
Chest		
Assess respiratory rate, rhythm, depth. Respiratory rate varies with age.	Look for symmetry of chest movement	Altered respiratory rate and pattern

Respiratory Patterns

When assessing a patient's respirations, the nurse should determine their rate, rhythm, and depth. These schematic diagrams show different respiratory patterns.

EUPNEA

Normal respiratory rate and rhythm.

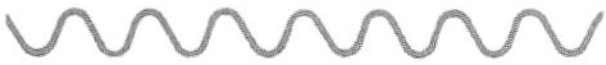

APNEA

Absence of breathing (may be periodic).

APNEUSTIC

Prolonged, gasping inspiration followed by extremely short, inefficient expiration.

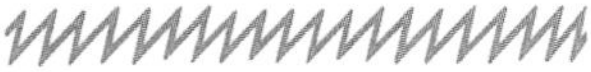

BIOT'S

Faster and deeper respirations than normal, with abrupt irregular pauses between them.

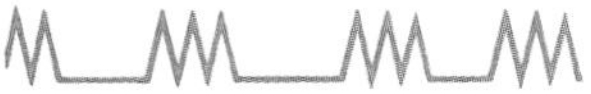

BRADYPNEA

Slow but regular respirations.

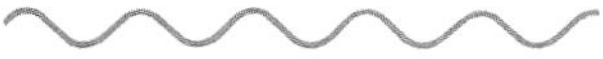

CHEYNE-STOKES

Respirations that gradually become faster and deeper than normal, then slower; alternates with periods of apnea.

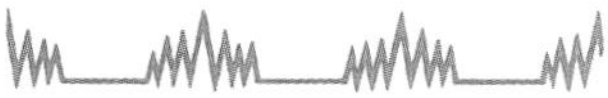

HYPERVENTILATION

Deeper respirations; normal rate.

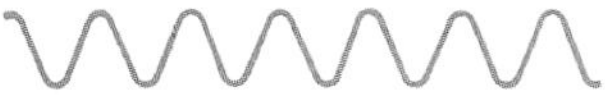

KUSSMAUL'S

Faster and deeper respirations without pauses.

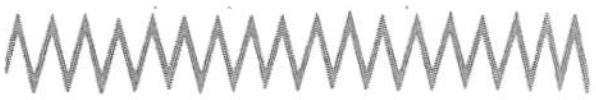

TACHYPNEA

Increased respiratory rate.

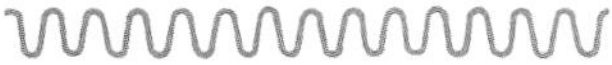

AREA/PA SKILL	NORMAL FINDINGS	ABNORMAL FINDINGS
	Respirations quiet, symmetrical, with regular rhythm and depth.	
Check AP: lateral ratio, costal angle.	AP:lateral ratio 1:2; costal angle 90 degrees.	
Inspect for spinal deformities.	No barrel chest or spinal deformities.	Altered shape—Barrel chest 1:1 with costal angle > 90 degrees: Chronic obstructive pulmonary disease (COPD).

(box continued on page 166)

Physical Assessment (continued)

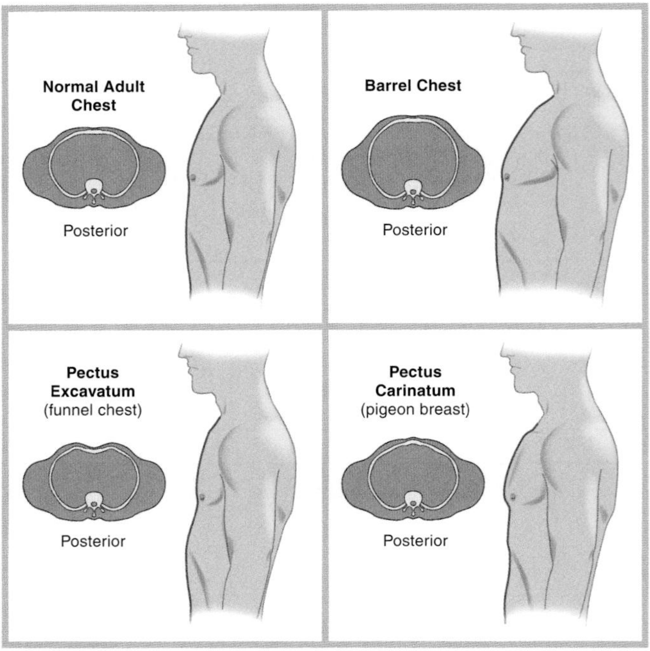

Chest shapes

AREA/PA SKILL	NORMAL FINDINGS	ABNORMAL FINDINGS
	No retraction or use of accessory muscles.	*Altered chest symmetry:* Spinal deformities, kyphosis, scoliosis.
Note muscles used for breathing.	Women are more thoracic breathers, men and infants are more abdominal breathers.	*Altered breathing symmetry:* Fractured ribs, flail chest, pneumothorax, atelectasis. *Sternal and intercostal retraction:* Hypoxia and severe respiratory distress, especially with airway obstruction. *Intercostal bulging:* COPD.
Note condition of skin.	Skin intact.	*Blue skin color (cyanosis):* Hypoxia or extreme cold temperature. *Scars:* Previous trauma or surgery.

AREA/PA SKILL	NORMAL FINDINGS	ABNORMAL FINDINGS
Palpation		
Trachea		
Note position.	Midline, no deviation.	*Tracheal deviation:* Tumor or thyroid enlargement; tension pneumothorax deviates trachea to unaffected side, severe atelectasis to affected side.
Chest		
Palpate for tenderness, masses, crepitus.	Chest nontender, no masses or crepitus.	*Crepitus:* Subcutaneous emphysema.

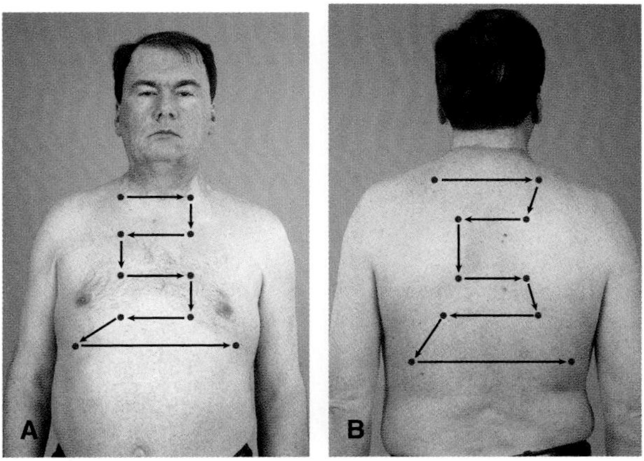

Palpation sequences

AREA/PA SKILL	NORMAL FINDINGS	ABNORMAL FINDINGS
Note excursion.	Symmetrical excursion at bases anterior and posterior, no lags.	*Asymmetrical* excursion: Thoracotomy, complete or partial obstruction, effusion, or pneumothorax.
Assess for tactile fremitus.	Equal tactile fremitus anterior and posterior.	*Increased fremitus:* Consolidating pneumonia, atelectasis, fibrosis, pulmonary edema, or infarction.
Use balls or ulnar surface of your hand as patient says "99."		*Decreased fremitus:* Emphysema, asthma, effusion, pneumothorax, or airway obstruction.

(box continued on page 168)

Physical Assessment (continued)

AREA/PA SKILL	NORMAL FINDINGS	ABNORMAL FINDINGS
Percussion Use indirect (mediate) percussion.		
Chest		
Assess density of underlying lung tissue.	*Anterior chest:* Resonance to second intercostal space (ICS) on left, to 4th ICS on right.	*Dullness:* Tumors, fluid, pleural effusion, pneumonia, pulmonary edema.

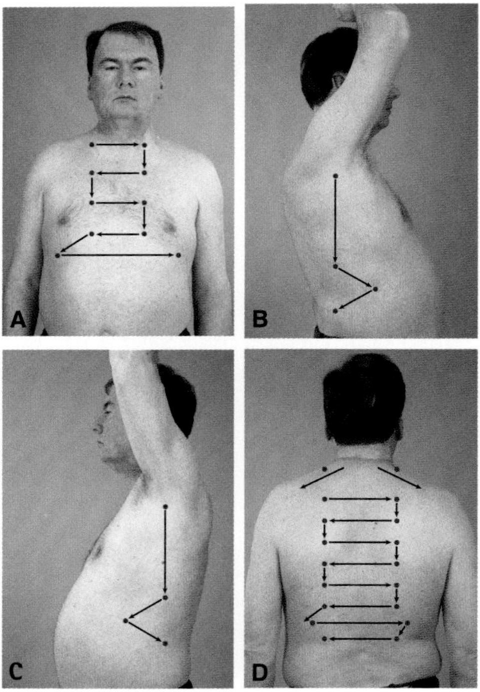

Percussion sequences

AREA/PA SKILL	NORMAL FINDINGS	ABNORMAL FINDINGS
Identify extent of lung fields.	*Lateral:* Resonance to eighth ICS. *Posterior:* Resonance to T10 and T12 on deep inspiration.	*Hyperresonance:* Air trapping of emphysema.
Assess diaphragmatic excursion.	Diaphragmatic excursion 3 to 6 cm.	*Decreased excursion:* Paralyzed diaphragm, atelectasis, COPD.

AREA/PA SKILL	NORMAL FINDINGS	ABNORMAL FINDINGS
Auscultation Use the diaphragm of the stethoscope. Have patient take slow deep breaths through mouth.		
Chest (Listen through one full respiratory cycle.)		
Note relationship of inspiration to expiration, pitch, intensity, and location of sound.		
Assess breath sounds.	Lungs clear to auscultation (CTA).	*Decreased breath sounds:* Poor inspiratory effort, emphysema, pleural effusion.

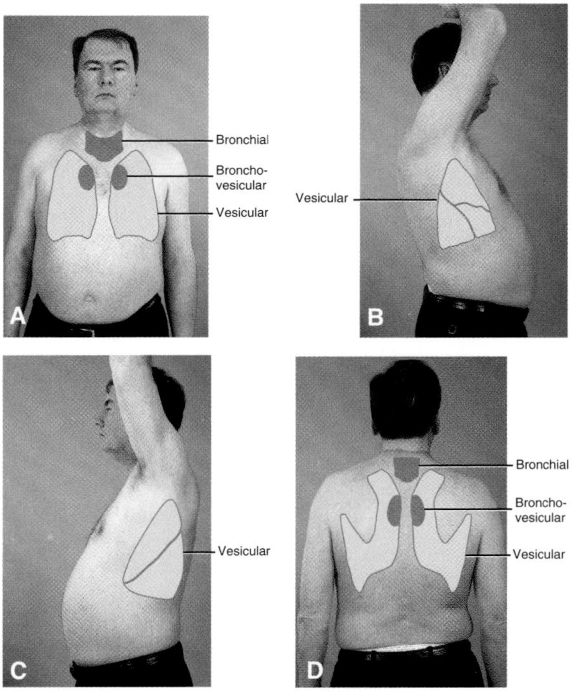

Normal breath sounds

(box continued on page 170)

Physical Assessment (continued)

AREA/PA SKILL	NORMAL FINDINGS	ABNORMAL FINDINGS
Note abnormal and adventitious breath sounds.	Bronchial sounds over trachea; broncho-vesicular over manubrium; vesicular over most of lung fields. 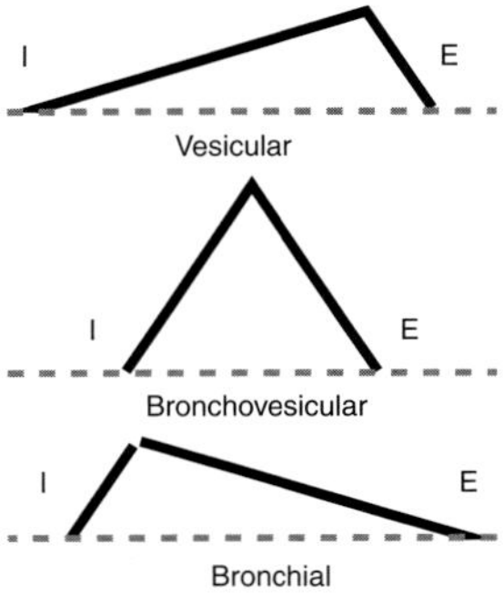	*Absent breath sounds:* Airway obstruction, pneumothorax.
	No adventitious sounds.	*Displaced bronchial breath sounds:* Pneumonia. *Crackles/rales:* Pulmonary edema, pneumonia, atelectasis, fibrosis. *Wheezes:* Asthma, COPD. *Rhonchi:* Pneumonia, bronchitis. *Stridor:* Laryngeal or tracheal obstruction, epiglottitis, viral croup. *Pleural friction rub:* Inflamed pleura, pleuritis.

AREA/PA SKILL	NORMAL FINDINGS	ABNORMAL FINDINGS
Auscultation *Chest (cont'd)*		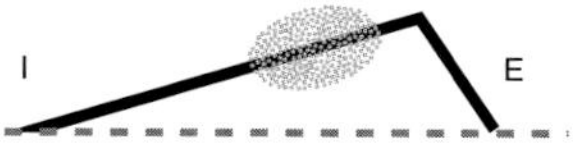 Crackles 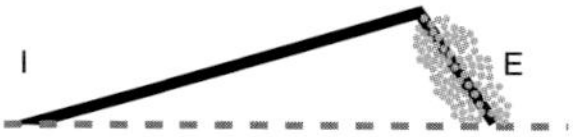 Rhonchi 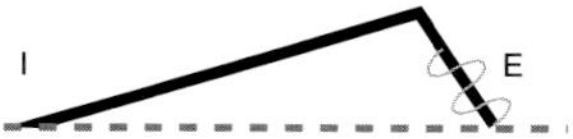 Mild Wheeze 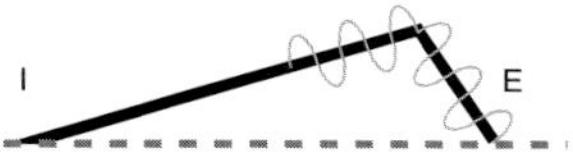 Moderate Wheeze 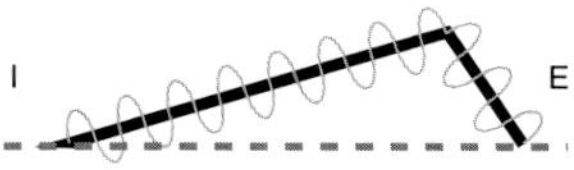 Severe Wheeze 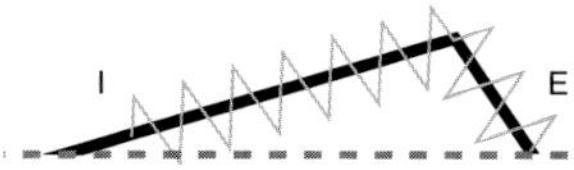 Friction Rub
Note abnormal voice sounds.	No abnormal voice sounds.	*Abnormal voice sounds (egophony, bronchophony, whispered pectoriloquy):* Consolidated lung tissue, pulmonary edema, pulmonary hemorrhage.

PA = Physical assessment.

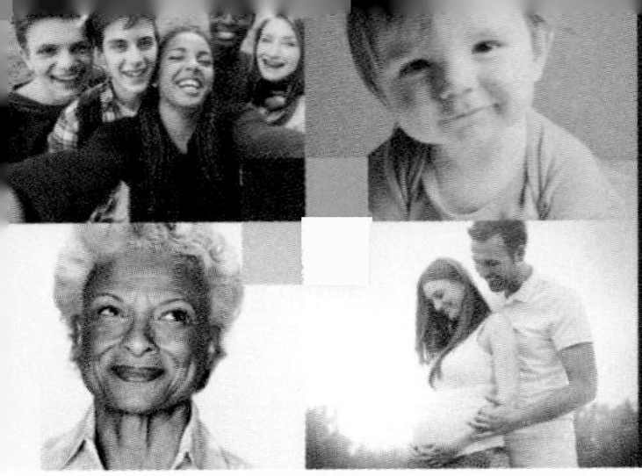

CHAPTER 6

Assessing the Cardiovascular System

Primary Functions

- Delivery of oxygenated blood throughout body
- Removal of metabolic wastes

Developmental Considerations

Infants and Children

- Change from fetal circulation with closure of foramen ovale and ductus arteriosus shortly after birth.
- Innocent systolic murmur commonly heard.
- Sinus arrhythmia with respirations common.
- Point of maximal impulse (PMI) at fourth intercostal space (ICS) to age 7, to left midclavicular line(MCL) until age 4, at MCL at age 6, to right MCL at age 7.

Pregnant Patients

- Mammary soufflé.
- Systolic murmur common.
- Displace PMI up and lateral.
- Blood pressure lower during first and second trimesters with slight increase in rate.

Older Adults

- Postural hypotension.
- Auscultatory gaps.
- Incidence of coronary vascular disease (CVD) increases with age.

Cultural Considerations

- Japanese have a lower incidence of hypertension (HTN) and high cholesterol.
- Hispanics have a lower mortality rate from heart disease than non-Hispanics.
- Middle-aged whites have the highest incidence of coronary artery disease (CAD).
- African Americans have an earlier onset and greater severity of CAD than other groups.
- African American women have a greater incidence of CAD than white women.
- Native Americans under age 35 have twice the mortality rate from heart disease as other groups.

Assessment

History

Symptoms ("PQRST" Any + Symptom)

- Chest pain
  - When did the pain begin?
  - What were you doing before the pain began?
  - Did anything you do make it better or worse?
  - Can you tell me what it feels like?
  - Point to where it hurts.
  - Are you having any breathing difficulties?
- Palpitations
  - Do you ever feel that your heart is racing or skipping beats?
  - Does your heart feel as if there is a butterfly in your chest?
- Syncope
  - Have you ever had a fainting or "blackout" spell?
  - Do you ever feel light-headed or dizzy?
- Edema
  - Have you noticed any swelling in your ankles or feet?
  - Are your shoes tight?
  - Have you noticed any recent changes in your weight?
- Fatigue
  - Have you noticed any changes in your energy level?
  - Do you find you don't have enough energy to get through the day?
  - Do you need to take naps throughout the day?

- Extremity changes
  - Do you ever experience numbness or tingling of your arms or legs?
  - Do your hands or feet feel cold?
  - Do you get pain or cramps in your legs while walking?
- Related symptoms
  - Do you have any breathing difficulties?
  - Do you wake up during the night short of breath?
  - How many pillows do you sleep on?
  - Do you get short of breath with activity?
  - Do you have a cough?
  - Is the cough productive? If yes, what color is the mucus?

Focused Cardiac History

- Are you having any chest discomfort? If yes, when did it start?
- What were you doing before the pain?
- Did anything make it better or worse?
- Have you ever had this pain before?
- What does it feel like?
- Show me where it hurts.
- On a scale from 1 to 10, how bad is the pain?
- Do you have a history of CVD? If yes, are you taking any medications, prescribed or over-the-counter (OTC) for it? If yes, what are you taking and why?
- Do you have any other medical problems?
- Are you taking any other medications, prescribed or OTC (Table 6.1)?
- Are you having any breathing difficulties?
- Do you have any allergies? If, yes, describe reaction.

TABLE 6.1 Drugs That Adversely Affect the Cardiovascular System

DRUG CLASS	DRUG	POSSIBLE ADVERSE REACTIONS
Antidepressants	Trazodone hydrochloride	Hypotension, HTN, syncope, tachycardia, palpitations, electrocardiogram (ECG) changes
	Tricyclic antidepressants	Postural hypotension, HTN, ECG changes, dysrhythmias, syncope

DRUG CLASS	DRUG	POSSIBLE ADVERSE REACTIONS
Antineoplastics	Daunorubicin, doxorubicin	Dose-dependent cardiomyopathy manifested by CHF, ECG changes, dysrhythmias
Antipsychotics	Phenothiazines, ziprasidone, haloperidol, risperidone, quetiapine, olanazapine, aripiprazole	Hypotension, postural hypotension, tachycardia, syncope, ECG changes, dysrhythmias
Anxiolytics	Diazepam	Hypotension, bradycardia, cardiac arrest, dysrhythmias (with intravenous route)
	Lorazepam	Hypotension
Antifungal	Midazolam	Hypotension, cardiorespiratory arrest
Bronchodilators, antiasthmatic agents	Aminophylline, theophylline	Palpitations, sinus tachycardia, extrasystoles, ventricular dysrhythmias, hypotension
Cerebral stimulants	Amphetamine	Tachycardia, palpitations, dysrrhythmias, HTN
	Caffeine	Tachycardia, HTN
Hormones	Oral contraceptives	HTN, fluid retention, increased risk of stroke, MI, thromboembolism
	Conjugated estrogens, estradiol, oral contraceptives	HTN, thromboembolism, thrombophlebitis
	Vasopressin	Angina in patients with vascular disease; in large doses, HTN, MI
Narcotic agents	Morphine	Hypotension, bradycardia
Miscellaneous agents	Bethanechol	Hypotension, tachycardia
	Hydralazine	Tachycardia, angina pectoris
	Levodopa-carbidopa	Orthostatic hypotension
	Levothyroxine	With excessive doses, angina pectoris, dysrhythmias, tachycardia, HTN
	Phenytoin	Hypotension, bradycardia, ventricular fibrillation (with intravenous route)
	Erectile dysfunction medications such as sildenafil	ERD medications may cause chest pain, irregular heart beat

Assessment of the Cardiovascular System's Relationship to Other Systems

Remember, all systems are related. As you assess the cardiovascular system, look at the relationship between it and all other systems.

(text continues on page 182)

Assessment of the Cardiovascular System's Relationship to Other Systems

SUBJECTIVE DATA/RATIONALE	OBJECTIVE DATA/RATIONALE
Area/System: General *Ask about:*	*Inspect for:*
Fatigue: Chronic CVD (chronic CHF) causes decreased cardiac output, impaired circulation, and decreased oxygen and often leads to early fatigue and difficulty performing activities of daily living (ADLs). Increasing fatigue and activity intolerance may correlate with disease's progression.	Signs of chest pain. Changes in mental status. *Confusion, restlessness, irritability, short attention span:* Early signs of hypoxia and impaired cerebral circulation caused by decreased cardiac output.
Dyspnea on exertion (DOE).	Shortness of breath (SOB).
Activity intolerance.	Posture.
Recent illness or flu: Influenza or other recent illness can cause cardiomyopathy.	Orthopnea.
Weight changes: Sudden weight gain may indicate fluid retention.	Changes in vital signs. *Measure:* Height and weight.
Area/System: Integumentary *Ask about:*	*Inspect for:*
Skin changes: May indicate vascular insufficiency.	*Color changes (e.g., cyanosis or pallor):* If cyanosis is present, differentiate between central and peripheral. • *Central cyanosis:* Suggests a cardiopulmonary problem, such as CHF, MI, or pulmonary edema. Look for central cyanosis in the oral mucosa or the conjunctiva. • *Peripheral cyanosis in absence of cold:* Hypovolemia, shock, or peripheral vascular disease caused by vasoconstriction, vascular occlusion, or decreased cardiac output. • *Ashen color:* MI.

SUBJECTIVE DATA/RATIONALE	OBJECTIVE DATA/RATIONALE
Poor wound healing: May signal diabetes, which is a risk factor for CAD.	Color changes in legs (e.g., red or brown). *Dependent rubor and pallor with elevation of extremities:* Arterial insufficiency. *Pallor:* Anemia and high-output failure. *Jaundice:* Hepatic congestion secondary to right CHF. *Cyanosis when dependent and brown pigmentation:* Venous insufficiency. *Petechiae:* Bacterial endocarditis. *Thin, shiny, hairless, cool skin with decreased or absent pulses:* Arterial insufficiency. *Peripheral edema, leathery skin with cyanosis and brownish discoloration:* Venous insufficiency. *Peripheral edema:* Right-sided CHF *Cool, clammy skin:* Shock, MI, CHF, arterial insufficiency, or occlusion as a result of vasoconstriction in response to decreased cardiac output. This is a compensatory mechanism to shunt blood to vital organs. *Taunt, shiny skin:* Edema caused by CVD such as right CHF or vascular insufficiency. *Anasarca (generalized body edema):* Right CHF.
Skin temperature changes.	Lesions (e.g., petechiae or leg wounds).
Nail color changes	Taut, shiny, hairless skin.
Clubbing and cyanosis: May reflect chronic cardiopulmonary problem	Arterial insufficiency.
Ankle swelling or tight shoes: Edema is associated with vascular disease and CHF.	*Clubbing:* May reflect chronic cardiopulmonary disease. *Splinter hemorrhages:* Bacterial endocarditis. *Palpate:* Skin temperature, turgor, edema. Capillary refill.

(continued)

Assessment of the Cardiovascular System's Relationship to Other Systems (continued)

SUBJECTIVE DATA/RATIONALE	OBJECTIVE DATA/RATIONALE
Area/System: HEENT **Head and neck** *Ask about:*	*Inspect:*
Headaches: May indicate HTN, a risk factor for CAD.	*Facial expression:* A struggling, frightened look may indicate pulmonary edema; an apprehensive look may indicate CAD or MI.
Dizzy spells: Syncopal attacks may occur with vascular disease or cardiac arrhythmias or may be a medication side effect.	*Palpate:* *Thyroid:* An enlarged thyroid may indicate hyperthyroid disease, which can affect the cardiac system, resulting in CHF. Neck vein distension.
Eyes *Ask about:*	*Test:*
Blurred or double vision: Double vision and temporary loss of vision are associated with HTN, transient ischemic attack (TIA), cerebrovascular insufficiency, and digitalis toxicity.	Visual acuity.
Yellow spots.	*Inspect for:* *Periorbital edema:* Suggest cardiovascular disorders. Edema is also associated with CHF. *Xanthelasma:* Lipid deposits that may indicate hyperlipidemia. *Arcus senilis in patients under age 65:* Hyperlipidemia. *Sclera icterus:* Right-sided CHF (cardiac cirrhosis). *Exophthalmos:* May indicate hyperthyroidism, which can result in supraventricular tachycardia (SVT), angina, or high-output failure. *Examine:* Fundus for atrioventricular nicking, exudates, cotton wool spots, hemorrhages: **HTN and diabetes are risk factors for CAD, so it is important to note fundoscopic changes.**

SUBJECTIVE DATA/RATIONALE	OBJECTIVE DATA/RATIONALE
Ears, nose, and throat *Ask about:*	*Note:*
Ringing in ears: Tinnitus is associated with cerebrovascular insufficiency.	Gross hearing.
Frequent "strep" throat: Beta-hemolytic streptococcal infection is associated with rheumatic heart disease.	*Inspect:*
Nosebleeds: Epistaxis is associated with HTN.	Oropharynx. Tonsils: red tonsils with exudate may be often strep.
Area/System: Respiratory *Ask about:*	*Inspect for:*
Breathing difficulties (e.g., SOB, DOE, paroxysmal nocturnal dyspnea).	Chest deformities • *Barrel chest:* Chronic obstructive pulmonary disease (COPD). Chronic COPD often has right-sided cardiac involvement. • *Pectus excavatum (depressed sternum), scoliosis (lateral deviation of spine), and kyphosis (accentuated convex thoracic curve):* If severe, may affect cardiac functioning by impairing chest expansion and cardiac movement.
Dry cough: Dry cough, SOB, DOE, paroxysmal nocturnal dyspnea (PND), orthopnea, and cough are symptoms of left-sided CHF.	Respiratory rate. *Breathing difficulties, such as dyspnea, DOE, PND, and tachypnea:* Associated with CHF, pulmonary edema, MI. *Cheyne-Stokes respiratory pattern:* Severe CHF. In patients with CHF, further assessment reveals crackles and wheezes. Cardiac asthma can develop with CHF.
History of COPD: Chronic COPD can result in cardiac involvement, such as pulmonary HTN and right-sided CHF.	*Retraction or use of accessory muscles:* Respiratory difficulty caused by a respiratory disorder, congenital heart defect, or CHF. *Auscultate:* Adventitious sounds such as crackles.

(continued)

Assessment of the Cardiovascular System's Relationship to Other Systems (continued)

SUBJECTIVE DATA/RATIONALE	OBJECTIVE DATA/RATIONALE
Area/System: Gastrointestinal *Ask about:* *Right upper quadrant pain, nausea, and gastrointestinal (GI) upset:* GI upset. GI upset and right upper quadrant (RUQ) pain may accompany right-sided CHF. GI complaints are associated with medications such as digitalis.	*Inspect for:* *Ascites:* Right-sided CHF. *Palpate for:* *Hepatomegaly:* Right-sided CHF. *Auscultate:* *Positive bruit or wide, diffuse pulsation in epigastric area:* Abdominal aortic aneurysm.
Area/System: Genitourinary/Reproductive *Ask about:* *Awakening to urinate (nocturia):* CHF leads to decreased renal perfusion during the day. But at night, when patient is in a recumbent position, fluid moves from interstitial spaces back into circulatory system, increasing renal blood flow and causing diuresis (nocturia). *For men:* *Sexual performance problems:* Impotence/erectile dysfunction may be caused by vascular disease, diabetes, or medication. Sexual activity increases the heart's workload and can precipitate an angina attack. *For women:* *Pre- or postmenopausal:* Postmenopausal women have increased CAD risk.	

SUBJECTIVE DATA/RATIONALE	OBJECTIVE DATA/RATIONALE
Birth control pills: Oral contraceptives/estrogen supplements are associated with thrombus formation.	
Hormone replacement therapy (HRT): HRT is associated with increased risk of CVD.	
Area/System: Musculoskeletal	
Ask about:	*Test:*
Weakness: Chronic CVD may result in weakness secondary to decreased use.	*Muscle strength:* Muscle weakness may indicate chronic cardiac disease, resulting in muscle atrophy from lack of use.
Muscle cramps: Intermittent claudication is associated with arterial insufficiency.	*Inspect for:* Atrophy. Wasting.
Area/System: Neurologic	
Ask about:	*Check:*
Fainting episodes: Syncopal attacks may signal vascular problems or cardiac arrhythmias.	Mental status (AAO x 3).
Behavioral changes: HTN or chronic CHF may cause hypoxia and impair cerebral circulation.	*Immediate, recent, and remote memory:* Memory loss may indicate hypoxia.
Confusion.	Judgment.
Memory loss.	*Decreased sensation and diminished deep tendon reflex (DTR):* Peripheral neuropathy associated with diabetes, which is a risk factor for CAD.
Area/System: Endocrine	
Ask about:	*Palpate:*
History of diabetes or thyroid disease: Diabetes is a known risk factor for CAD. Hyperthyroid disease can lead to hypertrophic cardiomyopathy.	Thyroid.
	Auscultate: Bruits over thyroid.

(continued)

Assessment of the Cardiovascular System's Relationship to Other Systems (continued)

SUBJECTIVE DATA/RATIONALE	OBJECTIVE DATA/RATIONALE
Area/System: Lymphatic/ Hematological	
Ask about:	*Inspect:*
Bleeding: Anemia increases the heart's workload. Polycythemia increases risk for thrombus, HTN, and cardiopulmonary disease.	Skin for ecchymosis, petechiae.
Recent infections: Can cause cardiomyopathy.	*Palpate for:*
	Enlarged lymph nodes.

HEENT = Head, eyes, ears, nose, and throat.

Physical Assessment

Anatomical Landmarks

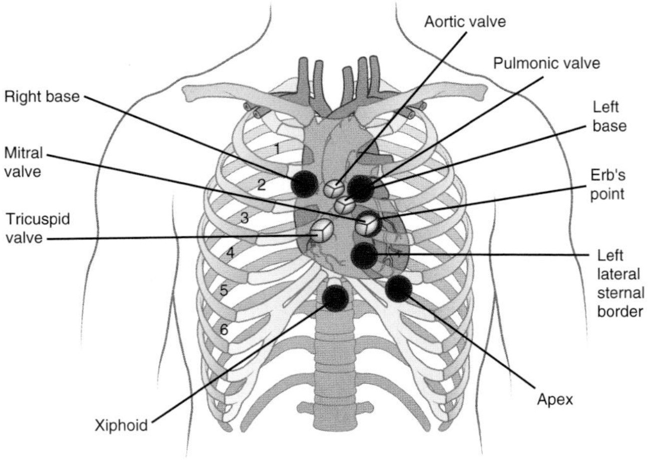

Anatomical site of heart

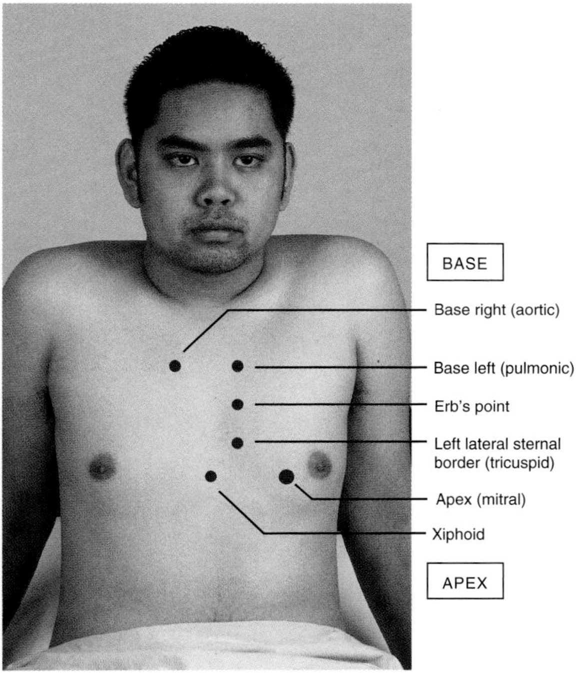

Sites for cardiac assessment

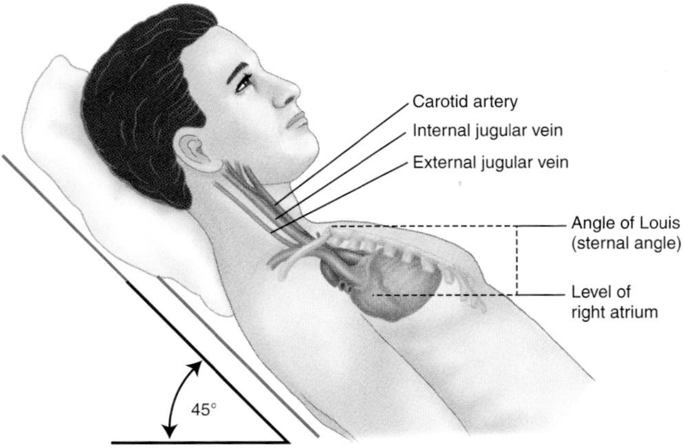

Neck structures

APPROACH: Inspection, palpation, percussion, auscultation.

POSITION: Supine, left lateral recumbent, sitting.

TOOLBOX: Stethoscope, sphygmomanometer, thermometer, ruler, marker, scale, penlight.

Cardiac Auscultation Sites

TRADITIONAL SITES	ALTERNATIVE SITES
Apex/mitral area	Apex
Left lateral sternal border (LLSB)/tricuspid area	Lower left sternal border
Erb's point	
Base left/pulmonic area	Left base
Base right/aortic area	Right base, xiphoid

Physical Assessment

AREA/PA SKILL	NORMAL FINDINGS	ABNORMAL FINDINGS
Inspection *Neck Vessels: Carotid Arteries and Jugular Veins*		
Differentiate carotid and jugular pulsation. 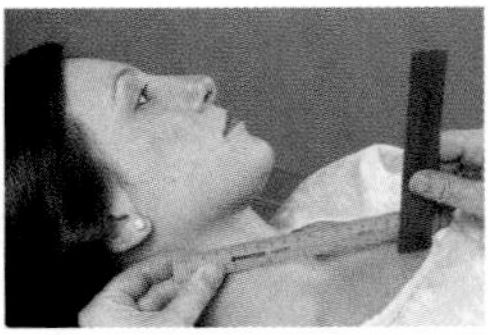 *Inspecting the neck*	Visible carotid pulsations. No neck vein distension.	*Large, bounding, visible pulsations in neck or at suprasternal notch:* HTN, aortic stenosis, or aneurysm.
Measure jugular venous pressure (JVP).	JVP at 45-degree angle < 3 cm.	*Elevated JVP:* Right-sided congestive heart failure (CHF), constrictive pericarditis, tricuspid stenosis, or superior vena cava obstruction.

AREA/PA SKILL	NORMAL FINDINGS	ABNORMAL FINDINGS
Jugular pulsations are easily obliterated, affected by position and respirations, and have undulating waves.	Carotid pulsation with one positive wave; jugular pulsation undulated.	
		Low JVP: Hypovolemia. Abnormal venous wave forms. *Giant A waves:* Tricuspid stenosis, right ventricular hypertrophy, or corpulmonale. *Absent A wave:* Atrial fibrillation.
Precordium Note pulsations in apex, left lateral sternal border, bases, and xiphoid or epigastric areas.	Positive pulsation noted at apex. Slight pulsation noted at the bases in thin adults and children. Slight epigastric pulsations may be noted.	*Pulsations to right of sternum or at epigastric area or sternoclavicular areas:* Aortic aneurysm. *Apical pulsation displaced toward axillary line:* Left ventricular hypertrophy.
Palpation *Neck Vessels: Carotid Arteries and Jugular Veins* **(Palpate Each Carotid Separately)** Note rate, rhythm, amplitude, contour, symmetry, and elasticity.	*Carotids:* Rate is age dependent. Regular rhythm + 2 amplitude (+ 3 in high-output states). Pulses equal. Contour has smooth upstroke with less acute descent. (Large pulse wave may be seen in older adults and during exercise.)	*Cardiac rates >100 beats per minute (BPM):* Sinus tachycardia, supraventricular tachycardia, paroxysmal atrial tachycardia, uncontrolled atrial fibrillation, ventricular tachycardia. Causes: CHF, drugs (e.g., atropine, nitrates, epinephrine, isoproterenol, nicotine, caffeine), hypercalcemia.

(box continued on page 186)

Physical Assessment (continued)

AREA/PA SKILL	NORMAL FINDINGS	ABNORMAL FINDINGS
Palpation *Neck Vessels: Carotid Arteries and Jugular Veins (cont'd)*		
	Carotids soft and pliable. (May be stiff and cordlike in older adults.)	
Note any thrills.	No thrills.	*Cardiac rates < 60 BPM:* Sinus bradycardia, heart block. Causes: myocardial infarction (MI), drugs (e.g., digoxin, quinidine, procainamide, beta-adrenergic inhibitors), hyperkalemia.
If you feel a carotid thrill, listen for a bruit.		*Irregular rhythm:* Arrhythmia. Abnormal pulses. *Bounding, + 3:* HTN, aortic regurgitation. *Absent or weak, + 1:* Arterial insufficiency or occlusion or decreased cardiac output, as in shock. *Pulsus paradoxus:* Chronic obstructive pulmonary disease, cardiac tamponade, CHF. *Pulsus alternans:* CHF, digoxin toxicity. *Pulsus bisferiens:* Aortic regurgitation. *Pulsus bigeminus:* Heart failure, hypoxia. *Small pulse wave:* CHF, hypovolemia, aortic stenosis. *Large pulse wave:* HTN, exercise, aging. *Corrigan pulse:* Aortic regurgitation. *Unequal pulses:* Obstruction or occlusion.

AREA/PA SKILL	NORMAL FINDINGS	ABNORMAL FINDINGS
		Stiff, cordlike arteries: Atherosclerosis.
Palpate jugular veins and check direction of fill.	Jugulars are easily obliterated and fill appropriately.	
Check for abdominojugular (hepatojugular) reflux (HJR).	Negative HJR.	*Positive abdominojugular reflux:* Right-sided CHF, tricuspid regurgitation, tricuspid stenosis, constrictive pericarditis, cardiac tamponade, inferior vena cava obstruction, hypervolemia.
Precordium		
Palpate apex, left lateral sternal border, bases, and xiphoid or epigastric areas.	PMI at apex 1-2 cm, nonsustained, or may normally be nonpalpable.	*Enlargement and displacement of PMI to midaxillary line:* Left ventricular hypertrophy with dilation.
Note size, duration, and diffusion of impulses.	Slight epigastric pulsation, no diffusion.	*Apical impulse on right side of precordium:*

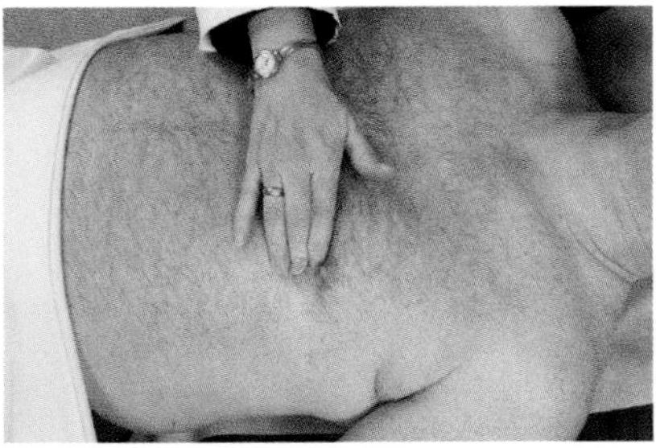

Palpating apex of heart

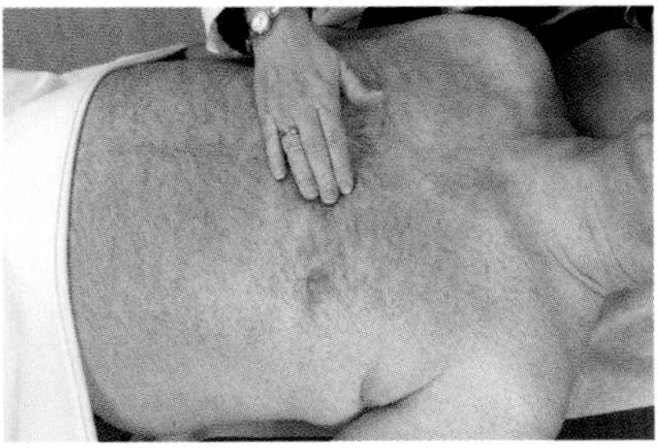

Palpating LLSB

(box continued on page 188)

Physical Assessment (continued)

AREA/PA SKILL	NORMAL FINDINGS	ABNORMAL FINDINGS
Palpation *Precordium (cont'd)*		

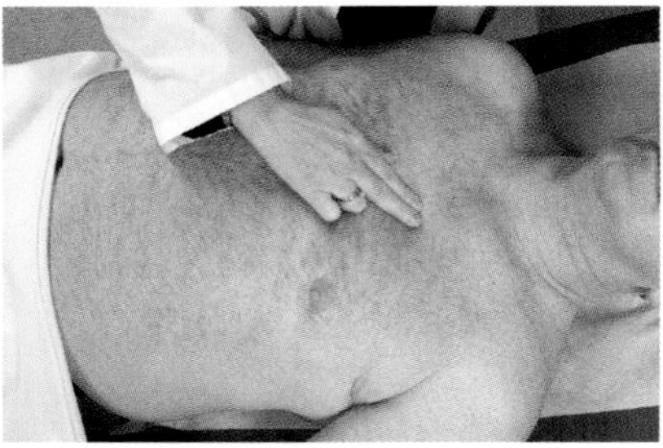

Palpating base left

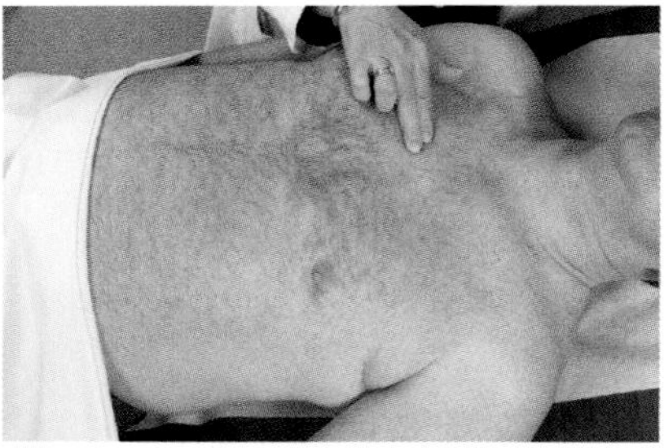

Palpating base right

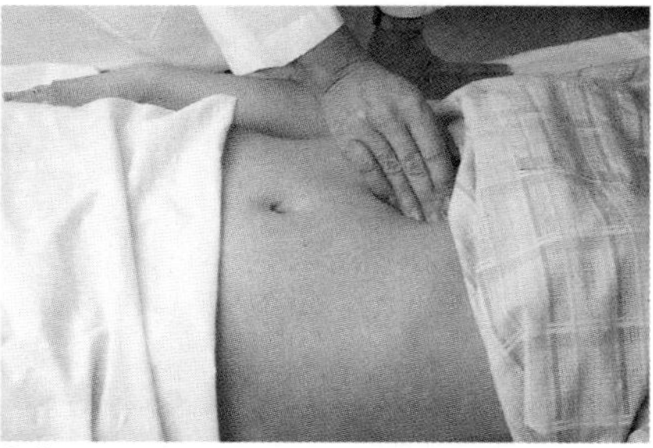

Palpating epigastric area

AREA/PA SKILL	NORMAL FINDINGS	ABNORMAL FINDINGS
	No pulsations noted at base and lower left lateral sternal border (LLSB).	Dextrocardia, often associated with congenital heart disease. *Enlarged apical pulsation without displacement > 2-2.5 cm with patient supine or > 3 cm with the patient in the left lateral recumbent*

AREA/PA SKILL	NORMAL FINDINGS	ABNORMAL FINDINGS
		position: Ventricular enlargement, HTN, aortic stenosis.
	Small nonsustained impulses may be palpable at base and LLSB of thin patients and children. PMI may be displaced laterally and to left during last trimester of pregnancy. Increased amplitude in high-output states.	*Sustained pulsation:* Hypertrophy, HTN, overload, cardiomyopathy. *Presystolic impulse:* S_4, may be seen with aortic stenosis. *Early diastolic impulse:* S_3, may be seen with CHF. *Diffuse, sustained impulse displaced downward and laterally:* Congestive cardiomyopathy.
Note thrills, lifts, or heaves. **If you palpate a thrill, listen for a murmur.**	No thrills, lifts, or heaves.	*Thrills:* Murmur. *Right ventricular impulse with increased amplitude and duration:* Pulmonary stenosis or pulmonary HTN. *Palpable lifts or heaves:* Right ventricular hypertrophy. *Pulsations felt on fingertips:* Right ventricular hypertrophy. *Large diffuse epigastric pulsation:* Abdominal aortic aneurysm. *Accentuated pulsation in pulmonic area:* Pulmonary HTN. *Accentuated pulsation in the aortic area:* HTN or aneurysm.

(box continued on page 190)

Physical Assessment (continued)

AREA/PA SKILL	NORMAL FINDINGS	ABNORMAL FINDINGS
Percussion		
Precordium (cont'd)		
Percuss from anterior axillary line to sternum at fifth ICS.	Dullness noted at third, fourth, and fifth ICS to left of sternum at MCL.	*Left sternal border extends to midaxillary lines:* Enlarged, dilated heart.
Auscultation		
Listen with both bell (light pressure) and diaphragm (heavy-pressure) at all sites.		

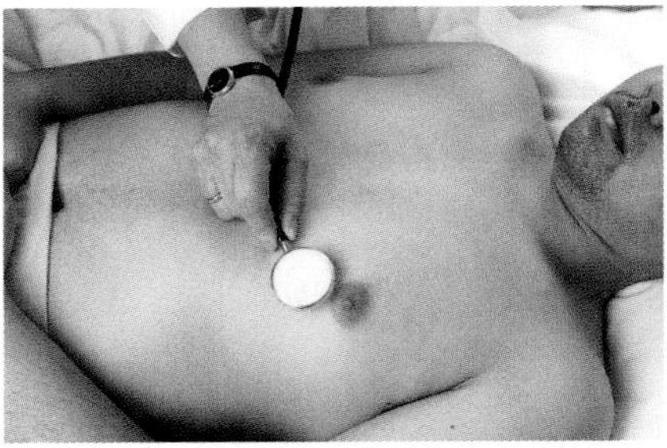

Auscultation with bell of stethoscope

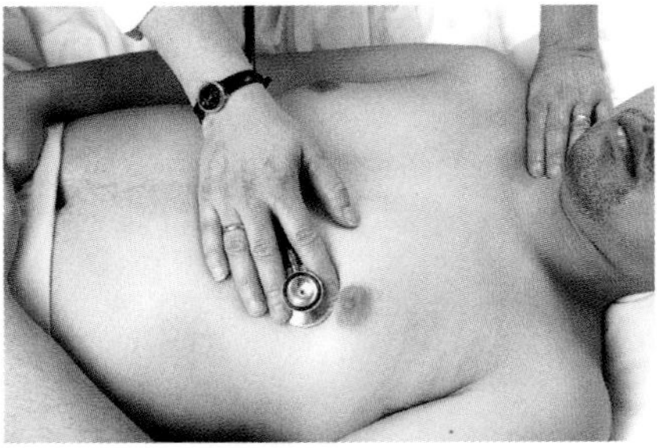

Auscultation with diaphragm of stethoscope

AREA/PA SKILL	NORMAL FINDINGS	ABNORMAL FINDINGS
Neck Vessels: Carotid Arteries and Jugular Veins		
Listen for carotid bruits and venous hums with the bell.	Negative carotid bruits.	*Bruit:* Carotid stenosis.

AREA/PA SKILL	NORMAL FINDINGS	ABNORMAL FINDINGS
Have patient hold breath when auscultating for carotid bruits and venous hums.	Carotid bruit may be normal in children and with high-output states. Negative venous hum. Venous hum may be normal in children.	Murmurs can also radiate up to neck from heart, as with aortic stenosis.

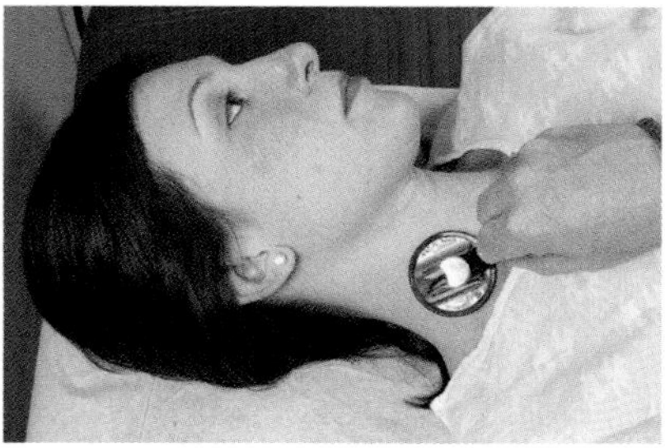

Auscultating carotid

AREA/PA SKILL	NORMAL FINDINGS	ABNORMAL FINDINGS
To differentiate venous hum from a transmitted murmur, venous hum disappears when pressure is applied to jugular vein.		
Precordium Auscultate the following sites:		*Bradycardia or tachycardia:* (See above-abnormal pulses under Palpation of Neck Vessels.)
• Apex: fifth ICS, left MCL. • LLSB: Fourth to fifth ICS, left sternal border (LSB). • Erb's point: Third ICS, LSB. • Base left: Second ICS, LSB. • Base right: Second ICS, right sternal border (RSB). • Xiphoid area.	Apex: Rate is age dependent, rhythm regular, high-pitched systolic, short duration, 3/6 intensity, $S_1 > S_2$, accentuated S_1 in high-output states.	*Irregular rhythm:* Arrhythmia. *Accentuated S_1:* High-output states, mitral or tricuspid stenosis. *Diminished S_1:* First-degree heart block, CHF, CAD. *Variable S_1:* Atrial fibrillation.

(box continued on page 192)

Physical Assessment (continued)

AREA/PA SKILL	NORMAL FINDINGS	ABNORMAL FINDINGS
Auscultation *Precordium (cont'd)* **Auscultate with patient in sitting, supine, and left lateral recumbent positions.**		
Listen to S_1, S_2 splits.	LLSB: $S_1 = S_2$, split S_1 possible. Base left: $S_1 < S_2$, split S_2 during inspiration. Base right: $S_1 < S_2$.	S_3, low-pitched early diastolic sound: CHF. S_4, low-pitched late diastolic sound: CAD, HTN, MI.
Note extra sounds: S_3, S_4, opening snap, ejection clicks.	No extra sounds. S3 and S4 may be normal in children and young adults. Not considered normal over the age of 30 years.	Quadruple rhythm, $S_3 + S_4$, with fast rate is called a summation gallop.
Note murmurs and pericardial rubs.		*Wide split:* Right bundle branch block (RBBB).
Note rate, rhythm, pitch, intensity, duration, timing in the cardiac cycle, quality, location, and radiation. (See Tables 6.2 and 6.3.)		*Midsystolic ejection click (high-pitched systolic sound):* Mitral valve prolapse (MVP).
Erb's point: Abnormal aortic murmurs heard best.		*Opening snap (high-pitched diastolic sound):* Mitral or tricuspid stenosis, ventricular septal defect (VSD), patent ductus arteriosus (PDA).
Grade murmurs on 1 to 6 scale.		*Early systolic murmur:* VSD. *Mid-systolic murmur:* MVP.
A diastolic murmur or a murmur > grade 3/6 is never innocent.		*Late systolic murmur or pansystolic (or holosystolic) murmur:* Mitral or tricuspid regurgitation.

AREA/PA SKILL	NORMAL FINDINGS	ABNORMAL FINDINGS
		Pansystolic murmur: VSD. *Mid- and late diastolic murmurs:* Mitral and tricuspid stenosis. *Pericardial friction rub (high-pitched systolic and diastolic sound):* Pericarditis or postoperative cardiac surgery. *Diminished S_2:* Incompetent aortic or pulmonic valves and low-output states. *Ejection click (high-pitched systolic sound):* Aortic or pulmonic stenosis. *Accentuated S_2:* HTN or pulmonary HTN. *Wide split S_2:* RBBB, pulmonic stenosis, atrial septal defect (ASD), VSD. *Fixed split S_2 (split with no respiratory variation):* ASD, VSD, CHF. *Paradoxical split S_2 (split occurs during expirations):* Left bundle branch block or aortic stenosis. *Midsystolic murmur:* Aortic or pulmonic stenosis. *Early diastolic murmur, heard best at Erb's point:* Aortic regurgitation. *Early diastolic murmur, heard best at base left:* Pulmonic regurgitation. *Pandiastolic murmur:* PDA.

PA = Physical assessment.

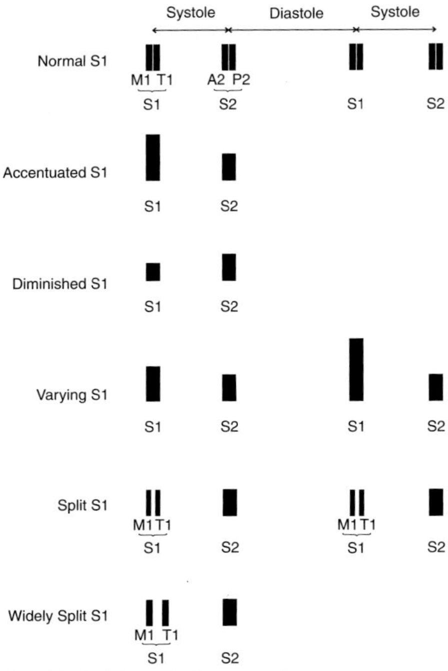

Graphic depiction of S_1 heart sounds

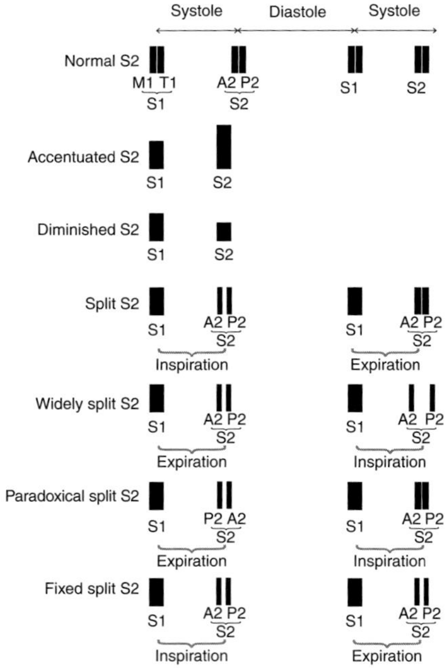

Graphic depiction of S_2 heart sounds

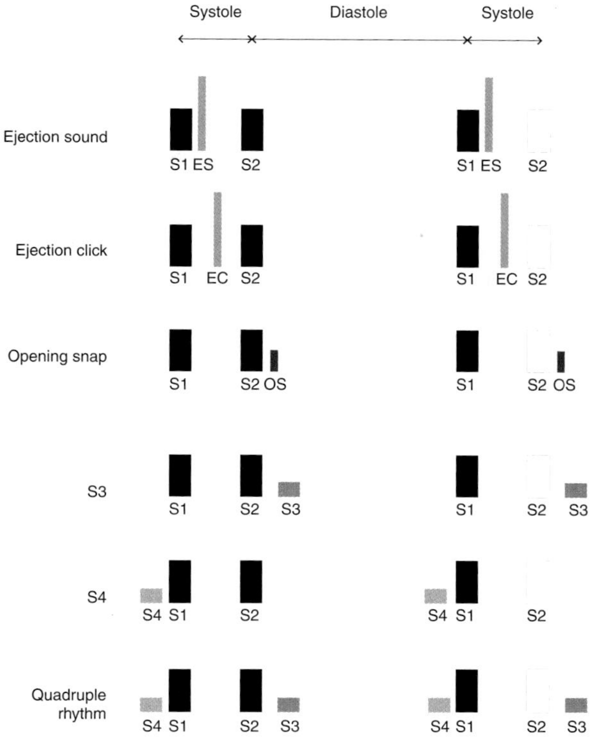

Graphic depiction of extra heart sounds

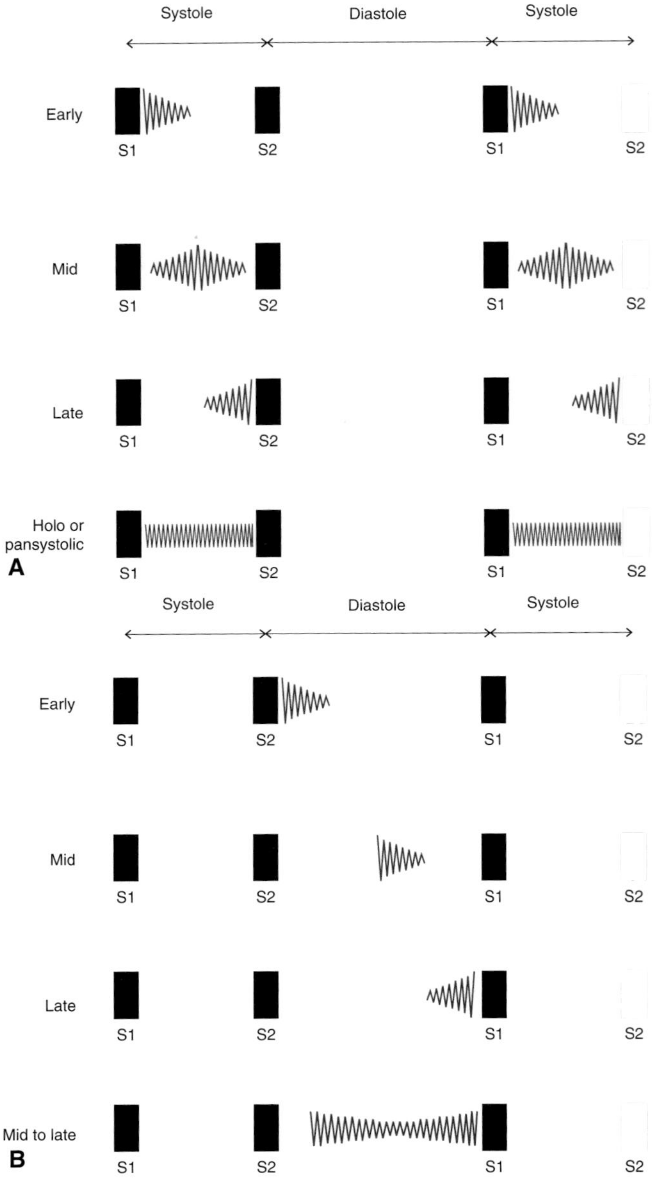

A. Graphic depiction of systolic murmurs. B. Graphic depiction of diastolic murmurs

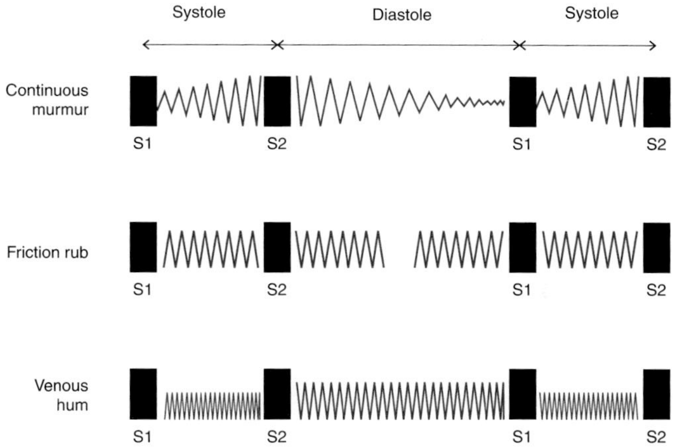

Graphic depiction of continuous sounds

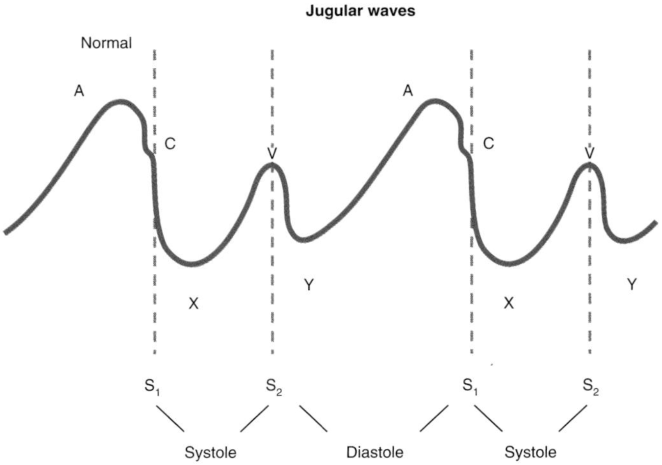

Correlation of jugular wave-form with cardiac cycle

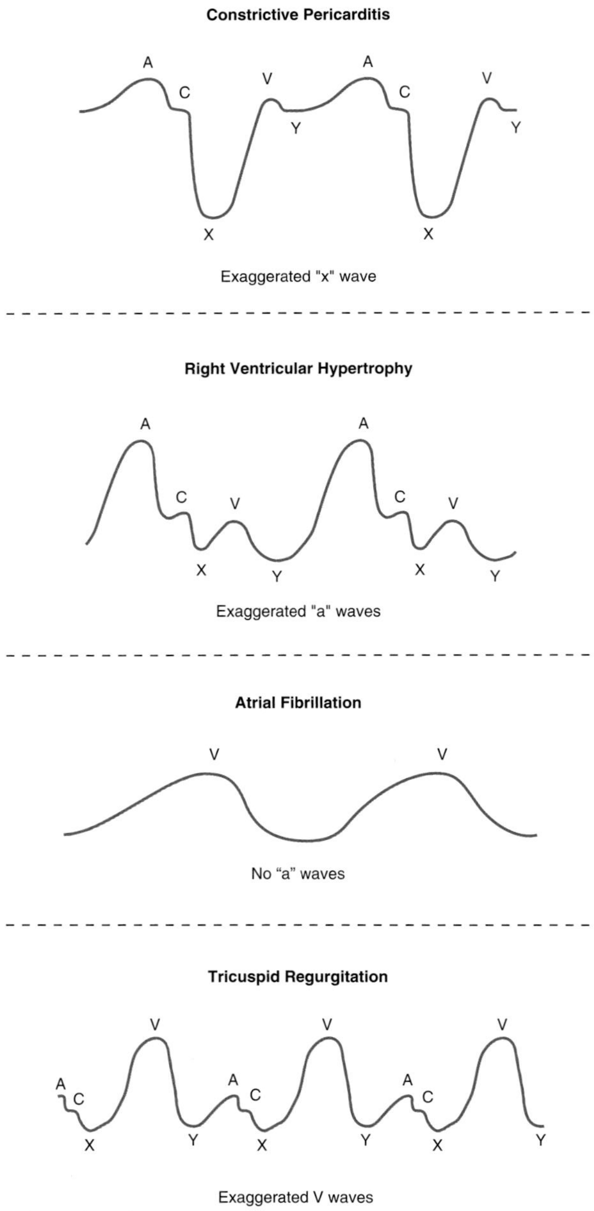

Abnormal jugular venous waves

Description	Possible Cause
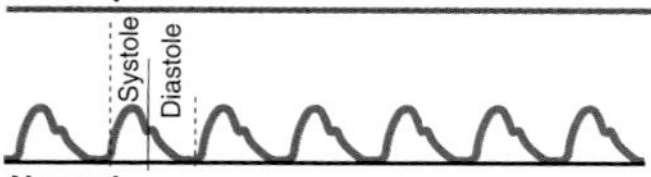 **Normal**	
 **Small, Weak Pulse** Decreased pulse pressure with a slow upstroke and prolonged peak	Increased peripheral vascular resistance such as occurs in cold weather or severe congestive heart failure; decreased stroke volume such as occurs in hypovolemia or aortic stenosis
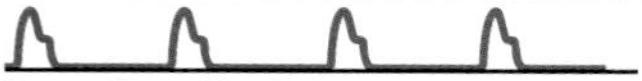 **Large, Bounding Pulse** Bounding pulse in which a great surge precedes a sudden absence of force or fullness	Increased stroke volume, as in aortic regurgitation; increased stiffness of arterial walls, as in atherosclerosis or normal aging; exercise; anxiety; fever; hypertension
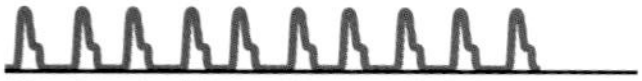 **Corrigan's (Water-Hammer) Pulse** Increased pulse pressure with a rapid upstroke and downstroke and a shortened peak	Aortic regurgitation, patent ductus arteriosus, systemic arteriosclerosis
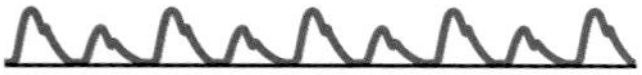 **Pulsus Alternans** Regular pulse rhythm with alternation of weak and strong beats (amplitude or volume)	Left ventricular failure
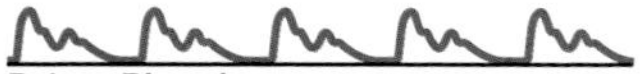 **Pulsus Bigeminus** Irregular pulse rhythm in which premature beats alternate with sinus beats	Premature ventricular beats caused by heart failure, hypoxia, or other condition
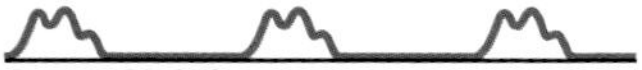 **Pulsus Bisferiens** A strong upstroke, downstroke, and second upstroke during systole	Aortic insufficiency, aortic regurgitation, aortic stenosis
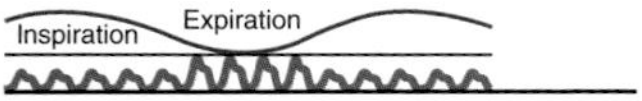 **Pulsus Paradoxus** Pulse with a markedly decreased amplitude during Inspiration	Constrictive pericarditis, pericardial tamponade, advanced heart failure, severe lung disease

Abnormal pulses

Auscultating Valvular Heart Sounds

DISEASE	DESCRIPTION/ ASSESSMENT FINDINGS
Mitral regurgitation 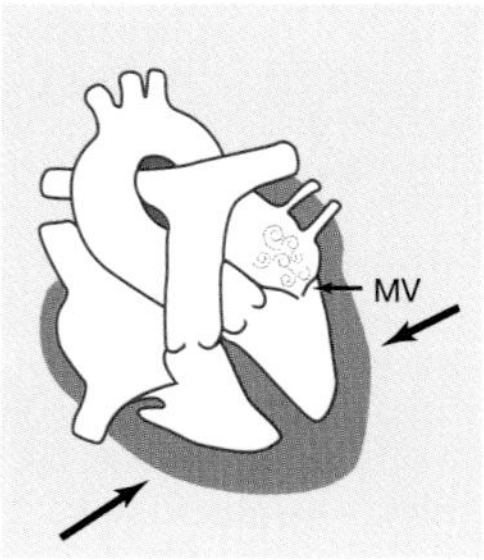	• Holosystolic; extends from S_1 to S_2. • Loudness constant throughout systole. • Heard best at apical area. • May radiate to left lateral chest or, less commonly, to base. • Blowing, rough (harsh), or musical. • If very loud, it may mask S_1.

(box continued on page 200)

Auscultating Valvular Heart Sounds (continued)

DISEASE	DESCRIPTION/ ASSESSMENT FINDINGS
Mitral stenosis 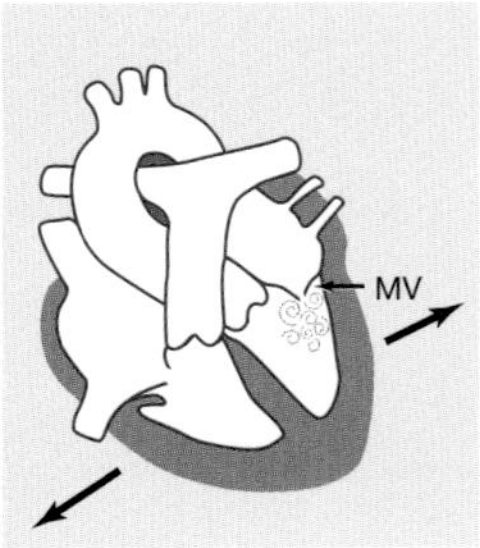 	• Occurs in diastolic phase of cardiac cycle. • With normal sinus rhythm, characteristically a low-pitched rough or harsh murmur beginning immediately after opening snap. • Extends to sharp S_1. • Demonstrates presystolic (late diastolic) accentuation with normal sinus rhythm and just before termination. • Presystolic accentuation of mid-late diastolic murmur disappears with atrial fibrillation. • Best heard in apical area with patient in left lateral position and with bell portion of stethoscope. • Localized to a very small (quarter-sized) area, so may be hard to find.
Aortic stenosis 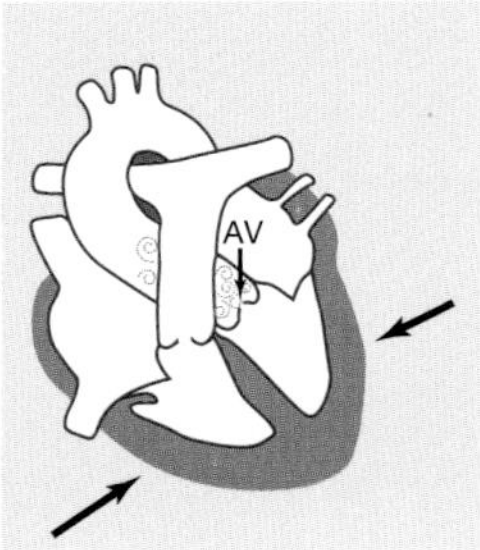 	• Midsystolic; characterized by crescendo/decrescendo pattern. • Begins shortly after S_1 and ends before S_2. • Rough (low-pitched). • S_2 at base markedly diminished or absent as a result of poor movement of severely calcified valve leaflets. • When transmitted to apex, may have musical overtone in addition to rough quality (Gallavardin effect). • If congenital (represented by two valve leaflets instead of three), early ejection click is often heard shortly after S_1. • Both acquired and congenital murmurs heard best at base in second right interspace. May also be transmitted to apex and neck.
Aortic regurgitation 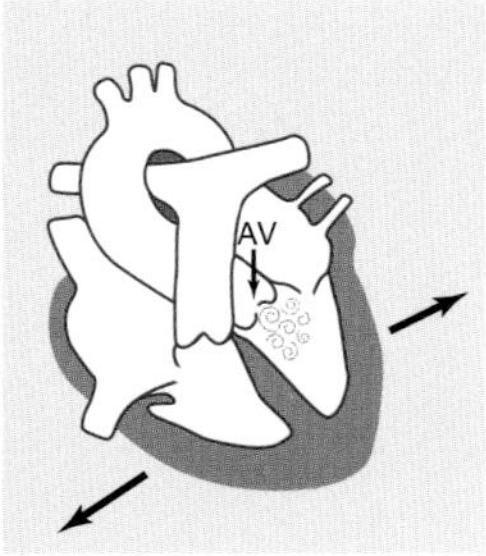 	• Onset early in diastole. • Decrescendo, ending before S_1. • Usually blowing. • Heard best at base of heart in third left interspace in parasternal line. • Often transmitted toward apex, if loud enough. • Loudness varies from grade 1 to grade 3 or 4. • Often is only grade 1 intensity. If so, to facilitate identification of murmur, have patient sit forward, exhale, and hold his or her breath while you listen in third left interspace in parasternal line.

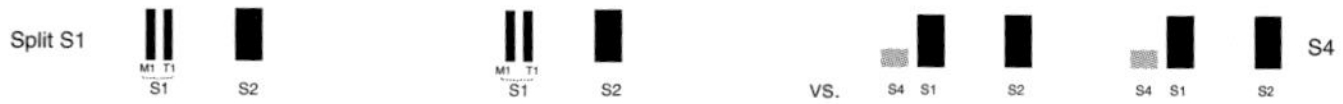

Split S_1: systolic, high pitch heard best at tricuspid area with diaphragm; S_4: diastolic, low pitch heard best at apex with the bell.

Split S_1: systolic, high pitch heard best at tricuspid area with diaphragm; Ejection sound: systolic (mid-late), high pitch heard best at base if aortic or pulmonic stenosis, with the diaphragm, or at the apex with MVP.

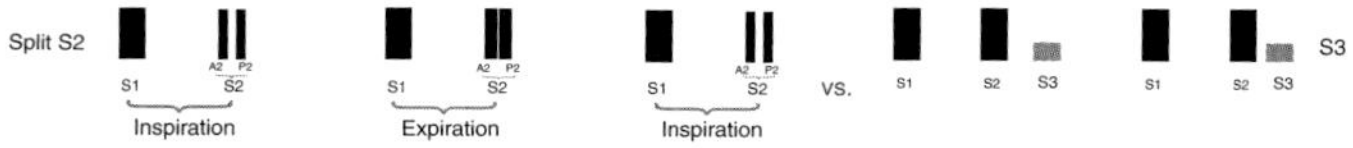

Split S_2: systolic, high pitch heard best at pulmonic area during inspiration with the diaphragm; S_3: diastolic, low pitch heard best at apex with the bell.

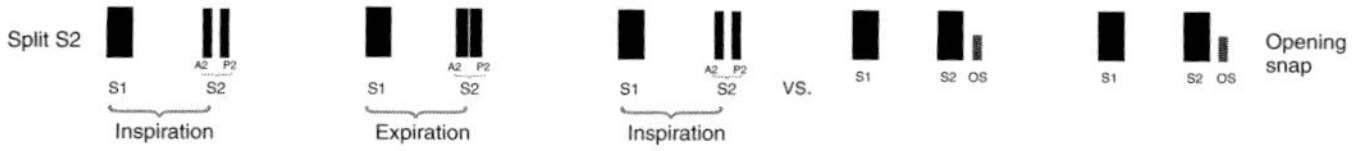

Split S_2: systolic, high pitch heard best at pulmonic area during inspiration with the diaphragm; OS: diastolic, high pitch heard best at apex with the diaphragm.

S_3: diastolic, low pitch heard best at apex with the bell; OS: diastolic, high pitch heard best at apex with the diaphragm.

How to differentiate sounds

TABLE 6.2 Heart Sounds

HEART SOUND	LOCATION	PITCH	TIMING IN CARDIAC CYCLE	INTERPRETATION
S_1	Apex/mitral area	High	Systolic	Normal
S_1 split	LLSB/tricuspid area	High	Systolic RBBB	Normal
S_2	Base right/aortic area	High	Systolic	Normal
S_2 split	Base left/pulmonic area	High	Systolic BBB, ASD, VSD, pulmonary emboli, pulmonic stenosis	Normal
S_3 (left ventricular origin)	Apex	Low	Diastolic	May be normal under age 30 Left-sided CHF
S_3 (right ventricular origin)	LLSB	Low	Diastolic	Right-sided CHF
S_4 (Left ventricular origin)	Apex, LLSB	Low	Diastolic	May be normal in children and young adults MI, HTN, CAD
S_4 (right ventricular origin)	Apex, LLSB	Low	Diastolic	Pulmonary HTN
Opening snap	Apex	High	Diastolic	Mitral stenosis
Ejection click	Base Apex	High High	Early systolic Midsystolic	Aortic stenosis, pulmonic stenosis MVP
Friction rub	LLSB	High	Systolic, diastolic, or both	Pericarditis, pericardial effusion

TABLE 6.3 Murmurs

TYPE	LOCATION	PITCH	QUALITY	INTERPRETATION
Early systolic	LLSB	High/low	Rough	VSD (muscular site)
Midsystolic	Base right Base left	High	Harsh	Aortic stenosis Pulmonic stenosis
Late systolic	Apex LLSB	High	Blowing	MVP Tricuspid regurgitation
Holosystolic	Apex LLSB	High		Mitral regurgitation, VSD Tricuspid regurgitation
Early diatolic	Erb's point Base left	High	Blowing	Aortic regurgitation Pulmonic regurgitation
Mid-diastolic	Apex LLSB	Low	Rumbling	Mitral stenosis Tricuspid stenosis
Late diastolic	Apex LLSB	Low	Rumbling	Mitral stenosis Tricuspid stenosis
Pandiastolic	Base left	Low	Continuous	PDA

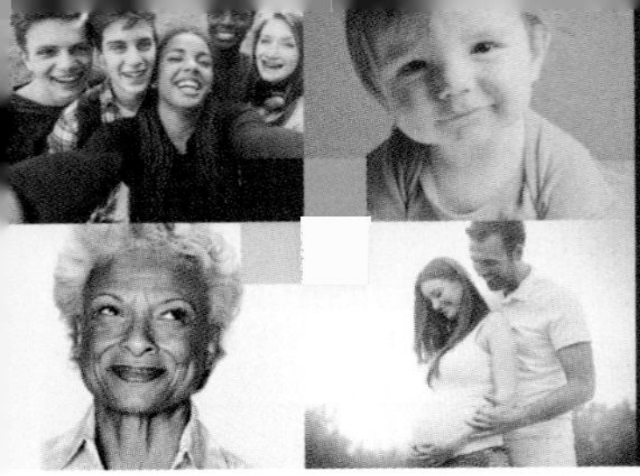

CHAPTER 7

Assessing the Peripheral-Vascular and Lymphatic Systems

Primary Functions

Primary function of the peripheral-vascular (PV) system:

- Transport of oxygenated blood to all organs and tissue and return of unoxygenated blood to the heart

Primary functions of the lymphatic system:

- Movement of lymph fluid in a closed circuit with the cardiovascular system
- Development and maintenance of the immune system
- Reabsorption of fat and fat-soluble substances from the small intestine

Developmental Considerations

Infants and Children

- Infants have immature immune systems, increasing risk for infection; they rely on mother's immunity.
- Amount of lymphatic tissue greatest between ages of 6 and 10 years.
- Thymus largest at birth.
- Tonsils larger during childhood than after puberty.
- Blood pressure (BP) at birth 70/50; slowly increases to adult level, 120/80, during adolescence.

Pregnant Clients

- Increase in leukocytes and decrease in immunoglobulin G (IgG) occur during pregnancy.

- Altered host defense results from decrease in chemotaxis that delays response to infection.
- Decreased systemic vascular resistance results in vasodilation, which may lead to palmar erythema and spider telangiectasis.
- BP decreases during second trimester then increases to prepregnant level.
- 30-mm systolic or 15-mm diastolic increase in BP may indicate preeclampsia supine hypotension.

Older Adults

- Number and size of lymph nodes decrease with age.
- Ability to resist infection decreases.
- Increased fibrosis and decreased elasticity of vessels result in increased peripheral-vascular resistance.

Cultural Considerations

- Hypertension (HTN) is a serious health problem for African Americans.
- High incidence of HTN in Puerto Ricans, Cubans, and Mexican Americans.
- One-sixth of Iranians have HTN, with stress as a major contributing factor.
- Navajo Native Americans have a high incidence of severe combined immunodeficiency syndrome (SCIDS), failure of antibody response, and cell-mediated immunity, unrelated to acquired immunodeficiency syndrome (AIDS).
- African Americans account for 30 percent of AIDS cases in the United States.

Assessment

History

Symptoms ("PQRST" Any + Symptom)

- Swelling
  - Where is the swelling located? Does it affect both arms or legs? Does it involve the entire extremity or just a certain area? How far up the extremity does the swelling go?
  - Is the swelling marked or slight? Has the swelling occurred before? If so, is it more or less severe?

- When does the swelling occur? On awakening or at the end of the day? Is it constant or intermittent? How long does it last?
- Do you have an imprint of a sock line or shoe when you take your shoes and socks off?
- Is the swelling associated with pain, warmth, or redness?
- Does anything, such as sitting for long periods of time or eating salty foods, make the swelling worse?
- Does anything, such as elevating your feet or using support hose, reduce the swelling?

■ Limb pain

- Where is the pain? Is it localized or generalized? Point to where you feel the pain. Is it deep or superficial? Does it radiate to another location?
- How bad is the pain? On a scale of 0 to 10, with 0 being no pain and 10 being the worst pain, how would you rate your pain? Does the pain interfere with your lifestyle? Can you walk without pain?
- In what setting does the pain occur? Does it occur only after walking long distances? Does it occur when going up and down stairs? Does it occur after repetitive movements? Does it occur only at night?
- When did the pain first begin? Did it begin suddenly or gradually? Is it intermittent or continuous? How long does the pain last?
- Can you describe the pain in your own words? Throbbing, burning?
- Is the pain associated with any other problems, such as swelling, tingling, or redness?
- Does anything make the pain worse? Does anything make it better?

■ Change in sensation

- Where is the sensation? Is it in just one part of the extremity? Does it involve the entire extremity? Does it involve one or both extremities?
- How intense is the sensation?
- When or where does it occur? Does it occur when your legs are elevated? When you are bending over?
- When did this problem begin? Was it sudden or gradual? Is this a new or chronic problem?

  - Can you describe the type of sensation? Is it associated with weakness or pain?
  - What makes the sensory change worse? Cold temperatures? Sitting for long periods?
  - What makes the sensation better, rest or leg elevation?
- Fatigue
  - How long have you noticed that you are fatigued?
  - Do you wake up tired or do you become tired during the day?
  - Is your fatigue related to exertion?
  - Have you been overworked at your job or with family commitments?
  - Have you been sleeping well? How many hours do you sleep per night?
  - Do you have trouble getting to sleep or staying asleep?
  - Have you noticed any other associated symptoms along with your fatigue?
  - Does your fatigue interfere with your lifestyle? Does it affect your ability to work or take care of your family?

Focused Peripheral-Vascular History

Arterial occlusion of an extremity can become a situation requiring rapid assessment. Be sure to ask the following questions:

- Have you noticed pain, pallor, pulselessness, polar sensation (cold), paresthesias, or paralysis (the six Ps of acute occlusion) in an extremity?
- Have you noticed aching, heaviness, throbbing or burning pain, itching, or cramping in your legs?
- Have you noticed ankle swelling? Is it difficult to fit into your shoes or wear your wedding band lately?
- Do you have leg pain when walking? Do you have leg pain at rest? What makes the leg pain better?
- Have you noticed any sores or ulcers on your feet or legs? How long have they been there? What have you used to treat them?
- Do you have a history of high BP?
- Do you have a history of a high cholesterol level?
- Do you have diabetes mellitus?
- Do you have a history of cardiovascular or peripheral-vascular disease?
- Do you smoke? If so, how long and how much?

Focused Lymphatic System History

Generally, there is no need to assess this system rapidly. However, these questions will help you narrow your assessment focus.

- Have you noticed any swelling in your neck, armpits, or groin? If so, are the swollen areas sore, hard, or red? Do they appear on both sides of your body?
- Are you unusually tired? If so, are you tired all the time or only after exertion? Do you need frequent naps, or do you sleep an unusually long time at night?
- Have you had a fever recently? If so, how high was it? Was it constant or intermittent? Did it follow a pattern?
- Do you ever have joint pain? If so, which joints are affected? Does swelling, redness, or warmth accompany the pain? Do your bones ache?
- Have you noticed any sores that heal slowly?
- Do you have a history of blood transfusions?
- Have you ever been diagnosed with a chronic infection?
- Are you taking any medications, prescribed or over-the-counter (OTC) (Table 7.1)?

TABLE 7.1 Drugs That Adversely Affect the Lymphatic System

For information on drugs that affect the cardiovascular system, see text Chapter 14, Assessing the Cardiovascular System.

DRUG CLASS	DRUG	POSSIBLE ADVERSE REACTIONS
Antiarrhythmics	Procainamide	Positive antinuclear antibody (ANA) titer; systemic lupus erythematosus (SLE)-like syndrome
	Quinidine	Thrombocytopenia, hemolytic anemia, agranulocytosis
Anticonvulsants	Carbamazepine	Aplastic anemia (characterized by decreased levels of all formed elements of blood), leukopenia (decreased leukocyte levels), agranulocyto-sis (severely decreased agranulocyte levels),

DRUG CLASS	DRUG	POSSIBLE ADVERSE REACTIONS
		eosinophilia (increased eosinophil levels), leukocytosis (increased leukocyte levels), thrombocytopenia (decreased thrombocyte levels)
	Phenytoin	Thrombocytopenia, leukopenia, granulocytosis, pancytopenia (decreased levels of all blood cells), megaloblastic anemia (characterized by increased, immature, enlarged erythrocytes)
Antidiabetics	Acetohexamide, chlorpropamide, glipizide, glyburide, tolbutamide	Leukopenia, thrombocytopenia, pancytopenia, agranulocytosis, aplastic anemia, hemolytic anemia (characterized by premature erythrocyte destruction)
Antihypertensives	Captopril	Neutropenia (decreased neutrophil levels), agranulocytosis
	Hydralazine	Positive ANA titer that occurs when the immune system creates antibodies against some of the body's own cells; SLE-like syndrome
	Methyldopa	Positive Coombs' test, indicating that some type of immunoglobulin coats the red blood cells
Anti-infectives	Cephalosporins	Positive Coombs' test, hypothrombinemia (decreased thrombin levels), with or without bleeding

(continued)

TABLE 7.1 Drugs That Adversely Affect the Lymphatic System (continued)

DRUG CLASS	DRUG	POSSIBLE ADVERSE REACTIONS
	Chloramphenicol	Bone marrow depression, pancytopenia, aplastic anemia
	Penicillins	Eosinophilia, hemolytic anemia, leukopenia, neutropenia, thrombocytopenia, positive Coombs' test
	Pentamidine isethionate	Leukopenia, thrombocytopenia
	Sulfonamides	Granulocytopenia, leukopenia, eosinophilia, hemolytic anemia, aplastic anemia, thrombocytopenia, methemoglobinemia (increased levels of an oxidative compound of hemoglobin)
Antineoplastics	Busulfan	Severe leukopenia, anemia, severe thrombocytopenia
	Chlorambucil	Leukopenia, thrombocytopenia, anemia
	Cisplatin, cyclophosphamide, doxorubicin	Leukopenia, granulocytopenia, thrombocytopenia, anemia
	Methotrexate	Leukopenia, thrombocytopenia, anemia
	Mitomycin	Anemia
Antipsychotic agents	Chlorpromazine, thioridazine	Agranulocytosis, mild leukopenia
Gold compounds	Auranofin, gold sodium thiomalate	Leukopenia, thrombocytopenia, anemia, eosinophilia, aplastic anemia
Nonsteroidal anti-inflammatory agents	Ibuprofen	Neutropenia, agranulocytosis, aplastic anemia, thrombocytopenia, decreased hemoglobin and hematocrit
Miscellaneous agents	Furosemide	Anemia, leukopenia, thrombocytopenia
	Lithium	Leukocytosis

Assessment of the Peripheral-Vascular and Lymphatic Systems' Relationship to Other Systems

Remember, all systems are related. As you assess the PV and lymphatic systems, look at the relationship between them and all other systems.

Assessment of the Peripheral-Vascular and Lymphatic Systems' Relationship to Other Systems

SUBJECTIVE DATA/RATIONALE	OBJECTIVE DATA/RATIONALE
Area/System: General	
Ask about:	*Inspect for:*
PV changes, infection.	Signs of distress.
Unexplained fever, night sweats, weight loss: AIDS or cancer involving lymphatic system.	*Measure:* Vital signs. Weight.
Area/System: Integumentary	
Ask about:	*Inspect for:*
Skin lesions, rashes.	Skin color, texture, lesions. *Cyanosis:* Impaired circulation. *Pallor or rubor:* Vascular problems. *Thin, shiny skin:* Arterial insufficiency. *Thick, leathery skin:* Venous insufficiency. *Rash:* Immune disorders such as the butterfly rash of SLE. *Poor wound healing:* Vascular insufficiency or immune deficiency.
Color changes/hair loss: Chronic arterial or venous insufficiency. *Ankle swelling/tight shoes:* Fluid retention associated with PV disease or lymphadenopathy.	Hair distribution. *Alopecia and short broken hair above forehead:* SLE. *Decreased hair on extremities:* Arterial insufficiency. Edema.
Area/System: HEENT	
Ask about:	*Inspect:*
Mouth lesions.	Oral mucosa, gums, tonsils.
Bleeding gums.	Nasal mucosa. *Pale nasal mucosa, boggy turbinates:* Chronic allergies.
Neck swelling or masses: Enlarged lymph nodes associated with infection or malignancy.	*Enlarged, red, inflamed tonsils with exudates:* Infection. *Oral lesions (e.g., lacy leukoplakia):* AIDS. *Bleeding gums:* Leukemia.

(continued)

Assessment of the Peripheral-Vascular and Lymphatic Systems' Relationship to Other Systems (continued)

SUBJECTIVE DATA/RATIONALE	OBJECTIVE DATA/RATIONALE
Area/System: HEENT *(cont'd)*	
Sore throat/difficulty swallowing: Bacterial or viral infection of lymphoid tissue.	*Enlarged nodes:* Infection or malignancy. *Enlarged thyroid:* Chronic thyroiditis (Hashimoto's), an autoimmune disorder.
Vision problems:	*Ptosis, extraocular movement deficits:*
PV disease such as HTN	Myasthenia gravis.
Area/System: Respiratory	
Ask about:	*Auscultate:*
History of asthma, allergies, difficulty breathing. *Dyspnea with sputum production:* Respiratory infection such as pneumonia. Dyspnea is also associated with CV problems.	*Adventitious breath sounds (such as wheezes):* Associated with asthma or allergic responses.
Area/System: Cardiovascular	
Ask about:	*Palpate:* Enlarged, displaced point of maximal impulse (PMI) associated with ventricular hypertrophy such as occurs with HTN.
Chest pain/dyspnea: Cardiac involvement.	*Auscultate:* Heart sounds.
History of murmurs.	Murmurs, rubs.
Area/System: Gastrointestinal	
Ask about:	*Auscultate:* *Hyperactive bowel sounds:* Ulcerative colitis, an autoimmune disorder. *Hypoactive bowel sounds:* Scleroderma, an autoimmune disorder.
Diarrhea, abdominal tenderness and pain, weight loss: Infections occurring with immunodeficiency disorders.	*Palpate:* Organs for enlargement. *Enlarged liver:* Infection, cardiovascular problem, immune disorder, malignancy. *Enlarged spleen:* Infection or cancer.
History of abdominal trauma.	

SUBJECTIVE DATA/RATIONALE	OBJECTIVE DATA/RATIONALE
Area/System: Genitourinary/ Reproductive	
Ask about:	*Inspect for:* *Lesions:* Associated with sexually transmitted diseases (STDs) and may cause lymphadenopathy.
Nocturia: Congestive heart failure (CHF).	
Urinary tract infections (UTIs).	Discharge.
Safe sex practices and STDs: Unprotected sexual activity increases risk for STDs.	STDs, lesions.
Impotence: PV disease.	
Area/System: Musculoskeletal	
Ask about:	*Palpate:*
Weakness.	Muscle strength.
Exercise-induced limb pain: Peripheral arterial disease. *Bone tenderness:* Leukemic or immunoproliferative disorder.	*Joint pain, deformity, limited range of motion, muscle weakness:* PV disease, multiple sclerosis, or autoimmune disorder such as rheumatoid arthritis.
Area/System: Neurologic	
Ask about:	*Test:*
Changes in mental status: Changes in mental status may indicate impaired cerebral circulation or an autoimmune disease such as SLE, which can cause mental status changes, including depression or even psychosis.	
Loss of sensation (paresthesia): Arterial insufficiency	*Sensation* *Decreased sensation: Vascular insufficiency* *Decreased DTR:* Peripheral neuropathies

HEENT = Head, eyes, ears, nose, and throat.

Physical Assessment

Anatomical Landmarks

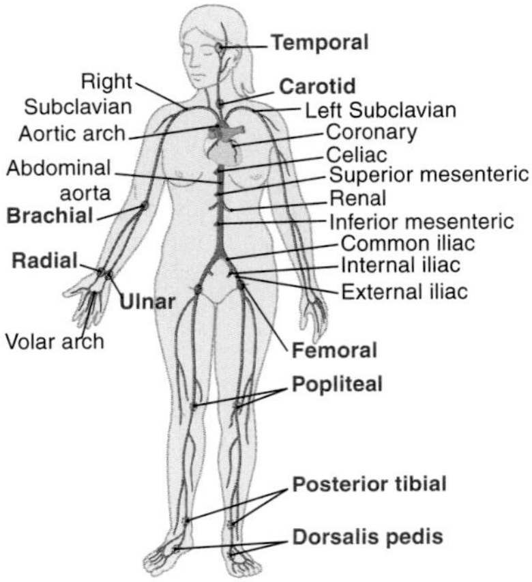

PV system. Pulse sites labeled in red.

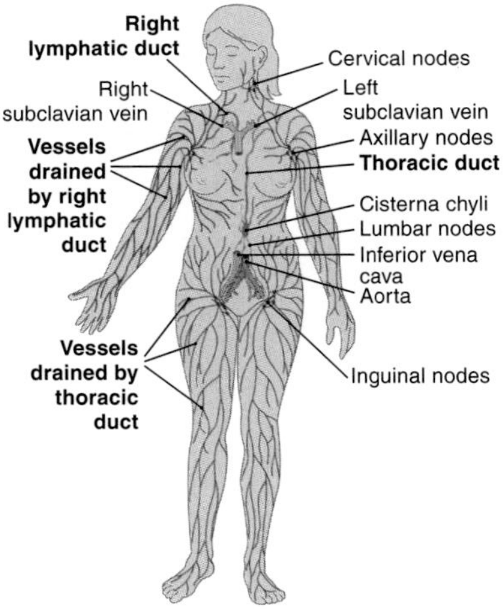

Lymphatic system

APPROACH: *PV system:* Inspection, palpation, auscultation
Lymphatic system: Inspection, palpation

POSITION: Supine and sitting

TOOLBOX: Stethoscope, sphygmomanometer, flashlight, ruler, tape measure

Physical Assessment

AREA/PA SKILL	NORMAL FINDINGS	ABNORMAL FINDINGS
Inspection *Upper Extremities*		
Inspect for color, edema, erythema, red streaks, lesions.	Skin color uniform, no erythema, red streaks, edema, or lesions.	*Edema:* Cellulitis, lymphedema, venous obstruction (thrombophlebitis). 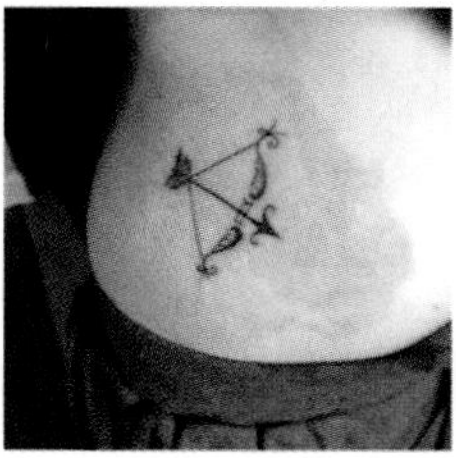 *Cellulitis*
Look for edema on most dependent parts of body.		*Intermittent pallor and cyanosis of hands and fingers:* Episodic constriction of peripheral small arteries or arterioles caused by Raynaud's phenomenon or Raynaud's disease. Constriction causes hyperemia and rubor (redness).
If edema is present, grade it and weigh patient daily.		*Ischemic changes and gangrene of hands and fingers:* Buerger's disease (thromboangiitis obliterans).
Abdomen		
Note shape, arterial pulsation, increased venous pattern, ascites.	Abdomen flat or slightly rounded	*Tense, shiny abdominal skin:* Ascites or edema.

(box continued on page 216)

Physical Assessment (continued)

AREA/PA SKILL	NORMAL FINDINGS	ABNORMAL FINDINGS
If ascites is present, do fluid wave test or test for shifting dullness.	No increased venous pattern or ascites	*Upward or centrifugal venous flow:* Inferior vena cava obstruction or portal HTN
If large, diffuse arterial pulsation is present, do not palpate the abdomen.	Slight arterial pulsation noted in epigastric area at midline.	*Visible, large, diffuse pulsations:* Aneurysm.
Lower Extremities		
Note color, condition of skin, hair distribution, edema, erythema, red streaks, lesions.	Skin color uniform; no erythema, red streaks, edema, or lesions.	*Streaky redness, tenderness, warmth along course of a vein:* Thrombophlebitis.
If edema is present, measure calf circumference.	Skin intact, even hair distribution.	*Hair loss:* Arterial insufficiency.
If varicosities are present, check venous valve competence with Trendelenburg test or manual compression test.		*Eczema, stasis dermatitis:* Chronic venous insufficiency. *Prominent leg veins, possibly with rope-like, dilated appearance or purplish spider-like appearance:* Chronic venous insufficiency. *Edema:* Injury, cellulitis, venous/lymph obstruction, thrombophlebitis, varicosities. 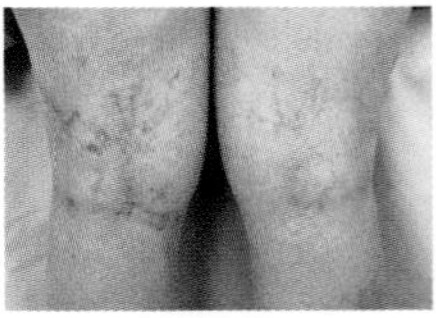 *Superficial varicosities*

AREA/PA SKILL	NORMAL FINDINGS	ABNORMAL FINDINGS
Inspection *Lower Extremities (cont'd)*		*Skin ulcers:* Trauma or venous/arterial insufficiency. Venous insufficiency stasis ulcers on ankle.

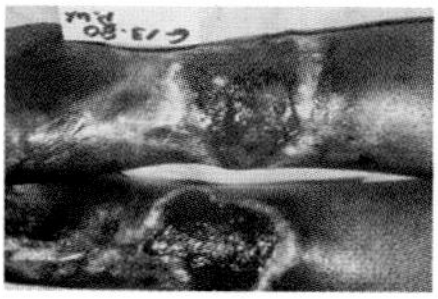

Venous stasis ulcer

Arterial insufficiency ulcers on toes.

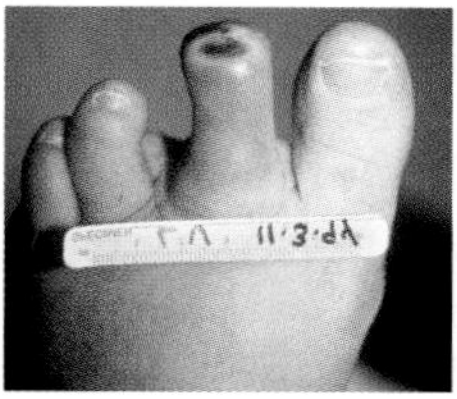

Arterial insufficiency

Difference in leg circumference ≥ 1 cm above ankle or 2 cm at calf: Edema.

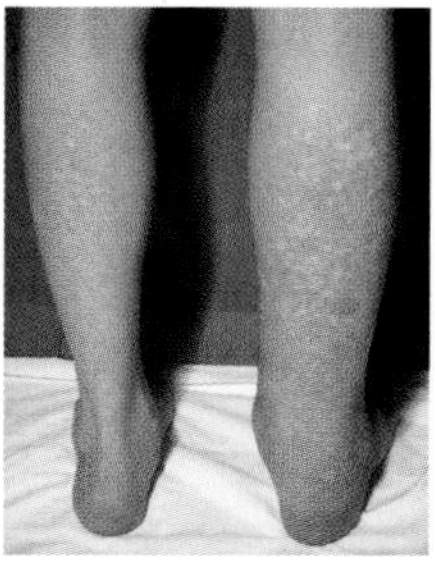

Lymphedema

(box continued on page 218)

Physical Assessment (continued)

AREA/PA SKILL	NORMAL FINDINGS	ABNORMAL FINDINGS

Assessing Edema

To assess edema, press your index finger over the bony prominence of the tibia or medial malleolus. Orthostatic (pitting) edema results in a depression that does not rapidly refill and resume its original contour. It is not usually accompanied by thickening or pigmentation of the overlying skin. The severity of edema can be graded on a scale of +1 to +4.

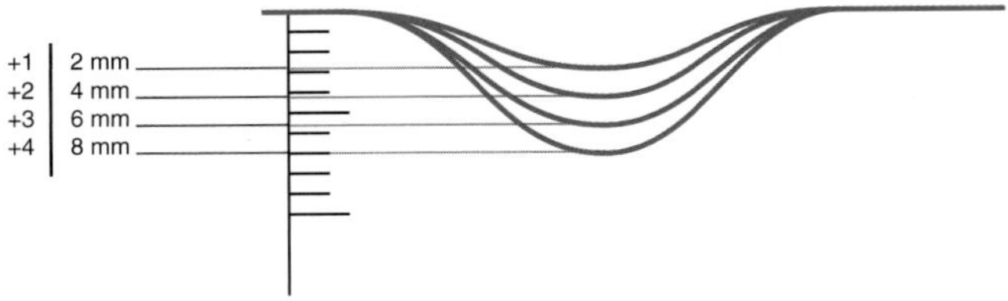

- +1: Slight pitting with about 2-mm depression that disappears rapidly. No visible distortion of extremity.
- +2: Deeper pitting with about 4-mm depression that disappears in 10 to 15 seconds. No visible distortion of extremity.
- +3: Depression of about 6 mm that lasts more than a minute. Dependent extremity looks swollen.
- +4: Very deep pitting with about 8-mm depression that lasts 2 to 3 minutes. Dependent extremity is grossly distorted.

Palpation

Upper and Lower Extremities

AREA/PA SKILL	NORMAL FINDINGS	ABNORMAL FINDINGS
Palpate for capillary refill, temperature.	+ Capillary refill < 3 seconds.	*Delayed capillary refill time:* Arterial occlusion, hypovolemic shock, hypothermia; also, environmental influences (e.g., decreased ambient temperature), suggesting a problem that may not exist.
	Extremities warm bilaterally.	*Cold feet:* Arterial insufficiency, especially if unilateral. *Cool extremities:* Decreased circulation, vasoconstriction, Raynaud's disease, Buerger's disease, response to cold external temperature.

AREA/PA SKILL	NORMAL FINDINGS	ABNORMAL FINDINGS
	Absence of Homans' sign.	*Presence of Homans' sign:* Deep vein thrombosis (DVT) in 50 percent of clients. Negative sign does not rule out DVT.
Pulse Sites: Carotid, Temporal, Brachial, Radial, Ulnar, Femoral, Popliteal, Dorsalis Pedis, Posterior Tibialis		
Note rate, rhythm, equality, thrills, amplitude.	Pulse rate is age dependent.	*Alterations in pulse rate/rhythm:* Cardiac arrhythmia.
Pulse amplitude scale: **0 = absent.** **1 = weak.** **2 = normal.** **3 = full.** **4 = bounding.**	Pulse regular, equal, +2. Arteries soft and pliable.	*Unequal pulses:* Arterial narrowing or obstruction on one side. *Diminished or absent pulse:* Arterial spasm, partial or complete arterial occlusion of proximal vessel, often caused by arteriosclerosis obliterans.
If thrill is present, listen for bruit. If indicated, do Allen's test to assess arterial flow to hands.	No thrills.	*Sudden absent pulse with cold, mottled extremity:* Arterial occlusion, a medical emergency.

(box continued on page 220)

Physical Assessment (continued)

AREA/PA SKILL	NORMAL FINDINGS	ABNORMAL FINDINGS
Palpation *(cont'd)* If indicated, do color change test or measure ankle-brachial index to assess arterial flow to legs.	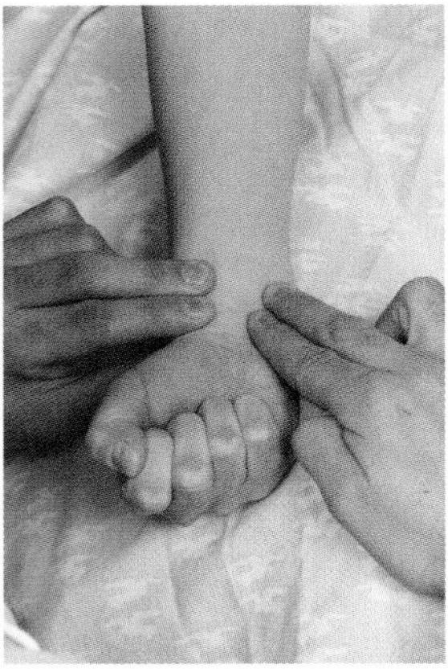 *Compressing the radial and ulnar arteries* 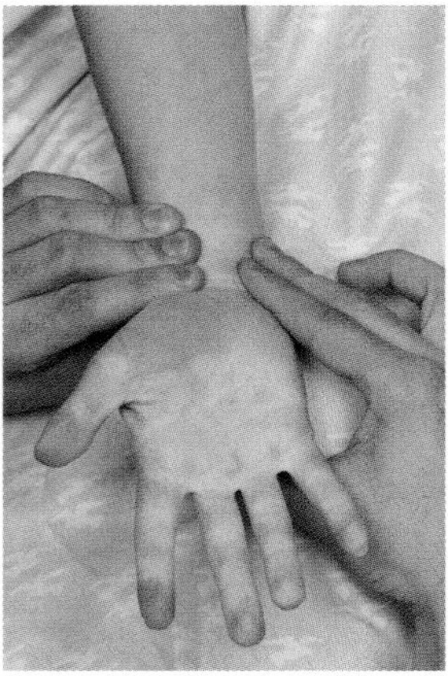 *Observing for pallor*	

AREA/PA SKILL	NORMAL FINDINGS	ABNORMAL FINDINGS
	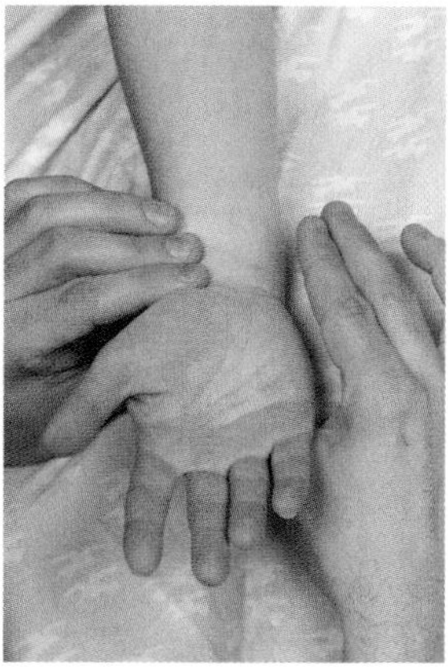 *Releasing pressure and observing for return of normal color*	
Ankle-Brachial Index Purpose: Assess circulation in the feet Technique: Measure ankle B/P using a Doppler at the dorsalis pedis or posterior tibialis pulse site, then measure brachial B/P. Normally leg pressures are equal or higher than arm pressures. This test is limited in diabetics with vascular calcification because the findings are falsely high. Calculate ABI by: *Ankle systolic pressure divided by brachial systolic pressure = ABI.* For example: if ankle pressure is 140 and brachial pressure is 110, ABI = 1.25	ABI = 1 or greater	Minimal disease: ABI = 0.8 to 0.95 Moderate disease: ABI = 0.4 to 0.8 Severe disease: ABI = 0 to 0.4

(box continued on page 222)

Physical Assessment (continued)

AREA/PA SKILL	NORMAL FINDINGS	ABNORMAL FINDINGS
Ankle-Brachial Index *(cont'd)* Manual Compression Test Purpose: assesses valve in patients with varicose veins. Technique: Have patient stand and then compress first the distal portion of the vein and then the proximal portion.	Normally, no backflow should occur, and you should not feel a wave with your distal hand	If the valves are incompetent, you will feel a wave with you lower hand as a result of backflow.
Trendelenberg Test Purpose: assesses valve competence in patients with varicose veins. Technique: With patient supine, elevate the leg to promote venous return, place tourniquet around thigh and have patient stand.	Veins should fill slowly from lower leg up.	After 30 seconds, release tourniquet. If veins fill rapidly from the upper leg down, the saphenous valves are incompetent.
Color Change Test Purpose: evaluates arterial insufficiency Technique: With the patient supine, elevate the legs to increase venous return and then have The patient sits and dangle legs. Note the color change. If thrombus or thrombophlebitis is suspected, test Homans' sign. *Lymph Node Sites: Cervical, Axillary, Epitrochlear, Inguinal (Horizontal and Vertical), Popliteal*	Normally, color returns to the feet within 10 seconds.	Elevation pallor and dependent rubor are associated with arterial insufficiency.

AREA/PA SKILL	NORMAL FINDINGS	ABNORMAL FINDINGS
Note size, shape, symmetry, tenderness, mobility, consistency, delineation, location, erythema, warmth, increased vascularity.	Lymph nodes not palpable, or if palpable, < 1 cm, firm, nontender, round, well-defined borders; no erythema, warmth, or increased vascularity.	*Tender, palpable lymph nodes:* Recent infection. *Large, well-defined nodes:* Acute infection. *Less-defined node borders:* Chronic infection. *Hard, enlarged, nontender, immobile nodes:* Malignancy. *Involvement of three or more node groups (generalized lymphadenopathy):* Autoimmune disease or neoplasm.
Auscultation **Use the bell of the stethoscope.**		
Arteries and Veins		
Listen for bruits and venous hums. **Have client hold breath when auscultating for bruits or hums over the neck.**	No bruits or venous hums.	*Soft, low-pitched, rushing sound during cardiac cycle:* Bruit in temporal or carotid artery. Signifies narrowing of artery.
Check the patient's BP. Measure BP in both arms, with patient supine, sitting, and standing. **Avoid auscultatory gap by palpating brachial pulse and inflating cuff until obliterated, then reinflating cuff 30 mm Hg above point where pulse was obliterated.**	Normal BP is age dependent; for adults: Systolic < 120 mm Hg diastolic < 80 mm Hg.	*Hypotension:* Heart failure, dehydration, endocrine disorders (hypothyroidism), neurogenic vena cava obstruction, cardiac tamponade.

(box continued on page 224)

Physical Assessment (continued)

AREA/PA SKILL	NORMAL FINDINGS	ABNORMAL FINDINGS
Auscultation *(cont'd)* Bell of stethoscope is best for detecting Korotkoff sounds.		
If BP heard down to "0," retake BP and listen for Korotkoff sounds 1, 4 (first diastolic), and 5; then record all 3.		
Check pulse pressure (difference between the systolic and the diastolic pressure).	Pulse pressure is one-third of systolic pressure.	
Note orthostatic drops.	No orthostatic drop.	*Decrease in systolic BP of 20 mm Hg and drop in diastolic BP on standing, with rise in pulse rate:* Orthostatic hypotension caused by antihypertensive medications, volume depletion, peripheral neurovascular disease, or bed rest. A systolic reading of 120 to 139 mm Hg and a diastolic reading of 80 to 89 mm Hg is considered pre-HTN; a systolic of 140 to 159 with a diastolic of 90 to 99, stage 1 HTN; a systolic of ≥ 160 with a diastolic of ≥ 100, stage 2 HTN. *Auscultatory gap:* Normal variation or sign of systolic HTN *Korotkoff sounds down to zero:* Cardiac valve

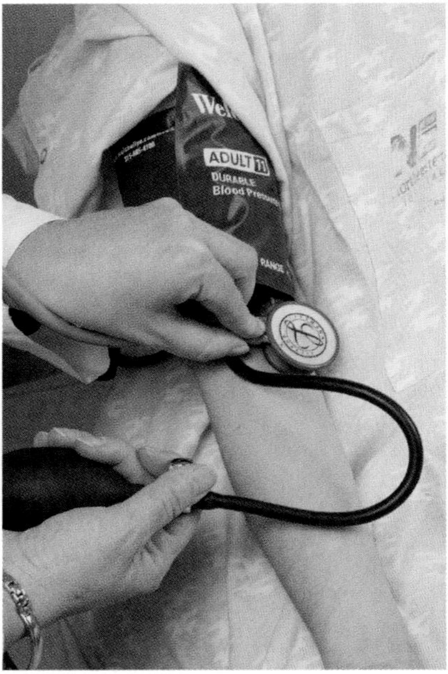

Taking BP with bell of stethoscope

AREA/PA SKILL	NORMAL FINDINGS	ABNORMAL FINDINGS
		replacement, hyperkinetic states, severe anemia, thyrotoxicosis, or following strenuous exercise. *Difference of > 10 mm Hg between arms:* Arterial compression on side of lower reading, aortic dissection, arm pressure > leg pressure, coarctation of aorta. *Widened pulse pressure with increased systolic BP:* Exercise, arteriosclerosis, severe anemia, thyrotoxicosis, increased intracranial pressure. *Narrowed pulse pressure with decreased systolic BP:* Shock, cardiac failure, pulmonary embolus.

PA = Physical assessment.

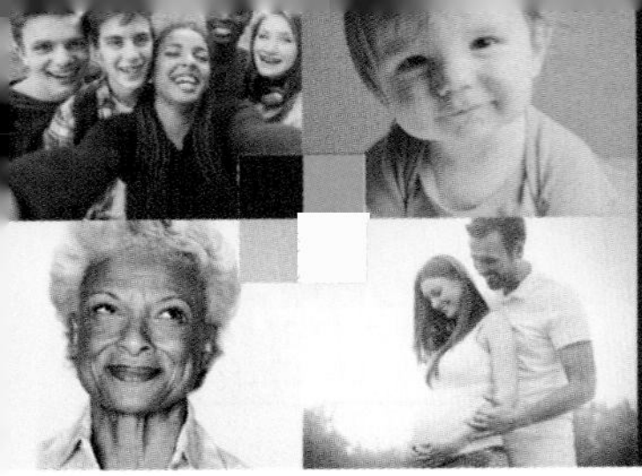

CHAPTER 8

Assessing the Breasts

Primary Functions

- Lactation
- Female sexuality

Developmental Considerations

Infants

- At birth, there is an elevation of the nipple.
- Slight secretion of milky material (witch's milk) may occur for 5 to 7 days.
- Palpable breast tissue during infancy is normal; however, not beyond this period.

Children

- A child's breast is underdeveloped compared with the mature breast. Growth of breast tissue generally begins in the prepubertal period.

Tanner Stages of Breast Development

- Stage 1. Prepuberty, elevation of papilla

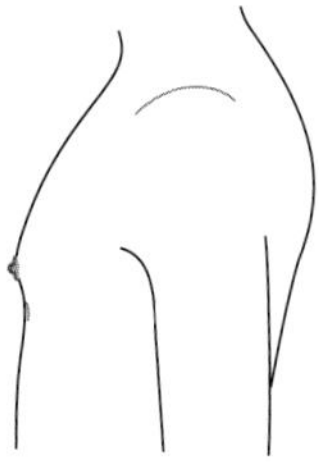

- Stage 2. "Breast-bud" stage. There is elevation of breast and nipple and increased diameter of areola.

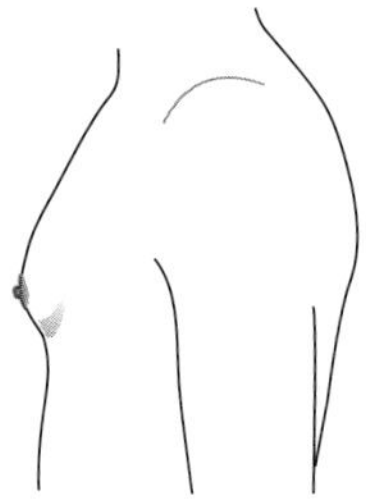

- Stage 3. Areola deepens in color and enlarges further. Glandular tissue begins to develop beneath areola.

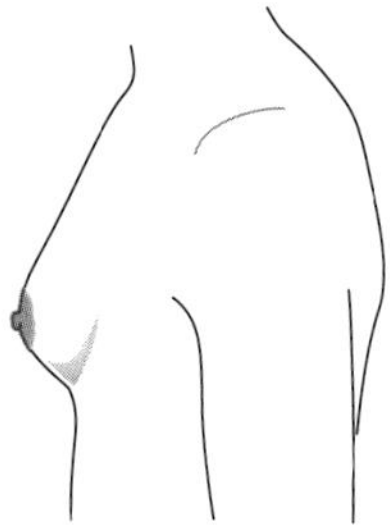

- Stage 4. Areola appears as a mound; breast appears as a mound.

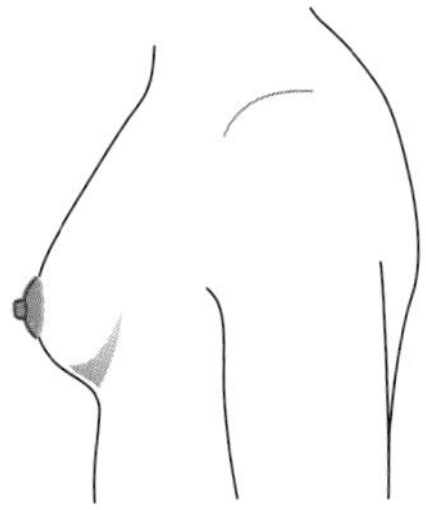

- Stage 5. Mature stage. Areola recesses to general contour of breast; nipple projects forward.

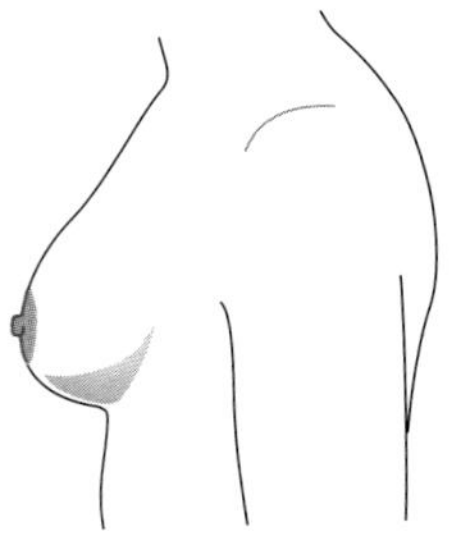

- Adolescent girls may have asymmetrical breasts as they go through puberty.
- Adolescent boys may have gynecomastia.

Pregnant Patients

- Breasts become fuller, firmer; areola and nipples darken and enlarge, and venous pattern increases.
- In the third trimester, colostrum occurs. It continues to be secreted after the birth of a baby until milk is produced.

Older Adults

- Ducts become more fibrous.
- Breasts lose elasticity and are less firm and more pendulous.

Cultural Considerations

- Ashkenazi Jews have a greater incidence of breast cancer than other groups.
- African American women in the South have been known to treat breast lesions with home remedies, which has delayed diagnosis until a more advanced stage.
- African American men appear to be at greater risk than white men for breast cancer.
- African American women have lower breast cancer survival rates than white women.
- White women have a higher incidence of breast cancer than nonwhite women.

Assessment

History

Symptoms ("PQRST" Any + Symptom)

- Lump or mass
  - Where is the lump or mass located?
  - Is there a "mirror" lesion in the opposite breast?
  - Is there pain or tenderness associated with the lump or mass?
  - When did you notice the lump?
  - Have you ever had a similar lump or mass before? When?
  - Does the lump or mass change in size during your menstrual cycle?
  - Have you had a recent injury to the breast?

Breast self-examination needs to be done when the breasts are not under hormonal influence—5 to 7 days after menstruation begins or 3 to 5 days after menstruation ceases. See Box 8.1.

- Pain
  - Is there pain on palpation?
  - Is there pain in one or both breasts?
  - Can you point to the area of pain?
  - Is the pain associated with a lump or mass?
  - Is pain related to the menstrual cycle? When did you first experience this pain?

BOX 8.1 Teaching Breast Self-Examination

1. First, teach the patient how to look at herself in a mirror and, with her arms at her sides, check for any visible abnormalities. She should observe for dimpling, retraction, or breast flattening as she first elevates her arms slowly, then presses her hands against her hips, and finally, bends forward.

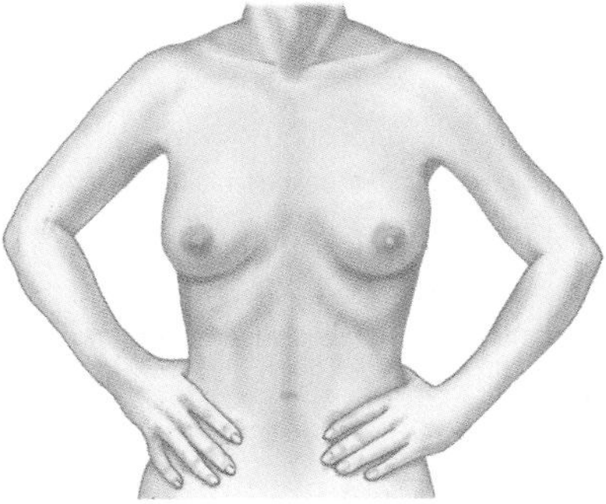

(box continued on page 230)

BOX 8.1 Teaching Breast Self-Examination (continued)

2. Next, by placing your hand over the patient's, show her how to use the pads of the middle three fingers of the opposite hand to palpate the breast systematically by compressing the breast tissue against the chest wall. She should palpate all portions of the breast, areola, nipple, tail of Spence, and axilla when she is in the shower or standing before a mirror. She should repeat the procedure lying down with a pillow or folded towel under the shoulder of the side she is examining.

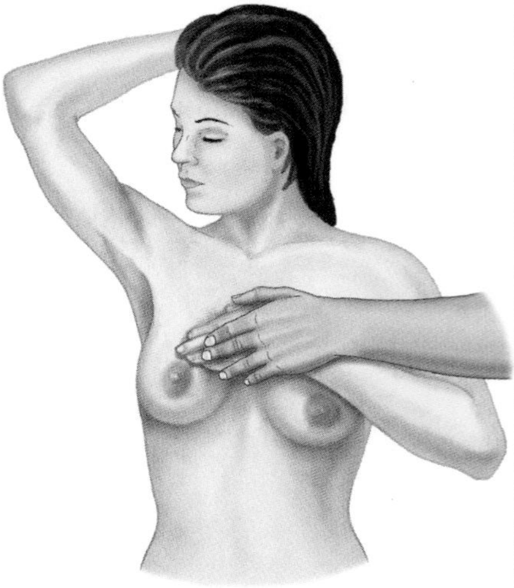

3. Next, show her how to compress the nipple gently between the thumb and the index finger as she observes for any discharge.

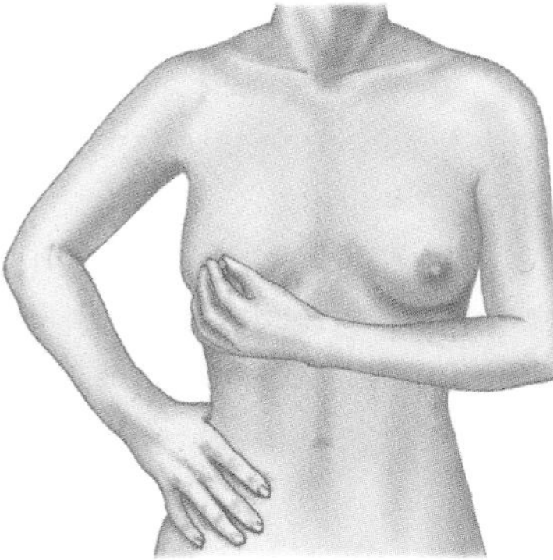

4. Finally, explain that she should report any redness or inflammation, swelling, masses, flattening, puckering, dimpling, retraction, sunken areas, asymmetrical nipple direction, discharge, bleeding, lesions, or eczematous nipple changes to her physician.

- Do you have any other symptoms? What started first? Second?
- When was your last menstrual period?
- Are you nursing?
- Did you recently complete a pregnancy?
- How would you describe the pain (sharp or dull)?
- Does the pain change, getting better or worse?
- Is it constant or intermittent? (If intermittent, how long does the pain last? How frequent are the episodes of pain?)
- Are there changes in the character of pain with your menstrual cycle?
- How would you rate the pain on a 0 to 10 scale, with 10 being the worst pain?
- What makes the pain worse? What makes it better?
- What have you tried to get rid of the pain? How well did that work?
- Has there been a change in your bra size?
- Have you had nipple piercing?
- Have you lost or gained weight? If yes, how much weight have you lost or gained and over what period of time?

Breast pain (or tenderness) is often a result of the normal physiological cycle. A lump associated with breast cancer is generally painless. Rapidly enlarging cysts may be painful.

■ Nipple discharge

- Are you having any problems with nipple discharge (color, amount, odor) or nipple retraction?
- When did the discharge start?
- How frequent is the discharge (continuous, or number of times per day or week)?
- When was the last discharge?
- Discharge from one or both breasts?
- What color is the discharge (clear, bloody, white, yellow)?
- Any changes in the appearance of the discharge (color, consistency)?
- How much discharge each time?
- Do you have any other symptoms (pain in your breast or nipple, change in the direction in which the nipple points, nipples becoming everted or inverted)?
- If you are premenopausal, any change in menstrual cycle?
- What have you tried to relieve this problem? How well has that worked?
- Has anything made it worse?

- Is the discharge spontaneous or when expressed?
- What medical illnesses do you have?
- Have you ever had this problem before? When? How was it treated?

Focused Breast History

- Address the warning signs and symptoms of breast cancer:
  - Lump or thickening in or near the breast or in the underarm that persists through the menstrual cycle.
  - Redness of the skin on the breast or nipple.
  - Change in the direction in which one nipple points; inversion, eversion, or discharge from the nipple.
  - Change in the size, shape, or contour of the breast.
  - Skin changes on the breast or nipple (dimpled, puckered, scaly, or inflamed).
- Ask whether the patient is taking any medications, prescribed or over-the-counter (Table 8.1).

TABLE 8.1 Drugs That Adversely Affect the Breasts

DRUG CLASS	DRUG	POSSIBLE ADVERSE REACTIONS
Androgens	Danazol, fluoxymesterone, methyltestosterone, testosterone	*Female:* Decreased breast size *Male:* Gynecomastia
Antidepressants	Tricyclic antidepressants	*Female:* Breast engorgement and galactorrhea (spontaneous milk flow) *Male:* Gynecomastia
Antipsychotics	Chlorpromazine hydrochloride, fluphenazine, haloperidol, perphenazine, prochlorperazine maleate, thioridazine, thiothixene	*Female:* Galactorrhea, moderate engorgement of the breast with lactation, mastalgia (breast pain) *Male:* Gynecomastia, mastalgia
Cardiac glycosides	Digitoxin, digoxin	*Male:* Gynecomastia
Estrogens	Conjugated estrogens, esterified estrogens, estradiol, estrone, ethinyl estradiol	*Female:* Breast changes, tenderness, enlargement, secretions *Male:* Breast changes, tenderness, gynecomastia
	Dienestrol	*Female:* Breast tenderness

DRUG CLASS	DRUG	POSSIBLE ADVERSE REACTIONS
Oral contraceptives	Estrogen-progesterone combinations	*Female:* Breast changes, tenderness, enlargement, secretions
Progestins	Medroxyprogesterone acetate, norethindrone, norgestrel, progesterone	*Female:* Breast tenderness or galactorrhea
Miscellaneous agents	Isoniazid	*Male:* Gynecomastia
	Reserpine	*Male:* Gynecomastia
	Spironolactone	*Female:* Breast tenderness *Male:* Painful gynecomastia
	Cimetidine	*Female:* Galactorrhea *Male:* Gynecomastia

Assessment of the Breasts' Relationship to Other Systems

Remember, all systems are related. Even though the breasts are not a system, as you assess the breasts, look at the relationship between them and all other systems. The relationship of the breasts to other systems is associated with breast disorders.

SUBJECTIVE DATA	OBJECTIVE DATA
Area/System: General	
Ask about:	*Observe:*
General health: Provides an indicator of general overall health.	*Level of consciousness (LOC):* If patient has breast cancer, changes in LOC, dyphasia, or hemiparesis may indicate brain metastasis.
Fever: Associated with mastitis, abscess, infection, and sometimes metastatic disease.	*Affect:* If patient has breast lump, mood may be depressed or anxious.
Weight changes: Unexplained weight loss may be associated with malignancy.	*Measure:* Vital signs. Weight.

(continued)

SUBJECTIVE DATA	OBJECTIVE DATA
Area/System: Integumentary	
Ask about:	*Inspect for:*
Rashes and lesions.	*Axillary rashes:* Allergies.
Scaly erosion of areola and nipple: Paget's disease (breast malignancy of areola and nipple).	*Breast lesions/redness:* Malignancy or mastitis.
Redness over affected area: Mastitis.	
Allergies.	Color changes.
Area/System: HEENT	
If patient has breast cancer, ask about:	*If patient has breast cancer:*
Headaches: May be related to metastatic breast cancer.	*Test vision:* Visual changes and papilledema may indicate brain metastasis.
Changes in mentation: May be due to metastatic breast cancer.	
Area/System: Respiratory	
If patient has breast cancer, ask about:	*If patient has breast cancer:*
Shortness of breath, cough, and breathing difficulty: Lung is common site for metastasis.	*Auscultate and percuss lungs:* Adventitious breath sounds, decreased chest excursion, and dullness to percussion seen with pleural effusion and may indicate metastasis to lungs.
Area/System: Cardiovascular	
Ask about:	*Inspect for:*
Cardiovascular medications: Some medications such as digoxin have side effect of gynecomastia.	*Increased vascularity of breasts:* Increased venous pattern, especially asymmetrical in nonpregnant patient may indicate breast cancer.
Area/System: Gastrointestinal	
If patient has breast cancer, ask about:	*If patient has breast cancer:*
Increase in size of abdominal girth: Liver is common site for metastasis. Liver disease can cause gynecomastia in men.	*Palpate abdomen:* Ascites and hepatomegaly may indicate metastasis to liver.
Area/System: Genitourinary/ Reproductive	
Ask about:	*Inspect:*
Age of menarche, last menstrual period, whether patient is pregnant, number of pregnancies, year of first pregnancy, whether patient is pre- or	*Perform pelvic exam:* Endometrial and ovarian cancer increase risk for breast cancer.

SUBJECTIVE DATA	OBJECTIVE DATA
postmenopausal: Early menarche and late menopause are risk factors for breast cancer. Nulliparity, first pregnancy after age 30, and infertility have been linked to breast cancer.	
Breast feeding decreases risk for breast cancer.	
Medications (birth control pill [BCP], hormone replacement therapy [HRT]): BCP can cause breast changes, such as tenderness, enlargement and secretions. HRT has been linked with increased incidence of breast cancer.	
Area/System: Musculoskeletal	
If patient has breast cancer, ask about:	*If patient has breast cancer:*
Weakness, bone pain, fractures: Musculoskeletal problem may be due to metastatic breast cancer.	*Test muscle strength:* Weakness and ataxia may indicate metastasis to bone and brain.
Area/System: Neurologic	
	If patient has breast cancer:
	Test LOC, sensory and motor function: Unilateral sensory loss and hemiparesis may indicate metastasis.
Area/System: Endocrine	
Ask about:	*Palpate:*
History of thyroid disease: Hyperthyroidism can cause gynecomastia in men.	*Thyroid:* Hyperthyroidism can cause gynecomastia in men.
Area/System: Lymphatic/Hematological	
Ask about:	*Palpate:*
Infection or malignancy.	*Lymph nodes:* Enlarged lymph nodes may indicate infection or metastasis.

HEENT = Head, eyes, ears, nose, and throat.

Physical Assessment

Anatomical Landmarks

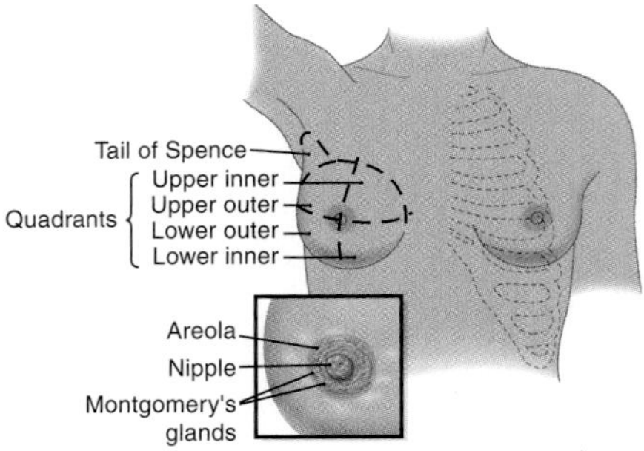

External breast structures and quadrants

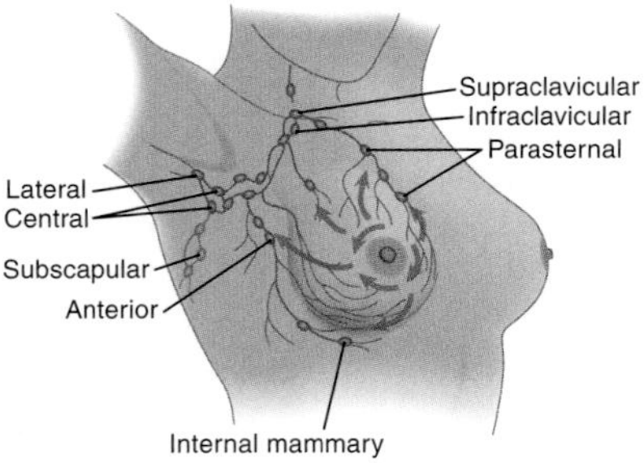

Lymph nodes

APPROACH: Inspection, palpation; vertical strip, pie wedge, or concentric circles

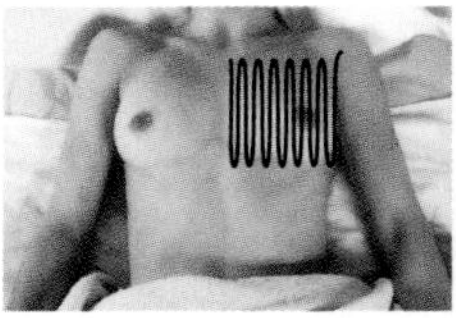

Vertical strip method

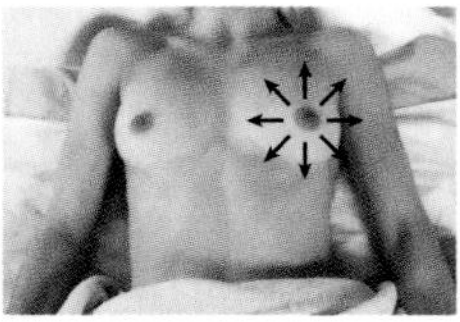

Pie wedge method

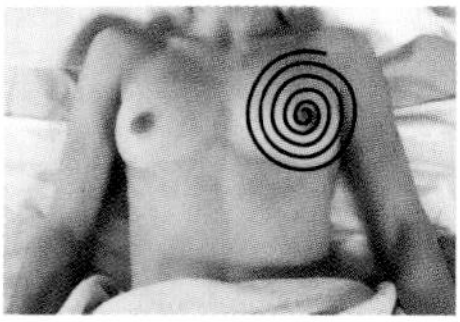

Concentric circles method

POSITION: Supine with pillow under shoulder of breast being examined, sitting with arms at side, sitting with arms over head, sitting with hands on hip or pushed together, sitting leaning forward

TOOLBOX: Small pillow or towel, mirror, centimeter ruler, nonsterile gloves, specimen slide, specimen culture slide

Physical Assessment

AREA/PA SKILL	NORMAL FINDINGS	ABNORMAL FINDINGS
Inspection *Breast*		
Assess size, shape, symmetry, color with the patient in a sitting position.	Breasts lobular, symmetrical, color consistent with body color.	*Change in breast symmetry:* Warrants further investigation.
Note visible masses, lesions, edema, and venous pattern.	No masses, lesions, edema, dimpling, retraction, or orange-peel skin. Breasts may normally be slightly asymmetrical.	*Edema and orange-peel skin appearance:* Lymphatic obstruction. *Erythema:* Infection, abscess, or inflammatory carcinoma of the breast.
Have patient press hands together or press hands on hips to check for dimpling or retraction. For very large, pendulous breast, have the patient lean forward.		*Dimpling or puckering:* Sign of retraction phenomena or abnormal traction on Cooper's ligaments—or attachment to fascia and pectoralis muscle—caused by neoplasm.

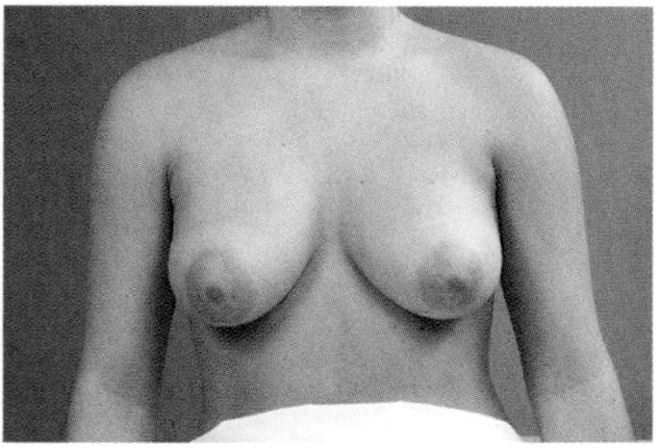

Sitting, arms at side

(box continued on page 238)

Physical Assessment (continued)

AREA/PA SKILL	NORMAL FINDINGS	ABNORMAL FINDINGS
Inspection *Breast (cont'd)*		

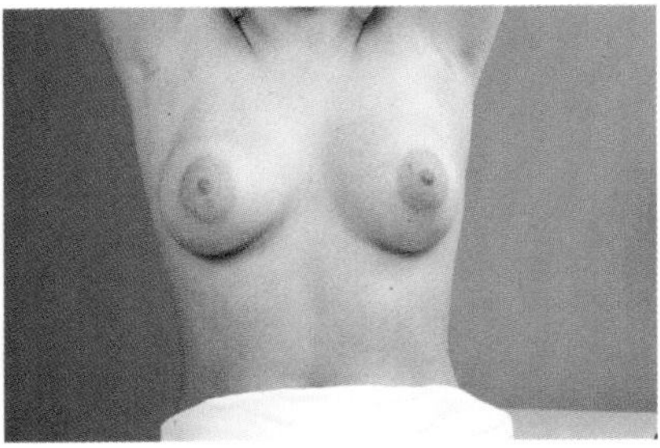

Sitting, arms over head

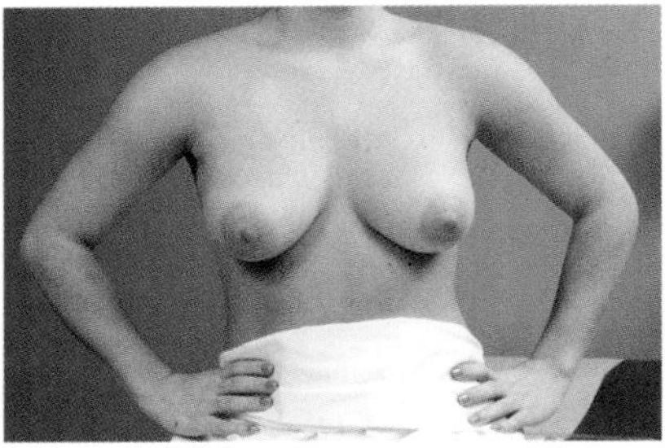

Sitting, hands on hips

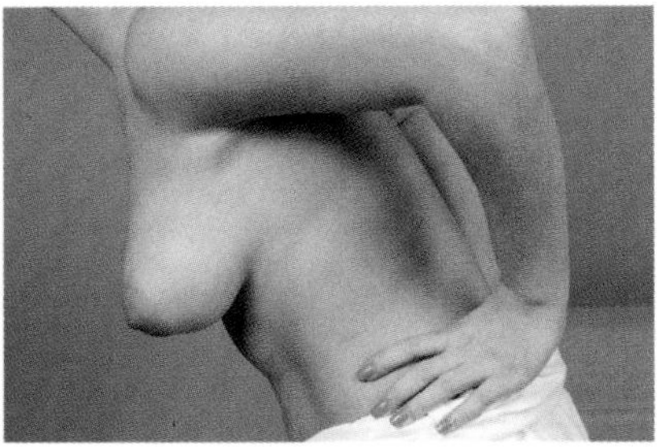

Sitting, leaning forward

AREA/PA SKILL	NORMAL FINDINGS	ABNORMAL FINDINGS

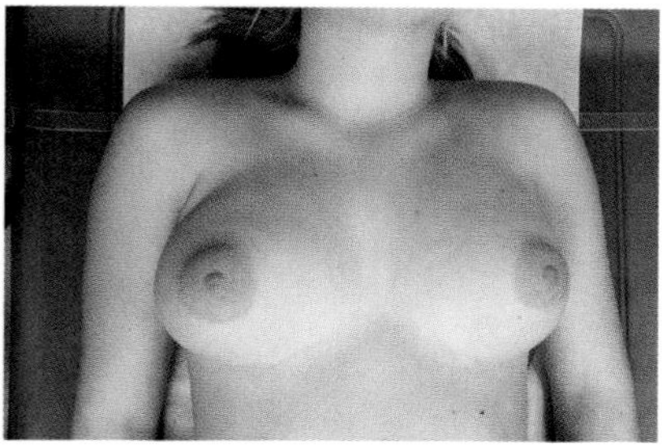

Supine, with pillow under shoulder of breast being examined

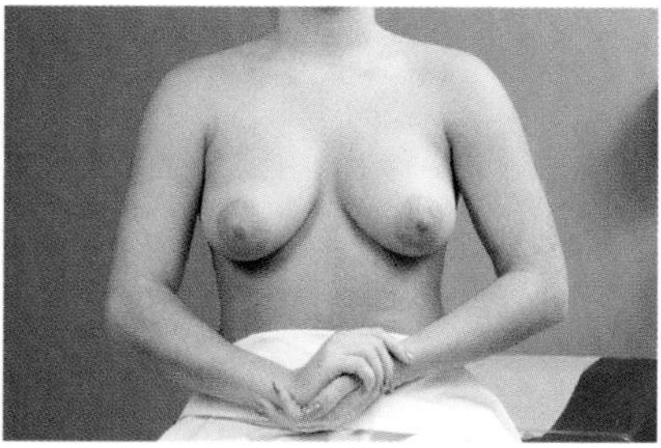

Sitting, pushing hands together

AREA/PA SKILL	NORMAL FINDINGS	ABNORMAL FINDINGS
Note dominant side.		*Lesions and asymmetrical increased venous pattern:* Signs of breast cancer.
Nipple and Areola		
Note color, shape, symmetry, inversions or eversions, discharge, masses, lesions.	Nipples and areola symmetrical, round, and darker than breast tissue. Color lighter in fair-skinned and darker in dark-skinned women. No masses, lesions, or discharge.	**Inverted nipples may make breast-feeding difficult.** *Change in nipple from everted to inverted, or in the direction in which it is pointing:* Underlying mass. *Flattened or inverted nipples:* Shortening of mammary ducts.
Note direction of nipples.	Spontaneous discharge normal during pregnancy and lactation. Symmetrical nipple direction, usually lateral and upward. Nipples	**Spontaneous discharge not associated with pregnancy or breast-feeding warrants follow-up. Obtain**

(box continued on page 240)

Physical Assessment (continued)

AREA/PA SKILL	NORMAL FINDINGS	ABNORMAL FINDINGS
Inspection *Nipple and Areola (cont'd)*	may be everted, flat, or inverted, but should be symmetrical.	**a specimen for evaluation.** *Lesions or erosion and ulceration of areola and nipple:* Paget's disease.
Inspect for supernumerary nipples.	No supernumerary nipples.	Discoloration of areola and nipple that is not associated with pregnancy warrants follow-up. Cracks and redness of nipple can occur with breast-feeding.
Axilla		
Note color, lesions, masses, and hair distribution.	Skin intact, no lesions or rashes. Hair growth appropriate for patient's age and sex.	*Rashes, redness, unusual pigmentation:* Infection, allergy. Malignant acanthosis nigricans, a rare cancer, causes dark pigmentation and velvety skin texture of axilla.
Palpation **Use finger pads of three middle fingers, make small circles with light, medium, and deep pressure.**		
Breasts		
Palpate from the clavicle to the 6th and 7th intercostal spaces and the sternum to the midaxillary line. Use vertical strip, pie wedge, or circular method.	Breast consistency depends on developmental stage of woman. Premenopausal breast is more firm and elastic, during pregnancy and lactation is firm and tender, postmenopausal is less firm and elastic with stringy ducts.	*Fibroadenoma:* Benign breast lumps; usually smooth, firm, round, movable, nontender, 1 to 5 cm in size.

AREA/PA SKILL	NORMAL FINDINGS	ABNORMAL FINDINGS
Note texture, consistency, tenderness, masses.	Nontender, but premenstrual breast may be tender and nodular.	*Fibrocystic breast:* Benign breast lumps; nodular, tender, movable, soft to firm, change in size with menstrual cycle, increasing before menstruation, and multiple in number.

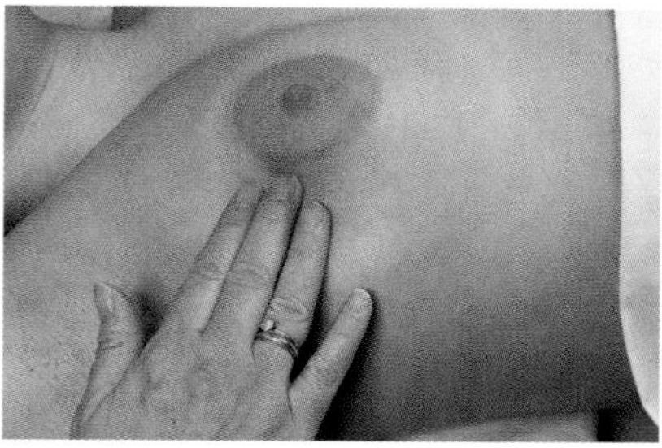

Palpating the breast

Do not remove finger pads from the skin surface or jump from area to area. Most breast lesions in women are found in the upper outer quadrant. (This area includes the tail of the breast and contains a greater amount of breast tissue than the other quadrants.) Although the incidence of breast cancer in men is about 1 percent, you still need to assess the breast. Breast cancer in men most frequently occurs in the areola.	No masses or lesions.	*Breast cancer:* Irregular shape, borders irregular and not well defined, nontender, immovable, increases in size as disease progresses. *Breast warm and indurated (hard):* Mastitis.

(box continued on page 242)

Physical Assessment (continued)

AREA/PA SKILL	NORMAL FINDINGS	ABNORMAL FINDINGS
Nipple and Areola		
Note elasticity, discharge, tenderness.	Nipple elastic, nontender, no discharge or white sebaceous secretion with nipple compression. Pregnant or lactating women may have milky discharge.	*Bloody, purulent discharge:* Infection. *Serous, serosanguineous, or bloody drainage:* Intraductal papilloma. *Thick, gray drainage and fixation of nipple:* Ductal ectasia. *Loss of elasticity:* Underlying malignancy.

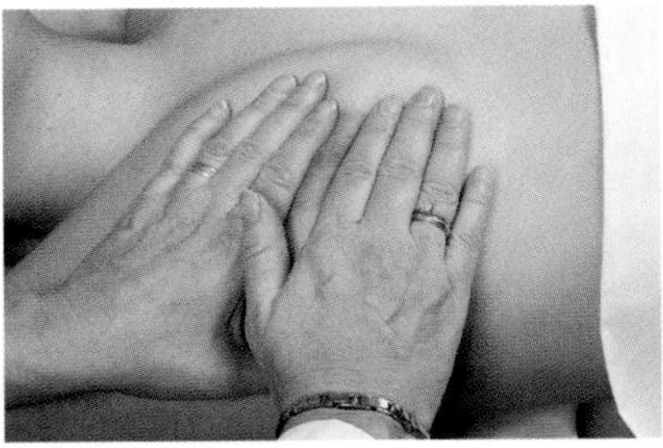

Palpating the nipple

AREA/PA SKILL	NORMAL FINDINGS	ABNORMAL FINDINGS
Axilla and Clavicular Nodes: Central, Anterior, Posterior, Lateral, Epitrochlear, Supra- and Infraclavicular		
Note palpable nodes, location, tenderness, size, shape, consistency, mobility, borders, temperature.	Lymph nodes nonpalpable, nontender.	*Palpable nodes:* Infection or metastatic disease. Lymph node enlargement caused by infection usually tender; by malignancy, nontender.

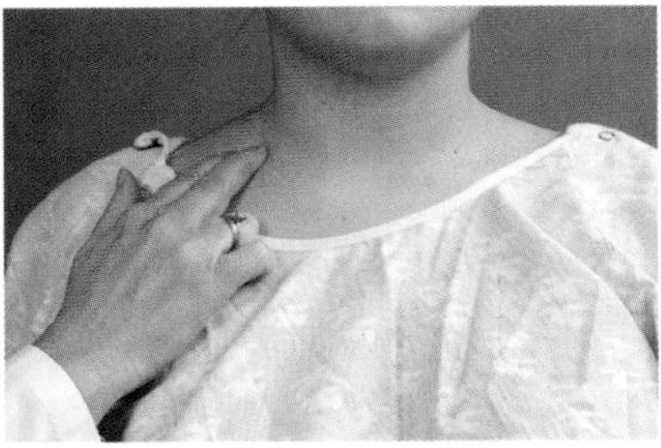

Palpating supraclavicular nodes

AREA/PA SKILL	NORMAL FINDINGS	ABNORMAL FINDINGS

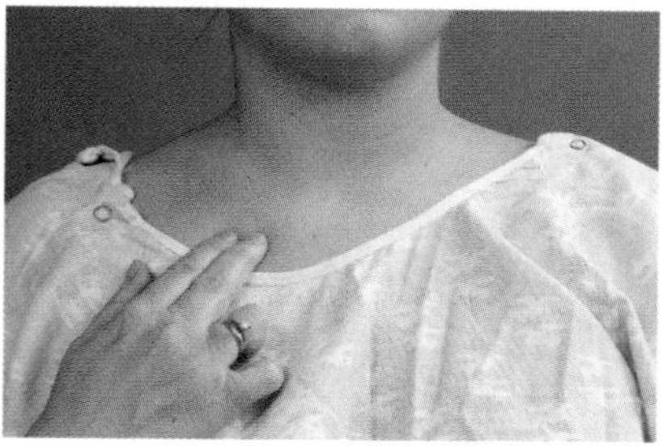

Palpating infraclavicular nodes

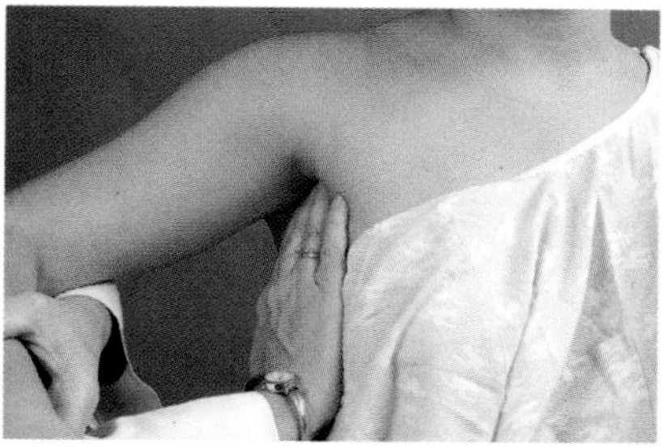

Palpating central nodes

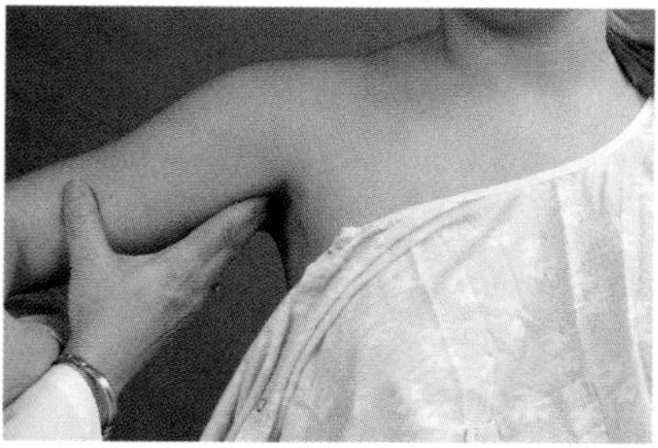

Palpating lateral nodes

(box continued on page 244)

Physical Assessment (continued)

AREA/PA SKILL	NORMAL FINDINGS	ABNORMAL FINDINGS
Palpation *Nipple and Areola (cont'd)*		

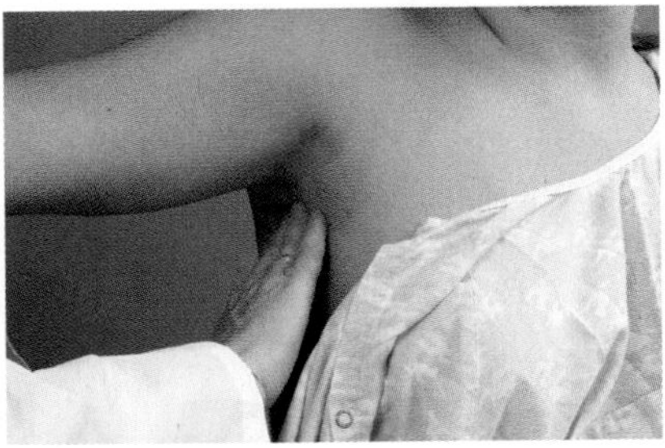

Palpating posterior nodes

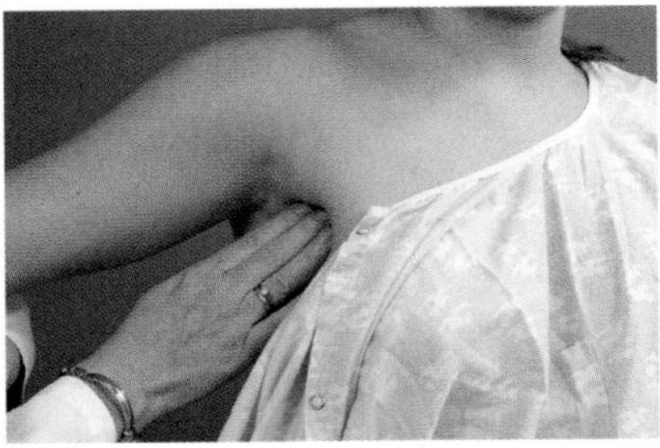

Palpating anterior nodes

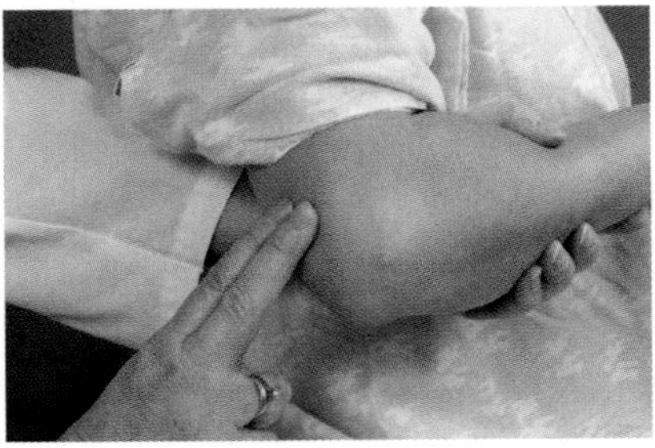

Palpating epitrochlear nodes

PA = Physical assessment.

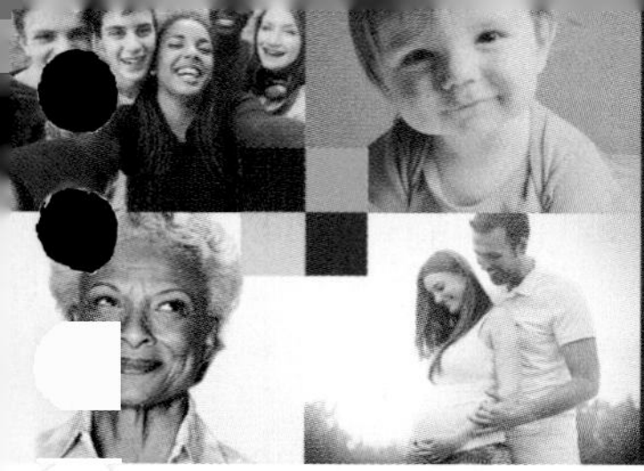

CHAPTER 9

Assessing the Abdomen

Primary Functions

- Every system, except the respiratory system, is found within the abdomen: the gastrointestinal (GI), cardiovascular, reproductive, neuromuscular, and genitourinary systems.
- The primary system is the digestive system, which is responsible for the ingestion and digestion of food, the absorption of nutrients, and the elimination of waste products.

Developmental Considerations

Infants

- The newborn's bladder is located above the symphysis pubis.
- The liver proportionally takes up more space in the abdomen and may extend 2 cm ($^{3}/_{4}$ inch) below the rib cage.
- The infant's abdominal muscles are weak, so the abdomen normally protrudes.

Children

- A child's abdomen is proportionally larger than an adult's and has a slightly protuberant appearance because of the curvature of the back.
- Abdominal respiration is common in most children.
- Children's abdominal muscles are underdeveloped, so the organs are more easily palpated.
- Children may have diastasis recti.

Pregnant Patients

- For women having multiple pregnancies or a multiple birth, the rectus abdominal muscles may become separated (diastasis recti abdominis).

- As the fetus grows, the stomach rises up and impinges on the diaphragm.
- Bowel sounds are diminished in the pregnant patient because the bowels are compressed by the fetus.
- Decreased activity in the lower GI tract, along with ingestion of prenatal vitamins containing large amounts of iron, contributes to constipation.
- Increased venous pressure in the lower abdomen may cause hemorrhoids to develop and create further problems with elimination.
- During pregnancy, the appendix is displaced upward and laterally to the right.
- Linea nigra is a characteristic skin change in most pregnant patients.
- Near the end of pregnancy, the umbilicus may become everted and striae may develop.

Older Adults

- Changes in dentition may affect chewing ability and digestion.
- Poorly fitted dentures may result in painful mastication.
- Reduced saliva, stomach acid, gastric motility, and peristalsis cause problems with swallowing, absorption, and digestion. These changes, along with a general reduction of muscle mass and tone, also contribute to constipation.
- Fat accumulates in the lower abdomen in women and around the waist in men, making physical assessment of the organs a little more challenging.
- The liver becomes smaller and liver function declines, making it harder to process medications.
- Older adults have a diminished response to painful stimuli that may mask abdominal health problems.

Cultural Considerations

- African Americans have a high incidence of sickle cell anemia, lactose intolerance, and obesity.
- Asian Americans have a high incidence of GI cancer and lactose intolerance.
- Jewish Americans have a high incidence of Crohn's disease, ulcerative colitis, and colon cancer.
- Mediterranean Americans have a high incidence of lactose intolerance and thalassemia anemia.

- Native Americans have a high incidence of alcoholism, liver disease, pancreatitis, diabetes, and gallbladder disease.

Assessment

History

Symptoms ("PQRST" Any + Symptom)

- Abdominal pain
  - Where is the pain? Would you point to where you feel the pain? (Box 9.1.)
  - Does the pain stay in one place or does it move (radiate)? Where does the pain go?
  - When did it start (date)? What were you doing when it started? Gradually or suddenly?
  - Do you have any other symptoms? What started first? Second?

BOX 9.1 Significance of Pain by Abdominal Quadrant

LEFT UPPER QUADRANT	RIGHT UPPER QUADRANT
Heart: Myocardial infarction (MI)/ischemia	*Heart:* MI/ischemia
Lungs: Pulmonary embolism, pneumonia	*Lungs:* Pneumonia
Pancreas: Pancreatitis	*Gallbladder:* Cholelithiasis, cholecystitis
Spleen: Ruptured spleen	*Liver:* Hepatitis, cancer
Stomach: Gastric ulcer, esophagitis, gastroesophageal reflux disease (GERD), hiatal hernia, varices	*Intestines:* Duodenal ulcer
LEFT LOWER QUADRANT	**RIGHT LOWER QUADRANT**
Ovary/Uterus: Ectopic pregnancy, ovarian cyst, pelvic inflammatory disease (PID)	*Ovary/Uterus:* Ectopic pregnancy, ovarian cyst, PID
Intestines: Perforation, constipation, diverticulitis, hernia, ulcerative colitis	*Intestines:* Perforation, obstruction, constipation, Crohn's disease, diverticulitis, hernia, ulcerative colitis, appendicitis
Kidney: Nephrolithiasis (kidney stones), infection	*Kidney:* Nephrolithiasis, infection

- Have you ever had this pain before?
- When was your last menstrual period (LMP)?
- How would you describe the pain (sharp or dull)? (Table 9.1.)
- Is the pain getting better or worse?
- Is it constant or intermittent? (If intermittent, how long does the pain last and how frequent are the episodes of pain?)
- What makes it worse? What makes it better?
- What have you tried to get rid of the pain? How well did that work?

TABLE 9.1 Pain Intensity Rating Scales

SCALE	APPROPRIATE PATIENTS
0–10 Numeric Pain Intensity Scale Horizontal line with 11 marks associated with numbers 0–10 0 = no pain; 5 = moderate pain; 10 = worst possible pain *Nurse asks patient to rate pain on 0–10 scale, either using written instructions on a card or verbally explaining scale.*	Patient must be able to: • Process verbal information • Communicate verbally or by body movements • Understand numbers 0–10
18 foreign language versions available at:http://www.partnersagainstpain.com/html/assess/as_scale.htm	Used with children age 8 and up, teens, and adults.
Wong-Baker FACES Pain Rating Scale (1999) Card with six faces with expressions ranging from happy to very sad and crying. Happy face indicates no pain (0); very sad face (5) indicates most severe pain.	Patient must be able to see and process information.
Nurse explains process first, then shows patient card and asks patient to pick face that best reflects pain.	Originally designed for use with children age 3 and over, but is used with adults as well.
Simple Descriptive Verbal Pain Intensity Scale Horizontal line with six demarcations from left to right with words that describe pain: No Pain—Mild Pain—Moderate Pain—Severe Pain—Very Severe Pain—Worst Possible Pain. *Nurse asks patient to select word best describing pain.*	Patient must be able to: • Speak or understand English. • Process information. • Communicate.

- Do you have a fever? Has your appetite changed?
- Have you lost weight? If so, how much weight have you lost and over what period of time?
- Are you having any problems with your bowels? Are there any changes in urination (frequency, burning, color, amount)?
- Have you noticed any bloating in your stomach?
- Are you having any discharge from your private parts (color, amount, odor).

■ Weight changes
- How is your appetite? Have you had any changes in your appetite recently?
- What have you had to eat in the last 24 hours (note 24-hour intake)?
- What is your present weight? What is your usual weight?
- Has your weight changed recently?
- How much weight have you lost or gained? Over what period of time?
- Were you trying to lose or gain weight? How did you lose or gain the weight?
- Are you satisfied with your present weight?
- Do you ever eat large amounts of food at one time (like a half gallon of ice cream)?

■ Bowel pattern changes
- When did the changes start?
- How frequent are your bowel movements usually (per day or week)? Presently?
- When was your last bowel movement?
- Do you wake up in the night to have a bowel movement?
- What color is your stool (black, dark brown, light brown, tan, gray, yellow)? Have there been any changes?
- Is it soft, hard, formed, loose, liquid? Have there been any changes in consistency?
- Any mucus or blood?
- How much are you eliminating at one time (especially important in diarrhea)?
- Do you have any other symptoms (fullness or pain in your abdomen, bloating, gas, indigestion, nausea, vomiting, fever, weight loss)?
- What have you tried to relieve this problem? How well has that worked?
- Has anything made it worse?

- Is there anything you eat that upsets your stomach or causes changes in your bowel movements? Has your diet changed recently?
- What medications do you take (medicines, antacids, laxatives, enemas, stool softeners)? Frequency of medications?
- What medical illnesses do you have?
- Have you ever had this problem before? When? How was it treated?
- Does anyone you know have similar symptoms (diarrhea)?
- Have you traveled out of the country recently (diarrhea)?

■ Indigestion
- Where do you feel the indigestion (point with one finger)?
- Do you have pain anywhere else?
- Does the pain stay in one place or does it radiate?
- When did it start?
- What were you doing at that time?
- Have you ever had this before? How long does it last?
- Would you describe the feeling to me (sharp, dull, burning, crushing)?
- Is it constant or intermittent?
- How would you rate the discomfort on a scale of 1 to 10, with 10 being the worst?
- What have you tried to make it better? How did that work?
- What makes it worse?
- Do you have any other symptoms?
- Do you have any difficulty swallowing?

■ Nausea
- When did the nausea start?
- What were you doing at the time?
- Does it come on at any particular time of the day?
- What have you eaten in the last 24 hours? Does anyone in your family have similar symptoms?
- How would you describe it?
- Does it come over you in a wave and then dissipate? Or is it constant?
- Does the nausea interfere with your daily activities?
- Have you been so nauseated that you have vomited?
- Have you lost weight?
- Is there any chance that you are pregnant?
- Do you have any other symptoms or health problems?
- What medicines do you take?

- What have you tried to relieve the nausea? How has that worked?
- Do you have any other symptoms with the nausea, such as fever, chills, headache?

- Vomiting
  - When did the vomiting start?
  - What were you doing at the time?
  - In the last few days, have you been hit on the head?
  - Does anyone else in your house have similar symptoms?
  - What color is the vomit?
  - What is its consistency?
  - How much have you been vomiting at one time?
  - How many times a day are you vomiting?
  - Have you been able to keep any food or fluids down?
  - What have you tried to stop the vomiting?
  - Did it work? Does anything make it better (lying still, eating crackers, ginger ale)?
  - What makes it worse (for example, eating)?
  - What other symptoms do you have (retching, nausea, pain, fever, distention, diarrhea, weakness, stiff neck, headache)?

Focused Abdominal History

- Do you have any abdominal pain?
- Have you ever had the following: stomach ulcer, hemorrhoids, hernia, bowel disease, cancer, hepatitis, cirrhosis, or appendicitis?
- Have you had abdominal surgery? If so, when, what type, and were there any subsequent problems?
- Do you have a family history of ulcer, gallbladder disease, bowel disease, or cancer?
- Do you have any problems with swallowing, heartburn, nausea, yellowing of your skin, gas, bloating, or vomiting (note onset, quality, and quantity)?
- Do you have any food allergies or lactose intolerance?
- Have you noticed any recent weight changes? What is your usual weight and height?
- How is your appetite? What did you eat in the last 24 hours?
- How is your health usually?
- Are you currently being treated for a health problem? If so, what?
- How often do you usually have a bowel movement? Have you noticed any changes in your bowel movements?
- Are you having problems with diarrhea, constipation, hemorrhoids, or fecal incontinence? Have you ever noticed blood in your stool or had black, tarry stools?

- How often do you urinate? Do you have incontinence or burning when you urinate?
- When was your LMP?
- Do you smoke? How many packs a day? (Calculate pack-years.)
- Do you drink alcohol? If so, how often? Do you use street drugs?
- How many cups of coffee, tea, or caffeinated soda do you drink every day?
- Have you been exposed to an infectious disease recently?
- What is your occupation?
- Have you been immunized against hepatitis B?
- Have you ever had a blood transfusion? If so, when?
- Are you taking any medications, prescribed or over the counter (Table 9.2)?
- Do you have any allergies to medications?
- What herbal preparations do you use?
- Do you use antacids, laxatives, enemas, nonsteroidal anti-inflammatory agents (NSAIDs), or aspirin?
- What home remedies do you use?

TABLE 9.2 Drugs that Adversely Affect the Gastrointestinal System

DRUG CLASS	DRUG	POSSIBLE ADVERSE REACTIONS
Analgesics	Acetaminophen	Hepatic necrosis with high (toxic) doses
	Aspirin	GI disturbances, GI bleeding, ulceration
Antacids	Aluminum hydroxide	Constipation
	Calcium carbonate	Constipation, gastric hypersecretion, acid rebound
	Magnesium hydroxide, magnesium oxide	Diarrhea
Anticholinergic agents	All anticholinergics	Nausea, vomiting, constipation, xerostomia (dry mouth), bloated feeling, paralytic ileus
Antidepressants	Amitriptyline hydrochloride, nortriptyline hydrochloride	Constipation, adynamic ileus, elevated liver enzyme concentrations
	Selective serotonin reuptake inhibitors	Nausea, vomiting, diarrhea, constipation
Antidiabetic agents	Acetohexamide	Nausea, vomiting, diarrhea, heartburn, cholestatic jaundice
	Chlorpropamide	Nausea, vomiting, diarrhea

DRUG CLASS	DRUG	POSSIBLE ADVERSE REACTIONS
Anti-infectives	Ampicillin	Diarrhea, nausea, vomiting, pseudomembranous colitis
	Ciprofloxacin	Nausea, vomiting, diarrhea
	Clindamycin	Nausea, vomiting, diarrhea, pseudomembranous colitis
	Erythromycin	Abdominal pain and cramping, nausea, vomiting, diarrhea, hepatic dysfunction, jaundice
	Griseofulvin	Nausea, vomiting, diarrhea, flatulence
	Metronidazole	Taste disturbances, abdominal discomfort, diarrhea, nausea, vomiting
	Sulfonamides	Nausea, vomiting, hepatic changes
	Tetracycline hydrochloride	Nausea, vomiting, diarrhea, stomatitis
Antihypertensives	Clonidine	Nausea, vomiting, constipation
	Methyldopa	Elevated liver function tests
Antineoplastic agents	All antineoplastics	Nausea, vomiting, stomatitis
Antituberculosis agents	Isoniazid	Increased liver enzyme concentrations
	Rifampin	Heartburn, nausea, vomiting, diarrhea, increased liver enzyme concentrations
Biphosphonates	Alendronate	Esophagitis, heartburn
Cardiac agents	Digoxin	Nausea, vomiting, diarrhea, anorexia with toxicity
	Quinidine	Nausea, vomiting, diarrhea, abdominal cramps, colic
Narcotic analgesics	Codeine, meperidine, methadone, morphine, oxycodone	Nausea, vomiting, constipation, biliary spasm or colic
NSAIDs	Ibuprofen, indomethacin, salicylates	Nausea, vomiting, dyspepsia, GI bleeding, peptic ulcer
Phenothiazines	Prochlorperazine, thioridazine	Constipation, dyspepsia, paralytic ileus, cholestatic jaundice (hypersensitivity reaction)
Miscellaneous agents	Acarbose	Diarrhea, flatulence, abdominal pain
	Allopurinol	Altered liver function, nausea, vomiting, diarrhea
	Aminophylline, theophylline	GI irritation, epigastric pain, nausea, vomiting, anorexia
	Barium sulfate	Cramping, diarrhea

(continued)

TABLE 9.2 Drugs that Adversely Affect the Gastrointestinal System (continued)

DRUG CLASS	DRUG	POSSIBLE ADVERSE REACTIONS
	Colchicine	Diarrhea, nausea, vomiting, abdominal pain
	Estrogen-progestin combinations	Nausea, vomiting, diarrhea, abdominal cramps, altered liver function tests, cholestatic jaundice
	Iron preparations	Constipation, nausea, vomiting, black stools
	Gold sodium thiomalate, auranofin	Changes in bowel habits, diarrhea, abdominal cramping, nausea, vomiting
	Levodopa	Nausea, vomiting, anorexia
	Lithium	Nausea, vomiting, diarrhea
	Phenytoin sodium	Nausea, vomiting, constipation, dysphagia
	Potassium supplements	Nausea, vomiting, diarrhea, abdominal discomfort, small-bowel ulceration (with enteric-coated tablets)
	Prednisone	Epigastric pain, gastric irritation, pancreatitis
	Zidovudine	Nausea, vomiting, anorexia

Assessment of the Abdomen's Relationship to Other Systems

Remember, all systems are related. As you assess the abdomen, look at the relationship between it and all other systems.

Assessment of the Abdomen's Relationship to Other Systems

SUBJECTIVE DATA/RATIONALE	OBJECTIVE DATA/RATIONALE
Area/System: General	
Ask about:	*Inspect for:*
Weight changes.	Orientation. • *Diminished mental status:* Can occur with hemorrhaging. Confusion or other nervous system problems may relate to liver's inability to detoxify medications or toxins or kidneys' inability to rid body of harmful wastes.

SUBJECTIVE DATA/RATIONALE	OBJECTIVE DATA/RATIONALE
Diet.	Facial expression.
Fever or chills: Seen with infections.	*Posture:* Fetal position often assumed with acute abdominal pain.
Dizziness, weakness, fatigue: May reflect poor nutritional state, anemia related to blood loss in the GI tract, or vitamin B_{12} deficiency. Malaise is commonly associated with GI diseases.	Nutritional status. *Measure:* Weight. *Cachexic appearance with dry, brittle hair, thin hair, dry skin:* **Anorexia nervosa** and/or **malnutrition.** Vital signs.
Area/System: Integumentary *Ask about:*	*Inspect:*
Changes in skin, hair, and nails: Jaundice associated with liver disease.	Skin, hair, and nails for changes in color and texture, lesions, and edema or ascites *Yellow skin:* Jaundice, associated with liver disease or biliary obstruction *Lower extremity edema:* Can be caused by iliac obstruction, pelvic mass, or renal disease. *Linear lesions on one-half of the abdomen:* Shingles, an infection of herpes zoster that follows the dermatome of the nervous system. • *Curved fingernails:* Cirrhosis or some type of bowel disease.
Rashes, itching, lesions: Pruritus associated with liver disease. Complaints of pruritus or pain along a dermatomally distributed vesicular rash located on the lower aspects of the rib cage indicates herpes zoster (shingles). Other rashes may reflect reactions to an antibiotic, which may also cause pain, nausea, cramping, and diarrhea.	*Dry skin and mucous membranes/poor skin turgor with tenting:* Dehydration. GI diseases may cause dehydration with fluid and electrolyte disturbances. For example, **ulcerative colitis** causes frequent, loose diarrhea and deficits in sodium, potassium, chloride, magnesium, zinc, copper, and other minerals. **Gastroenteritis** causes severe fluid and electrolyte imbalances from vomiting and diarrhea that result in loss of water, sodium, chloride, potassium, and bicarbonate. **Peptic ulcer disease** may cause bleeding, resulting in hematemesis and melena. Besides dehydration and fluid and electrolyte,

(continued)

Assessment of the Abdomen's Relationship to Other Systems (continued)

SUBJECTIVE DATA/RATIONALE	OBJECTIVE DATA/RATIONALE
Area/System: Integumentary *(cont'd)*	imbalances, severe blood loss (>1 L) may cause hypovolemic shock, with symptoms including hypotension, weak pulse, chills, palpitations, and cold, clammy skin.
Area/System: HEENT **Head and neck** *Ask about:*	*Inspect for:*
Thyroid disease: Associated with weight changes.	Neck masses.
Neck masses: History of goiter (hypothyroidism) may be related to iodine deficiency in diet.	*Palpate:*
Recent infections: Infections, such as mononucleosis, can cause spleen enlargement.	*Thyroid:* Goiter and other masses may reflect thyroid disease and impair swallowing. *Lymph nodes:* Cervical lymphadenopathy may indicate a systemic infection or malignancy, such as mononucleosis or Hodgkin's disease, and cause splenomegaly.
Eyes *Ask about:*	*Inspect for:*
History of diabetes, renal disease, liver disease: Icteric sclera are seen with liver disease.	Edema. Color of sclera. • *Icteric sclera:* Liver disease or biliary obstruction. *Conjunctivitis, uveitis, episcleritis:* Extraintestinal complications of ulcerative colitis. *Periorbital edema:* Renal disease. Retinal changes.
Ears, nose, and throat *Ask about:*	*Inspect:*
Problems swallowing: May be a sign of esophageal mass, muscular or neurologic problems, or benign diagnoses.	Mouth. • *Dry lips/mucous membranes:* Dehydration. • *Red, beefy tongue:* Pernicious anemia. *Parotitis, dental problems, irritated pharynx:* Bulimia.
Sore throat: Infections,such as strep throat, often cause abdominal discomfort.	Throat. *Absence of gag/swallowing reflex:* Neurologic diseases such as stroke may alter nutritional status.

SUBJECTIVE DATA/RATIONALE	OBJECTIVE DATA/RATIONALE
Dizziness: A sign of Ménière's disease, which causes nausea.	Condition of teeth. *Dental caries/mouth lesions (aphthous ulcers):* Affect nutritional intake. Mouth lesions associated with ulcerative colitis.
Last dental examination.	*Test:* Cranial nerves I, VII, VIII, IX, X, XII. Balance using Romberg's test.
Area/System: Respiratory *Ask about:*	*Measure:*
Breathing problems, shortness of breath (SOB): Dyspnea may be caused by edema in the abdomen or large tumors of the liver, esophagus, or stomach, which impinge on respiratory structures, or may be by portal HTN from liver congestion.	Respiratory rate and depth. *Hypoxia:* May be caused by distended abdomen, which raises diaphragm and inhibits respiration. • *Shallow respirations:* Voluntary guarding, an attempt to avoid abdominal pain caused by movement in patients with peritonitis.
History of chronic obstructive pulmonary disease (COPD): Patients with COPD often have right-sided heart failure that may cause liver enlargement.	*Auscultate:* Breath sounds.
Area/System: Cardiovascular *Ask about:*	*Measure:*
History of cerebrovascular disease (CVD), HTN, CHF: Cardiac disease often mimics GI complaints. CHF can cause liver enlargement and ascites.	Vital signs.
Abdominal pain: Pain associated with a pulsating mass may indicate an abdominal aortic aneurysm.	*Palpate:* Pulses for thrills. *Auscultate:* *Heart for extra sounds (S_3) and bruits:* S_3 sign of CHF; bruits and thrills may be a sign of an abdominal aortic aneurysm.
Area/System: Genitourinary/ Reproductive *Ask about:*	*Inspect:*
Color of urine: Dark yellow, orange, or brown urine can be caused by excessive breakdown of red blood cells or liver problems. Blood in the urine is caused by renal calculi, renal infarct,	Color of urine. External genitalia for lesions or discharge. *Sexually transmitted disease (STD):* May cause painful oral lesions that affect patient's nutritional status.

(continued)

Assessment of the Abdomen's Relationship to Other Systems (continued)

SUBJECTIVE DATA/RATIONALE	OBJECTIVE DATA/RATIONALE
Area/System: Genitourinary/ Reproductive *(cont'd)*	
glomerulonephritis, or pyelonephritis. *Urinary burning, frequency, hesitancy:* Urinary tract infections can cause flank pain and costovertebral angle tenderness. *History of STDs:* Unprotected sex increases the risk for STDs for both men and women, which in turn may affect the GI system.	*Acquired immunodeficiency syndrome (AIDS):* Associated with weight loss and viral and fungal infections that affect the GI tract, causing diarrhea, abdominal pain, stomatitis, esophagitis, and gastritis. *Palpate:*
Women:	Bladder for distension.
LMP: Important to rule out pregnancy in women of childbearing age. After menopause, bleeding may signal a gynecological problem. Amenorrhea may indicate an eating disorder such as anorexia nervosa.	Kidneys. Prostate. *Percuss:* Costovertebral angle for tenderness.
Vaginal discharge: May indicate vaginal infection that could lead to pelvic inflammatory disease (PID).	
Men:	
Prostate problems: Difficulty starting urine stream or urinary hesitancy indicates possible prostate disease in men.	*Women:* Perform pelvic examination. *Men:* Perform rectal examination.
Penile discharge: Related to STDs.	
Area/System: Musculoskeletal *Ask about:*	*Measure:*
History of fractures, joint pain, weakness: Arthritis and osteoporosis are extraintestinal complications of ulcerative colitis. Splenomegaly is associated with rheumatoid arthritis.	Height for loss. *Inspect:* Spinal curves. Joints. Range of motion (ROM). *Palpate:* Muscle strength. *Arthritis and osteoporosis:* Extraintestinal complications of ulcerative colitis. • *Rheumatoid arthritis:* Associated with splenomegaly. • *Muscle weakness:* Lack of protein intake or absorption problems.

SUBJECTIVE DATA/RATIONALE	OBJECTIVE DATA/RATIONALE
	Muscle twitching: Associated with loss of electrolytes from diarrhea.
Area/System: Neurologic *Ask about:*	*Test:*
Alcohol use: A deficiency of vitamin B_1 (thiamine) may present with numbness or paresthesias in the extremities and is commonly seen in alcoholics and people with long-standing diarrhea.	Sensation. *Numbness/paresthesias in extremities:* Vitamin B_1 deficiency, commonly seen in alcoholics and people with long-standing diarrhea. ***Disc problems such as cauda equina syndrome:* Loss of bowel and bladder control. This is a medical emergency; patient should seek immediate medical attention.**
Numbness.	Deep tendon reflex (DTR).
Back problems.	
Loss of bowel/bladder control: Can occur with disk problems, such as cauda equina syndrome.	
Area/System: Endocrine *Ask about:*	
History of diabetes: Diabetes can result in gastroparesis, polyuria, and polydipsia.	
Thyroid problems: Thyroid disease can affect weight, appetite, and bowel patterns.	
Area/System: Immunological/ Hematological *Ask about:*	*Inspect:*
Food allergies: May cause GI tract pain and changes in bowel habits.	Lymph nodes for enlargement.
Infection: Patients with AIDS have problems maintaining their weight. Risk of an enlarged tender spleen.	*Palpate:* Lymph nodes. Spleen.
Sickle cell anemia: Often causes abdominal pain.	

HEENT = Head, eyes, ears, nose, and throat.

Physical Assessment

ANATOMICAL LANDMARKS: Four quadrants; nine regions (Boxes 9.2 and 9.3).

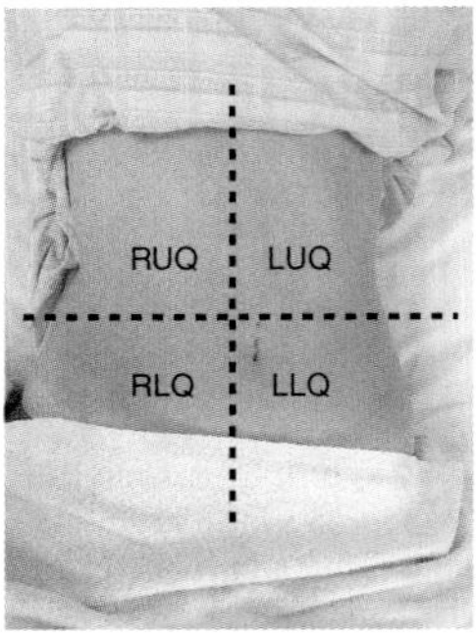

Four-quadrant method

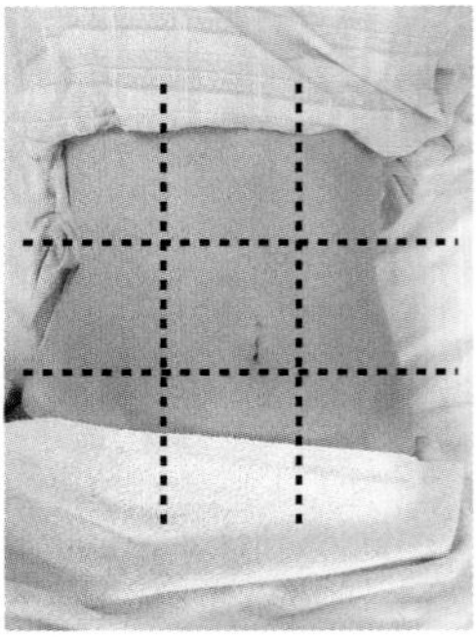

Nine regions of the abdomen

BOX 9.2 Four-Quadrant Method

RIGHT UPPER QUADRANT	LEFT UPPER QUADRANT
Liver	Left lobe of liver
Gallbladder	Spleen
Pylorus	Stomach
Duodenum	Body of pancreas
Head of pancreas	Left adrenal gland
Right adrenal gland	Portion of left kidney
Portion of right kidney	Splenic flexure of colon
Hepatic flexure of colon	Portions of transverse and descending colon
Portions of ascending and transverse colon	

RIGHT LOWER QUADRANT	LEFT LOWER QUADRANT
Lower portion of right kidney	Lower section of left kidney
Cecum and appendix	Sigmoid colon
Portion of ascending colon	Descending colon
Bladder (if distended)	Bladder (if distended)
Ovary and salpinx	Ovary and salpinx

RIGHT LOWER QUADRANT	LEFT LOWER QUADRANT
Uterus (if enlarged)	Uterus (if enlarged)
Right spermatic cord	Left spermatic cord
Right ureter	Left ureter

MIDLINE
Aorta
Uterus (if enlarged)
Bladder (if enlarged)
Spine

BOX 9.3 Nine Regions of the Abdomen

RIGHT HYPO-CHONDRIAC	EPIGASTRIC	LEFT HYPO-CHONDRIAC
Right lobe of liver	Pylorus	Stomach
Gallbladder	Duodenum	Spleen
Duodenum	Head of pancreas	Pancreas tail
Hepatic flexure	Portion of liver	Splenic flexure
Portion of right kidney	Aorta	Upper portion of left kidney
Suprarenal gland	Spine	Suprarenal gland
RIGHT LUMBAR	**UMBILICAL**	**LEFT LUMBAR**
Portion of right kidney	Lower duodenum	Descending colon
Hepatic flexure of colon	Jejunum and ileum	Lower half of left kidney
Ascending colon	Aorta	Jejunum and ileum
Duodenum	Spine	
Jejunum		
RIGHT INGUINAL	**HYPOGASTRIC**	**LEFT INGUINAL**
Cecum	Ileum	Sigmoid colon
Appendix	Bladder	Left ureter
Ileum	Uterus (if enlarged)	Left spermatic cord
Right ureter	Aorta	Left ovary
Right spermatic cord	Spine	
Right ovary		

APPROACH: Inspection, auscultation, percussion, palpation.

POSITION: Supine, or with knees slightly flexed with a pillow under knees to relax abdominal muscles.

TOOLBOX: Stethoscope (bell and diaphragm), pen, metric ruler, reflex hammer or tongue blade to assess abdominal reflexes. *Remember: Always listen before palpating!*

Physical Assessment

AREA/PA SKILL	NORMAL FINDINGS	ABNORMAL FINDINGS
Inspection **Inspect from side and foot of bed. Have patient void before examination.**		
Abdomen		
Note size, shape, and symmetry of abdomen. 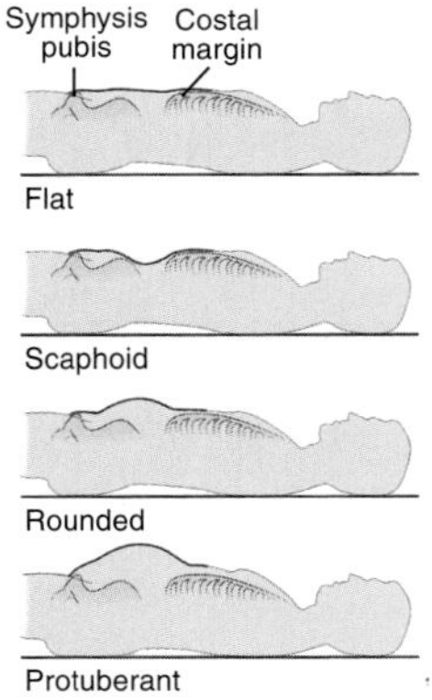 *Shapes of abdomen*	Skin color consistent or slightly lighter than exposed areas. No lesions, striae, superficial veins, scars, rashes, or discoloration.	*Jaundice:* Liver disease.
Note condition of skin, color, lesions, scars, striae, superficial veins, and hair distribution.	Hair distribution appropriate for age and gender of patient.	*Redness:* Inflammation. *Cyanosis:* Hypoxia.
Note abdominal movements: respiratory, peristalsis, and pulsations.	Abdomen flat or slightly rounded and symmetrical, no bulges or hernias.	

AREA/PA SKILL	NORMAL FINDINGS	ABNORMAL FINDINGS
Note position, contour, color, and herniation of the umbilicus.	+ Respiratory movements, slight pulsation noted in epigastric region, no peristaltic waves.	*Cullen's sign around umbilicus:* Hemorrhagic pancreatitis or intraperitoneal bleeding.
Have patient raise head off bed and look for bulges (hernias). 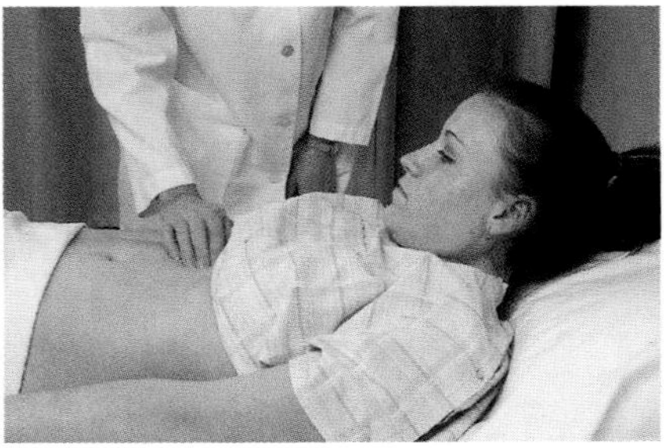 *Lifting head to accentuate hernia*	Umbilicus midline, inverted, no discoloration or discharge.	*Grey-Turner's sign in flank areas:* Pancreatitis or extraperitoneal bleeding. *Bruises:* Recent trauma. *Pink-purple striae:* Cushing's syndrome. *Spider angioma:* Liver failure. *Caput medusa:* Liver failure. *Dermatomally distributed vesicular rash on lower rib cage in upper quadrants:* Herpes zoster. Hernias are caused by weakness of abdominal muscles. Seen as bulges that occur when patient bears down. Occur on old surgical incisions, around umbilicus, or in inguinal area. Epigastric or linea alba hernias occur when intestine protrudes through opening in midline of abdomen above umbilicus. Diastasis recti occurs in pregnant women and newborns. *Protrusion of umbilicus:* Umbilical hernia. Underlying mass causes umbilicus to deviate from midline.

(box continued on page 264)

Physical Assessment (continued)

AREA/PA SKILL	NORMAL FINDINGS	ABNORMAL FINDINGS
Inspection *Abdomen (cont'd)*		*Asymmetry:* Tumors, cysts, bowel obstruction, organomegaly, or scoliosis. *Abdominal distention is caused by "Nine Fs":* Fat, fluid, feces, fetus, flatus, fibroid, full bladder, false pregnancy, or fatal tumor. Area of abdomen that is distended can pinpoint cause: • *Right lower quadrant and left lower quadrant:* Pregnancy, ovarian or uterine tumor, bladder enlargement. • *Left and right upper quadrants:* Pancreatic cyst or tumor or gastric distension. • *Asymmetrical:* Tumor, hernia, cyst, bowel obstruction. *Concave abdomen:* Malnutrition. *Increased peristaltic waves:* Intestinal obstruction. *Reverse peristaltic waves:* Pyloric stenosis. *Shallow respirations in male patients:* Abdominal pain. *Increased/diffuse pulsations:* Aortic aneurysm.

AREA/PA SKILL	NORMAL FINDINGS	ABNORMAL FINDINGS
Auscultation **Use the diaphragm of the stethoscope for bowel sounds and friction rubs. Use the bell for vascular sounds.** *Abdomen, Liver, and Arteries*		
Listen for bowel sounds in each quadrant.	Soft, medium-pitched bowel sounds every 5 to 15 seconds in all four quadrants.	*Bowel sounds more than 30 clicks/min:* Hyperactive bowel sounds or hyperperistalsis; caused by irritable bowel disease, bowel infection, early bowel obstruction, diarrhea, resolving paralytic ileus, or laxative use.
Listen for at least 5 minutes before saying that bowel sounds are absent.	No borborygmi, bruits, hums, or rubs.	Types of hyperperistalsis include borborygmi and succussion splash.
If you are having difficulty hearing bowel sounds, listen over ileocecal valve to the right of the umbilicus in the right lower quadrant.		*Bowel sounds < 5 clicks/min but present:* Hypoactive bowel sounds or hypoperistalsis; caused by peritonitis, medications such as opioids, bowel obstruction, or postoperative occurrence.
Use scratch test to locate the inferior edge of the liver. 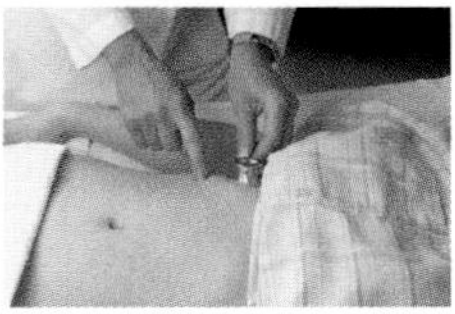 *Scratch test*	Lower edge of liver located at costal margin by scratch test.	*Absent bowel sounds:* Late bowel obstruction, peritonitis, paralytic ileus following manipulation of the bowel during surgery.

(box continued on page 266)

Physical Assessment (continued)

AREA/PA SKILL	NORMAL FINDINGS	ABNORMAL FINDINGS
Auscultation *(cont'd)* Auscultate for bruits over the aorta and renal, iliac, and femoral arteries. If indicated, auscultate for venous hum over liver. If indicated, auscultate for friction rubs over organs.		A bruit with a systolic and diastolic component is abnormal. Cause depends on area where it is heard: • *Aortic:* Aortic aneurysm. • *Epigastric:* Renal artery stenosis. • *Aortic, iliac, or femoral:* Arterial insufficiency. *Venous hums:* Venous portal hypertension (HTN) and liver disease. *Cruveilhier-Baumgarten murmur:* Portal HTN. *Friction rub:* Inflammation of peritoneal surface of an organ from tumor, infection, or infarct. • *Splenic friction rubs:* Infection, abscess, infarction, or tumor; best heard at lower rib cage in left anterior axillary line. • *Liver friction rubs:* Liver cancer or abscess; can be auscultated over lower right sternal border.

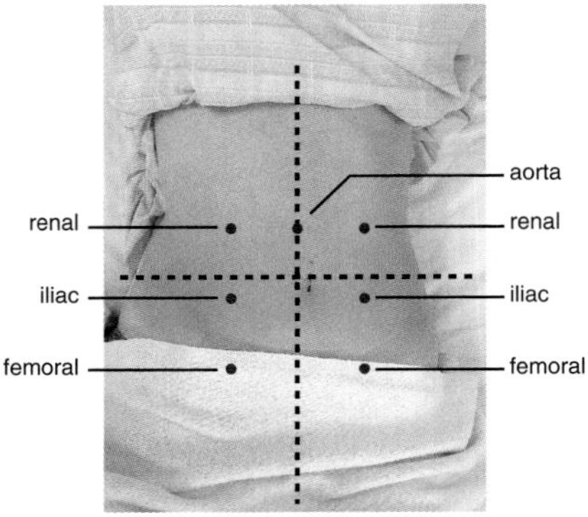

Auscultating sites for vascular sounds

AREA/PA SKILL	NORMAL FINDINGS	ABNORMAL FINDINGS
Percussion Use indirect (mediate) percussion in all four quadrants. 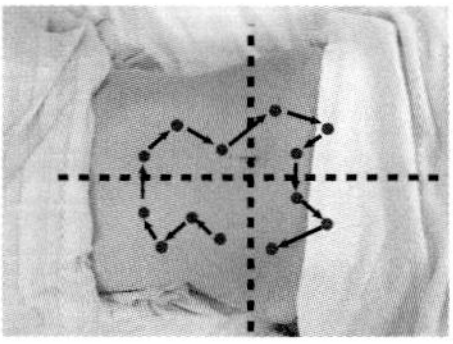 *Percussion sites*		
Abdomen, Organs (Liver, Gallbladder, Spleen, Kidneys) Note areas of tympany, dullness, tenderness.	Tympany in all four quadrants, dullness over organs.	*Extremely high-pitched tympanic sounds:* Distension.
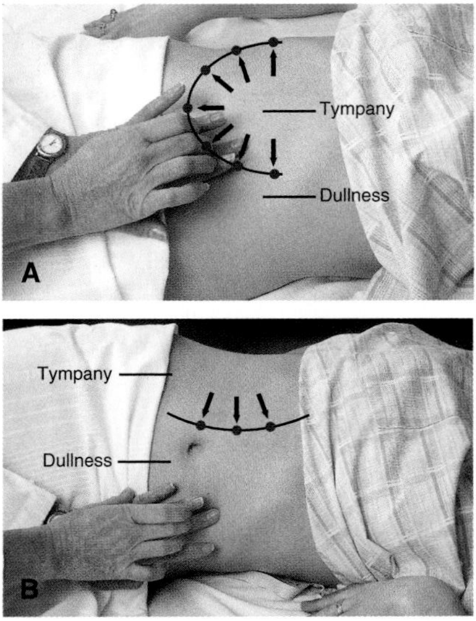 *A. Percussing shifting dullness with patient supine, B. Percussing shifting dullness with patient on side*		

(box continued on page 268)

Physical Assessment (continued)

AREA/PA SKILL	NORMAL FINDINGS	ABNORMAL FINDINGS
Percussion *Abdomen, Organs (Liver, Gallbladder, Spleen, Kidneys) (cont'd)*		
Percuss tender areas last.		*Extensive dullness:* Organ enlargement or underlying mass.
Measure liver size at the right midclavicular line (RMCL). If enlarged, do measurement at midsternal line. Locate gastric bubble over stomach.	Liver 6 to 12 cm at RMCL. Liver 4 to 8 cm at the midsternal line	*Liver span > 12 cm:* Hepatomegaly.
Locate splenic dullness at left midaxillary line (LMAL). Another way to assess the spleen is to percuss the left anterior axillary line. Have patient take deep breath and note percussion sound.	Splenic dullness at 9th, 10th, 11th ribs at LMAL, < 7 cm. LAA line remains tympanic with deep inspiration.	*Splenic upper border percussed beyond 8 cm above costal margin:* Enlarged spleen caused by portal HTN, thrombosis, stenosis, atresia, deformities of splenic vein, cysts, cancer, mononucleosis, trauma, and infection (as long as patient does not have a full stomach or intestines). Dullness with inspiration at the LAA line suggest enlargement.

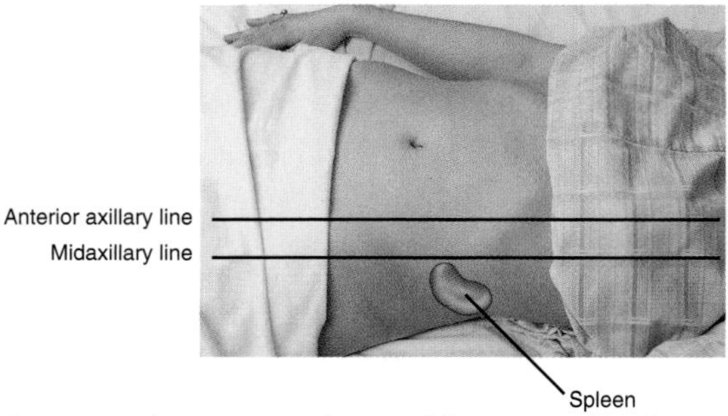

Percussing at lowest intercostal space at left anterior axillary line

AREA/PA SKILL	NORMAL FINDINGS	ABNORMAL FINDINGS
Bladder		
If indicated, percuss for bladder dullness at the midline above the symphsis pubis. If ascites is present, percuss for shifting dullness.	Normally not percussed.	*Dullness in suprapubic area:* Full bladder (for other causes, see section on abdominal contour and distension).
If indicated, use fist (blunt) percussion to assess for organ (liver or gallbladder) tenderness. Check for kidney tenderness at posterior costovertebral angle.	Organs nontender.	*Severe pain or costovertebral angle tenderness:* Kidney infection or musculoskeletal problem.

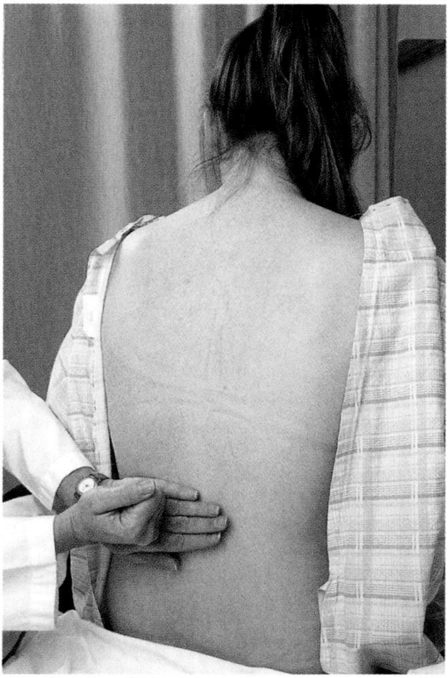

Checking for CVA tenderness

(box continued on page 270)

Physical Assessment (continued)

AREA/PA SKILL	NORMAL FINDINGS	ABNORMAL FINDINGS
Palpation **Begin with light palpation, then deep, bimanual in all four quadrants.** **If patient is tense (voluntary guarding), have patient slightly flex knees or let patient hold your hand as you palpate.**		
Abdomen, Organs, and Aorta		
Use light palpation to identify surface characteristics, tenderness, muscular resistance, and turgor, and to put patient at ease. Assess the umbilicus for bulges or nodules.	Abdomen soft and nontender, no masses, + skin turgor, no umbilical bulges.	*Involuntary guarding and rigidity:* Peritonitis.
Do not palpate abdomen if large, diffuse pulsations are present or if patient has history of organ transplant or known or suspected Wilms' tumor.		*Areas of tenderness:* Underlying problem.
Use deep palpation with bimanual technique to palpate organs (liver, spleen, kidneys) and masses. Note tenderness, consistency, pulsations, enlarged organs. Palpate aorta; note pulsation, size, and diffusion. 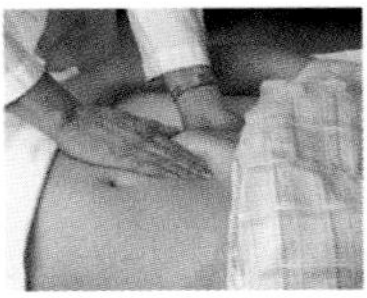 *Palpating the liver*	Liver nonpalpable or liver's edge may be palpable at costal margin, firm, smooth, and nontender. Spleen nontender, nonpalpable. Kidneys nonpalpable. Right kidney may be palpable in thin women. + Nonpalpable aortic pulsation or slight aortic pulsation, no diffusion, aorta 2.5 cm.	*Masses:* Underlying tumor, enlarged uterus, feces-filled colon. *Enlarged liver:* Cirrhosis, tumor, hepatitis. *Enlarged spleen:* Malignancy, infection, trauma to spleen. *Lateral diffuse pulsation:* Abdominal aortic aneurysm. *Aortic width > 3 cm:* Abdominal aortic aneurysm. *Liver palpable below costal margin:* Congestive heart failure (CHF), hepatitis,

AREA/PA SKILL	NORMAL FINDINGS	ABNORMAL FINDINGS
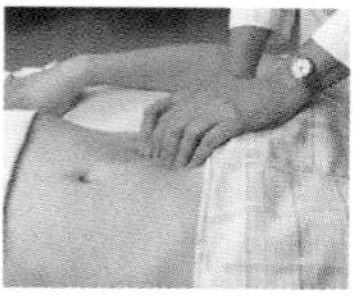 *Hooking technique* 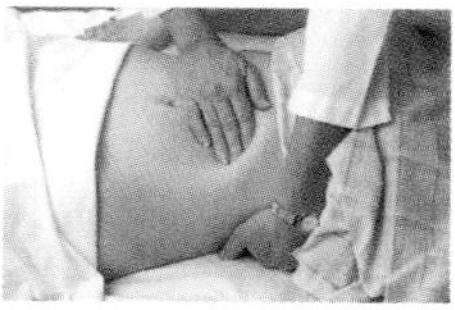 *Palpating the spleen* 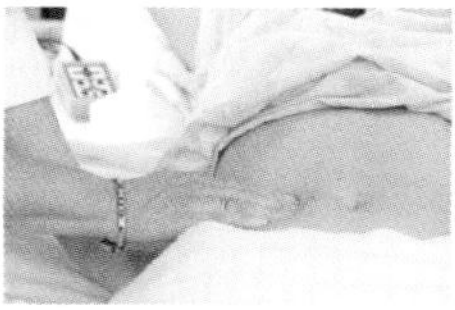 *Palpating the kidneys*		encephalopathy, cirrhosis, cysts, cancer. If liver is enlarged, tender, firm, and nodular or has an irregular border, suspect liver cancer. *Splenic enlargement and tenderness:* Infection, CHF, cancer, cirrhosis, trauma. *Enlarged kidneys:* Hydronephrosis, neoplasm, polycystic disease. *Kidney tenderness:* Trauma or infection. *Nodular or asymmetrical bladder:* Possible malignancy.
If indicated, assess for rebound tenderness at McBurney's point and perform the iliopsoas test and the obturator test. 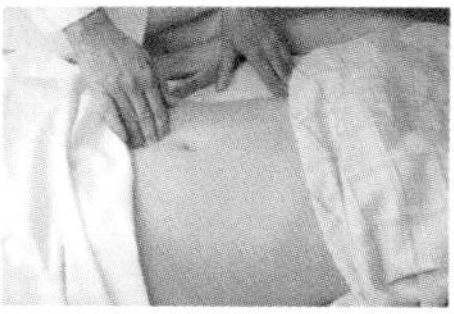 *McBurney's point* 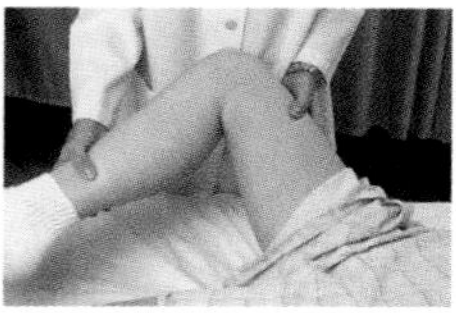 *Obdurator muscle test*	Negative rebound.	*+ Rebound tenderness, iliopsoas, and obturator signs:* Peritoneal inflammation, peritonitis, appendicitis.

(box continued on page 272)

Physical Assessment (continued)

AREA/PA SKILL	NORMAL FINDINGS	ABNORMAL FINDINGS
Palpation *Abdomen, Organs, and Aorta (cont'd)* 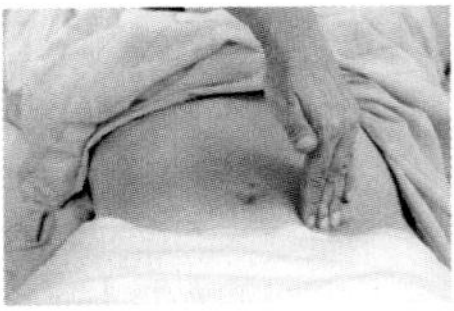 *Rovsing's sing* 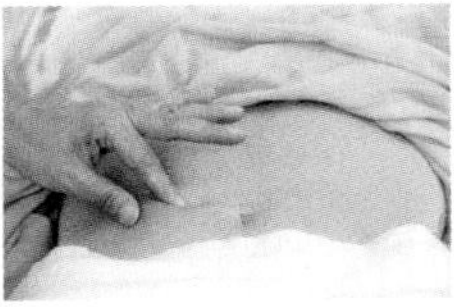 *Cutaneous hypersensitivity* 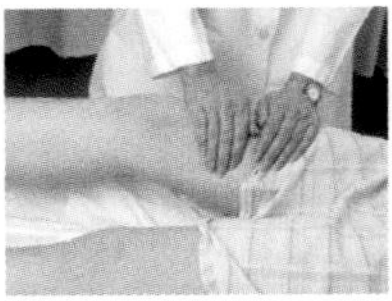 *Iliopsoas muscle test*		
To test for fluid, perform the fluid wave test. 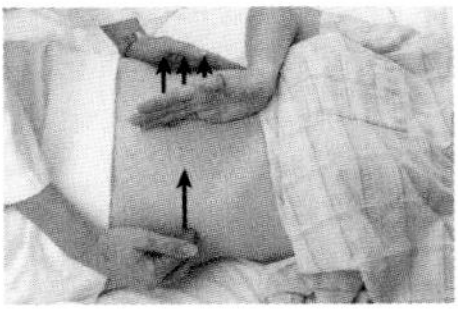 *Fluid wave test*		*+ Fluid wave, shifting dullness, puddle sign:* Ascites.
Use ballottement to assess fetal position or masses. 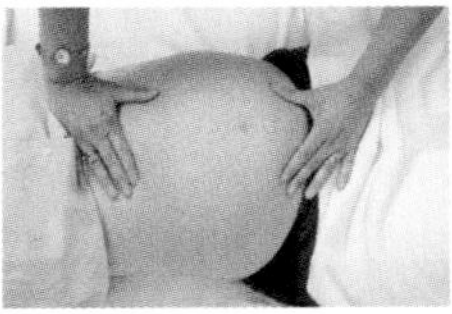 *Ballottement*		*Free-floating mass in abdomen:* Malignant or benign tumor. *+ Kehr's sign:* Splenic injury, renal calculi, ectopic pregnancy. *+ Ballance's sign:* Peritoneal irritation, splenic injury. *+ Murphy's sign:* Cholecystitis.

AREA/PA SKILL	NORMAL FINDINGS	ABNORMAL FINDINGS
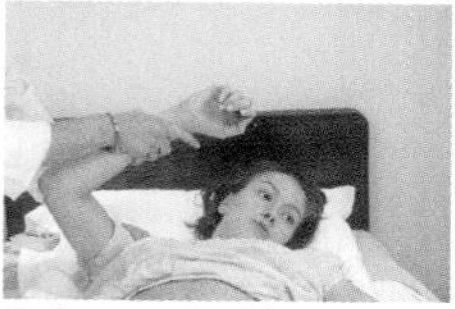 *Palpating shoulder to elicit Kehr's sign*		
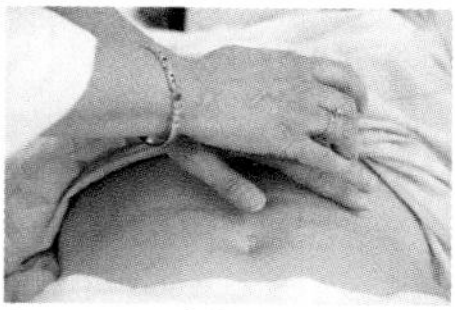 *Percussing left upper quadrant to elicit Balance's sign*		
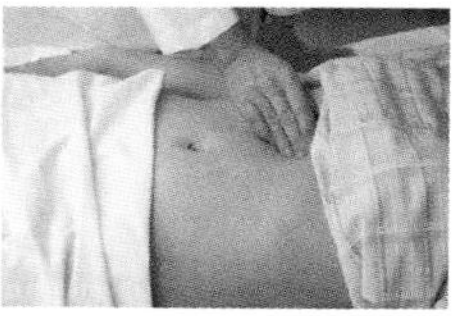 *Palpating at RMCL to elicit Murphy's sign*		
Test abdominal reflexes by lightly stroking each quadrant toward the umbilicus. 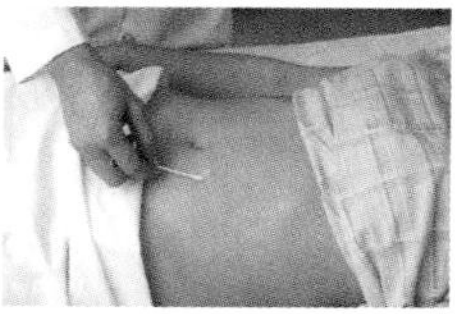 *Assessing abdominal reflexes*	+ Abdominal reflexes.	*Absent abdominal reflexes:* Pyramidal tract lesion. *Absent upper abdominal reflexes:* Problems at spinal levels T8 through T10. *Absent lower abdominal reflexes:* Problems at spinal levels T10 through T12.

(box continued on page 274)

Physical Assessment (continued)

AREA/PA SKILL	NORMAL FINDINGS	ABNORMAL FINDINGS
Palpation *Abdomen, Organs, and Aorta (cont'd)* If patient is ticklish, have him or her place a hand over the abdomen, and then place yours over it and do light palpation. When the patient starts to feel more relaxed, slip your hand underneath. If you detect a mass, have patient tighten his or her abdominal muscles. This helps you feel the mass better. But if the mass is deep in the abdomen below the muscles, it will be difficult to palpate.		
Inguinal Lymph Nodes Use light palpation to palpate horizontal and vertical inguinal nodes. Note size, shape, consistency, tenderness, mobility.	Inguinal nodes nonpalpable, nontender.	*Tender, unmovable nodes > 1 cm:* Infection, cancer, lymphoma.

PA = Physical assessment.

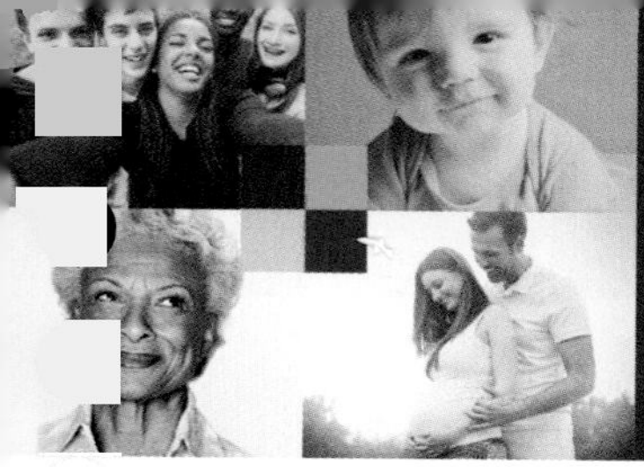

CHAPTER 10

Assessing the Female Genitourinary System

Primary Functions

- Manufacturing and protecting ova for fertilization
- Transporting the fertilized ovum for implantation and embryonic/fetal development
- Housing and nourishing the developing fetus
- Regulating hormonal production and secretion of several sex hormones
- Providing sexual stimulation and pleasure
- Providing a drainage site for the excretion of urine (urinary structures)

Developmental Considerations

Infants

- Female infant's genitals are enlarged at birth in response to maternal estrogen.
- Hormonal effect may also cause pseudomenstruation.

Children and Adolescents

- The female child begins puberty changes any time from 8 to 13 years of age (Table 10.1).

Pregnant Patients

- The uterus becomes hypertrophied, and its capacity increases to 500 to 1000 times its nonpregnant state.
- The vascularity of the cervix increases and contributes to softening of the cervix.

TABLE 10.1 Maturation States in Girls

Stage 1

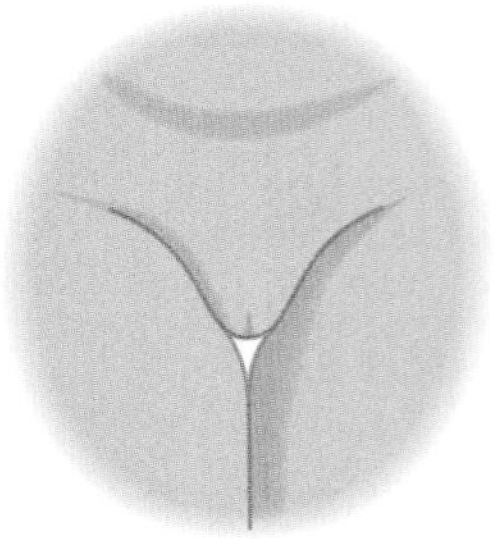

Hair distribution in the preadolescent: There is no pubic hair except for fine body hair similar to hair on the abdomen.

Stage 2

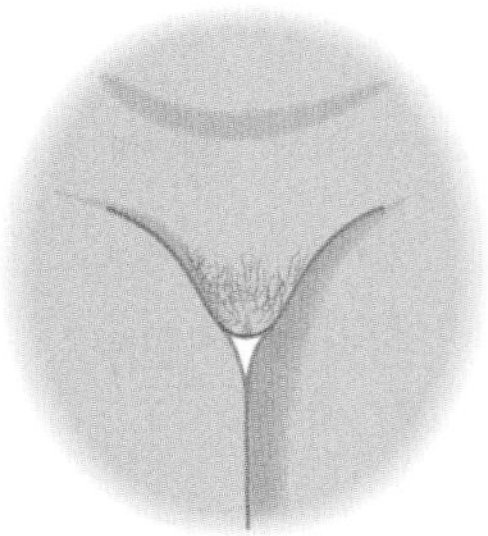

Sparse growth of long, slightly pigmented, downy hair, straight or only slightly curled, mostly along the labia.

Stage 3

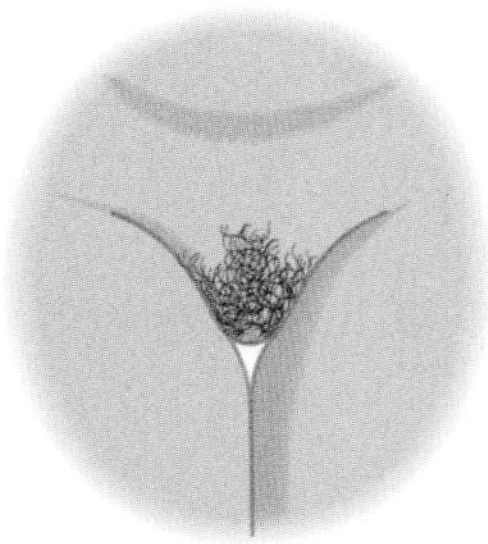

Hair is darker, coarser, and curly and spreads sparsely over the pubic symphysis.

Stage 4

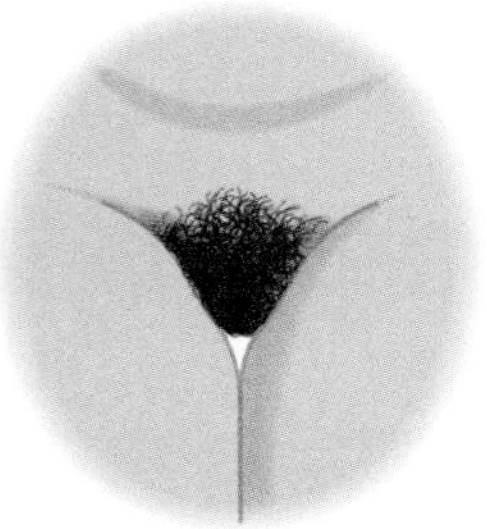

Pubic hair is coarser and curlier, as in adults. It covers more area than in stage 3, but not as great as in the adult.

Stage 5

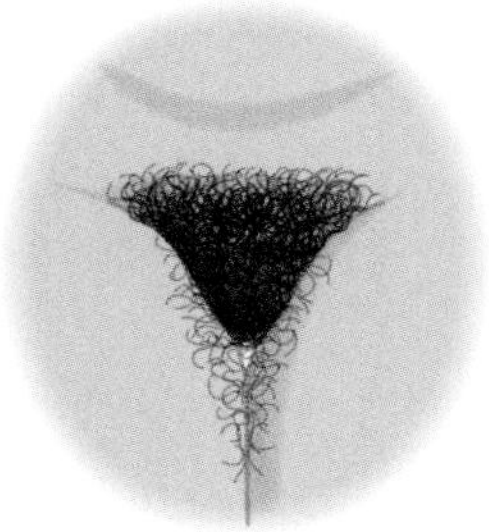

The quality and quantity are consistent with adult pubic hair distribution and spread over medial surfaces of thighs but not over the abdomen.

- The vascular congestion creates a blue-purple blemish or change in the cervical color (Chadwick's sign).
- Estrogen causes the glandular cervical tissue to produce a thick mucus, which builds up and forms a mucus plug at the endocervical canal.
- The vaginal wall softens and relaxes to accommodate the movement of the infant during birth.

Older Adults

- Around the age of 46 to 55 years, menstrual periods become shorter and less frequent until they stop entirely.

- Menopause is said to have occurred when the woman has not experienced a menstrual period in more than a year.
- Sexual organs atrophy; the clitoris becomes smaller; and vaginal secretions are not as plentiful. Painful intercourse may result.
- Vaginal changes increase the risk for vaginal infections.

Cultural Considerations

Cultural/Ethnic Views of Women

CULTURE	VIEW OF WOMEN
Amish	High status associated with role of wife and mother. Responsibilities include feeding, clothing, and caring for family.
Appalachian	High status associated with motherhood. Having children associated with fulfillment. Responsible for child rearing. Older women preserve culture. Responsible for preparing herbal medicines and folk medicine.
Arab American	Women gain status with age. Responsible for caring and educating children and tending to husband's needs.
Chinese American	Woman's role is to perpetuate male dominance.
Cuban American	Women expected to stay at home and care for children.
Egyptian American	Status and power increase with pregnancy and birthing, especially of a son. This is expected within 1 year of marriage.
Filipino American	Women have equal role with men in health, welfare, and family finance.
Greek American	Pregnancy seen as a time of great respect.
Iranian American	Prestige associated with having children.
Jewish American	Woman runs home and is responsible for children.
Mexican American	Woman maintains home and health of family.
Navajo Native American (Indian)	Mother is the center of Indian society.
Vietnamese American	Women expected to be dutiful and respectful of husband and to make healthcare decisions.

Assessment

History

Symptoms ("PQRST" Any + Symptom)

- Vaginal discharge
  - When did you first notice the vaginal discharge?
  - Do you have any itching in the genital area?
  - What color is the discharge? Is there an odor to the discharge?
  - Is the amount of discharge small, moderate, or large?
- Lesions
  - When did you first notice the rash, blisters, ulcers, sores, or warts on your genital area or surrounding area?
  - Does your sex partner have any of the same symptoms?
  - Is the lesion painful?
  - Have you ever had a sexually transmitted disease (STD)? If so, what was it? What treatment did you have for it?
- Vaginal bleeding
  - How often do you have any vaginal bleeding outside the time of your normal menstrual period?
  - When did/does it occur?
  - How would you describe the bleeding? Spotty, small, moderate, large amount?
  - Is it more than your normal period?
  - How much bleeding occurs? (Clarify by asking numbers of pads or tampons used in 24 hours.)
  - What method of birth control do you use?
  - When was your last menstrual period (LMP)?
  - Describe your "normal flow."
- Pain (dysmenorrhea)
  - Describe the pain: Is it dull, sharp, radiating, intermittent, continuous?
  - When did the pain start?
  - Are you having any pain in the area now?
  - What makes the pain better or worse?
  - Do you have any associated symptoms of headache, vomiting, or diarrhea?

- Amenorrhea
  - What is your menstrual history?
  - What is your pregnancy history?
  - What is your sexual history?
  - Do you use prescription or over-the-counter (OTC) drugs? If so, what?
  - Do you exercise every day? What type of exercise and what is the duration of the activity?
  - Can you describe any emotional stresses you have?
  - What are your eating habits?
- Urinary symptoms
  - Do you have pain when voiding?
  - Describe the pain.
  - How often do you void and how much at one time?
  - Do you take showers or tub baths (bubble baths)?
  - How many times do you get up at night to void?
  - How long have you had the symptoms?
  - Do you have pain in any other area?

Sexual History

- Have you ever been sexually active?
- Are you currently sexually active? That is, have you had sex with anyone in the past few months? If the answer is yes, answer next question.
- Do you have sex with men, women, or both (heterosexual, homosexual, or bisexual)?
- Type of sexual activity (oral, vaginal, or anal)?
- Do you have more than one partner? How many partners have you had in the last 6 months? Number of lifetime partners? Do you trade sexual favors for drugs or money?
- Are you using birth control? What kind? How often?
- Are you worried about the acquired immunodeficiency syndrome (AIDS) virus or other STDs?
- Do you take any precautions to avoid infections? If so, what?
- Do you have any problems or concerns about your sexual function?
- Have you had surgery on any of your reproductive organs? If so, what and when?
- Are you taking any medications, prescribed or OTC (Table 10.2)?

Reproductive/Menstrual/Sexuality History

AREAS TO INVESTIGATE	RATIONALE/ SIGNIFICANCE
Menstrual Period	
Age of menarche, LMP, length of cycle, regularity of cycle, duration of menses, character and amount of flow, amenorrhea, menorrhagia, dysmenorrhea, spotting.	Late onset of menarche (by age 16–18) can result from inadequate nutrition caused by eating disorders, chronic diseases such as Crohn's disease, environmental stresses, intensive athletic training, hypothyroidism, or the use of opiates or steroids.
Premenstrual Syndrome	
Breast tenderness; bloating; moodiness; cravings for salt, sugar, or chocolate; fatigue; weight gain; headaches; joint pain.	Uncomfortable signs and symptoms may be alleviated by offering instruction about stress-reducing techniques and avoidance of certain foods.
Obstetrical History	
LMP, use of fertility drugs, previous pregnancies, number of living children, number of abortions or miscarriages, complications with pregnancy, duration of labor, postpartum complications.	Past obstetrical health is a predictor of future reproductive health.
Perimenopause	
Spotting, hot flashes, palpitations, numbness, tingling, drenching sweats, mood swings, vaginal dryness, itching, use of estrogen replacement therapy, feelings about menopause.	Women may have various discomforting signs and symptoms associated with menopause. Hormonal and physical changes relate to changes in self-concept. Identifying symptoms can help plan appropriate interventions for your client.
Sexual Functioning History	
Frequency of intercourse; number of sexual partners; ability to achieve orgasm; heterosexual, bisexual, homosexual; sexual practices; trading of sex for drugs or money.	Changes in sexual functioning may indicate pain, infection, hormonal changes, disease, change in mental status, or altered role and relationship patterns. Sexual preferences and practices may increase risk for certain diseases or cross-contamination to other areas. Risk of STDs, HIV/AIDS, hepatitis, cervical carcinoma, and dysplasias increases with increase in number of partners.

(continued)

Reproductive/Menstrual/Sexuality History (continued)

AREAS TO INVESTIGATE	RATIONALE/ SIGNIFICANCE
Contraceptive History	
Use of contraceptives (if used, types used, frequency, methods used to prevent STDs, problems with contraceptive use, smoking history).	Intrauterine devices increase the risk of PID. Diaphragms may cause urinary discomfort. A client may be allergic to spermicides or latex. Oral contraceptives have a variety of side effects. Smokers' use of oral contraceptives increases the risk for cardiovascular problems. Obtaining this history is an opportunity to provide the client with education about the methods used for contraception.

TABLE 10.2 Drugs That Adversely Affect the Female Reproductive System

DRUG CLASS	DRUG	POSSIBLE ADVERSE REACTIONS
Androgens	Danazol	Vaginitis with itching, dryness, burning, or bleeding; amenorrhea
	Fluoxymesterone, methyltestosterone, testosterone	Amenorrhea and other menstrual irregularities; virilization, including clitoral enlargement
Antidepressants	Tricyclic antidepressants	Changed libido, menstrual irregularity
	Selective serotonin reuptake inhibitors	Decreased libido, anorgasmia
Antihypertensives	Clonidine, reserpine	Decreased libido
	Methyldopa	Decreased libido, amenorrhea
Antipsychotics	Chlorpromazine, perphenazine, prochlorperazine, thioridazine, trifluoperazine, haloperidol	Inhibition of ovulation (chlorpromazine only), menstrual irregularities, amenorrhea, changed libido
Beta-blockers	Qtenolol, labetalol hydrochloride, nadolol, propranolol hydrochloride, metoprolol	Decreased libido
Cardiac glycosides	Digoxin	Changes in cellular layer of vaginal walls in postmenopausal women

DRUG CLASS	DRUG	POSSIBLE ADVERSE REACTIONS
Corticosteroids	Dexamethasone, hydrocortisone, prednisone	Amenorrhea and menstrual irregularities
Cytotoxics	Busulfan	Amenorrhea with menopausal symptoms in premenopausal women, ovarian suppression, ovarian fibrosis and atrophy
	Chlorambucil	Amenorrhea
	Cyclophosphamide	Gonadal suppression (possibly irreversible), amenorrhea, ovarian fibrosis
	Methotrexate	Menstrual dysfunction, infertility
	Tamoxifen	Vaginal discharge or bleeding, menstrual irregularities, pruritus vulvae (intense itching of the female external genitalia)
	Thiotepa	Amenorrhea
Estrogens	Conjugated estrogens, esterified estrogens, estradiol, estrone, ethinyl estradiol	Altered menstrual flow, dysmenorrhea, amenorrhea cervical erosion or abnormal secretions, enlargement of uterine fibromas, vaginal candidiasis
	Dienestrol	Vaginal discharge, uterine bleeding with excessive use
Progestins	Medroxyprogesterone acetate, norethindrone, norgestrel, progesterone	Breakthrough bleeding, dysmenorrhea, amenorrhea, cervical erosion, and abnormal secretions
Thyroid hormones	Levothyroxine sodium, thyroid USP, and others	Menstrual irregularities with excessive doses
Miscellaneous	Lithium carbonate,	Decreased libido
	L-tryptophan	Decreased libido
	Spironolactone	Menstrual irregularities, amenorrhea, postmenopausal bleeding
	Valproic acid	Menstrual irregularities, amenorrhea, possible polycystic ovarian syndrome

Assessment of the Female Genitourinary System's Relationship to Other Systems

Remember, all systems are related. As you assess the female genitourinary system, look at the relationship between it and all other systems.

Assessment of the Female Genitourinary System's Relationship to Other Systems

SUBJECTIVE DATA	OBJECTIVE DATA
Area/System: General	
Ask about:	*Measure:*
Changes in energy level: Fatigue or activity intolerance is often a sign of underlying health problem. For example, fatigue from HIV/AIDS would interfere with activity tolerance; fatigue influences desire and ability to perform sexual intercourse and may also be associated with anemia.	*Height and weight:* Height loss may occur in postmenopausal women and may be associated with osteoporosis. Weight loss resulting from anorexia can cause amenorrhea. Weight gain is associated with pregnancy. Unexplained weight loss may be associated with malignancy.
Weight changes: Unexplained weight loss may indicate an endocrine problem or malignancy.	Vital signs, checking for temperature elevations, hypertension (HTN).
Pregnancy	*Inspect:* Signs of discomfort.
Fevers: May be sign of infection.	*Affect:* Depression can affect sexual functioning.
Area/System: Integumentary	
Ask about:	*Inspect for:*
Changes in hair growth: Changes in hair texture, moisture, and distribution occur during pregnancy and menopause.	*Skin lesions:* Rashes and skin lesions are associated with many STDs. • *Systemic rash:* Secondary syphilis. • *Vesicles:* HSV types 1 and 2. • *Increased skin pigmentation:* Increased hormones during pregnancy.
Rashes, lesions: Rashes, growths, and lumps may indicate pathology. Pruritus in hair or on labia may indicate scabies, kidney or liver problems. Estrogen and progesterone can cause changes in skin, hair, and nails, such as those seen during pregnancy and menopause.	Hair distribution • *Alopecia:* Secondary syphilis. • *Abnormal increase in body hair (hirsutism):* Decrease in female hormones.
Area/System: HEENT **Head and neck**	
Ask about:	*Palpate:*
Headaches: A common side effect of oral contraceptives.	*Lymph node enlargement:* Palpable lymph nodes may indicate systemic infection or malignancy.

SUBJECTIVE DATA	OBJECTIVE DATA
Swollen glands, nodes: Swelling of lymph nodes associated with infection, malignancy. Enlarged thyroid may affect sexual function.	*Enlarged thyroid (hypo- or hyperthyroidism):* May affect reproductive and sexual functioning.
Eyes, mouth, and throat *Ask about:*	*Inspect:*
Eye drainage: Gonorrheal eye infections occur in newborns (ophthalmia neonatorum) and gonorrheal conjunctivitis in adults.	*Oral mucosa for redness and lesions:* Oral lesions may be associated with STDs.
Oral lesions, sore throat: Secondary syphilis can result in oral mucous patches.	*Conjunctiva for drainage:* Conjunctivitis can be caused by gonorrhea.
Tearing, photophobia, eyelid edema, conjunctival edema: Chlamydia trachomatis.	
Oropharynx and eyes are sites for STDs, such as HSV 2 and gonorrhea.	
Area/System: Respiratory *Ask about:*	*Inspect:*
History of respiratory disease: Respiratory disease such as chronic obstructive pulmonary disease (COPD) may affect sexual activity.	Signs of respiratory distress. *Auscultate:* *Abnormal breath sounds:* Chronic lung disease may impair sexual functioning.
Area/System: Cardiovascular *Ask about:*	*Inspect:*
History of cardiovascular disease, HTN, thrombophlebitis, heart murmurs: Some heart murmurs are associated with anemia. Cardiovascular symptoms are associated with oral contraceptive use. Chronic cardiovascular disease can affect ability to perform sexually.	Signs of impaired circulation. Skin changes. *Palpate:* Pulses, edema, presence of Homans' sign. **Oral contraceptives associated with increased risk of thrombus formation.** *Auscultate:* *Extra heart sounds:* Anemia can cause tachycardia and a systolic flow murmur.

(continued)

Assessment of the Female Genitourinary System's Relationship to Other Systems (continued)

SUBJECTIVE DATA	OBJECTIVE DATA
Area/System: Breasts	
Ask about:	*Inspect/Palpate:*
Changes in breast, tenderness: Cyclical hormonal changes are associated with breast tenderness. Female hormones are associated with fibrocystic disease and breast cancer.	*Breasts:* Cyclical hormonal changes may cause breast fullness and tenderness.
Area/System: Gastrointestinal	
Ask about:	*Inspect:*
History of liver disease: Associated with gynecological malignancy may cause ascites.	Ascites.
Loss of appetite: May indicate underlying eating disorder, malignancy, or AIDS.	*Palpate/percuss:*
Abdominal pain: May indicate pathology of reproductive organs.	*Liver enlargement:* Enlarged liver and ascites associated with metastasis of gynecological cancers. *Masses:* Palpable abdominal masses may be a fetus or fibroid tumor.
Area/System: Musculoskeletal	
Ask about:	*Test:*
Weakness/limitations.	*Muscle strength:* Weakness or joint pain may limit sexual functioning; weakness or paralysis may indicate neurosyphilis.
Joint pain, swelling.	*Inspect:*
The physical act of sexual intercourse requires the musculoskeletal system to be functional.	*Joint swelling and deformity:* Charcot joints may indicate late syphilis. *Spinal deformities:* Unexplained fractures or spinal changes (dowager's hump) may indicate osteoporosis in postmenopausal women.
Unexplained fracture: Postmenopausal women are at greater risk for developing osteoporosis.	
Area/System: Neurologic	
Ask about:	*Test:*
History of neurologic problems: Amenorrhea may result from problems with hypothalamus of diencephalon.	*Changes in mental status and affect:* May be associated with late syphilis. Post-partum depression.
Paralysis. Tremors. Personality changes.	Sensory deficits.

SUBJECTIVE DATA	OBJECTIVE DATA
Neurosyphilis occurs in late syphilis and can cause paresis, tremors, personality changes, and psychosis.	
Depression: Hormonal fluctuations may affect emotional state (e.g., during pregnancy).	
Area/System: Endocrine	
Ask about:	*Palpate:*
History of diabetes and thyroid disease: Diabetes increases risk for candidal vaginal infections. Hypothyroidism causes menorrhagia, decreased libido, and infertility.	*Thyroid:* May be palpable normally during pregnancy. Enlarged thyroid may indicate thyroid disease and affect menstrual cycle.
Area/System: Lymphatic/ Hematological	
Ask about:	*Palpate:*
History of malignancies, HIV, AIDS: AIDS affects the immune system. Gynecological cancers can metastasize to local lymphatic tissue.	*Lymph nodes:* Palpable lymph nodes may indicate infection or metastatic disease.
Abnormal menses: Heavy menses (menorrhagia) can lead to anemia.	

HEENT = Head, eyes, ears, nose, and throat.

Physical Assessment

APPROACH: Inspection, palpation; external and internal exam

POSITION: Lithotomy

TOOLBOX: Large hand mirror, gooseneck lamp, disposable exam gloves, drape, vaginal specula (Graves' size medium and large are adequate for most sexually active adult women; Pederson size small and medium are useful for non–sexually active women and children), cytological materials (Ayre spatula, cytobrush, cotton-tipped applicators, OB swabs, microscope slides), Thayer-Martin culture plate labeled, cytology fixative spray, reagents (normal saline solution or potassium hydroxide [KOH]), Hemoccult slide and developer, acetic acid, warm water, water-soluble lubricant

Physical Assessment

AREA/PA SKILL	NORMAL FINDINGS	ABNORMAL FINDINGS
Inspection Have patient void before the examination.		
External Genitalia		
Note color, hair distribution, condition of skin, swelling, lesions, polyps, discharge or odor, prolapse, and pediculosis.	External genitalia intact, pink, and moist; color depends on client's pigmentation. Hair distribution depends on age and development of client. No lesions, edema, discharge, odor, or prolapse (bladder, uterus, or rectum). *Normal cervical discharge depends on menstrual cycle:* Clear and stretchy before ovulation, white and opaque after, bloody during menstruation.	Diamond-shaped hair distribution pattern is abnormal if not associated with cultural or familial differences. May indicate hirsutism, an endocrine disorder. *Pubic lice, nits, or flecks of residual blood on skin:* Pediculosis pubis. *Ecchymosis over mons pubis:* Blunt trauma. *Labial varicosities:* Pregnancy or uterine tumor. *Edema:* Hematoma formation, obstruction of lymphatic system, or Bartholin's cyst. *Broken areas of skin surface:* Ulcerations or abrasions from infection or trauma. Rash over mons pubis and labia is abnormal. *Painless, reddish, round ulcer with depressed center, raised with indurated edges (chancre):* Primary stage of syphilis. *White, dry, painless growths with narrow bases:* Condylomata acuminata (venereal warts) caused by human papillomavirus (HPV).

AREA/PA SKILL	NORMAL FINDINGS	ABNORMAL FINDINGS
		Small, red, painful vesicles that progress to the ulcer stage: Herpes simplex virus (HSV). Pruritus may be present. 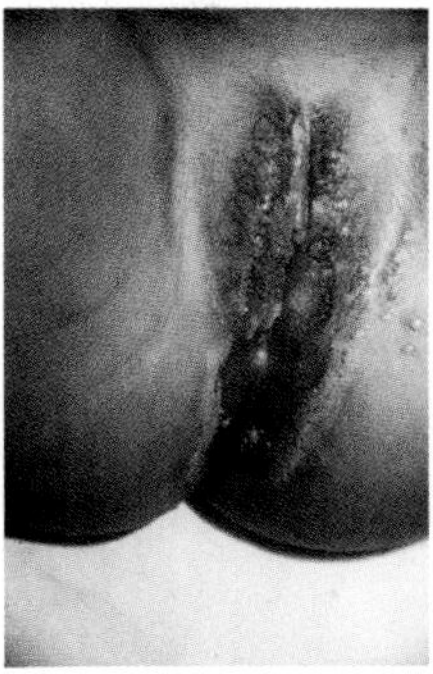 *Herpes vulvovaginitis*
Examine clitoris.	Clitoris about 2 cm long and 0.5 cm in diameter. No redness or lesions.	*Hypertrophy of clitoris:* Female pseudohermaphroditism from androgen excess. Female circumcision is widespread in many African countries and among some Muslim groups.
Inspect urethral meatus for shape, color, and size.	Urethral opening is slitlike, midline, and free of discharge, swelling, redness, or lesions.	*Discharge of any color from urethral meatus:* Urinary tract infection. *Swelling or redness around meatus:* Infection of Skene's glands, urethral caruncle, urethral carcinoma, or prolapse of urethral mucosal.
Inspect introitus for color and moistness of mucosa, discharge or odor, patency, bulging, or tenderness.	Introitus mucosa is pink, moist. Normal discharge is clear to white with no foul odors. Introitus is patent, with no bulging or tenderness.	*Pale color and dryness of introitus mucosa:* Atrophy from topical steroids and aging. Foul-smelling discharge that is not clear to slightly pale white is abnormal.

(box continued on page 290)

Physical Assessment (continued)

AREA/PA SKILL	NORMAL FINDINGS	ABNORMAL FINDINGS
Inspection *External Genitalia (cont'd)*		
		Gonorrhea, chlamydia, Candida, Trichomonas, bacterial vaginosis, atrophic vaginitis, and cervicitis are possible infectious processes that produce an abnormal vaginal discharge. *External tear:* Trauma from sexual activity or abuse. *Fissure:* Congenital malformation or childbirth trauma. *Bulging of anterior vaginal wall:* Cystocele. *Bulging of anterior vaginal wall, bladder, and urethra into vaginal introitus:* Cystourethrocele. *Bulging of posterior vaginal wall:* Rectocele.
Rectal Area		
Note condition of skin, inflammation, rashes, excoriation, rectal prolapse, external hemorrhoids, polyps, lesions, fissures, bleeding, discharge.	Rectal area intact, no inflammation, lesions, prolapse, hemorrhoids, discharge, or bleeding.	*Fissure or tear of perineum:* Trauma, abscess, or unhealed episiotomy. *Venous prominences around anal area:* External hemorrhoids.
Pelvic Examination With Speculum (Use Warm Speculum)		
Note color, lesions, discharge, bleeding, position, size, shape, and symmetry of cervix, shape and patency of os.	Cervix round, midline, pink, no lesions or discharge; os is slit in parous women, round and closed in nulliparous women. Bluish color seen with pregnancy (Chadwick's sign), paler color seen in postmenopausal women.	*Cyanosis without pregnancy:* Venous congestion or systemic hypoxia as in congestive heart failure (CHF).

AREA/PA SKILL	NORMAL FINDINGS	ABNORMAL FINDINGS
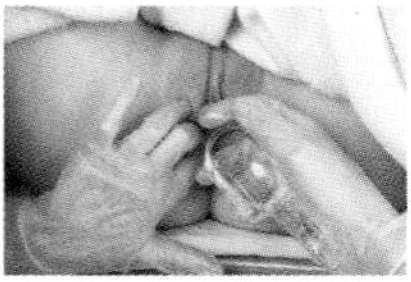 *Inserting speculum* 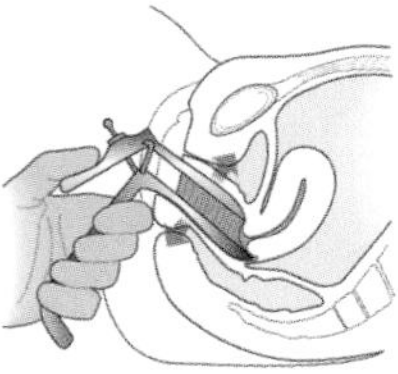 *Proper position of speculum in vagina* 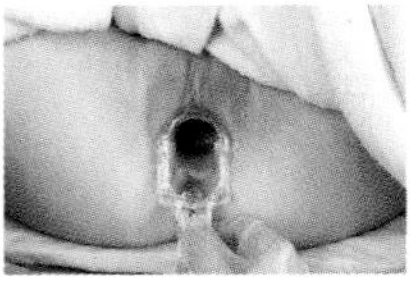 *Opening speculum* 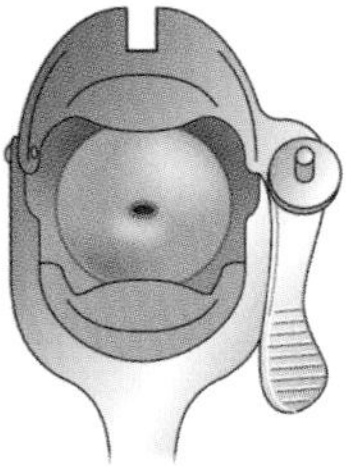 *View through speculum* 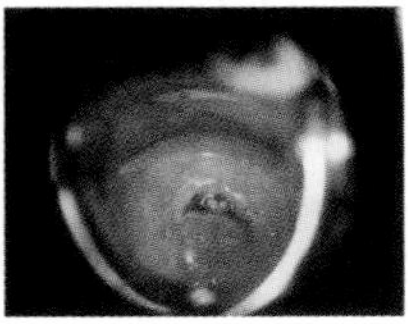 *Chadwick's sign*		

(box continued on page 292)

Physical Assessment (continued)

AREA/PA SKILL	NORMAL FINDINGS	ABNORMAL FINDINGS
Inspection *Pelvic Examination With Speculum (Use Warm Speculum) (cont'd)* 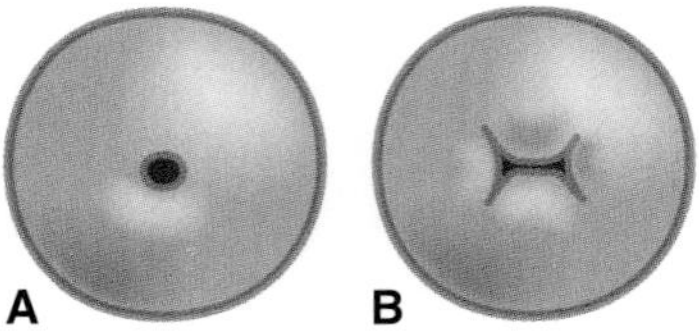 *A. Nulliparous cervical os; B. Parous cervical os*		
Obtain specimens as indicated. 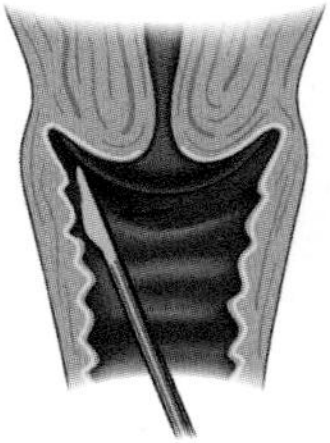 *Taking a vaginal pool smear* 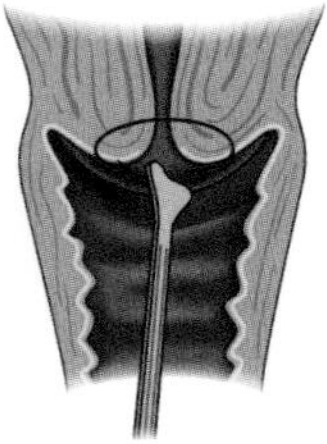 *Taking a cervical smear*		*Redness or a friable cervix:* Infection and inflammation (e.g., chlamydia or gonorrhea). *Lateral positioning of cervix:* Tumor or adhesions. *Projection of cervix into vaginal vault > 2.5 cm:* Uterine prolapse. *Cervical size > 4 cm:* Hypertrophy from inflammation or tumor. A reddish circle around the os may be abnormal. *Ectropion or eversion:* Lacerations during childbirth or congenital variation. *Small, round, yellow lesions:* Nabothian cysts, benign cysts from obstruction of cervical glands. *Bright red, soft protrusions through the cervical os:* Polyps; they are abnormal. *Hemorrhages over the surface:* Strawberry spots, associated with trichomonal infection.

AREA/PA SKILL	NORMAL FINDINGS	ABNORMAL FINDINGS
		Unilateral transverse, bilateral transverse, stellate, or irregular cervical os: Caused by cervical tears occurring during rapid second-stage childbirth delivery, forceps delivery, or trauma. *Greenish-yellow mucopurulent discharge that adheres to vaginal walls, with pus in os:* Gonococcal infection. *White, cottage-cheese–like discharge that adheres to vaginal walls, with patches of discharge on os:* *Candida* infection. *Grayish-yellow, purulent, often bubbly discharge that smells fishy and often pools in fornix: Trichomonas;* cervix may show red spots.
Inspect the vaginal walls while withdrawing the speculum.	Vaginal walls pink with rugae, no lesions.	*White spots on vaginal wall:* Leukoplakia from *Candida albicans.* Repeated occurrences may indicate human immunodeficiency virus (HIV) infection. *Pallor of vaginal walls:* Anemia or menopause. *Redness of vaginal walls:* Inflammation, hyperemia, or trauma from tampon insertion or removal. *Vaginal lesions or masses:* Carcinoma, tumors, and diethylstilbestrol (DES) exposure.

(box continued on page 294)

Physical Assessment (continued)

AREA/PA SKILL	NORMAL FINDINGS	ABNORMAL FINDINGS
Palpation		
Lubricate index and middle fingers of gloved hand. Vaginal exam performed first, then rectovaginal exam can be performed.		
Skene's Glands and Bartholin's Glands		
Usually performed before speculum insertion.		
Skene's Gland: Insert index finger into vagina with finger pad upward, milk urethra and Skene's gland.		
Bartholin's Glands: Insert index finger into vagina with finger pad downward toward perineum.		
Note any masses, swelling, discharge, or tenderness.	Area smooth, no swelling, discharge, masses, or tenderness.	*Swelling, redness, induration, or purulent discharge from labial folds with hot, tender areas:* Bartholin's gland infection from gonococci and *Chlamydia trachomatis.* *Pain and discharge from urethra:* Skene's gland infection or urinary tract infection.
Vagina/Walls		
Note texture, swelling, lesions, tenderness.	Vaginal walls have rugae; no swelling, lesions, nodules, or tenderness. Fewer rugae in postmenopausal women.	*Significantly diminished or absent vaginal muscle tone and bulging of vagina:* Injury, age, childbirth, medication. *Bulging:* Cystocele, rectocele, or uterine prolapse.

AREA/PA SKILL	NORMAL FINDINGS	ABNORMAL FINDINGS
		Lesions, masses, scarring, or cysts: Benign lesions (e.g., inclusion cysts, myomas, or fibromas) or malignant ones. Most common site for malignant lesions of vagina in upper one third of posterior wall.
Assess tone and texture.	Perineum is smooth, firm, and homogeneous in nulliparous women; thinner in parous women.	*Thin perineum, fissures, or tears:* Atrophy, trauma, or unhealed episiotomy.
Cervix		
Note size, shape, consistency, position, mobility, tenderness.	Cervix round, smooth, firm, midline, mobile, and nontender.	*Pain on palpation or when assessing mobility (presence of chandelier sign or cervical motion tenderness):* PID or ectopic pregnancy.
	Cervix smaller in older women.	*Irregular surface, immobility, or nodular surface of cervix:* Malignancy, nabothian cysts, or polyps.
	Cervix softer and enlarged during pregnancy. Softening of cervix (Goodell's sign) seen at the 5th to 6th week of pregnancy.	*Nodules or irregularities on fornices:* Malignancy, polyps, herniations.
Uterus		
Note size, shape, symmetry, position, masses, tenderness. 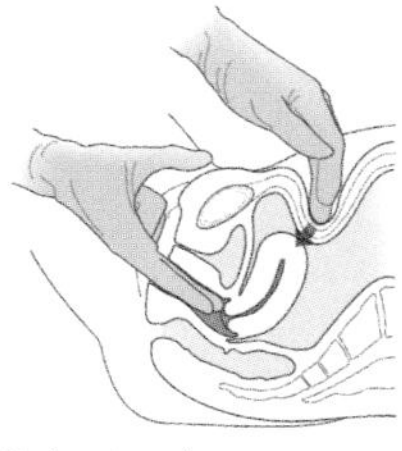 *Palpating the uterus*	Uterus midline; may be anteflexed or anteverted, midplane, retroflexed or retroverted. Size and shape depend on parity: Pear-shaped in nongravid, more rounded in parous women; size increases with pregnancy. Firm, mobile, slightly tender. No masses.	*Enlargement and changes in uterine shape:* Intrauterine pregnancy or tumor. *Nodule:* Myomas, tumors containing muscle tissue. A retroverted and retroflexed uterus can only be assessed rectovaginally.

(box continued on page 296)

Physical Assessment (continued)

AREA/PA SKILL	NORMAL FINDINGS	ABNORMAL FINDINGS
Palpation *(cont'd)* *Ovaries*		
Note size, shape, symmetry, tenderness. 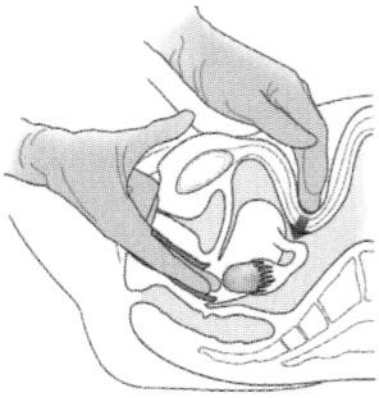 *Palpating the ovaries*	Ovaries nonpalpable; or if palpable, almond shape, firm, smooth, about 3 x 2 x 1 cm, mobile, sensitive to palpation. Ovaries are not palpable in postmenopausal women or prepubertal girls.	*Enlarged, irregular, nodular, painful, immobile ovaries:* Ectopic pregnancy, ovarian cyst, PID, or malignancy.
Anus and Rectum **Vaginal exam performed first, then rectovaginal exam. Remember to change gloves before rectovaginal exam to prevent cross-contamination.**		
Perform rectal examination and note sphincter tone, pain, tenderness, nodules, lesions, masses, hemorrhoids, polyps, bleeding. 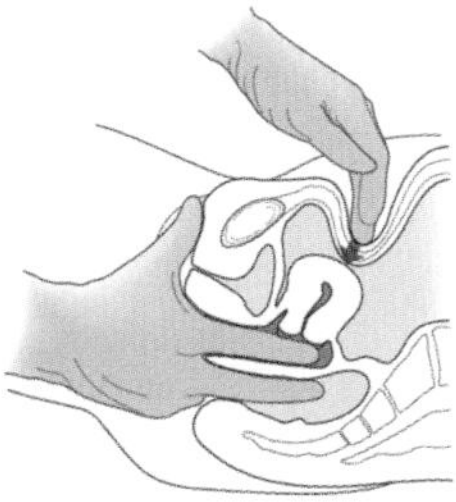 *Proper position of hands*	+ Sphincter tone, nontender, no masses, polyps, lesions, hemorrhoids, or bleeding.	*Masses or lesions:* Malignancy or internal hemorrhoids.
Note color of stool; test for occult blood.	Stool brown; negative for occult blood.	*Lax sphincter tone:* Perineal trauma from childbirth or anal intercourse, or neurologic disorders.

PA = Physical assessment.

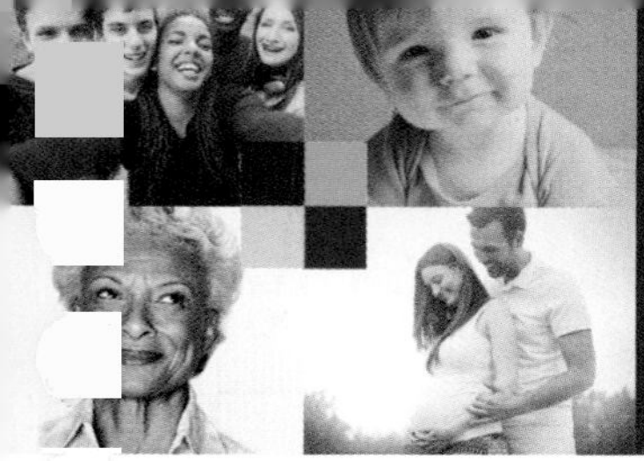

CHAPTER 11

Assessing the Male Genitourinary System

Primary Functions

- Manufacturing and protecting sperm for fertilization
- Transporting sperm
- Regulating hormonal production and secretion of male sex hormones
- Providing sexual pleasure
- Excreting urine

Developmental Considerations

Infants

- Premature infants may have undescended testes and few rugae.
- Breech-delivered infants may have scrotal edema and ecchymoses.
- Hydroceles and hernias are common findings in boys younger than age 2.
- Decision to circumcise is culturally based.

Children and Adolescents

- Tanner staging, characterizing pubic hair distribution and penile and testicular size, is used to track sexual maturation during puberty (Table 11.1).

TABLE 11.1 Maturation States in Boys

STAGE	PUBIC HAIR	PENIS	TESTES AND SCROTUM
Stage 1: Preadolescent 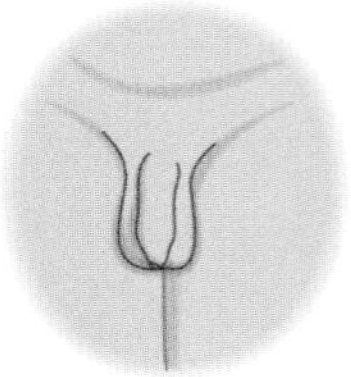	No pubic hair except for fine body hair similar to that on abdomen.	Same size and proportions as in childhood.	Same size and proportions as in childhood.
Stage 2 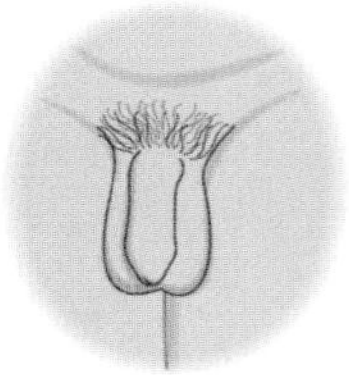	Sparse growth of long, slightly pigmented, downy hair, straight or only slightly curled, chiefly at base of penis.	Slight or no enlargement.	Testes larger; scrotum larger, somewhat reddened, and altered in texture.
Stage 3 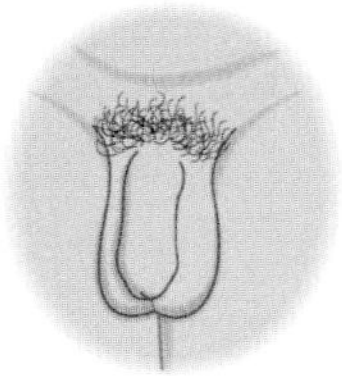	Darker, coarser, curlier hair spreading sparsely over pubic symphysis.	Larger, especially in length.	Further enlarged.
Stage 4 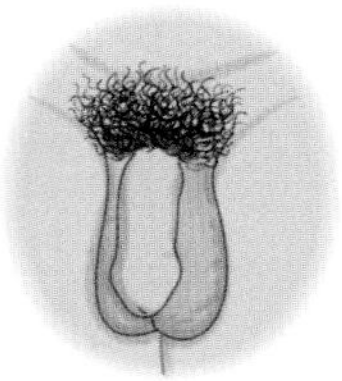	Coarse and curly hair, as in adult; area covered greater than in stage 3 but not as great as in adult.	Further enlarged in length and breadth, with development of glans.	Further enlarged; scrotal skin darkened.
Stage 5 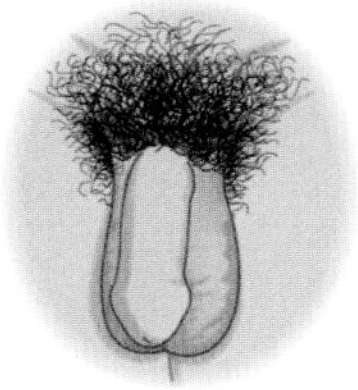	Hair same as adult in quantity and quality, spread to medial surfaces of thighs but not up over abdomen.	Adult in size and shape.	Adult in size and shape.

Older Adults

- Pubic hair thins on the external genitalia.
- Penis appears atrophic and testicles smaller and slightly softer than in a younger man.
- Prostate may feel larger than in a younger patient.
- Scrotal sac loses its elasticity.
- Reduction in testosterone levels occurs by age 50.
- Although sperm output may be decreased, normal spermatogenesis is present in most men until age 70.
- Prevalence of impotence increases markedly with aging.

Cultural Considerations

- Decision to circumcise is culturally based.
- United States has a higher rate of newborn male circumcisions than Canada, England, or Sweden, where circumcision is considered unnecessary.
- Native Americans and Hispanics have no tradition to practice circumcision.
- Jews and Muslims practice circumcision as part of their religious value system.

Assessment

History

Symptoms ("PQRST" Any + Symptom)

- Pain
  - Do you have pain in your penis, scrotum, testes, or groin? If so, please describe the pain (pain assessment pattern).
  - Have you noticed any pain or burning when urinating?
  - When did the pain first begin?
- Lesions
  - Have you noticed any blisters, ulcers, sores, warts, or rashes on your penis, scrotum, or surrounding areas?
    If so, please describe them.
  - When did you first notice the lesion?
  - Has the appearance of the lesion changed?
  - Is the lesion painful?
  - Did you have a painful lesion that healed?
  - Has anyone you have been intimate with told you they had a sexually transmitted disease (STD)?

- Swelling
  - Have you felt any lumps, swelling, or masses in the scrotum, genital, or groin area? If so, describe it and its location. Was the onset gradual or sudden?
  - Have you noticed any heaviness or dragging feeling in the scrotum?
  - When did you first notice the lumps, swelling, or masses?
  - Is tenderness present?
  - If you exert pressure on the lumps or masses, do they disappear?
- Discharge
  - Have you noticed any unusual discharge from your penis? If so, what color is the discharge?
  - Is there any odor to the discharge?
  - Is it a small, moderate, or large amount?
  - Is there any burning or pain with the discharge?
- Genitourinary symptoms
  - Do you ever have blood in your urine? If so, when or how often?
  - Describe the color of your urine.
  - How many times do you wake during the night to urinate?
  - Have you had any changes in your voiding pattern (e.g., frequency)?
  - Have you ever had kidney stones?

Sexual History

- Have you ever been sexually active?
- Are you currently sexually active? That is, have you had sex with anyone in the past few months? If the answer is yes, answer next question.
- Do you have sex with men, women, or both (heterosexual, homosexual, or bisexual)?
- Type of sexual activity (oral, genital, or anal)?
- Do you have more than one partner? How many partners have you had in the last 6 months?
- Are you using birth control? What kind? How often?
- Are you worried about the acquired immunodeficiency syndrome (AIDS) virus or other STDs?
- Do you take any precautions to avoid infections? If so, what?
- Do you have any problems or concerns about your sexual function?

- Have you had surgery on any of your reproductive organs? If so, what and when?
- Have you been taught to examine your testes?
- Are you taking any medications, prescribed or over-the-counter (Table 11.2)?

Erectile Dysfunction

- Have you maintained an interest in sex?
- Are you able to achieve and maintain an erection?
- Do you have morning erections?

TABLE 11.2 Drugs That Adversely Affect the Male Genitourinary System

CLASSIFICATION	MEDICATION	EFFECT
Antiandrogen	Finasteride	Impotence
Antianxiety/Sedative	Benzodiazepines, chlordiazepoxide	Changes in libido
Anticholinergic	Atropine	Impotence
Antidepressants	Tricyclic antidepressants	Increased/decreased libido and impotence
	Trazodone	Decreased libido, impotence, priapism, retrograde ejaculation
	Selective serotonin reuptake inhibitors	Decreased libido, delayed orgasm, anorgasmia, ejaculatory dysfunction
Antiepileptic	Primidone	Impotence
Antihypertensive	Methyldopa	Ejaculatory failure
	Prazosin	Impotence, priapism
	Clonidine	Impotence, decreased sexual activity, decreased libido
	All beta blockers	Impotence, decreased libido
Antipsychotics	All antipsychotics	Priapism, impotence, ejaculatory inhibition
Diuretics	Chlorothiazide, spironolactone	Impotence
Estrogen	Conjugated estrogen	Impotence, testicular atrophy
Tranquilizers	Diazepam, alprazolam	Changes in libido

- Were there any changes in your relationship with your partner or in your life situation when the problem began?
- How long does intercourse last?
- Do you sometimes feel that you cannot ejaculate?
- Are you satisfied with your sex life as it is now?

Assessment of the Male Genitourinary System's Relationship to Other Systems

Remember, all systems are related. As you assess the male genitourinary system, look at the relationship between it and all other systems.

Assessment of the Male Genitourinary System's Relationship to Other Systems

SUBJECTIVE DATA/ RATIONALE	OBJECTIVE DATA/ RATIONALE
Area/System: General	
Ask about:	*Measure:*
Changes in energy level, weight: Scrotal abnormalities may cause discomfort and affect activity tolerance. Fatigue influences desire and ability to perform sexual intercourse.	Vital signs, checking for temperature elevations, hypertension (HTN). *Note:* Signs of discomfort. *Affect:* Depression can affect sexual function.
Fevers.	
Fatigue, activity intolerance, fever, and weight loss are often signs of underlying health problems, such as human immunodeficiency virus (HIV)/AIDS or prostatitis.	
Area/System: Integumentary	
Ask about:	*Inspect for:*
Changes in hair growth: Male hormones affect body hair growth. Secondary syphilis can cause alopecia.	*Skin lesions:* Rashes and skin lesions are associated with many STDs. • *Systemic rash:* Secondary syphilis. • *Vesicles:* HSV 1 and 2.
Rashes, lesions: May be associated with STDs, but not restricted to genitalia. Primary syphilis chancre found on lip as well as penis. Bilateral, symmetrical rash of secondary syphilis usually occurs on palms and soles.	Hair distribution. • *Areas of alopecia:* Associated with secondary syphilis. • *Decrease in body hair:* Possible decrease in male hormones.

SUBJECTIVE DATA/ RATIONALE	OBJECTIVE DATA/ RATIONALE
Area/System: HEENT	
Ask about:	*Palpate:*
Swollen glands/nodes or neck mass or thyroid disease: Associated with infection and malignancy.	*Lymph nodes:* Palpable lymph nodes may indicate systemic infection or malignancy.
Eye drainage: Gonorrheal eye infections occur in newborns (ophthalmia neonatorum) and adults (gonorrheal conjunctivitis).	*Thyroid:* An enlarged thyroid may affect sexual functioning.
	Inspect:
Tearing, photophobia, edema of eyelids, and conjunctival edema are symptoms of *Chlamydia trachomatis* infection.	*Conjunctiva for drainage:* Conjunctivitis can be caused by gonorrhea. *Oral mucosa for redness and lesions:* Associated with STDs.
Sore throat: STDs can be found in the oropharynx and are often not assessed in patient complaining of sore throat.	
Oral lesions: Secondary syphilis can result in oral mucous patches.	
Area/System: Respiratory	
Ask about:	*Inspect for:*
History of respiratory disease: Respiratory disease such as chronic obstructive pulmonary disease (COPD) may affect sexual activity.	Signs of respiratory distress. *Auscultate:* *Breath sounds:* Chronic lung disease indicated by abnormal breath sounds may impair sexual functioning.
Area/System: Cardiovascular	
Ask about:	*Inspect for:*
History of cardiovascular disease (CVD), HTN, congestive heart failure (CHF): May compromise sexual activity. Vascular problems and HTN medications may cause erectile dysfunction. Scrotal edema may accompany CHF.	Signs of impaired circulation. Skin changes. *Palpate:* Pulses, edema. *Auscultate:* Extra heart sounds.
Area/System: Breasts	
	Inspect: Gynecomastia.
Area/System: Gastrointestinal	
Ask about:	*Inspect for:*
History of liver disease: Liver disease associated with ascites may cause scrotal edema.	Ascites. *Palpate/percuss:*

(continued)

Assessment of the Male Genitourinary System's Relationship to Other Systems (continued)

SUBJECTIVE DATA/ RATIONALE	OBJECTIVE DATA/ RATIONALE
Area/System: Gastrointestinal *(cont'd)*	
Weight/appetite loss: May be associated with malignancy or AIDS.	Liver enlargement.
Area/System: Musculoskeletal *Ask about:*	*Test:*
Weakness, limitations. Joint pain, swelling.	*Muscle strength:* Weakness and paralysis may be associated with neurosyphilis.
Physical act of sexual intercourse requires functional musculoskeletal system.	*Inspect:*
Late-stage syphilis damages joints (Charcot's joint).	*Joint swelling and deformity:* Charcot's joints associated with late syphilis.
Area/System: Neurologic *Ask about:*	*Test for:*
History of neurological problems: May affect sexual function.	*Changes in mental status, affect:* May be associated with late-stage syphilis.
Paralysis. Tremors. Personality changes.	Sensory deficits.
Neurosyphilis occurs in late syphilis and can cause paresis, tremors, personality changes, and psychosis.	
Depression: Risk factor for erectile dysfunction.	
Area/System: Endocrine *Ask about:*	
History of thyroid disease and diabetes: Diabetic neuropathy can cause impotence. Hypothyroidism causes decreased libido and infertility. Hyperthyroidism can cause impotence and gynecomastia.	
Area/System: Lymphatic/ Hematological *Ask about:*	
History of HIV, AIDS, sickle cell anemia: AIDS, an STD, affects the immune system. Sickle cell anemia can cause priapism (painful, sustained erection without sexual desire).	

HEENT = Head, eyes, ears, nose, and throat.

Physical Assessment

APPROACH: Inspection, palpation, auscultation; external and rectal exam

POSITION: Standing

TOOLBOX: Nonsterile gloves, water-soluble lubricant, penlight, stethoscope, Culturette tube, sterile cotton swabs, 1½" to 2" gauze wrap, 5 percent acetic acid solution in a spray bottle, Thayer-Martin plate.

Physical Assessment

AREA/PA SKILL	NORMAL FINDINGS	ABNORMAL FINDINGS
Inspection		
Have patient void before examination.		
Penis		
Inspect dorsal, lateral, and ventral sides.		
Note condition of skin, color lesions, discharge.	Skin intact, color pink to light brown in whites, light to dark brown in African Americans; no lesions or discharge.	*Sparse or absent hair in genital area:* Genetic factors (e.g., developmental defects and hereditary disorders), aging, local or systemic disease (e.g., infection, neoplasms, endocrine diseases, nutritional or metabolic deficiencies), physical or chemical agents, destruction of or damage to hair follicles.
Note size in relation to physical development and age.	Urinary meatus midline at tip of glans.	*Painless, ulcerated, exudative, papular lesion with an erythematous halo, surrounding edema, and a friable base:* Chancre, the lesion of primary syphilis. 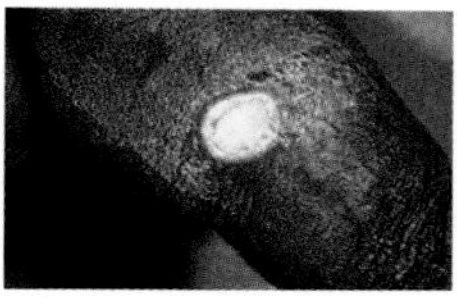 *Chancre*

(box continued on page 306)

Physical Assessment (continued)

AREA/PA SKILL	NORMAL FINDINGS	ABNORMAL FINDINGS
Inspection *Penis (cont'd)*		
Note position of urinary meatus.	Foreskin retracts easily.	*Pinhead papules to cauliflower-like groupings of painful, filiform, skin-colored, pink, or red lesions:* Chancroid; caused by *Haemophilus* through small breaks in epidermal tissue. 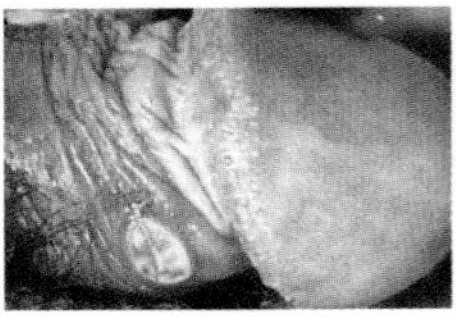 *Chancroid*
Note presence of foreskin or circumcised. If uncircumcised, retract foreskin; note ease of retraction and presence of lesions.		Multifocal, wartlike, maculopapular lesions—tan, brown, pink, violet, or white: Condylomata acuminatum (genital warts); caused by human papillomavirus (HPV) infection. 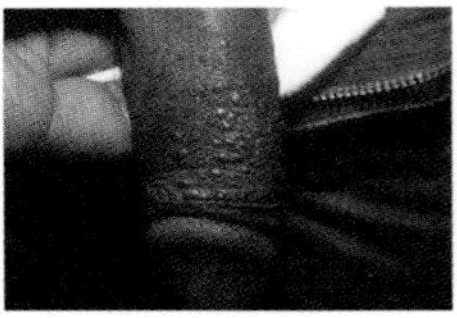 *Genital warts on penis* 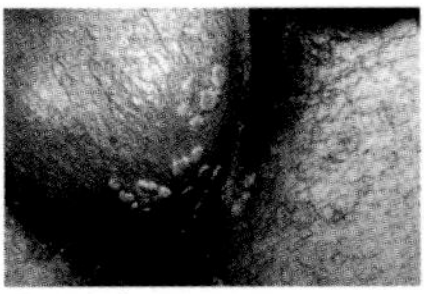 *Genital warts on scrotum* *Erythematous plaques with scaling, papular lesions with sharp margins and occasionally clear centers and pustules: Candida* infection.

AREA/PA SKILL	NORMAL FINDINGS	ABNORMAL FINDINGS
		Painful eruptions of pustules and vesicles that rupture: Herpes simplex virus (HSV) 1 and 2 (accompanying symptoms: Fever, headache, dysuria, dyspareunia, and urinary retention). 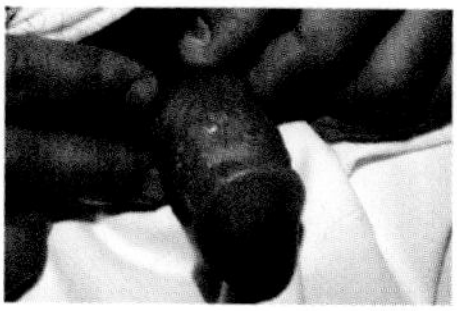 *Genital herpes* *Tinea cruris ("jock itch"):* Fungal infection of groin. 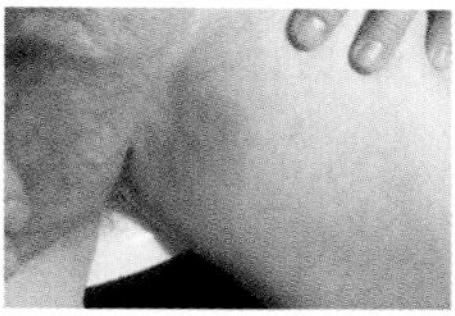 *Tinea cruris* *Foreskin unable to retract; may become swollen:* Phimosis. *Priapism:* Leukemia, metastatic carcinoma, or sickling hemoglobinopathies. *Ventral or dorsal curvature of penis:* Chordee (ventral chordee seen mostly with epispadias). *Urethral meatus opens on dorsal side of glans on shaft of penis:* Epispadias. *Urethral meatus opens on ventral side of glans on shaft of penis:* Hypospadias.

(box continued on page 308)

Physical Assessment (continued)

AREA/PA SKILL	NORMAL FINDINGS	ABNORMAL FINDINGS
Scrotum		
Note color, hair distribution, lesions, swelling, size, and position.	Skin color darker than rest of body. Hair distribution appropriate for age of patient.	*Scrotal swelling:* Inguinal hernia, hydrocele, varicocele, spermatocele, tumor, edema.
Note pubic pediculosis.	Testes hang freely, left testis slightly lower than right.	Erythema and swelling are abnormal.
	No lesions, pediculosis.	*Nontender accumulation of fluid between two layers of tunica vaginalis:* Hydrocele; idiopathic or from trauma, inguinal surgery, epididymitis, or tumor. Mass transilluminates. *Nontender, well-defined cystic mass on superior testis or epididymis:* Spermatocele; from blockage of efferent ductules of rete testis. *Varicose veins of spermatic cord that feel like a "bag of worms" and slowly collapse when scrotum is elevated:* Varicocele, caused by dilated veins in pampiniform plexus of spermatic cord. Right-sided may indicate obstruction at vena cava. *Round, firm, nontender cutaneous cyst confined to scrotal skin:* Sebaceous cyst from decrease in localized circulation and closure of sebaceous glands or ducts.

AREA/PA SKILL	NORMAL FINDINGS	ABNORMAL FINDINGS
Inguinal Area		
Note condition of skin, bulges. Have patient bear down, and inspect again for any bulges. Note enlarged lymph nodes.	Skin intact, no bulges, no palpable lymph nodes.	*Bulge:* Hernia or enlarged lymph node.

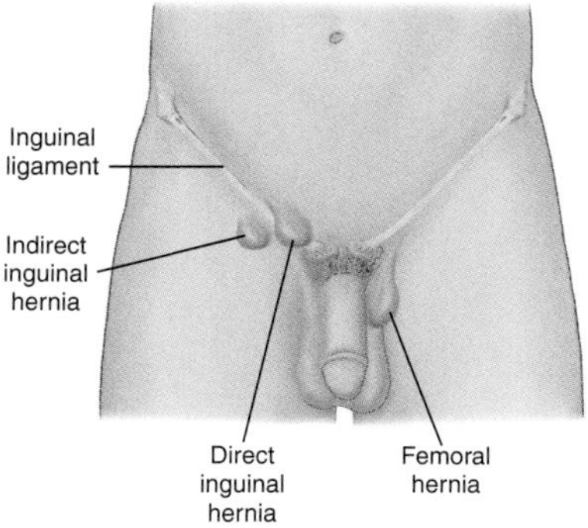

Location of indirect and direct femoral and inguinal hernias

AREA/PA SKILL	NORMAL FINDINGS	ABNORMAL FINDINGS
Rectal Area		
Note condition of skin, inflammation, rashes, excoriation, rectal prolapse, external hemorrhoids, polyps, lesions, fissures, bleeding, discharge.	Rectal area intact; no inflammation, lesions, prolapse, hemorrhoids, discharge, or bleeding.	STD lesions, warts, hemorrhoids, fissures, bleeding, rectal prolapse.
Palpation		
Maintain standard precautions; wear gloves.		
Penis		
Use thumb and two fingers to palpate shaft.		
Note consistency, tenderness, induration, masses, or nodules.	Nonerect penis soft, nontender, no nodules.	*Diminished/absent palpable pulse or pulsations:* Possible vascular insufficiency. Normal blood flow may be affected by systemic disease or localized trauma or disease.

(box continued on page 310)

Physical Assessment (continued)

AREA/PA SKILL	NORMAL FINDINGS	ABNORMAL FINDINGS
Palpation *Penis (cont'd)*		
		Priapism: Spinal cord lesions or sickle cell anemia. Phimosis or paraphimosis (foreskin retracts but does not return). **Seek immediate assistance if foreskin cannot be retracted. Prolonged constriction of vessels can constrict blood flow and lead to necrosis.** *Purulent discharge or mucus shreds:* Bacterial infection of genitourinary tract; causes inflammation with leukocytes, shedding tissue cells, and bacteria.
Use thumb and two fingers to palpate scrotum.		
Palpate surface characteristics of scrotum.	Scrotal skin rough without lesions. Testes rubbery, round, movable, smooth, 2 x 5 cm, slight tenderness with compression.	Unilateral mass within or above testicle is abnormal. Intratesticular masses are nodular and painless. They should be considered malignant until proven otherwise.
Note size, shape, consistency, mobility, masses, nodules, tenderness of testes.		*Testicle enlarged, retracted, in a lateral position, and extremely sensitive:* Testicular torsion. Abnormal for one or both testes to be undescended. *Absence of testes and epididymis in scrotal sac:* Cryptorchidism; related to testicular failure, deficient gonadotrophic stimulation, mechanical obstruction, or gubernacular defects. Because undescended testes have a histological change by age 6, referral should take place as early as possible.

AREA/PA SKILL	NORMAL FINDINGS	ABNORMAL FINDINGS
		Acute, painful onset of swelling of testicle, with warm scrotal skin: Orchitis. Testes may feel heavy in the scrotum. Atrophic testicle and scrotal edema are abnormal. *Red glow with transillumination:* Serous fluid within scrotal sac; seen in hydrocele and spermatocele.
Palpate epididymis and vas deferens on the posterolateral surface. Note swelling or nodules. Transilluminate any lumps, nodules, or edematous areas.	Ridge of epididymis noted, and vas deferens smooth and movable. No swelling or nodules.	Abnormal to palpate indurated, swollen, tender epididymis.
Inguinal Area		
Palpate for inguinal and femoral hernias or masses. Have patient bear down or cough as you palpate for a bulge or hernia.	No inguinal or femoral hernias or masses.	*Mass that comes down inguinal canal and is palpable at inguinal ring or in scrotum:* Indirect inguinal hernia.

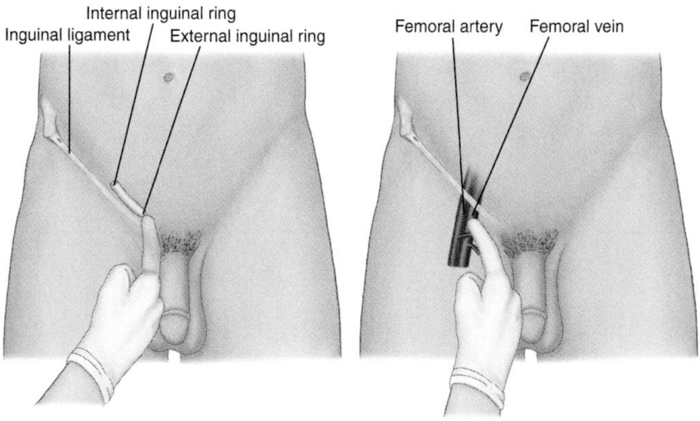

Palpating for inguinal and femoral hernias.

(box continued on page 312)

Physical Assessment (continued)

AREA/PA SKILL	NORMAL FINDINGS	ABNORMAL FINDINGS
Palpation *Inguinal Area (cont'd)*		
		Mass that enlarges with coughing: Direct inguinal hernia. *Mass palpated in medial to femoral vessels and inferior to inguinal ligament:* Femoral hernia. **A strangulated hernia is a surgical emergency.**
Palpate inguinal lymph nodes.	No palpable nodes.	*Unilateral enlargement of lymph nodes along with erythematous skin:* Bacterial infections. *Unilateral or bilateral enlargement of inguinal lymph nodes, tender or painless:* Bacterial infections or malignancy.
Anus and Rectum		
Have patient bend over exam table or assume side-lying position.		
Note sphincter tone, pain, tenderness, nodules, lesions, masses, hemorrhoids, polyps, bleeding.	+ Sphincter tone, nontender, no masses, polyps, lesions, hemorrhoids, or bleeding.	Fissure, warts, hemorrhoids, bleeding, rectal prolapse.
Note color of stool; test for occult blood.	Stool brown; negative for occult blood.	

AREA/PA SKILL	NORMAL FINDINGS	ABNORMAL FINDINGS
Prostate		
Note size, shape, symmetry, mobility, consistency, nodules, tenderness.	Prostate is shape and size of walnut, smooth, rubbery, nontender.	*Soft, nontender, enlarged prostate:* Benign prostatic hypertrophy; related to aging and presence of dihydroxytestosterone.

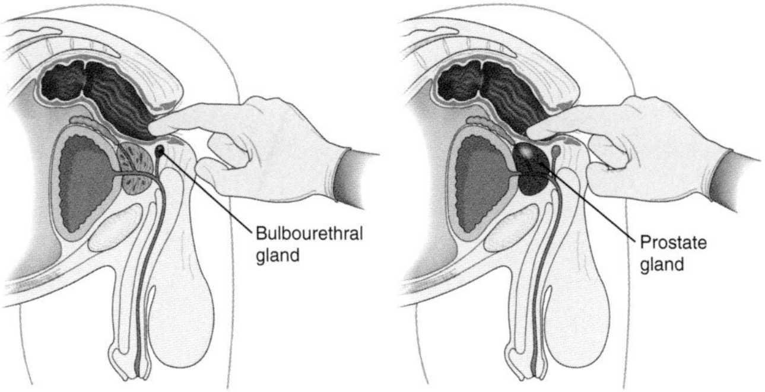

Palpating the prostate and bulbourethral glands

AREA/PA SKILL	NORMAL FINDINGS	ABNORMAL FINDINGS
Grading scale for prostate gland: • Grade I: <1-cm protrusion into rectum. • Grade II: 1- to 2-cm protrusion into rectum. • Grade III: 2- to 3-cm protrusion into rectum. • Grade IV: >3 cm protrusion into rectum.		*Firm, tender, or fluctuant mass on prostate:* Acute bacterial prostatitis or urinary tract infection; patient at risk for prostatic abscess. *Firm, hard, or indurated nodule(s) on prostate:* Possible prostate cancer. *Extremely tender, warm prostate:* Bacterial prostatitis. If suspected, do not vigorously palpate, because of possibility of bacteremia.
Auscultation *Scrotum*		
If scrotal mass detected, auscultate the scrotum for bowel sounds.	No bowel sounds.	*Bowel sounds in scrotum:* Indirect inguinal hernia.

PA = Physical assessment.

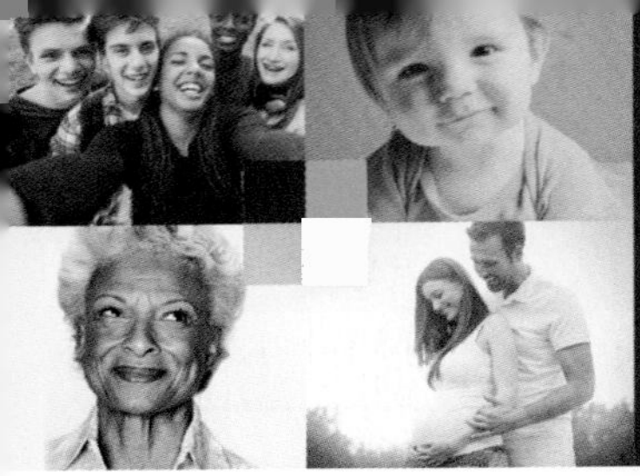

CHAPTER 12

Assessing the Motor-Musculoskeletal System

Primary Functions

- Provides shape and support to the body
- Allows for movement
- Protects the internal organs
- Produces red blood cells (hematopoiesis)
- Stores calcium and phosphorus in the bones

Developmental Considerations

Infants and Children

- Rapid growth periods occur during infancy and adolescence.
- Longitudinal bone growth continues until closure of the epiphyses, at age 20.
- Infant has C-shaped spine.
- Toddler has wide base of support while learning to walk.
- Toddlers with "potbellies" often have a postural lordosis.
- Common knee deviations include genu valgum (knock knees) and genu varum (bowlegs).
- Scoliosis often becomes apparent during adolescence; more common in girls than in boys.

Pregnant Patients

- Postural lordosis with anterior cervical flexion (kyphosis) occurs in latter part of pregnancy.
- Wide base of support compensates for shifting center of gravity.
- Low back pain is common late in pregnancy.

- Increased mobility of the sacroiliac, sacrococcygeal, and symphysis pubis joints in preparation for delivery contributes to "waddling" gait.

Older Adults

- Muscle changes cause a wider base of support.
- Older adults have increased risk for osteoporosis, especially women.
- Kyphosis occurs with aging.
- Height decreases.
- Body fat is redistributed to abdomen and hips.
- Loss of muscle mass occurs.
- Older adults have a high incidence of degenerative joint disease (DJD).

Cultural Considerations

- African Americans
  - Tendency toward hyperplasia of connective tissue accounts for increased incidence of lupus erythematosus.
  - Greater bone density than that of Europeans, Asians, and Hispanics accounts for decreased incidence of osteoporosis.
- Amish
  - Dwarfism syndrome is found in nearly all Amish communities.
- Chinese Americans
  - Generally shorter than Westerners.
  - Bone structure also differs from that of Westerners:
    - Ulna longer than radius.
    - Hip measurements smaller (women 4.14 cm smaller; men 7.6 cm smaller).
    - Bone length shorter.
    - Bone density less.
- Egyptian Americans
  - Relatively short in stature. Average height for men 5′10″; for women 5′4″.
- Filipino Americans
  - Short in stature. Average height ranges from 5′ to average American size.
- Irish Americans
  - Taller and broader than average European American and Asian.

- Hip width greater.
- Bone density less than that of African Americans.

■ Navajo Native Americans
- Taller and thinner than other American tribes.
- Noted for being good runners.

■ Vietnamese Americans
- Small in stature. Average height 5′ for women, with men being a few inches taller.

Assessment

History

Symptoms ("PQRST" Any + Symptom)

■ Pain
- When did you first become aware of the pain?
- Where do you feel the pain? Point to the area where you feel the pain.
- How would you describe the pain—for instance, dull, aching, burning, stabbing, or throbbing?
- When you have this pain, do you also have pain in any other location?
- When did the pain begin? What were you doing at the time it began?
- Did the pain occur suddenly?
- Does the pain occur daily?
- During what part of the day is your pain worse: morning, afternoon, or evening?
- Did a recent illness precede the pain?
- What makes the pain worse?
- What do you do to relieve the pain?
- What kind of medications—prescribed or over-the- counter (OTC)—have you taken to help with the pain?
- Does the pain change according to the weather?
- Do you have difficulty dressing?
- Does the pain interfere with your sleep?
- Does the pain move from one joint to another?
- Has there been an injury, strain, overuse?
- Have you noticed any swelling?
- Do you have any other unusual sensations, such as tingling, with the pain?

- Weakness
  - When did you first notice muscle weakness?
  - Do you have difficulty lifting objects?
  - Do you have difficulty writing with a pen or pencil?
  - Do you have trouble standing up after sitting in a chair?
  - Does the weakness worsen or improve as the day progresses?
  - Have your muscles decreased in size?
  - Is there any pain or stiffness with your weak muscles?
  - Do you have trouble with double vision, swallowing, or chewing?
- Stiffness
  - When did the stiffness begin?
  - Has the stiffness increased since it began?
  - Do you feel stiff only on awakening or all the time?
  - Is pain associated with the stiffness?
  - What methods have you tried to reduce the stiffness?

Focused Musculoskeletal History

- Do you have a history of musculoskeletal problems, pain, or disease? If yes, are you taking any medications or undergoing any treatments for these problems?
- Do you have any other medical problems?
- Have any accidents or trauma ever affected your bones or joints?
- Do your joint, muscle, or bone problems limit your usual activities?
- Do you have any occupational hazards that could affect your muscles and joints?
- Have you been immunized for tetanus and polio?
- Do you smoke or consume alcohol or caffeine? If yes, how much and how often?
- Are you taking any medications, prescribed or OTC (Table 12.1)?

TABLE 12.1 Drugs That Adversely Affect the Musculoskeletal System

DRUG NAME	DRUG	POSSIBLE ADVERSE REACTIONS
Adrenocorticotropic hormone (ACTH)	Corticotropin	Muscle weakness, muscle wasting, osteoporosis, vertebral compression fractures, aseptic necrosis of humeral or femoral heads
Anticonvulsants	Phenytoin	Ataxia
Antidepressants	Trazadone	Musculoskeletal aches and pains
Antigout agents	Colchicine	Myopathy with prolonged administration
Antilipemic agents	3-hydroxy-3-methylglutaryl coenzyme A (HMG-CoA) reductase inhibitors ("statins"), fibric acid derivatives, niacin	Myopathy, rhabdomyolysis, myalgias
Benzodiazepines	All benzodiazepines	Ataxia
Central nervous system stimulants	Amphetamine sulfate	Increased motor activity
Corticosteroids	Prednisone, dexamethasone, hydrocortisone	Muscle weakness, muscle wasting, osteoporosis, vertebral compression fractures, aseptic necrosis of humeral or femoral heads
Diuretics	Thiazides and loops	Muscle cramps
Phenothiazines	All phenothiazines	Extrapyramidal symptoms (dystonic reactions, motor restlessness, and Parkinsonian signs and symptoms)
Miscellaneous skin agents	Isotretinoin	Bone or joint pain, general muscle aches

Assessment of the Musculoskeletal System's Relationship to Other Systems

Remember, all systems are related. As you assess the musculoskeletal system, look at the relationship between it and all other systems.

Assessment of the Musculoskeletal System's Relationship to Other Systems

SUBJECTIVE DATA	OBJECTIVE DATA
Area/System: General	
Ask about:	*Measure:*
General health: Fatigue and activity intolerance may be associated with RA, systemic lupus erythematosus (SLE), and Lyme disease. Weight gain is a risk factor for DJD, osteoarthritis, and low back pain. Anorexia or weight loss may be associated with RA. *Height loss:* May be associated with osteoporosis. *Fever:* May be associated with RA or Lyme disease.	Vital signs. *Height and weight:* Loss of height associated with aging and osteoporosis. Obesity associated with osteoarthritis.
Area/System: Integumentary	
Ask about:	*Inspect for:*
Rashes • *Bull's-eye rash:* Lyme disease. • *Ulcers and subcutaneous rheumatoid nodules on forearm and elbow:* RA. • *Butterfly facial rash:* SLE. Hair loss • *Patchy alopecia and short broken hair above forehead:* SLE.	Rashes, lesions, alopecia • *Bull's-eye rash:* Lyme disease. • *Butterfly rash, patchy alopecia:* SLE.
Area/System: HEENT	
Ask about:	*Inspect:*
Enlarged lymph nodes: Systemic infection. *Lymphadenopathy:* RA. **(!) Enlarged thyroid as a result of thyroid disease can affect musculoskeletal system.** *Dry, red eyes:* Sjögren's syndrome causes dry mouth and eyes and is associated with RA. *Episcleritis and keratoconjunctivitis:* RA.	Eyes for redness • *Red eye (episcleritis):* RA. *Palpate:* *Lymph nodes:* Enlarged lymph nodes may indicate infection or RA.

(continued)

Assessment of the Musculoskeletal System's Relationship to Other Systems (continued)

SUBJECTIVE DATA	OBJECTIVE DATA
Area/System: HEENT ***(cont'd)***	
Weakness, pain with weight bearing, osteoporosis, decreased muscle tone: Hyperthyroidism.	
Muscle weakness and cramps, difficulty walking: Hypothyroidism.	
Area/System: Respiratory	
Ask about:	*Auscultate:*
Breathing difficulty • *Interstitial fibrosis and pleuritis:* RA. • *Pneumonitis and pleural effusion:* SLE.	Lungs • *Intersitial fibrosis:* RA. • *Pleural effusion, pneumonitis:* SLE.
Area/System: Cardiovascular	
Ask about:	*Auscultate:*
History of cardiovascular disease: Rheumatoid heart disease associated with RA. Pericarditis, myocarditis and Raynaud's disease associated with RA and SLE.	*Heart sounds:* Pericarditis, myocarditis, Raynaud's disease associated with RA and SLE.
Area/System: Gastrointestinal	
Ask about:	*Auscultate:*
Nausea, vomiting, diarrhea: Gastrointestinal (GI) complaints may be associated with SLE. Bowel problems, incontinence, and loss of bowel function may be associated with cauda equina syndrome caused by compression of sacral nerve, as can occur with a herniated disc or spinal stenosis.	*Bowel sounds:* GI problems associated with SLE.
Area/System: Genitourinary/ Reproductive	
Ask about:	*Inspect for:*
History of sexually transmitted diseases (STDs): Tertiary syphilis can cause ataxia and Charcot's joints.	*Lesions and diseases:* STDs, such as syphilis, can cause tabes dorsalis, ataxia, areflexia, and damaged joints (Charcot's joint).
Hormone replacement therapy, in menopausal women: Postmenopausal women at greater risk for osteoporosis.	
Area/System: Neurologic	
Ask about:	*Test:*
Changes in sensation: Loss of sensation associated with herniated disc.	*Sensory deficits, paralysis:* Decreased sensations and numbness associated with

SUBJECTIVE DATA	OBJECTIVE DATA
Numbness, tingling: Neuropathies may be associated with RA, SLE.	neuropathies. Paralysis can result in muscle atrophy.
Area/System: Endocrine *Ask about:*	
History of diabetes mellitus or thyroid disease: Diabetes can cause neuropathies and muscle wasting. Hypothyroidism can cause weakness, muscle aches, pain, and arthralgia. Hyperthyroidism can cause osteoporosis.	
Area/System: Lymphatic/Hematological *Ask about:*	
Sickle cell anemia: Can cause joint pain. *Bruising:* SLE can cause thrombocytopenia.	

HEENT = Head, eyes, ears, nose, and throat.

Physical Assessment

ANATOMICAL LANDMARKS: Types of joints (Table 12.2).

TABLE 12.2 Types of Synovial Joints

DESCRIPTION	EXAMPLE/MOVEMENT
Pivot Permits rotation in one axis. Axis is longitudinal, with bone moving around a central axis without any displacement from that axis.	*Proximal radioulnar joint* Supination, pronation, and rotation
Hinge Allows movement in only one axis, namely flexion or extension, with axis situated transversely.	*Elbow, knee* Flexion and extension
Condyloid Permits movement in two axes. Described as an "egg-in-spoon joint," with long diameter of oval serving as one axis and short diameter of oval serving as other axis.	*Wrist* Flexion, extension, abduction, adduction, and circumduction

(continued)

TABLE 12.2 Types of Synovial Joints (continued)

DESCRIPTION	EXAMPLE/MOVEMENT
Saddle Has two axis-like condyloid joints. Articular surfaces are saddle shaped and move in similar fashion to condyloid joint.	*Thumb* Abduction, adduction, opposition, and reposition
Ball and Socket Moves across many possible axes. Articular surfaces are reciprocal segments of a sphere.	*Shoulder and hip* Flexion, extension, internal rotation, external rotation, abduction, adduction, and circumduction
Plane/Gliding Moves across many axes. Articular surfaces are flat, and one bone rides over the other in many directions.	*Patellofemoral and acromioclavicular joints, some carpal and tarsal bones, and articular vertebral processes* Limited movement in many directions

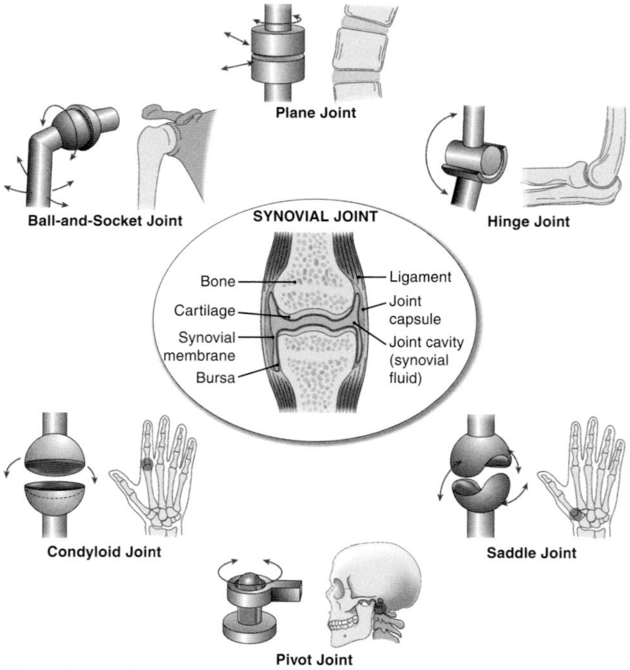

Types of synovial joints

APPROACH: Inspection, palpation.

POSITION: Standing, sitting, supine.

TOOLBOX: Tape measure, goniometer.

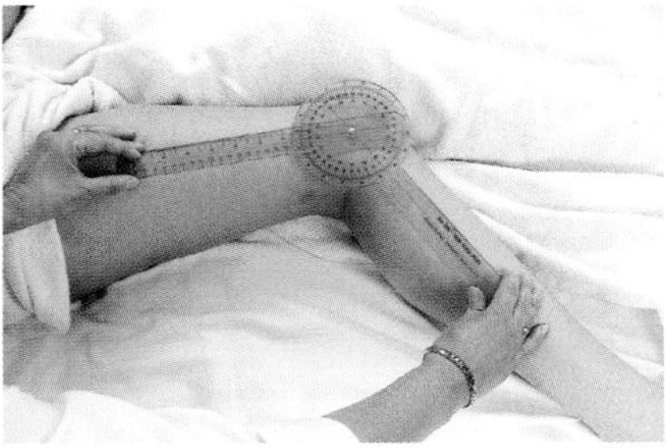

Using a goniometer

Physical Assessment

AREA/PA SKILL	NORMAL FINDINGS	ABNORMAL FINDINGS
Inspection *Posture and Spinal Curves*		
Note posture in relation to environment, head position, body alignment.	Posture erect, head midline.	
Note knee position, draw imaginary line from anterior superior iliac crest through knee to feet. 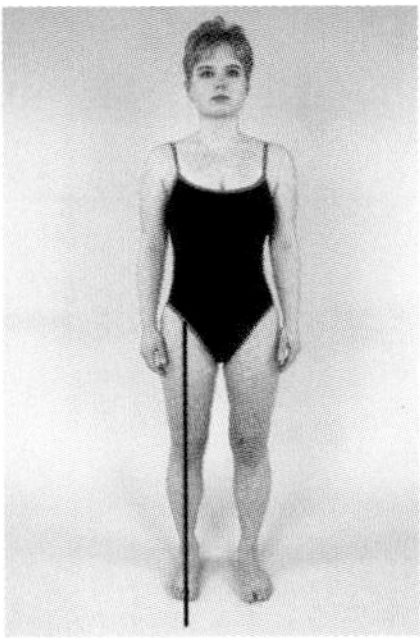 *Assessing for deviation of knees*	Knees aligned with no valgus or varus deviation.	*Knees touch and medial malleoli are 2 to 3 cm or more apart:* Genu valgum. *Knees are > 2.5 cm (1″) apart and medial malleoli touch:* Genu varum.

(box continued on page 324)

Physical Assessment (continued)

AREA/PA SKILL	NORMAL FINDINGS	ABNORMAL FINDINGS
Inspection *Posture and Spinal Curves (cont'd)*		
Inspect normal curves of the spine (cervical, thoracic, lumbar, and sacral). 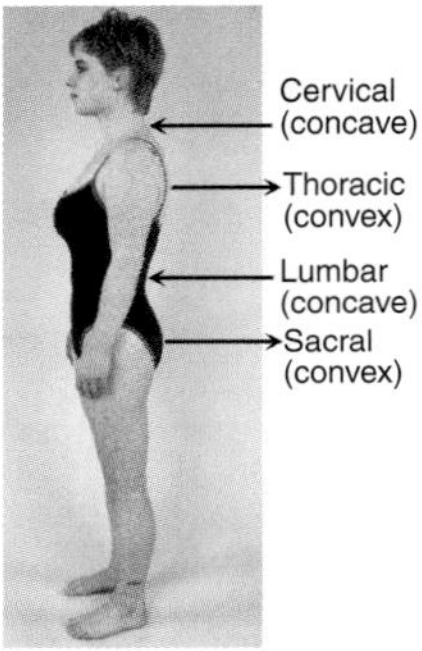 *Assessing for normal curves*	Normal spinal curves noted; no kyphosis, scoliosis, or lordosis.	Spinal deformities include: • *Kyphosis:* Accentuated thoracic curve. 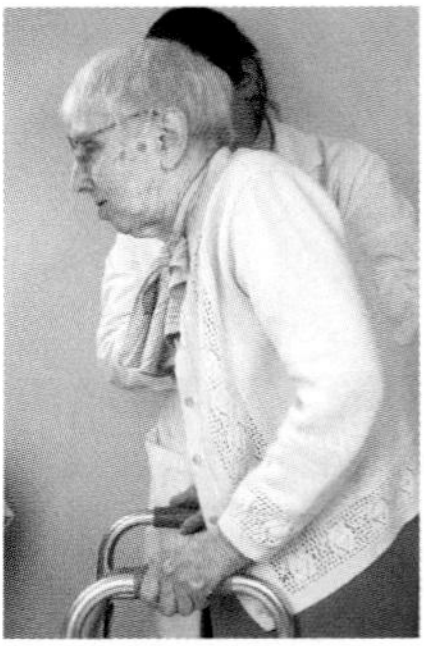 *Senile kyphosis*
Determine if spinal deformities are structural or functional (postural). Test for kyphosis and scoliosis by having patient bend from waist. **In true structural scoliosis, deviation is apparent when patient bends at waist. In functional scoliosis, deviation disappears.**		• *Scoliosis:* Lateral "S" spinal deviation. 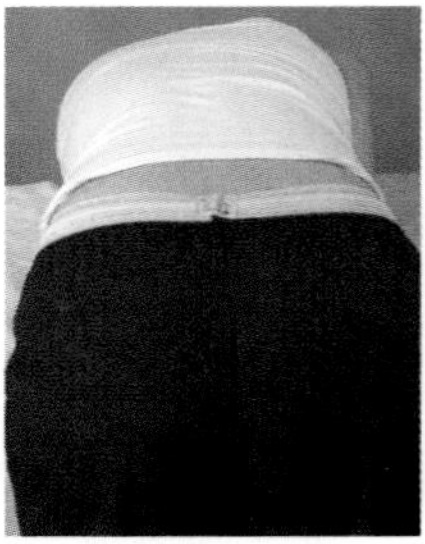 *Scoliosis*

AREA/PA SKILL	NORMAL FINDINGS	ABNORMAL FINDINGS
Test for lordosis by having patient flatten back against wall. 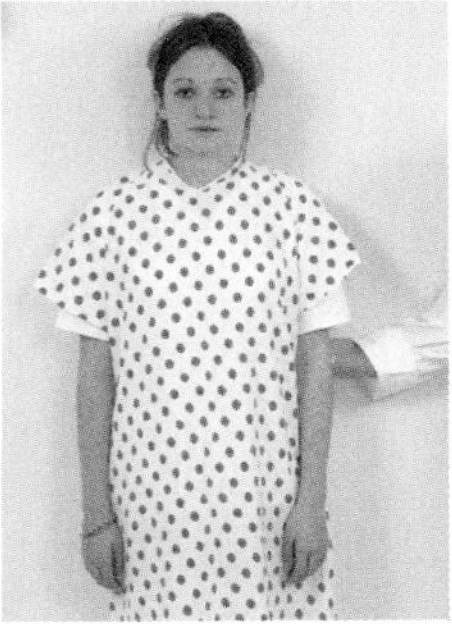 *Testing for lordosis*		• *Lordosis:* Accentuated lumbar curve. 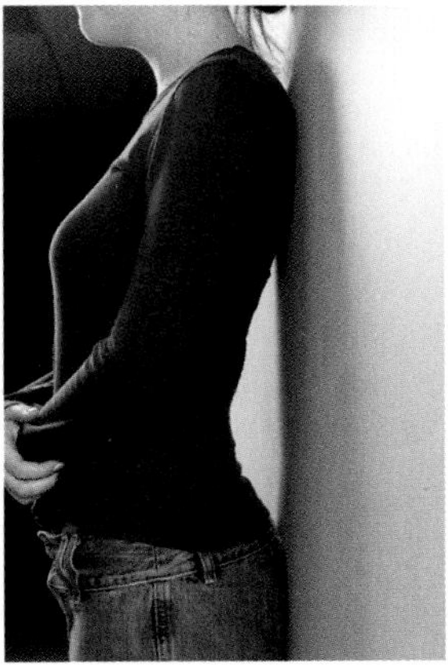 *Lordosis* 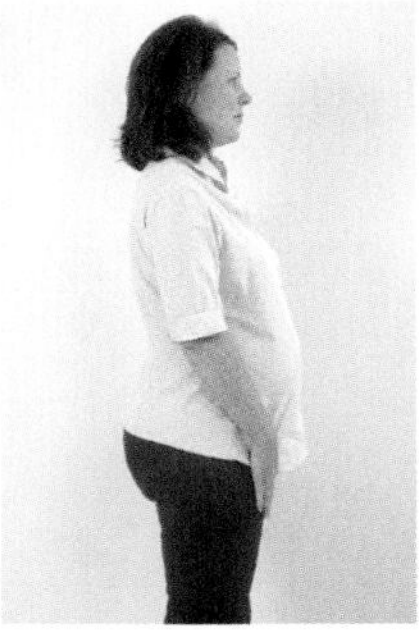 *Pregnancy lordosis*
Gait		
Inspect gait as patient walks [Table 12.3].		
Note wear of shoes.	Shoes worn evenly.	*Uneven weight bearing:* Associated with joint pain.

(box continued on page 326)

Physical Assessment (continued)

AREA/PA SKILL	NORMAL FINDINGS	ABNORMAL FINDINGS
Inspection		
Gait (cont'd)		
Note phases of gait, arm swing, cadence, base of support, stride length, toeing.	Phases of gait conform; gait smooth, fluid, rhythmic; arms swing in opposition; no toeing in or out; 2" to 4" base of support; 12" to 14" stride length.	
Wider base of support and shorter stride length often reflect balance problem.	Toddler, older adult, obese, or pregnant patient may have a wider base of support, shorter stride length, and uneven rhythm.	*Wide base of support:* Cerebellar dysfunction. *Ataxia, spasticity, and tremors:* Parkinson's disease, multiple sclerosis (MS), cerebral palsy (CP). *Scissors gait:* Disorders of motor cortex or corticospinal tracts (e.g., bilateral spastic paresis). *Spastic movements:* Upper motor neuron disorders. *Flaccidity:* Lower motor neuron disorders. *Flaccidity and foot drop:* Peripheral nerve disorders.
Cerebellar Function Balance		
Observe gait, tandem walk (heel to toe), heel-and-toe walk, deep knee bend.	Coordinated, balanced gait; + tandem walk, heel-and-toe walk, deep knee bend.	*Balance problems:* Cerebellar disorder.
Perform Romberg's test. Stand close to patient when performing	Negative results on Romberg's test.	*Positive results on Romberg's test:* Cerebellar disorder if patient has difficulty maintaining

AREA/PA SKILL	NORMAL FINDINGS	ABNORMAL FINDINGS
Romberg's test; patient's feet together, eyes opened then closed. Note swaying.		balance with eyes open or closed. If patient loses balance only when eyes are closed, damage to the dorsal column should be *suspected.*

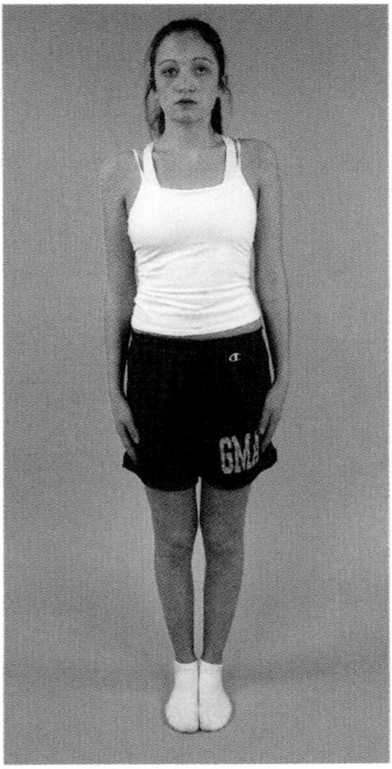

Romberg test. A. Eyes open

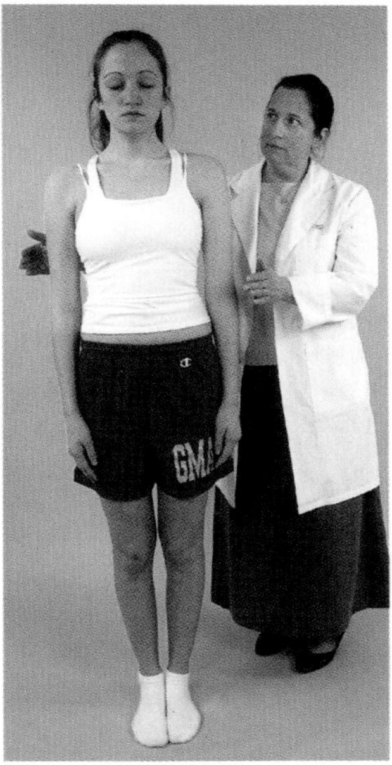

B. Eyes closed

(box continued on page 328)

Physical Assessment (continued)

AREA/PA SKILL	NORMAL FINDINGS	ABNORMAL FINDINGS
Inspection *(cont'd)* *Coordination*		
Test upper extremities using finger-thumb opposition and rapid alternating movements (RAM).	Coordination intact. RAM intact bilaterally; + finger-thumb opposition.	*Slowness and awkwardness in performing movements:* Cerebellar disorder or motor weakness associated with extrapyramidal disease.

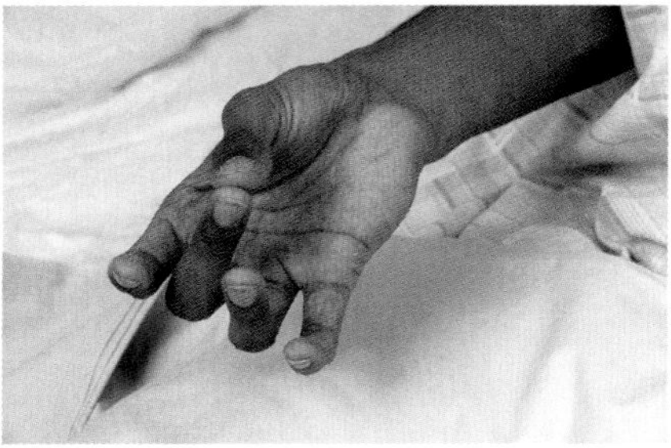

Finger-thumb opposition

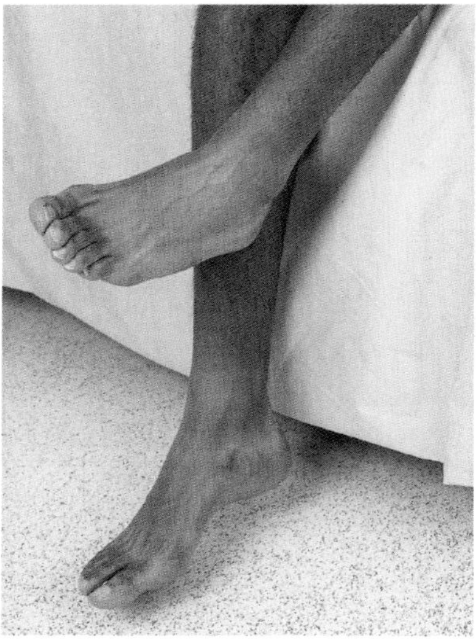

Running heel down shin

AREA/PA SKILL	NORMAL FINDINGS	ABNORMAL FINDINGS
Test lower extremities using toe tapping and running heel down shin. **Note dominant side; usually more coordinated.**	+ Toe tapping; able to run heel down shin bilaterally.	
Accuracy of Movements		
Assess point-to-point localization with eyes open, then closed.	Point-to-point localization intact bilaterally.	*Inaccurate movements:* Cerebellar disorder.

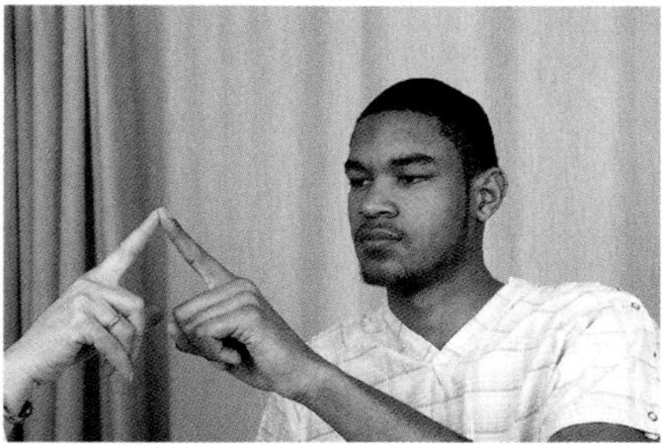

Finger to finger

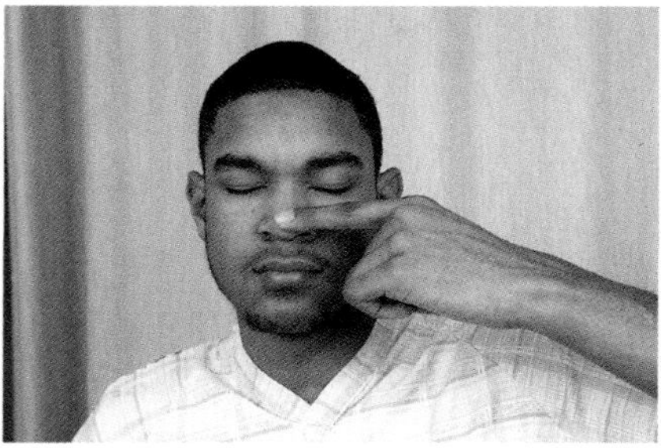

Finger to nose

(box continued on page 330)

Physical Assessment (continued)

AREA/PA SKILL	NORMAL FINDINGS	ABNORMAL FINDINGS
Inspection *(cont'd)* *Pronator Drift*		
Test with eyes open then closed. Note drifting.	Negative pronator drift.	*+ Pronator drift:* Weakness (e.g., hemiparesis, stroke).

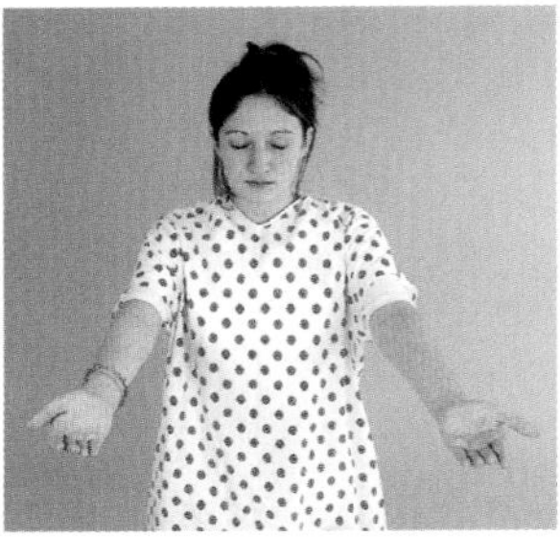

Assessing pronator drift

AREA/PA SKILL	NORMAL FINDINGS	ABNORMAL FINDINGS
Measurements		
Measure arm and leg lengths and circumferences in cm.	Equal arm and leg lengths, or differences not > 1 cm.	Leg length discrepancies can cause back and hip pain, gait problems, and pseudoscoliosis.
Arm lengths: Measure from the acromion process to tip of middle finger.	Equal arm and leg circumferences; note that dominant side may be greater, but not > 1 cm difference.	*Equal true leg lengths but unequal apparent leg lengths:* Hip and pelvic-area abnormalities.

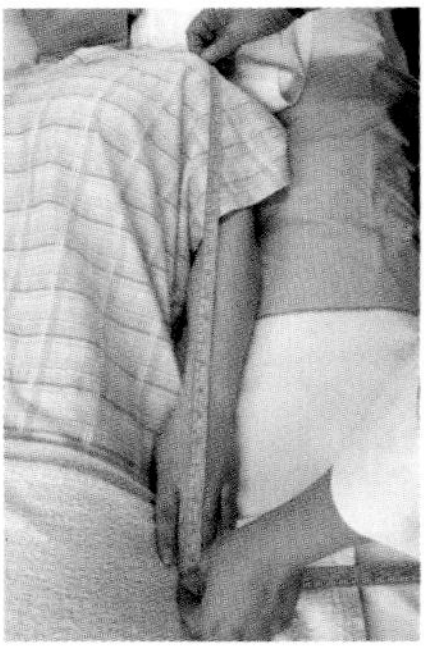

Measuring arm length

AREA/PA SKILL	NORMAL FINDINGS	ABNORMAL FINDINGS
Leg lengths: Measure from anterosuperior iliac crest to medial malleolus (true leg length). Measure from umbilicus to medial malleolus (apparent leg length).		*Circumference differences > 1 cm:* Muscular atrophy or hypertrophy.

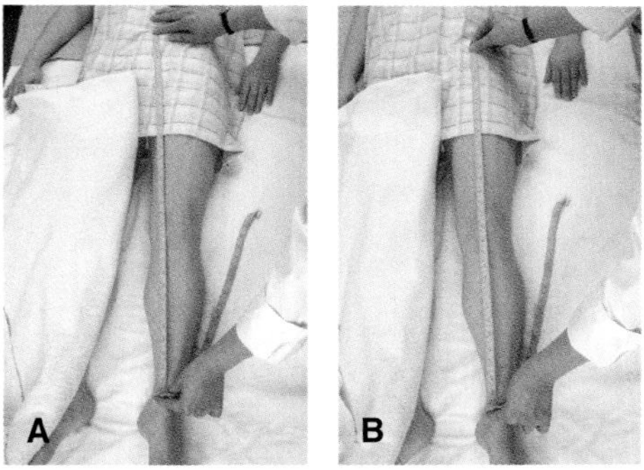

Measuring leg length. A. Apparent; B. True

To ensure accurate circumference measurements, determine midpoint of extremity.

Palpation

Muscle Tone

Palpate muscles of upper and lower extremities in relaxed and contracted state.	Muscles at rest soft and pliable; contracted, + muscle tone and firm.	Atrophy, unexplained hypertrophy, atony, weakness, fasciculations, tremors.
Note any involuntary movement or tenderness.	No involuntary movements or tenderness.	

(box continued on page 332)

Physical Assessment (continued)

AREA/PA SKILL	NORMAL FINDINGS	ABNORMAL FINDINGS
Palpation *Muscle Tone (cont'd)*		
Note atony, hypotony, or hypertony of muscles.	No atony, hypotony, or unexplained hypertony.	
Muscle Strength		
Screen strength with hand grip and foot push/leg raise.	All muscle groups 4/5 to 5/5 muscle strength. Hand grip strong and equal. Foot push and leg raise against resistance strong and equal.	*Weakness:* Paralysis, stroke, muscle disease, myasthenia gravis, Guillain-Barré syndrome.
Test muscle strength by noting ability to perform active range of motion (AROM) against resistance for face, neck, shoulders, arms, elbows, hands, wrists, hips, knees, ankles, and feet. Grade strength on 0–5 scale (Table 12.4). **Compare side to side. Note that dominant side may be stronger.**		

AREA/PA SKILL	NORMAL FINDINGS	ABNORMAL FINDINGS
Inspection/Palpation of Joints Test muscle strength as you assess range of motion (ROM) of joints.		

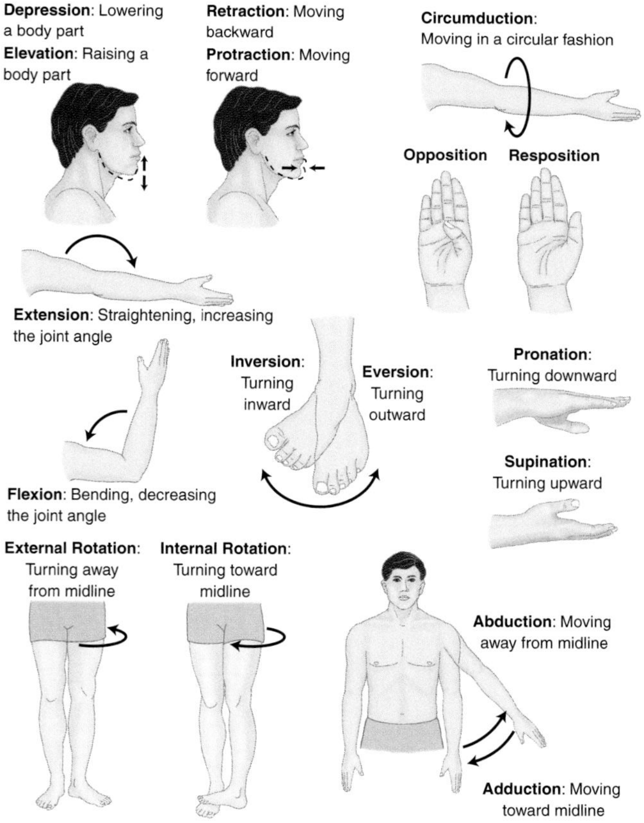

Body movement

AREA/PA SKILL	NORMAL FINDINGS	ABNORMAL FINDINGS
Assess all joints for ROM, condition of skin, erythema, edema, heat, deformity, crepitus, tenderness, and stability.		

(box continued on page 334)

Physical Assessment (continued)

AREA/PA SKILL	NORMAL FINDINGS	ABNORMAL FINDINGS
Inspection/Palpation of Joints *(cont'd)* *Temporomandibular Joint*		
Assess as for all joints, with attention to crepitus or clicks.	Full AROM (flexion, extension, side to side, protraction, retraction). No tenderness, deformity, crepitus, edema, or erythema.	*Decreased ROM, tenderness, swelling, crepitus:* Arthritis. *Pain, swelling, popping, clicking, or grating sounds:* Temporomandibular joint (TMJ) dysfunction. **TMJ dysfunction may present as ear pain and headache.** *Decreased muscle strength:* Muscle and joint disease. *Pain and spasms:* Myofacial pain syndrome. *Less-than-full contraction:* Lesion to cranial nerve V.
Cervical Spine (Neck)		
Assess as for all joints.	Full AROM (flexion, extension, hyperextension, rotation, lateral bend). No tenderness, crepitus, erythema, or deformity.	A neck not straight and erect is abnormal.
Note cervical curve.	Normal cervical curve.	*Inability to perform ROM because of pain:* Cervical disc degenerative disease, spinal cord tumor. Pain may radiate to back, shoulder, or arms. *Neck pain associated with weakness/loss of sensation in legs:* Cervical spinal cord compression. *Inability to perform ROM against resistance:* Muscle and joint disease.

AREA/PA SKILL	NORMAL FINDINGS	ABNORMAL FINDINGS
Scapulae		
Assess as for all joints. Note location and symmetry and winging.	Scapula equal over 2nd to 7th ribs, no winging.	Winging.
Ribs		
Assess as for all joints. Note condition of ribs.	Ribs firm, continuous, and nontender.	*Swelling, redness, enlargement, tenderness:* Inflammation.
Shoulders		
Assess as for all joints, with attention to stability.	Full AROM (flexion, extension, adduction, abduction, internal/external rotation, circumduction). Joint stable, no deformity, crepitus, or tenderness.	*Weakness and limited ROM:* Torn rotator cuff.
Elbows		
Assess as for all joints, with attention to nodules.	Full AROM (flexion, extension, supination, pronation). No nodules, crepitus, tenderness, or swelling.	*Redness, swelling and tenderness at elbow (olecranon process):* Bursitis. 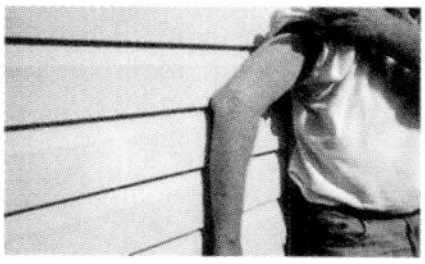 *Bursitis of elbow* *Tennis elbow (lateral epicondylitis):* Inflammation of forearm extensors or supinator muscles of fingers and wrist, or tendon attachment to lateral epicondyle or lateral collateral ligament caused by repetitive supination of forearm against resistance.

(box continued on page 336)

Physical Assessment (continued)

AREA/PA SKILL	NORMAL FINDINGS	ABNORMAL FINDINGS
Inspection/Palpation of Joints *Elbows (cont'd)*		
		Golf elbow (medial epicondylitis): Same as tennis elbow, except flexor and pronator muscles and tendons are affected.
Wrists		
Assess as for all joints.	Full AROM (flexion, extension, hyperextension, radial/ulnar deviation). Joint stable, no crepitus or tenderness.	*Swelling, tenderness, nodules, ulnar deviation, limited ROM:* Rheumatoid arthritis (RA). *Nontender, round, enlarged, swollen, fluid-filled cysts on wrists:* Ganglion cyst. *Pain with movement:* Tendinitis. *Pain on extension of wrist against resistance:* Epicondylitis. *Pain on flexion of wrist against resistance:* Medial epicondylitis. *Decreased muscle strength:* Muscle and joint disease.
If indicated, assess for carpal tunnel syndrome with Tinel's sign or Phalen's test.	Negative Tinel's and Phalen's tests.	*+ Tinel's or Phalen's test:* Carpal tunnel syndrome.

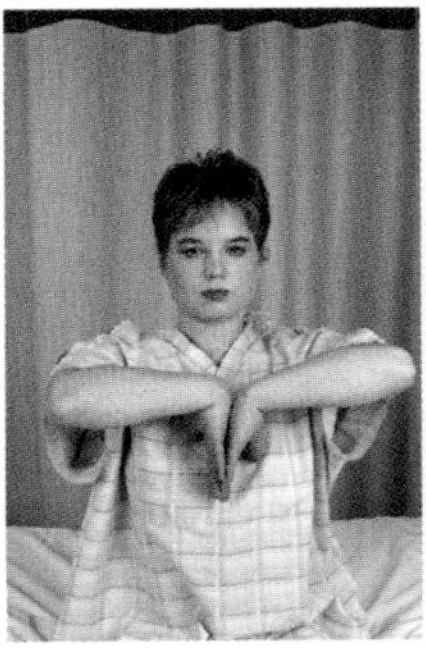

Phalen's test

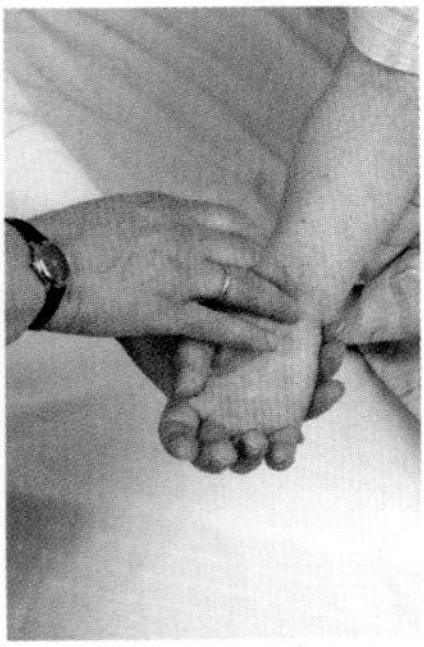

Tinel's test

AREA/PA SKILL	NORMAL FINDINGS	ABNORMAL FINDINGS
Fingers and Thumbs		
Assess as for all joints, with attention to deformities.	Full AROM (flexion, extension, hyperextension, abduction, adduction).	*Swollen, stiff, tender finger joints:* Acute RA.
Inspect palmar surface for shape and symmetry.	Nontender, no deformities.	*Boutonnière deformity and swan-neck deformity:* Long-term RA. 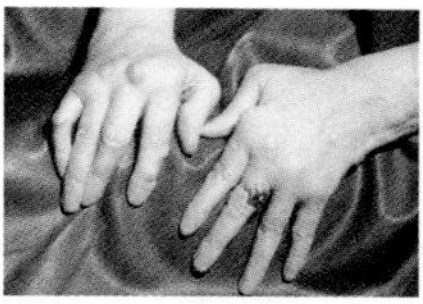 *Rheumatoid arthritis*
	Palms concave and symmetrical.	*Atrophy of thenar prominence:* Carpal tunnel syndrome. *Hard, painless nodules over distal interphalangeal joints:* Heberden's nodes. 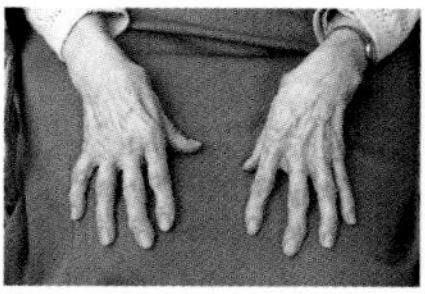 *Heberden's nodes* *Hard, painless nodules over proximal interphalangeal joints:* Bouchard's nodes. **Both types of nodes seen in osteoarthritis and RA.**

(box continued on page 338)

Physical Assessment (continued)

AREA/PA SKILL	NORMAL FINDINGS	ABNORMAL FINDINGS
Inspection/Palpation of Joints *Fingers and Thumbs (cont'd)*		*Gouty arthritis:* Deformities and nodules of hands. 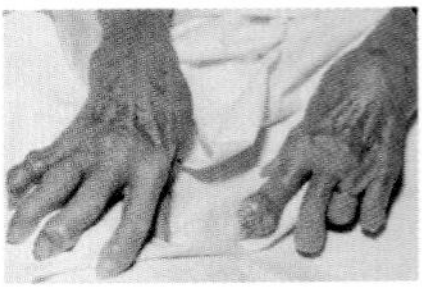 *Gouty arthritis* *Pain on extension of a finger:* Tenosynovitis. *Inability to extend ring finger:* Dupuytren's contracture. *Decreased muscle strength:* Muscle and joint disease.
Thoracic and Lumbar Curve		
Assess as for all joints. Note thoracic and lumbar curves.	Full AROM (flexion, extension, hyper-extension, lateral bends, rotation).	Limited ROM related to arthritis, DJD, disc disease of spine.
Hips		
Assess as for all joints, with attention to stability.	Full AROM (flexion, extension, hyper-extension, internal/external rotation, abduction, adduction). Joint stable, no crepitus, nontender.	*Unequal gluteal folds:* Dislocated hip. *Inability to abduct hip:* Common sign of hip disease. *Decrease in internal hip rotation:* Early sign of hip disease. *Decreased muscle strength against resistance:* Muscle and joint disease.
If indicated, perform Trendelenburg's test for hip dislocation.		*+ Trendelenburg's test:* Hip dislocation.

AREA/PA SKILL	NORMAL FINDINGS	ABNORMAL FINDINGS
If indicated, do Thomas's test for hip flexure contraction.		+ *Thomas's test:* Hip flexure contraction may be hidden by excessive lumbar lordosis.
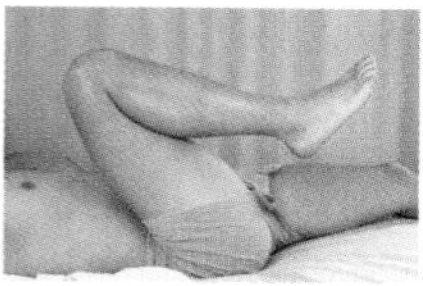 *Thomas's test*		
In newborn, do Ortolani's maneuver to test for hip dislocation.		+ *Ortolani's maneuver:* Hip dislocation.
If sciatica is present, do straight leg raise.		+ *Straight leg:* Herniated disc.
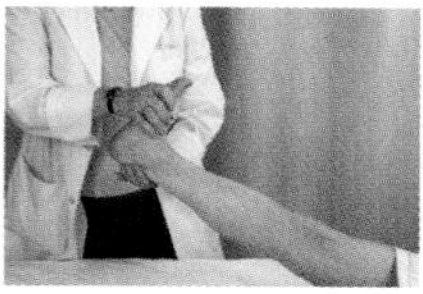 *Straight leg raising*		
Knees		
Assess as for all joints, with attention to crepitus and swelling.	Full AROM (flexion, extension). Knee stable. No swelling, tenderness, crepitus, nodules.	*Tenderness, warmth, boggy consistency:* Synovitis. *Crepitation:* Osteoarthritis. *Decreased ROM:* Synovial thickening. *Inability to extend knee fully:* Flexion contracture of knee.

(box continued on page 340)

Physical Assessment (continued)

AREA/PA SKILL	NORMAL FINDINGS	ABNORMAL FINDINGS
Inspection/Palpation of Joints *Knees (cont'd)*		*Decreased muscle strength against resistance:* Muscle and joint disease. 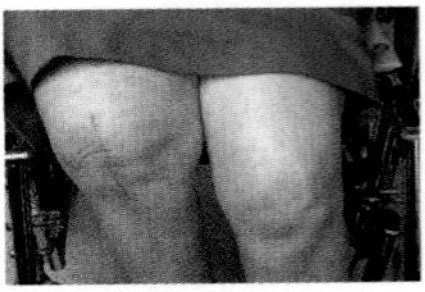 *DJD of knees*
If indicated, do McMurray's and Apley's tests for foreign body, torn meniscus. 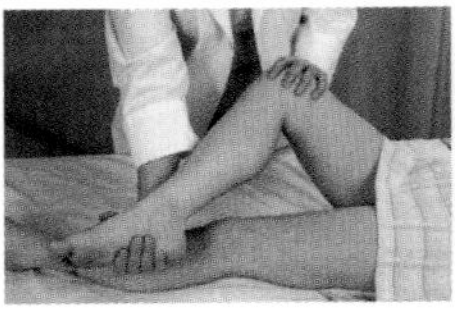 *McMurray's test*	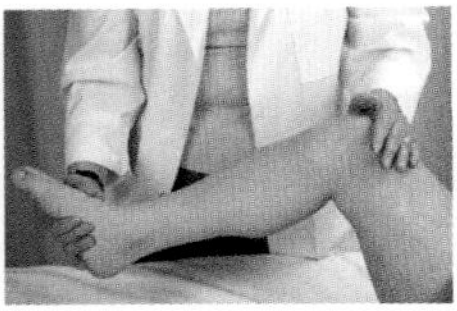 *Apley's test*	*+ Apley's and McMurray's tests:* Meniscus tear.
If indicated, do Lachman's test for anterior cruciate ligament (ACL)/posterior cruciate ligament (PCL) tears. 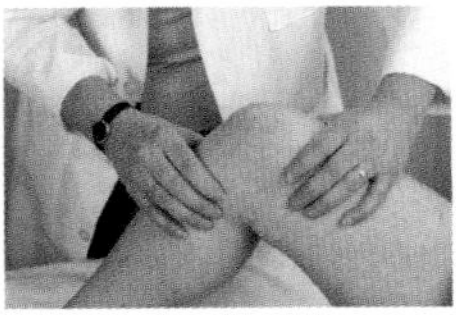 *Lachman's test*		*+ Lachman's test:* ACL or PCL tear.
If indicated, do bulge sign or patellar tap for fluid. 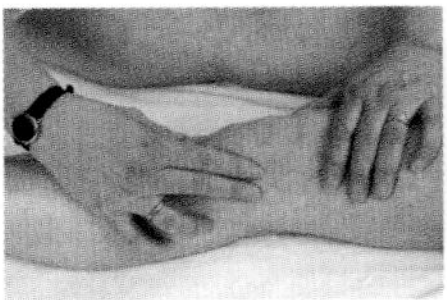 *Bulge test*	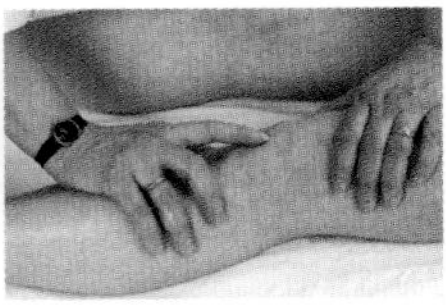 *Patellar ballottement*	*+ Bulge sign and patellar tap:* Fluid.

AREA/PA SKILL	NORMAL FINDINGS	ABNORMAL FINDINGS
Ankles		
Assess as for all joints, with attention to tenderness.	Full AROM (plantarflexion, dorsiflexion, eversion, inversion). No tenderness or crepitus.	*Nodules on posterior ankle:* RA.
Feet and Toes		
Assess as for all joints, with attention to deformities, corns, bunions, hammer toes, hallux valgus.	Full AROM (flexion, extension, hyperextension, dorsiflexion, abduction, adduction). No deformities; longitudinal arch; weight bearing on foot at midline.	Hallux valgus often on medial side, may present with laterally deviated great toe with overlapping of second toe. *Bunion:* Enlarged, painful, inflamed bursa, often occurs with hammer toe.
Note flat feet or high arches. **Look at type of shoes patient wears. Many foot problems are caused by poorly fitting shoes.**		*Hammer toe:* Hyperextension of metatarsophalangeal joint and flexion of proximal interphalangeal joint. 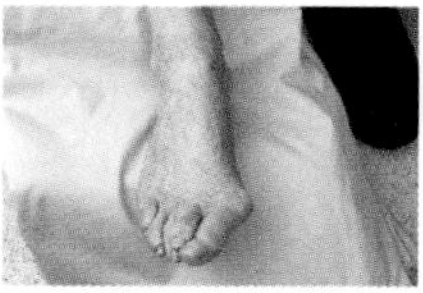 *Hallux vagus, bunion, and hammer toe* *Flat feet (pes planus):* No arches. High arches (pes cavus). *Corns:* Painful, thickened skin over bony prominences and pressure points. 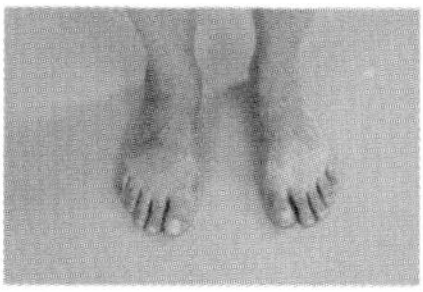 *Corns and bunions*

(box continued on page 342)

Physical Assessment (continued)		
AREA/PA SKILL	**NORMAL FINDINGS**	**ABNORMAL FINDINGS**
Inspection/Palpation of Joints *Feet and Toes (cont'd)*		*Callus:* Nonpainful, thickened skin over pressure points. 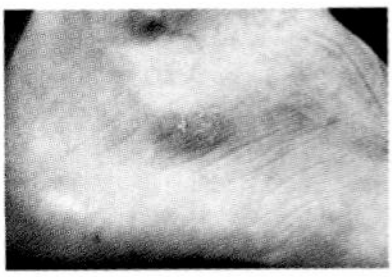 *Callus* *Plantar warts (verruca vulgaris):* Painful warts that occur under a callus. *Tender, painful, reddened, hot, swollen metatarsophalangeal joint of great toe:* Gouty arthritis. *Pain and tenderness of metatarsophalangeal joints:* DJD, RA, joint inflammation.

PA = Physical assessment.

TABLE 12.3 Abnormal Gaits

TYPE OF GAIT	DESCRIPTION/CAUSE
Propulsive gait 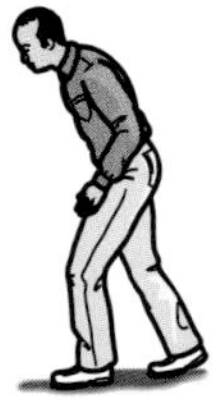	Rigid, stooped posture with head leaning forward and arms, knees, and hips stiffly flexed. Rapid, short, shuffling steps. *Causes:* Classic gait of Parkinson's disease.

TYPE OF GAIT	DESCRIPTION/CAUSE
Scissors gait 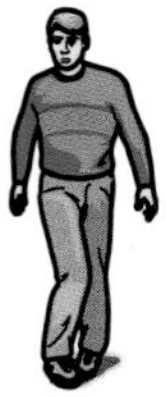	Bilateral spastic paresis of legs; arms not involved. Legs flexed at hip and knees. Knees adduct and meet or cross like scissors. Short steps, foot plantarflexed, walks on toes. *Causes:* CP, MS, spinal cord tumors.
Spastic gait (hemiplegic) 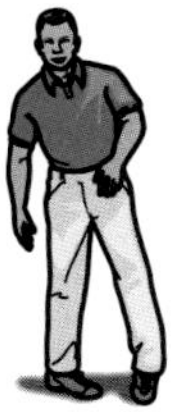	Unilateral stiff, dragging leg from leg, muscle hypertonicity. *Causes:* Stroke, MS, brain tumor.
Steppage gait (equine, prancing, paretic, or weak) 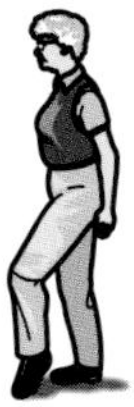	Foot drop with external rotation of hip and hip and knee flexion. Foot slaps when it hits ground. *Causes:* MS, herniated lumbar disk, Guillain-Barré syndrome, perineal muscle atrophy, or nerve damage.
Waddling gait 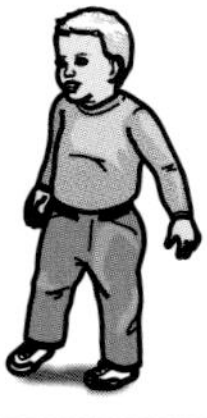	Ducklike walk with wide base of support, chest thrown back, exaggerated lumbar curve (lordosis), and protruding abdomen. *Causes:* Normal in toddlers and late stages of pregnancy. Weak pelvic girdle muscles (gluteus medius, hip flexors, and extensors). *Causes:* MS, hip dislocation.

TABLE 12.4 Rating Scale for Muscle Strength

RATING SCALE	EXPLANATION	CLASSIFICATION
5	Active motion against full resistance	Normal
4	Active motion against some resistance	Slight weakness
3	Active motion against gravity	Average weakness
2	Passive ROM (gravity removed and assisted by examiner)	Poor ROM
1	Slight flicker of contraction	Severe weakness
0	No muscular contraction	Paralysis

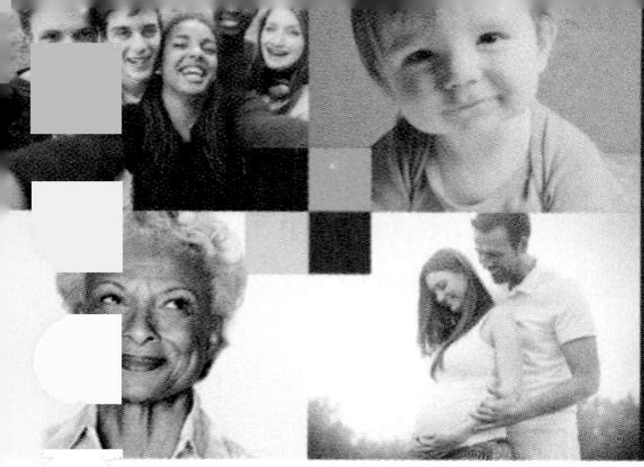

CHAPTER 13

Assessing the Sensory-Neurologic System

Primary Functions

- Acts as main "circuit board" of the body
- Allows interaction with the external environment
- Maintains activities of internal organs

Developmental Considerations

Newborns and Infants

- Reflexes are primitive because of immature neurologic system.
- Injury to the facial nerve during vaginal birth can cause a transient palsy.
- Down syndrome is a genetic disorder that causes mental retardation ranging from mild to severe.
- Maternal use of drugs (including alcohol) during pregnancy, dietary deficiencies, antepartal infections, systemic diseases, and birth trauma can result in neurologic disorders such as mental retardation, blindness, deafness, seizures, neuromuscular impairments, and other deficits.

Children and Adolescents

- Later-onset disorders, such as obsessive-compulsive disorder and hyperactivity, may become apparent only during the preschool years.
- Changes in behavior may also signal abuse.
- If the parent reports seizure activity, assess whether or not it is associated with signs of infection, such as a runny nose, high

temperature, or recent immunizations. Fevers in toddlers and preschoolers occasionally cause seizures. Repeated episodes of seizure activity may indicate epilepsy.
- Lead poisoning can cause neurologic problems in children.
- Diets high in caffeine and sugar may contribute to hyperactivity.

Pregnant Patients

- Folic acid deficiency, especially in the first trimester of pregnancy, is closely linked to neural tube defects, such as spina bifida, in the newborn.
- Transient episodes of neurologic pain occur, including carpal tunnel syndrome, foot and leg cramps, numbness or tingling in the thigh, and frequent headaches. They usually resolve after delivery.
- Hyperactive reflexes during pregnancy may suggest the presence of preeclampsia, a hypertensive disorder that can be accompanied by seizures.

Older Adults

- Neural impulses slow.
- Creative, critical, and abstract thinking, as well as problem-solving ability, is more typically *increased* in older adults.
- Neurologic deficits in older adults are commonly caused by:
  - Adverse effects of medications or medication interactions.
  - Nutritional deficiencies.
  - Dehydration.
  - Cardiovascular (CV) disease affecting cerebral perfusion.
  - Diabetes and other endocrine disorders.
  - Neurologic trauma
  - Degenerative neurologic diseases, such as Alzheimer's disease and Parkinson's disease.
  - Alcohol or drug abuse.
  - Stress, grief, isolation.
  - Psychiatric disorders.
  - Abuse or neglect.
- The number and sensitivity of sensory neurons decreases in older adults, leading to a diminished sense of touch.
- Reflexes are also diminished: The Achilles tendon reflex may be totally lost in older adults; other deep tendon reflexes (DTRs) should be present, but may be less brisk.

Cultural Considerations

- African Americans have a higher incidence of hypertension (HTN) and, subsequently, a higher incidence of stroke.
- Irish Americans have a high incidence of neural tube defects.
- Navajo Native Americans have a unique neuropathy that causes death by age 24.

Assessment

History

Symptoms ("PQRST" Any + Symptom)

- Headache
  - Any recent trauma?
  - Stress?
  - When does it occur; how long does it last?
  - Any medical problems?
  - Where does it hurt?
  - What does it feel like?
  - Any vision changes, nausea, vomiting, or numbness?
  - Recent infections?
- Change in mental status
  - Any medical problems?
  - Recent head trauma?
  - Psychiatric problems?
  - Are you taking any medications—prescribed or over-the-counter (OTC)?
  - Alcohol or drug use?
- Dizziness, vertigo, syncope
  - Any CV problems? HTN?
  - Are you taking any medications—prescribed or OTC?
- Numbness, loss of sensation
  - Do you have any vascular problems? Diabetes? Neurologic problems?
  - Any recent injury?
- Change in any of the five senses
  - Any changes in sense of sight, smell, touch, taste, or hearing?
  - Any other medical problems?
  - Are you taking any medications—prescribed or OTC?
  - Drug and alcohol use?

Focused Sensory-Neurologic History

- Do you have any neurologic problems?
- Do you have any other medical problems?
- Are you taking any medications, prescribed or OTC (Table 13.1)?
- History of head trauma, loss of consciousness, dizziness, headaches?
- History of seizures?
- Memory problems, changes in senses?
- Weakness, numbness, paralysis?
- Problems walking or performing activities of daily living (ADLs)?
- Mood problems, depression?
- Drug and alcohol use?
- Allergies?
- Ever treated for neurologic or psychiatric problem?
- Time of onset of symptoms?

TABLE 13.1 Drugs That Adversely Affect the Sensory-Neurologic System

DRUG CLASS	DRUG	POSSIBLE ADVERSE REACTIONS
Adrenergics	Albuterol sulfate, epinephrine, isoproterenol hydrochloride, terbutaline sulfate	Nervousness, tremors, dizziness, restlessness, insomnia
Adrenergic blockers	Ergotamine tartrate	Lightheadedness, vertigo, insomnia, euphoria, confusion, hallucinations, numbness and tingling of fingers and toes.
Antianginals	Diltiazem hydrochloride	Headache, fatigue
	Isosorbide dinitrate, nitroglycerin	Headache, dizziness, weakness, orthostatic hypotension
	Nifedipine	Headache, dizziness, lightheadedness, flushing
	Verapamil hydrochloride	Headache, dizziness
Antiarrhythmics	Lidocaine	Lightheadedness, dizziness, paresthesia, tremors, restlessness, confusion, hallucinations, headache
Anticonvulsants	Carbamazepine	Dizziness, drowsiness, ataxia, confusion, speech disturbances, involuntary movements

DRUG CLASS	DRUG	POSSIBLE ADVERSE REACTIONS
	Phenytoin	Dose-related headache, confusion, ataxia, slurred speech, lethargy, drowsiness, nervousness, insomnia, blurred vision, diplopia, nystagmus
Antidepressants	Tricyclic antidepressants	Drowsiness, weakness, lethargy, fatigue, agitation, nightmares, restlessness; confusion, disorientation (especially in elderly patients)
	Monoamine oxidase inhibitors	Restlessness, insomnia, drowsiness, headache, orthostatic hypotension, HTN
Antihypertensives	Clonidine	Drowsiness, sedation, dizziness, headache, nightmares, depression, hallucinations
	Hydralazine	Headache
	Methyldopa	Drowsiness, sedation, decreased mental acuity, vertigo, headache, psychic disturbances, nightmares, depression
	All beta-blockers	Fatigue, lethargy, vivid dreams, hallucinations, depression
Anti-infectives	Aminoglycosides	Neuromuscular blockade; ototoxicity causing vertigo, hearing impairment, or both
	Acyclovir	Myoclonus, seizures
	Isoniazid	Peripheral neuropathy
	Nitrofurantoin	Peripheral neuropathy
Antineoplastic agents	Fludarabine	Dysarthrias, paresthesias, weakness, seizures, paralysis
	Procarbazine	Paresthesis, neuropathy, confusion
	Vinblastine sulfate	Paresthesis
	Vincristine sulfate	Peripheral neuropathy, loss of DTRs, jaw pain
Antiparkinsonian agents	Amantadine	Psychic disturbances, nervousness, irritability, fatigue, depression, insomnia, confusion, hallucinations, difficulty concentrating
	Levodopa, pramipexole, ropinirole	Psychic disturbances, decreased attention span, memory loss, nervousness, vivid dreams, involuntary muscle movements

(continued)

TABLE 13.1 Drugs That Adversely Affect the Sensory-Neurologic System (continued)

DRUG CLASS	DRUG	POSSIBLE ADVERSE REACTIONS
Antipsychotics	Haloperidol, phenothiazines	Extrapyramidal reactions, tardive dyskinesia, headache, lethargy, confusion, agitation, hallucinations
Cholinergic blockers	Atropine sulfate, benztropine mesylate, glycopyrrolate	Blurred vision, headache, nervousness, drowsiness, weakness, dizziness, insomnia, disorientation
Corticosteroids	Dexamethasone, hydrocortisone, methylprednisolone, prednisone	Mood swings, euphoria, insomnia, headache, vertigo, behavior
Gastrointestinal agents	Cimetidine	Confusion (especially in elderly patients), depression
	Metoclopramide	Restlessness, anxiety drowsiness, lassitude, extrapyramidal reactions, tardive dyskinesia
Narcotic analgesics	Morphine sulfate, hydromorphone, meperidine, methadone, oxycodone	Sedation, dizziness, visual disturbances, clouded sensorium
	Butorphanol tartrate, nalbuphine, pentazocine	Sedation, headache, dizziness, vertigo, light-headedness, euphoria
Nonsteroidal anti-inflammatory agents	Ibuprofen, indomethacin	Drowsiness, dizziness
Sedatives and hypnotics	Barbiturates	Drowsiness, lethargy, vertigo, headache, depression, "hangover," paradoxical excitement in elderly patients, hyperactivity in children
	Benzodiazepines	Drowsiness, dizziness, ataxia, daytime sedation, headache, confusion
Skeletal muscle relaxants	Baclofen	Drowsiness
	Chlorzoxazone	Drowsiness, dizziness
	Cyclobenzaprine	Drowsiness, dizziness, headache, nervousness, confusion
Miscellaneous agents	Lithium	Lethargy, tremors, headache, mental confusion, dizziness, seizures, difficulty concentrating

Assessment of the Sensory-Neurologic System's Relationship to Other Systems

Remember, all systems are related. As you assess the sensory-neurologic system, look at the relationship between it and all other systems.

Assessment of the Sensory-Neurologic System's Relationship to Other Systems

SUBJECTIVE DATA/RATIONALE	OBJECTIVE DATA/RATIONALE
Area/System: General	
Ask about:	*Measure:*
General health: Ask about affective changes such as depression. Lethargy, emotional lability seen with stroke.	Vital signs: **Cushing's triad indicated by increased systolic pressure, widening pulse pressure and bradycardia sign of increased ICP.**
Fever: Associated with meningitis.	*Observe:*
	Mental status, grooming, affect, behavior, symmetry: Changes in level of consciousness may be an early sign of a developing central nervous system disorder. Inability to care for self as reflected by poor grooming may be caused by a neurologic problem, such as hemiparesis, or a psychiatric problem, such as depression.
Area/System: Integumentary	
Ask about:	*Inspect for:*
Rashes, petechiae: Meningococcal meningitis.	*Rashes or petechiae:* Meningitis.
Changes in sensations: Loss of sensation may indicate transient ischemic attack (TIA) or stroke.	*Test:*
	Superficial sensations: Peripheral neuropathies, spinal cord injuries, and stroke can cause sensory deficits.
Area/System: HEENT	
Ask about:	*Inspect:*
Changes in sense of smell, taste, sight, hearing, touch: Associated with TIA and stroke.	*Symmetry of facial features:* Asymmetrical facial features related to stroke. Masklike facial expression related to Parkinson's disease.
Headaches: HTN, intracranial bleeding.	*Palpate:*
	Lymph nodes, thyroid.
Changes in speech or swallowing: Impaired speech may indicate dysphasia. Lack of	*Examine:*
	Optic disc: *Papilledema:* Increased ICP.

(continued)

Assessment of the Sensory-Neurologic System's Relationship to Other Systems (continued)

SUBJECTIVE DATA/RATIONALE	OBJECTIVE DATA/RATIONALE
articulation of speech may indicate dysarthria. **Patients with dysarthria often have dysphagia (difficulty swallowing) as well.** *Thyroid disease:* Hypo- or hyperthyroidism can affect patient's mood.	*Test:* *CNs:* Abnormal CNs can indicate a neurologic problem. *Visual and pupillary changes:* Increased ICP. *Peripheral field deficits:* Neurologic problems, such as stroke.
Area/System: Respiratory *Ask about:* *Breathing difficulty:* Mental status changes can occur with chronic obstructive pulmonary disease (COPD) as a result of hypoxia or hypercapnia.	*Auscultate:* *Lungs:* An irregular breathing pattern may indicate increased ICP. Hypoxia can cause confusion and increased ICP.
Area/System: Cardiovascular *Ask about:* *History of CV problems:* Positive history of CV disease increases risk for stroke. Atrial fibrillation, a common dysrhythmia in older adults, increases risk for stroke. **Raynaud's and Buerger's diseases can cause paresthesia.**	*Auscultate:* *Heart sounds, noting rhythm:* Atrial fibrillation increases risk for embolic stroke. *Carotids for bruits and thrills:* Carotid bruits or thrills reflect carotid stenosis, increasing risk for thrombotic stroke.
Area/System: Gastrointestinal *Ask about:* *Nausea, vomiting:* Nausea is often seen with neurologic problems such as head trauma and increased ICP. Changes in bowel function. Difficulty swallowing. **Patients who have difficulty swallowing are at higher risk for aspiration.** Dysphagia: May occur with stroke, MS, myasthenia gravis (MG), ALS.	*Auscultate:* *Bowel sounds:* Constipation is most common bowel problem in stroke patients.

SUBJECTIVE DATA/RATIONALE	OBJECTIVE DATA/RATIONALE
Area/System: Genitourinary/ Reproductive	
Ask about:	*Inspect for:*
History of sexually transmitted diseases (STDs): Tertiary syphilis can cause neurosyphilis.	Lesions.
	Palpate:
Changes in sexual activity, desire, ability: Loss of sensation and inability to achieve erection may be neurologic in origin. Problems with erection can occur with neuropathies and central nervous system disease such as Parkinson's disease.	*Bladder distension:* Poor bladder control or incontinence frequently occurs during acute phase of stroke. Can also occur with spinal cord injuries and other neurologic disorders.
Menstrual cycle/birth control pills (BCP): Hypercoagulable states increase the risk for stroke.	
Bowel problems, incontinence, loss of bowel function: Cauda equina syndrome caused by compression of sacral nerve, can occur with herniated disc or spinal stenosis.	
This is a medical emergency.	
Transient loss of bowel and bladder function: Stroke or spinal cord dysfunction.	
Incontinence: Tonic-clonic seizures.	
Area/System: Musculoskeletal	
Ask about:	*Inspect:*
Muscle weakness: Associated with many neurologic disorders.	Gait.
	Test:
Paralysis: Paralysis can lead to muscle atrophy from disuse.	*Muscle strength:* Paralysis can result in muscle atrophy.
Problems walking.	ROM.
Balance problems.	*Cerebellar function:* Cerebellar dysfunctions can result in balance problems. Spatial perception problems can result from a stroke.
	(continued)

Assessment of the Sensory-Neurologic System's Relationship to Other Systems (continued)

SUBJECTIVE DATA/RATIONALE	OBJECTIVE DATA/RATIONALE
Area/System: Endocrine *Ask about:* *History of diabetes mellitus and thyroid disease:* Diabetes can cause neuropathies and muscle wasting. Hypothyroidism can cause weakness, lethargy, flat affect, and labile affect.	
Area/System: Lymphatic/ Hematological *Ask about:* Fever. *Bruising:* Bleeding disorders may increase risk for stroke.	

HEENT = Head, eyes, ears, nose, and throat.

Stroke Assessment Scales

CINCINNATI PREHOSPITAL STROKE SCALE: The Cincinnati Prehospital Stroke Scale can be used to quickly assess for signs of stroke. Presence of even one sign, either facial droop, motor weakness or slurred speech, warrants immediate medical evaluation.

- Facial droop – have client smile
- Test motor weakness – pronator drift
- Slurred speech – "Can't teach old dog new tricks"

NIH STROKE SCALE: The National Institute of Health Stroke Scale quantifies the severity of the stroke. This scale is used for initial evaluation, and then to monitor the patient's progress and response to treatment. It has 12 categories with scores - 0 (normal) to 42 (severely impaired). Categories include:

- LOC
- LOC question
- LOC commands
- Gaze abnormalities
- Visual loss
- Facial weakness
- Motor weakness arms and legs
- Limb ataxia

- Sensory loss
- Language
- Dysarthria
- Extinction and inattention

Glasgow Coma Scale

OBSERVATION	RESPONSE	SCORE
Eye Response	Opens spontaneously	4
	Opens to verbal command	3
	Opens to pain	2
	No response	1
Motor Response	Reacts to verbal command	6
	Reacts to painful stimuli	
	• Identifies localized pain	5
	• Flexes and withdraws	4
	• Assumes flexor posture	3
	• Assumes extensor posture	2
	No response	1
Verbal Response	Oriented and converses	5
	Disoriented but converses	4
	Uses inappropriate words	3
	Makes incomprehensible sounds	2
	No response	1
Best Score		15
Comatose		8 or less
Totally Unresponsive		3

Physical Assessment

APPROACH: Inspection, palpation; cerebral function, cranial nerves (CNs), sensory function, reflexes.

POSITION: Sitting.

TOOLBOX: Stethoscope, blood pressure (BP) cuff, penlight, nonsterile gloves, wisp of cotton, sharp object (e.g., toothpicks or sterile needle), objects to touch (e.g., a coin, button, key, or paper clip), something fragrant (e.g., rubbing alcohol or coffee), things to taste (e.g., lemon juice, for sour; sugar; salt; and quinine, for bitter), tongue blade, two test tubes or other vials, reflex hammer, ophthalmoscope.

Remember, if the right side of the brain has a problem, the clinical manifestations will be on the left side, and vice versa.

If your patient has a spatial perception problem, be aware that he or she may have neglect, a spatial perception problem in which the patient doesn't see the affected side as part of his or her body.

Physical Assessment

AREA/PA SKILL	NORMAL FINDINGS	ABNORMAL FINDINGS
Cerebral Function **Consider the age and the educational and cultural background of your patient.**		
Behavior		
Note facial expression, posture, affect, and grooming.	Well-groomed, erect posture, pleasant facial expression, affect appropriate. Normal findings vary depending on situation.	Lack of facial expression, or inappropriate expression for speech. *Content:* Psychiatric disorder (e.g., depression or schizophrenia) or neurologic impairment affecting CNs. *Masklike expression:* Parkinson's disease. *Poor grooming or slumped posture:* Psychiatric origin, as in depression; or physiological origin, as in stroke with hemiparesis. **Safety is an issue for patients with right-side brain injury because they tend to be impulsive and not know their own limits.**
Level of Consciousness		
Assess arousal state using minimal stimuli first, then increasing intensity as needed (Table 13.2). Document appropriately (Table 13.3). Test orientation to time, place, and person.	Awake, alert, and oriented (AAO) x 3 (time, place, and person). Older person may be disoriented to time, but note if patient reorients easily.	*Disorientation physical in origin:* Exhaustion, anxiety, hypoxia, fluid and electrolyte imbalance, drugs, or neurologic problem. *Disorientation psychiatric in origin:* Schizophrenia.

AREA/PA SKILL	NORMAL FINDINGS	ABNORMAL FINDINGS
Disorientation to time and place usually occurs before disorientation to person.		
Cerebral Function *Memory*		
Test immediate, recent, and remote memory. • *Immediate:* Ask patient to repeat series of numbers. • *Recent:* Name three objects and ask patient to recall later in exam. • *Remote:* Ask patient's birth date, major historical event. **If asking personal data, such as birth date, be able to validate information independently.**	Immediate, recent, and remote memory intact.	Memory problems can be benign or signal a more serious neurologic problem such as Alzheimer's disease. Forgetfulness—especially for immediate and recent events—is frequently seen in older adults. With benign forgetfulness, patient can retrace or use memory aids to help with recall. Pathological memory loss, as in Alzheimer's disease, is subtle and progressive until ability to function is impaired. *Temporary loss of memory:* Head trauma, concussion, minor head injury. Patient may experience amnesia for the event causing injury (retrograde amnesia). Postconcussion syndrome can occur anywhere from 2 weeks to 2 months after injury; may cause short-term memory deficits.
Mathematical and Calculative Ability		
Have patient perform simple mathematical problem, such as 4 + 5, serial 7s or 4s, subtraction from 100.	Calculative skills intact.	Inability to calculate at a level appropriate to age, education, and language ability requires evaluation for neurologic impairment.

(box continued on page 358)

Physical Assessment (continued)

AREA/PA SKILL	NORMAL FINDINGS	ABNORMAL FINDINGS
Cerebral Function *(cont'd)* *General Knowledge and Vocabulary*		
Assess vocabulary and general knowledge. Ask how many days in a week? Months in a year? Ask patient to define familiar words, such as apple, earthquake, chastise. **Begin with easy words and proceed to more difficult words.**	Vocabulary appropriate and general knowledge intact.	Inability to define familiar words requires further evaluation.
Thought Process		
Note attention span, logic of speech, ability to stay focused, appropriateness of responses.	Thought process clear; responds appropriately; speech coherent and logical.	*Incoherent speech, illogical or unrealistic ideas, repetition of words and phrases, markedly and/or repeatedly straying from the topic, and suddenly losing train of thought:* Examples of altered thought processes that warrant further evaluation. *Causes of alteration in thought process:* Physical disorder (e.g., dementia), psychiatric disorder (e.g., psychosis), or drugs and alcohol.
Abstract Reasoning		
Give patient a proverb to interpret. Have patient identify similarities, such as apples and oranges.	Abstract thinking intact.	*Impaired ability to think abstractly:* Dementia, delirium, mental retardation, psychoses.
Judgment		
Assess patient's response to hypothetical situations.	Judgment intact.	*Impaired judgment:* Dementia, psychosis, drug and alcohol abuse.

AREA/PA SKILL	NORMAL FINDINGS	ABNORMAL FINDINGS
Communication		
Note speech and language, enunciation, fluency. Note any dysarthria, dysphasia, dysphonia, neologisms, or circumlocution.	Speech clear, fluent, no dysarthria, dysphasia, dysphonia, neologisms, or circumlocution.	*Hesitancy, stuttering, stammering, unclear speech:* Lack of familiarity with language, deference or shyness, anxiety, or neurologic disorder.
The following, more specific tests assess for a variety of neurologic problems (Table 13.4).	*Communication skills intact:* Spontaneous speech, motor speech, automatic speech, sound recognition, auditory-verbal comprehension, visual recognition, visual-verbal comprehension, writing, and figure copying.	*Dysphasia or aphasia:* Neurologic problems such as stroke. Drugs and alcohol can also cause slurred speech. **In assessing a possible stroke patient, remember that if she or he has dysarthria, she or he probably also has dysphagia.** **If you suspect that your patient has had a stroke, test gag, swallow, and cough reflexes before allowing him or her to eat, to avoid aspiration.**
Test spontaneous speech: Have patient describe a picture.		*Impaired spontaneous speech:* Cognitive impairment.
Test motor speech: Have patient say "do, re, mi, fa, so, la, ti, do."		*Impaired motor speech:* Problem with CN XII.
Test automatic speech: Have patient recite days of the week.		*Impaired automatic speech:* Cognitive impairment or memory problem.
Test sound recognition: Have patient identify a familiar sound.		*Impaired sound recognition:* Temporal lobe affected.
Test auditory-verbal comprehension: Note patient's ability to follow directions.		*Impaired auditory-verbal comprehension:* Temporal lobe affected. *Expressive aphasia:* Frontal lobe affected. *Auditory-receptive aphasia:* Temporal lobe affected.

(box continued on page 360)

Physical Assessment (continued)

AREA/PA SKILL	NORMAL FINDINGS	ABNORMAL FINDINGS
Cerebral Function *Communication (cont'd)*		
Test visual recognition: Have patient identify object by sight.		*Impaired visual recognition:* Parieto-occipital lobe affected.
Test visual-verbal comprehension: Have patient read a sentence and explain meaning.		*Impaired visual-verbal comprehension:* Cognitive impairment.
Test writing: Have patient write name and address.		Impaired writing ability.
Test figure copying: Have patient copy circle, x, square, triangle, star.		Impaired figure copying ability.
Work from simple to complex.		
Cranial Nerves		
Compare side to side. Have patient close eyes when testing sensory nerves.		
CN I—Olfactory Nerve		
Check patency of nostrils before testing nerve function. Test each nostril separately.	CN I intact.	
Have patient identify a distinct odor (e.g., coffee, vanilla).	Sense of smell intact.	
Note anosmia.		*Anosmia:* Inherited and nonpathological, or from chronic rhinitis, sinusitis, heavy smoking, zinc deficiency, cocaine use, damage from facial fractures or head injuries, disorders of base of frontal lobe (e.g., tumor), or atherosclerotic changes.

AREA/PA SKILL	NORMAL FINDINGS	ABNORMAL FINDINGS
		Patients with anosmia usually also have a problem with sense of taste.
CN II—Optic Nerve		
Test visual acuity, visual fields, retinal structures.	CN II intact. Visual acuity intact.	*CN II deficit:* Stroke or brain tumor.
CNs III, IV, VI—Oculomotor, Trochlear, Abducens Nerves		
Test extraocular movement (EOM) with six cardinal fields; check pupillary reaction to light and accommodation.	CNs III, IV, VI intact.	CN III deficits are seen in changes in pupillary reactions. Increased intracranial pressure (ICP) causes changes in pupillary reaction.
If indicated, test oculocephalic ("doll's eyes") reflex. **Never perform oculocephalic reflex test on a patient with suspected neck injury.**	EOM intact in both eyes; pupils equal, round, react to light and accommodation—direct and consensual.	*Abnormal doll's eyes (eyes fixed):* Damage to oculomotor nerves (CNs III, IV, VI) or brainstem.
CN V—Trigeminal Nerve		
Test muscle of mastication strength by having patient bite down on tongue blade.	CN V intact Jaw muscle strength + 5.	*Weak or absent contraction unilaterally:* Lesion of the nerve, cervical spine, or brainstem.
Test sensations on face (forehead, cheeks and chin).	Facial sensations intact.	**Stroke patient may pocket food on affected side, increasing the risk for aspiration.**
Test corneal reflex.	+ Corneal reflex.	*Inability to perceive light touch and superficial pain:* Peripheral nerve damage.

(box continued on page 362)

Physical Assessment (continued)

AREA/PA SKILL	NORMAL FINDINGS	ABNORMAL FINDINGS
Cranial Nerves *(cont'd)* *CN VII—Facial Nerve*		
Test motor function of facial muscles: Have patient make faces, smile, frown, whistle.	CN VII intact. Facial movements symmetrical.	*Asymmetrical or impaired movement:* Nerve damage such as Bell's palsy or a stroke.
Test taste (sweet, sour, salty) on anterior portion of tongue.	Taste on anterior tongue intact.	*Impaired taste or loss of taste:* Damage to the nerve, chemotherapy, or radiation therapy to head and neck.
CN VIII—Acoustic Nerve		
Test hearing, balance.	CN VIII intact.	*Hearing loss, nystagmus, balance disturbance, dizziness/vertigo:* Acoustic nerve damage.
If indicated, do cold caloric test for oculovestibular reflex; look for nystagmus.	Hearing and balance intact. Negative Romberg.	*Nystagmus:* CN VIII, brainstem, or cerebellum problem; or phenytoin (Dilantin) toxicity. *Abnormal cold caloric test (no movement):* Damage to CNs III, VI, and VIII.
CNs IX, X—Glossopharyngeal and Vagus Nerves		
Note quality of voice, ability to swallow and cough. Look for symmetrical rise of the uvula.	CNs IX and X intact. Strong, clear voice, symmetrical rise of uvula, able to swallow and cough.	*Unilateral movement:* Contralateral nerve damage. *Impaired swallowing:* Damage to CNs IX, X.
Test gag reflex.	+ Gag reflex.	*Diminished or absent gag reflex:* Nerve damage. **Evaluate further; these patients are at increased risk for aspiration.** *Changes in voice quality (e.g., hoarseness):* Damage to CN X. CN X damage may also affect vital functions, causing arrhythmias because the vagus innervates most of the viscera through the parasympathetic system.

AREA/PA SKILL	NORMAL FINDINGS	ABNORMAL FINDINGS
Assess taste on posterior one-third of tongue.	Taste intact.	*Impaired taste on posterior portion of tongue:* Problem with CN IX.
CN XI—Spinoaccessory Nerve		
Test muscle strength of neck and shoulders.	CN XI intact. +5 muscle strength of neck and shoulders.	*Asymmetrical, diminished, or absent movement; pain; or unilateral or bilateral weakness:* Peripheral nerve damage.
CN XII—Hypoglossal Nerve		
Test mobility and strength of tongue. Note ability to say d, l, n, t. Note tongue position, atrophy, or fasciculation.	CN XII intact. Full range of motion (ROM) of tongue, midline, no atrophy or fasciculation.	*Asymmetrical, diminished, or absent movement; or tongue deviated from midline or protruded:* Peripheral nerve damage. Paralysis of the tongue results in dysarthria.
Sensory Function **When testing sensory function, have patient close eyes. Compare side to side.**		
Light Touch, Pain, and Temperature		
Test light touch, pain, and temperature on various areas of the body. **If touch sensation is intact distally, do not assume it is intact proximally.** **If pain sensation is intact, no need to test temperature.** **Avoid using pins, which could break skin. Use tooth-picks, sharp and dull sides, to test pain.**	Light touch, pain, and temperature intact in upper and lower extremities.	*Diminished or absent cutaneous perception:* Peripheral nerve damage, or damage to posterior column of spinal cord. Peripheral neuropathies can also cause sensory deficits. *Increased sensitivity:* Hyperesthesia. *Numbness and tingling:* Paresthesia. *Loss of sensation:* Aesthesia. *Diminished or absent temperature perception:* Peripheral nerve damage or damage to lateral spinothalamic tract.

(box continued on page 364)

Physical Assessment (continued)

AREA/PA SKILL	NORMAL FINDINGS	ABNORMAL FINDINGS
Sensory Function *Light Touch, Pain, and Temperature* (cont'd)		
Deep Sensations		
Vibratory: Place vibrating tuning fork on bony joint, great toe, and distal interphalangeal.	Vibratory sensation and kinesthetic sensation intact in upper and lower extremities.	*Diminished or absent vibration sense:* Peripheral nerve damage from alcoholism or diabetes, or damage to posterior column of spinal cord.

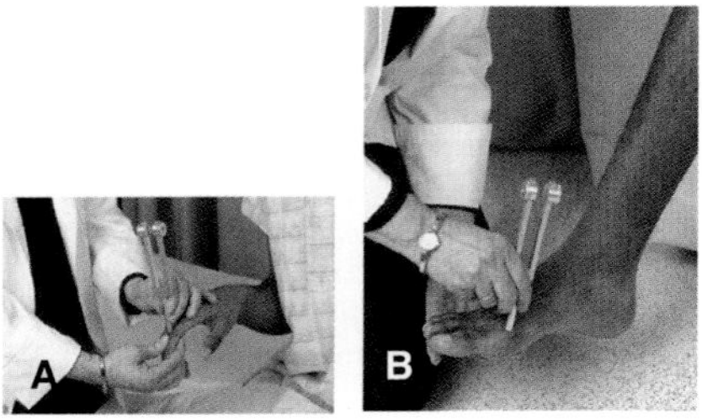

A. Vibrating upper extremity B. Vibrating lower extremity

AREA/PA SKILL	NORMAL FINDINGS	ABNORMAL FINDINGS
Kinesthetics (position sense): Move finger and toe up and down, and have patient identify direction of movement. **If intact distally, intact proximally.**		*Diminished or absent position sense:* Peripheral nerve damage, or damage to posterior column of spinal cord.

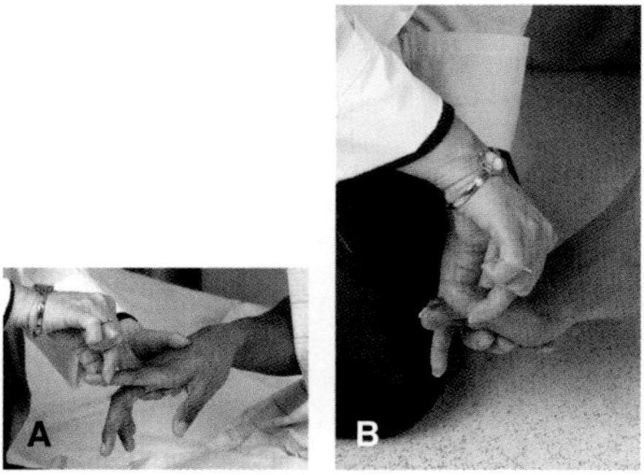

A. Testing position sense in finger B. Testing position sense in toe

AREA/PA SKILL	NORMAL FINDINGS	ABNORMAL FINDINGS
Discriminatory Sensations		
Stereognosis: Have patient identify familiar object (key, paper clip) by touch. 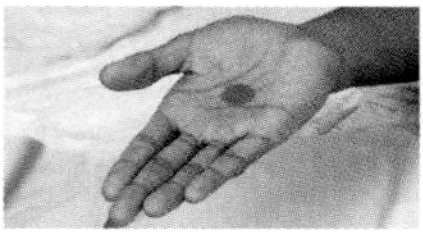 *Testing stereognosis* *Graphesthesia:* Draw number or letter in palm of hand and have patient identify it. 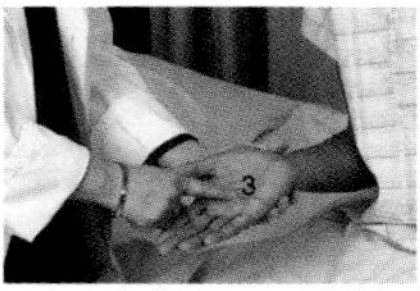 *Testing graphesthesia* *Two-point discrimination:* Note ability to differentiate being touched at one or two points simultaneously. Ability to discriminate depends on area tested; the fingertips are the most discriminatory. 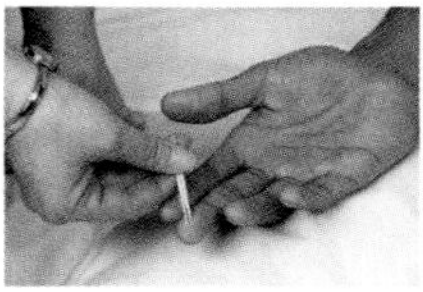 *Testing two-point discrimination*	Stereognosis, graphesthesia, point localization, and extinction intact; two-point discrimination < 5 mm on fingertips.	*Abnormal findings:* Lesion or other disorder involving sensory cortex, or disorder affecting posterior column.

(box continued on page 366)

Physical Assessment (continued)

AREA/PA SKILL	NORMAL FINDINGS	ABNORMAL FINDINGS
Sensory Function *Discriminatory Sensations (cont'd)*		
Point localization: Note ability to identify a point touched. 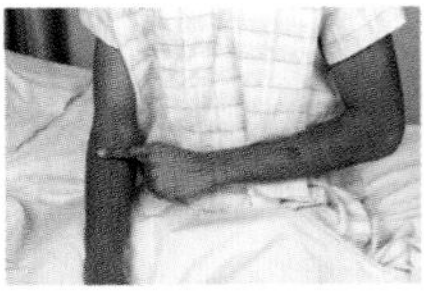 *Testing point localization*		
Extinction: Note ability to identify two corresponding areas touched simultaneously. 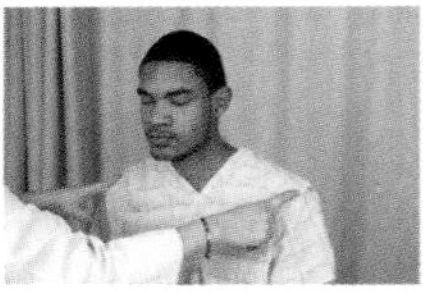 *Testing extinction*		*Extinction:* Identification of stimulus on only one side suggests lesion or other disorder involving sensory cortical region in opposite hemisphere.
Deep Tendon Reflexes		
Grade DTR on 0 to 4 scale.		*Absent or diminished reflexes:* Degenerative disease, damage to peripheral nerve (e.g., peripheral neuropathy), or lower motor neuron disorder (e.g., amyotrophic lateral sclerosis [LAS] and Guillain-Barré syndrome).

AREA/PA SKILL	NORMAL FINDINGS	ABNORMAL FINDINGS

Documenting Reflex Findings

Use these grading scales to rate the strength of each reflex in a deep tendon and superficial reflex assessment.

Deep tendon reflex grades

0 absent
+ present but diminished
+ + normal
+ + + increased but not necessarily pathologic
+ + + + hyperactive or clonic (involuntary contraction and relaxation of skeletal muscle)

Superficial reflex grades

0 absent
+ present

Use the patient's reflex ratings on a drawing of a stick figure. The figures here show documentation of normal and abnormal reflex responses.

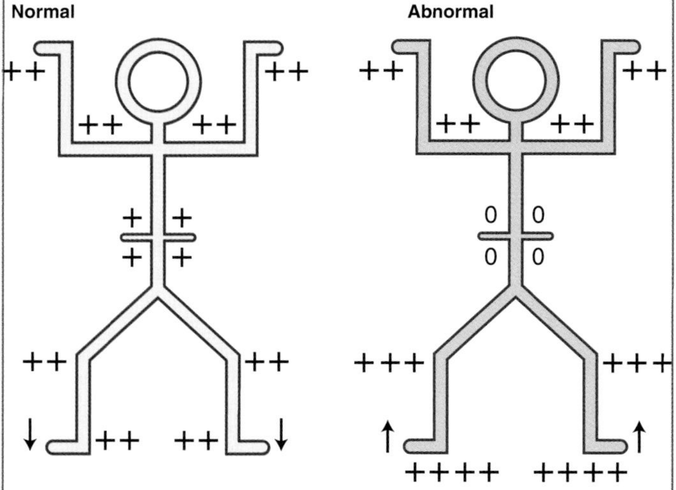

(box continued on page 368)

Physical Assessment (continued)

AREA/PA SKILL	NORMAL FINDINGS	ABNORMAL FINDINGS
Sensory Function *Deep Tendon Reflexes (cont'd)* If difficult to elicit reflex, use reinforcement techniques (e.g., clenching teeth, interlocking hands). 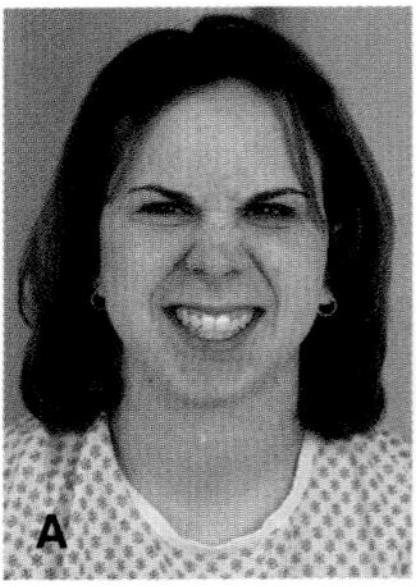 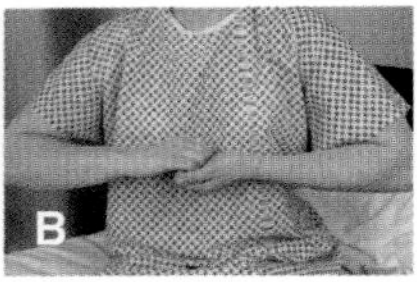 *Isometric maneuvers: A. Clenching teeth B. Interlocking hands*		
Use percussion hammer. Test for clonus. 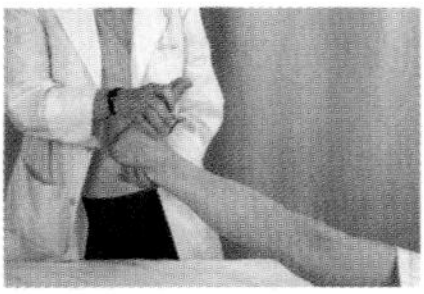 *Testing for clonus*		*Hyperactive reflexes with clonus:* Spinal cord injuries and upper motor neuron disease such as multiple sclerosis (MS).
Biceps Reflex Place your thumb on biceps tendon and strike. 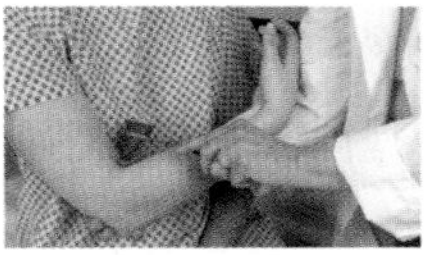 *Testing biceps reflex* *Response:* Flexion at elbow.	+2/4.	C5, C6 problem.

AREA/PA SKILL	NORMAL FINDINGS	ABNORMAL FINDINGS
Triceps Reflex		
Strike triceps tendon 1" to 2" above elbow.	+2/4.	C7, C8 problem.
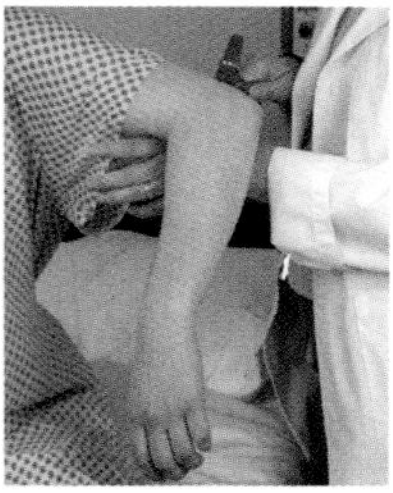 *Testing triceps reflex*		
Response: Extension at elbow.		
Brachioradialis Reflex		
Strike brachioradialis tendon 3 to 5 cm above wrist.	+2/4.	C5, C6 problem.
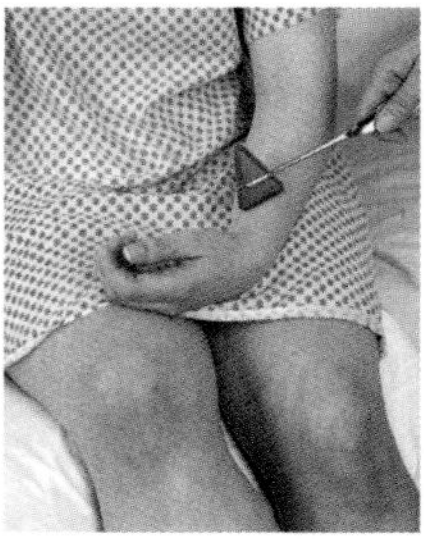 *Testing brachioradialis reflex*		
Response: Flexion at elbow and supination of hand.		
Patellar Reflex		
Strike patellar tendon below patella.	+2/4.	L2, L3, L4 problem.
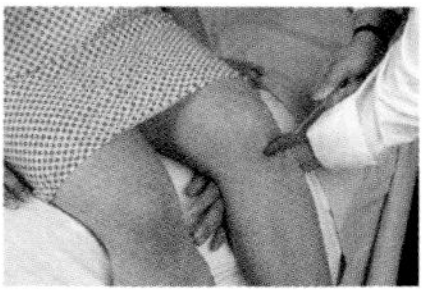 *Testing patellar reflex*		

(box continued on page 370)

Physical Assessment (continued)

AREA/PA SKILL	NORMAL FINDINGS	ABNORMAL FINDINGS
Sensory Function *Patellar Reflex (cont'd)*		
Response: Extension of knee.		
Achilles Reflex		
Strike Achilles tendon about 2 above the heel. 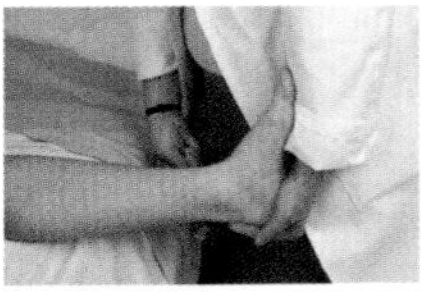 *Testing Achilles reflex*	+2/4.	S1, S2 problem.
Response: Plantar-flexion of foot.		
Superficial Reflexes		
Grade as positive or negative.		*Absence of superficial reflexes:* Pyramidal tract lesions.
Plantar Reflex		
Stroke sole of foot from heel laterally across ball of foot to great toe. 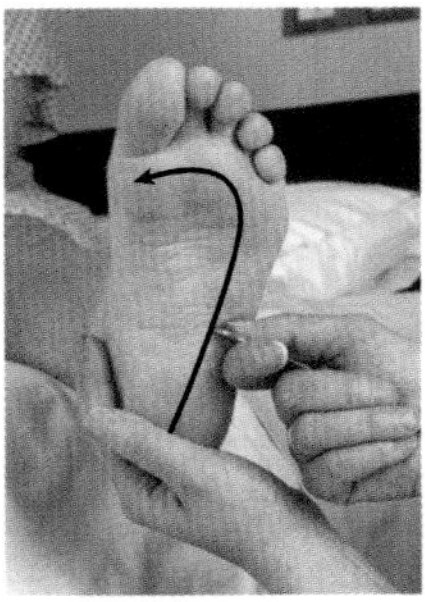 *Testing plantar reflex*	+ Plantar reflex.	*Babinski's response, dorsiflexion of great toe, with or without fanning of other toes:* In absence of drug or alcohol intoxication, suggests pathology involving upper motor neurons.
Response: Flexion of toes.	Babinski normal in infants.	L4 to S2 problem.

AREA/PA SKILL	NORMAL FINDINGS	ABNORMAL FINDINGS
Abdominal Reflex		
Stroke each quadrant of abdomen toward umbilicus.	+ Abdominal reflex.	T8, T9, T10 problem.
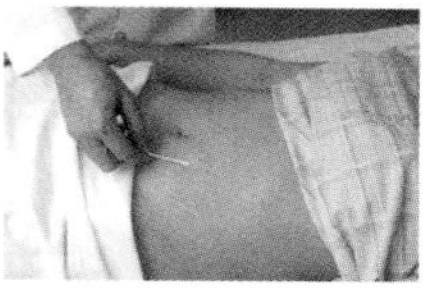 *Testing abdominal reflex*		
Response: Umbilicus moves toward stimulus.	May be absent in obese or pregnant patients.	
Anal Reflex		
Scratch side of anus.	+ Anal reflex.	S3, S4, S5 problem.
Response: Anus puckers.		
Cremasteric Reflex		
Stroke inner aspect of man's thigh.	+ Cremasteric reflex	L1, L2 problem.
Response: Elevation of testes.		
Bulbocavernosus Reflex		
Gently apply pressure over bulbocavernosus muscle and gently pinch foreskin or glans.	+ Bulbocavernosus reflex.	S3, S4 problem.
Response: Contraction of bulbocavernosus muscle.		
Primitive or Pathological Reflexes		
Grasp: Place your fingers in palm of patient's hand; patient will close fingers and grasp your fingers.		Usually indicate severe underlying neurologic problem reflecting cerebral degeneration or late-stage dementia.

(box continued on page 372)

Physical Assessment (continued)

AREA/PA SKILL	NORMAL FINDINGS	ABNORMAL FINDINGS
Primitive or Pathological Reflexes *(cont'd)*		
Sucking: Gently stimulate patient's lips with a mouth swab; patient will start sucking.		
Snout: Gently tap oral area with finger; patient's lips will pucker.		
Rooting: Gently stroke side of patient's face; patient will turn toward stimulated side.		
Glabellar: Gently tap on forehead; patient will blink.		
Babinski's sign: Stroke lateral aspect of sole of foot; patient will dorsiflect great toe and fan toes.		
Meningeal Signs		
If meningitis is suspected, assess for Kernig's and Brudzinski's signs.		Classic signs of meningitis include nuchal rigidity (extension of neck with resistance to flexion), fever, photosensitivity, headache, and nausea and vomiting.
To assess for Kernig's sign: With patient supine, flex leg and have patient attempt to extend while you apply pressure to knee. 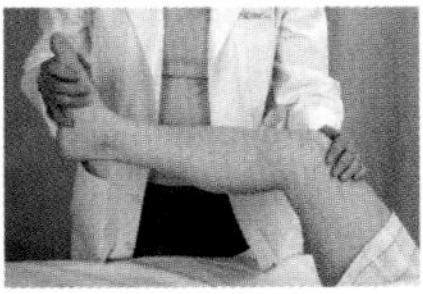 *Kernig's sign*		*Kernig's sign:* Contraction and pain of hamstring muscles and resistance to extension are positive signs of meningitis.

AREA/PA SKILL	NORMAL FINDINGS	ABNORMAL FINDINGS
To assess for Brudzinski's sign: With patient supine, flex head to chest. 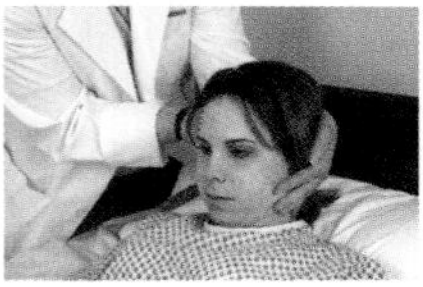 *Brudzinski's sign*		*Brudzinski's sign:* Flexion of hips is a positive sign of meningitis.

PA = Physical assessment.

TABLE 13.2 Painful Stimuli for Assessing Arousal State

STIMULUS	TECHNIQUE
Trapezius squeeze	Pinch 1 to 2 inches of trapezius muscle and twist. You should get movement if patient is going to respond.
Supraorbital pressure	Apply firm pressure with thumbs at notch at center of orbital rim below eyebrows. Because a nerve runs in notch, pressure to this area will cause sinus pain. If you use this stimulus, use it carefully to avoid damage to eyes.
Mandibular pressure	With index and middle finger apply inward and upward pressure at angle of jaw. If responsive, patient will experience pain where pressure is being applied.
Sternal rub	Use knuckles of dominant hand and apply pressure in a grinding motion to sternum. You will see movement if the patient responds. Repeated use of this site will likely cause bruising, so rotate sites and types of stimulus.
Nail pressure	Apply pressure over moon of fingernail with a pen or pencil. Movement will occur if patient responds.
Achilles pinch	Squeeze Achilles tendon between thumb and index finger. Movement will occur if patient responds.

TABLE 13.3 Terms Used to Describe Patient's Level of Consciousness

TERM	DESCRIPTION OF PATIENT'S RESPONSE
Alert	Follows commands in a timely fashion.
Lethargic	Appears drowsy, may drift off to sleep during the exam.
Stuporous	Requires vigorous stimulation (shaking, shouting) for a response.
Comatose	Doesn't respond appropriately to either verbal or painful stimuli.

TABLE 13.4 Neurologic Problems

PROBLEM	DEFINITION
Agnosia	Inability to recognize object by sight (visual agnosia), touch (tactile agnosia), or hearing (auditory agnosia).
Akinesia	Complete or partial loss of voluntary muscle movement.
Aphasia	Absence or impairment of ability to communicate through speech, writing, or signs.
Expressive aphasia	Inability to express language even though person knows what he or she wants to say (also called Broca's, or motor, aphasia).
Fluent aphasia	Words can be spoken but are used incorrectly.
Nonfluent aphasia	Slow, deliberate speech, few words.
Receptive aphasia	Inability to comprehend spoken or written words (also called Wernicke's, or sensory, aphasia).
Apraxia	Inability to carry out learned sequential movements or commands.
Circumlocution	Inability to name object verbally, so patient talks around object or uses gestures to define it.
Dysarthria	Defective speech; inability to articulate words; impairment of tongue and other muscles needed for speech.
Dysphagia	Difficulty swallowing.
Dysphasia	Impaired or difficult speech.
Dysphonia	Difficulty with quality of voice; hoarseness.
Neologisms	Made-up, nonsense, meaningless words.
Paraphrasia	Loss of ability to use words correctly and coherently; words are jumbled or misused.
Tremors	Involuntary movement of part of body.
Intention tremor	Involuntary movement when attempting coordinated movements.
Fasciculation	Involuntary contraction or twitching of muscle fibers.

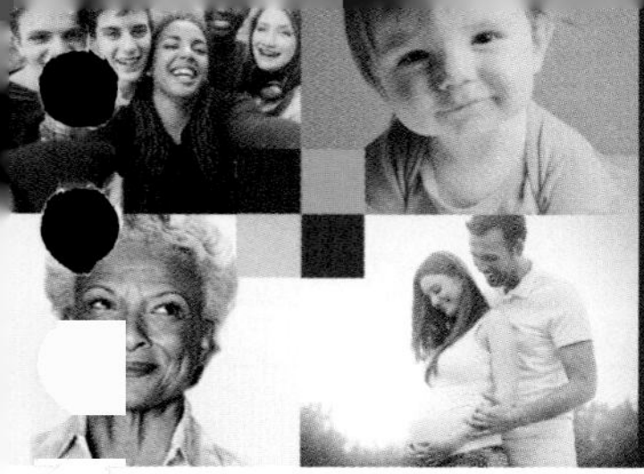

CHAPTER 14

Assessing the Mother-to-Be

Assessment of the mother-to-be entails assessing both the mother and the fetus throughout the perinatal period.

Developmental Considerations

Adolescents

- Careful attention to baseline blood pressure (BP) is necessary because teenagers have lower systolic and diastolic pressures than older women.
- Look for signs of physical and sexual abuse in the young adolescent, who may be ashamed or afraid to share this important information.
- The diets of adolescents are often lacking in essential nutrients, such as calcium and iron, needed during pregnancy.
- Mother and fetus are both growing, so they compete for nutrients.
- Cephalopelvic disproportion is a common problem for teen pregnancy because growth of the pelvis lags behind growth in stature.
- For all of these reasons, teen pregnancies are at increased risk for complications.

Older Women

- Risk for maternal or fetal complications increases with the patient's age (Table 14.1).
- Pregnant women older than age 35 have an increased risk of developing gestational diabetes, pregnancy-induced hypertension (PIH), gestational bleeding, abruptio placentae, and intrapartal fetal distress.
- Older women also have an increased risk for conceiving a child with chromosomal abnormalities.

TABLE 14.1 Complications of Pregnancy

SIGNS/SYMPTOMS	POSSIBLE CAUSES
First Trimester	
Severe vomiting	Hyperemesis gravidarum
Chills, fever	Infection
Burning on urination	Infection
Abdominal cramping, bloating, vaginal bleeding	Spontaneous abortion, miscarriage
Second and Third Trimesters	
Severe vomiting	Hyperemesis gravidarum
Leakage of amniotic fluid from vagina before labor begins	Premature rupture of membranes
Vaginal bleeding, severe abdominal pain	Miscarriage, placental separation
Chills, fever, diarrhea, burning on urination	Infection
Change in fetal activity	Fetal distress, intrauterine fetal demise
Uterine contractions before due date (expected date of delivery [EDD])	Preterm labor
Visual disturbances: Blurring, double vision, spots	Hypertensive disorders: PIH
Swelling of face, fingers, eye orbits, sacral area	PIH
Severe, frequent, or continuous headaches	PIH
Muscular irritability or convulsions (seizures)	PIH
Severe stomachache (epigastric pain)	PIH
Glucosuria, positive glucose tolerance test result	Gestational diabetes mellitus

- Older women are more likely to have preexisting medical conditions, such as diabetes and hypertension (HTN). In fact, preexisting conditions appear to pose a greater risk for maternal well-being and pregnancy outcome than the mother's age.

Cultural Considerations

- African Americans and Southeast Asians are at risk for sickle cell disease.

- Jewish women are at risk for Tay-Sachs disease.
- Mediterranean, Italian, and Greek women are at risk for beta-thalassemia.
- Asians are at risk for alpha-thalassemia.

Pregnancy and Childbearing Practices and Beliefs of Various Ethnic Groups*

African American

- Oral contraceptives most popular type of birth control.
- High rate of teen pregnancy.
- Primary advisors are grandmother and maternal relatives.
- Geophagia, eating of earth or clay, is a common practice.
- Taboos/beliefs:
  - If food cravings are not met, baby is marked.
  - Labor is induced by a bumpy ride, a big meal, castor oil, or sniffing pepper.
  - Photographing pregnant woman causes stillbirth or captures baby's soul.
  - Lifting hands over head causes cord to wrap around baby's neck.
  - Amniotic sac over baby's face denotes baby has special powers.
  - Child born after a set of twins, the seventh child, or a child born with a physical condition has special powers from God.

Amish

- Children are a gift from God.
- Average number of children per family is seven.
- Women have high status owing to their role as child producers.
- Birth control seen as interfering with God's will.
- Prenatal care by Amish lay-midwives.
- Fathers expected to be involved and present during delivery and to participate in prenatal classes.
- No major taboos, but showing emotions is considered inappropriate, so woman labors quietly without expressing discomfort.
- Childbirth is not viewed as medical condition, so few have health insurance, keeping hospitalizations very short.
- Family and community are expected to care for mother and baby.

*Adapted from Purnell, L.D., and Paulanka, B.J. (2012): *Transcultural Healthcare: A Culturally Competent Approach,* 4th ed. Philadelphia, F.A. Davis.

Appalachian

- Contraceptive practices similar to those of the general public, but a common belief is that laxatives facilitate abortion.
- Believe that healthy living during pregnancy leads to a healthy baby.
- Taboos/beliefs:
  - Boys are carried high, girls low.
  - Photo taking causes stillbirth.
  - Reaching over the head causes cord strangulation.
  - Wearing an opal ring may harm baby.
  - Birthmarks are caused by eating strawberries or citrus fruit.
  - Experiencing a tragedy during pregnancy leads to congenital anomalies.
- Birthing is considered a natural process to be endured.
- Family members are expected to care for mother and child during postpartum period.
- A band may be placed around the baby's abdomen to prevent umbilical hernias, and an asafetida bag around the neck to prevent contagious diseases.

Arab American

- Believe that God decides family size and God provides.
- Procreation is the purpose of marriage, resulting in high fertility rates.
- Irreversible means of contraception and abortions are considered unlawful. Sterility may lead to rejection or divorce. With emphasis on fertility and bearing a son, pregnancy occurs early in marriages.
- Pregnant women are pampered. Unmet cravings are thought to result in birthmarks. Pregnant women are excused from fasting during sacred days.
- Men are excluded from labor and delivery. Deliveries are often performed at home by midwives because of limited access to hospitals. Breathing and relaxation techniques are not practiced, and labor pain is openly expressed.
- Baby's stomach wrapped after birth to prevent exposure to cold. Male circumcision is a Muslim requirement.
- Postpartum bathing is avoided for fear of mother being exposed to cold.
- Breast-feeding delayed until 2nd or 3rd day to allow mother to rest.
- Postpartum foods include lentil soup to increase milk production and teas to cleanse the body.

Chinese American

- To control population, Chinese government has one-child law. Contraception is free; abortion is common.
- Pregnancy is seen as a positive experience. Men are not very involved in process. Female midwives are often preferred because of modesty of Chinese women.
- Dietary beliefs:
  - Adding meat to diet makes blood "strong" for fetus.
  - Shellfish cause allergies.
  - Iron makes delivery more difficult.
  - Avoid fruits and vegetables during postpartum period because they are "cold" foods.
  - Mother drinks rice wine to increase strength and has five to six meals a day with rice, soups, and seven to eight eggs.

! Wine may increase bleeding time.

- Five- to 7-day hospital stay after delivery, 1 month for recovery. Chinese government allows 6 months maternity leave with full pay. If mother is breast-feeding, time is allowed from work for feedings.
- Mothers avoid "cold"—don't go outside or bathe, and wear many layers of clothes even in warm weather.

Cuban American

- Cuba has lowest birth rate in Latin America because of high labor force participation for women and high divorce rate.
- Childbirth is a celebration.
- Beliefs:
  - Must eat for two during pregnancy (leads to excessive weight gain).
  - Eating coffee grounds cures morning sickness.
  - Eating fruit ensures that the baby will have smooth complexion.
  - Wearing necklaces causes umbilical cord to wrap around neck.
- During the postpartum period, family members care for mother for 4 weeks. Mother avoids ambulation and exposure to cold because this is seen as risk for infection.
- Prefer breast-feeding but wean at 3 months and start solid foods. Believe that a fat child is a healthy child.

Egyptian American

- Must have children to make family complete. Three children is the ideal number. Woman are expected to conceive within first year of marriage, and there is much stress until pregnancy occurs.

Inability to conceive is grounds for divorce. Pregnancy brings security and respect. Birthing, especially of a son, has status and power.

- Beliefs:
  - Curtail activities during pregnancy to prevent miscarriage.
  - Eat for two.
  - Cravings must be met or baby marked with the shape of the craved food.
  - Maternal mother is expectant mother's source of support during labor and delivery.
  - Men are excluded from the birthing process.
  - Postpartum, avoid cold, such as bathing. Postpartum period is 40 days, and family members tend to mother and baby.

Filipino American

- Fertility practices influenced by Catholic faith; rhythm is only acceptable method of contraception; abortion is a sin.
- Child-centered culture. Pregnancy is normal; expectant mothers are pampered. Maternal mother is great source of support and often serves as labor coach.
- Beliefs:
  - Use healthcare providers but also a massage therapist.
  - Cravings should be met to avoid harm to baby.
  - Baby takes on characteristics of craved foods (e.g., dark-colored foods, dark skin).
  - If mother has a sudden scare or stress, it can harm fetus.
- Postpartum beliefs:
  - Chicken soup stimulates milk production.
  - Showers may cause arthritis, but sponge baths are allowed.
- Family cares for new mother and baby during postpartum period.

French Canadian

- Fertility practices influenced by Catholic faith. Abortion considered morally wrong by many.
- Fear of labor and delivery. Fathers are encouraged to be present during delivery. Use of analgesia is high.
- Breast-feeding has regained popularity.
- Both maternity and paternity leaves are available.
- Beliefs:
  - Washing floors can trigger labor; so can full moon.
  - Hyperglycemia during pregnancy means you are likely to give birth to a boy. Hyponatremia during pregnancy means you are likely to give birth to a girl.

Greek American

- Limited family size because of desire to provide for family and ensure education for children.
- Greek Orthodox faith condemns birth control and abortion.
- Infertility causes great stress.
- Pregnant mother is greatly respected and protected.
- Birthing usually by midwife or female relatives; fathers remain uninvolved.
- Mother considered impure and susceptible to illness for 40 days postpartum. Remains at home. Breast-feeding is common.
- Beliefs:
  - Eat foods high in iron and protein.
  - Child will be marked if food cravings are unmet.
  - Breast-feeding mothers who shower may cause diarrhea or milk allergy in baby.
  - Silver objects or coins placed in crib bring good luck.

Iranian American

- Hot and cold influence pregnancy practices.
- Women are expected to have children early in marriage.
- Infertility blamed on woman.
- Breast-feeding used as method of contraception.
- Birthing a child, especially a boy, is prestigious.
- Beliefs:
  - Cravings must be met with balance for hot and cold foods.
  - Heavy work causes miscarriages.
  - Much support from female relatives. Father usually not present during delivery. The postpartum period is 30 to 40 days.
- Postpartum beliefs:
  - Baby boys are "hotter" than baby girls.
  - Baby may be kept at home for first 40 days until he or she is strong enough to defend against environmental pathogens.
  - Ritual baby bath given between 10th and 40th day.

Irish American

- Fertility practices influenced by Catholicism. Sexual relationships are often seen as a duty. Abstinence and rhythm are the only acceptable methods of birth control, and abortion is considered morally wrong.
- Beliefs:
  - Eating a well-balanced diet during pregnancy is important.
  - Not eating right leads to deformities.

- Lifting hands above the head wraps cord around baby's neck.
- Experiencing a tragedy during pregnancy results in congenital anomalies.
- Going to bed with wet hair or wet feet causes illness in pregnant woman.

Jewish American

- Children are a gift and duty; boys are more important. Sterility is a curse.
- Birth control pill is acceptable form of contraception.
- Orthodox Jews condone abortion if mother's health is at risk. Reform Jews believe women have control over their own bodies; therefore, it is their decision.
- Hasidic husbands are not allowed to touch the mother during delivery or view her genitals; therefore, they may give only verbal support or choose not to be present during delivery.
- Male circumcision performed the 8th day by a mohel—a person trained in circumcision, asepsis, and the religious ritual.

Mexican American

- Fertility practices influenced by Catholicism. Abstinence and rhythm are acceptable methods of birth control. Breast-feeding is also seen as method of birth control. Abortion is considered morally wrong.
- Multiple births are common; childbearing age between 19 and 24 years is seen as best time; woman older than 24 may be considered too old.
- A large family is a sign of a man's virility. Pregnancy is a natural and desirable condition, so many do not seek prenatal care; extended family provides advice and support.
- Beliefs:
  - Hot food provides fetus with warmth.
  - Cold foods should be eaten during postpartum period.
  - Pregnant women sleep on back to prevent harm to baby.
  - Frequent intercourse during pregnancy keeps vaginal canal lubricated and eases delivery.
  - Walking in moonlight and viewing lunar eclipses lead to deformities.
  - Pregnant women should avoid becoming cold.
  - Lifting hands over head causes cord to wrap around baby's neck.
  - The pregnant woman may wear a safety pin or metal object to prevent deformities.

- The father is not included in delivery. Mothers are very verbal during labor and do not practice breathing techniques. Mother puts legs together after delivery and wears cotton binder or girdle to prevent air from entering the womb.
- The postpartum period is 40 days, warmth preferred, showers avoided.
- Lactating mothers exposed to pesticides have decreased milk production and increased risk of breast cancer.
- Postpartum belief: Cutting baby's nails causes blindness and deafness.

Navajo Native American

- Large families are favorable; many do not practice birth control. Having twins is not favorable, and traditionally, one must die; now, however, one may be placed for adoption.
- Beliefs:
  - Mothers are reluctant to deliver in hospital because hospitals are associated with sickness and death.
  - Birthing necklaces are worn during labor to ensure a safe birth. Mother holds onto woven sash when ready to push.
  - Chanting may occur during delivery.
  - Baby clothes are not bought before baby's birth.
- Postpartum beliefs:
  - Placenta is buried after birth to protect the baby from evil spirits.
  - The baby is given special mixtures after birth to rid mouth of mucus.

Vietnamese American

- High fertility rate as a result of long period of childbearing (up to age 44).
- Taboos/beliefs:
  - Dietary practices influenced by hot/cold, wind/tonic. Wind foods are cold; tonic foods are hot and sweet. Maintaining balance between hot and cold restores bodily balance. First trimester, woman considered weak and cold, so she eats hot foods. Second trimester is neutral state. Third trimester, woman considered hot, so she eats cold foods.
  - Woman remains physically active but avoids heavy lifting and raising hands above the head (thought to pull on placenta).
  - Sexual intercourse late in pregnancy is believed to cause respiratory distress.
  - It is taboo to attend weddings and funerals while pregnant.

- Early prenatal care is not the norm. Labor is usually short, may prefer squatting or walking while in labor.
- Postpartum beliefs:
  - Head of mother and baby considered sacred, so cannot be touched.
  - Placenta buried to protect baby's health.
  - Ritual cleansing of mother without water. Showers avoided for a month after delivery because of cold influence.
  - Family helps care for mother and child.
  - Breast-feeding is a common practice, but the mother may discard colostrum. May alternate breast with bottle because of hot and cold influence (hot foods benefit mother's health, whereas cold foods promote healthy breast milk).

Assessment

History

Key points to remember when obtaining a prenatal history:

- Focus on the current pregnancy and the presenting presumptive symptoms. Take a detailed obstetrical and gynecological history.
- Use the past medical history to identify anything that would affect or be affected by pregnancy.
- Pay special attention to the nutritional history.
- Pay special attention to prescribed, over-the-counter (OTC), and illegal drug use because it may have a major impact on the developing fetus.
- Determine the patient's reaction to pregnancy—Was this a planned pregnancy?
- Identify major supports—family, spouse, significant other?
- Assess for history or risk of physical abuse.
- After you have completed your questions, ask the patient if she has any problems or concerns that have not been covered, and give her an opportunity to discuss them.

Diagnosis of Pregnancy

The diagnosis of pregnancy (Table 14.2) is based on the following indicators:

- Presumptive signs (experienced by the patient).
- Probable signs (observed by the examiner).
- Positive signs (attributed only to the presence of the fetus).

TABLE 14.2 Signs and Symptoms of Pregnancy

SIGNS AND SYMPTOMS	DESCRIPTION/TIME FRAME
Presumptive Signs	
Cessation of menses (amenorrhea)	Uterine lining does not slough off; women may experience spotting during implantation.
Nausea, vomiting	From weeks 2 to 12; usually subsides after 12 weeks.
Frequent urination	Bladder irritability caused by enlarging uterus.
Breast tenderness	Starts at 2 to 3 weeks; soreness; tingling.
Perception of fetal movement (quickening)	Occurs at 16 to 18 weeks; sensation of "fluttering" in abdomen perceived by mother-to-be.
Skin changes	Increased pigmentation; striae gravidarum.
Fatigue	Starts at 12 weeks.
Probable Signs	
Abdominal enlargement	Palpated at 12 weeks.
Piskacek's sign	Palpated at 4 to 6 weeks; uterus asymmetrical with soft prominence on implantation side.
Hegar's sign	6 weeks; palpable softening of the lower uterine segment.
Goodell's sign	Palpated at 8 weeks; softening of the cervix.
Chadwick's sign	Seen at 6 to 8 weeks; bluish hue on vulva, vagina, cervix from increased venous congestion.
Braxton Hicks contractions	Painless, irregular, intermittent uterine contractions that typically start after the 4th month and last through remainder of pregnancy.
Pregnancy test	Positive 7 to 10 days after conception.
Ballottement	Occurs at 16 to 18 weeks; passive movement of the unengaged fetus.
Positive Signs	
Fetal heartbeat	By ultrasound, fetal heart motion is noted by 4 to 8 weeks after conception; by Doppler, auscultated by 10 to 12 weeks; by fetal stethoscope, auscultated by 17 to 19 weeks.
Visualization of the fetus	By ultrasound, at 5 to 6 weeks; by radiograph, by 16 weeks (rarely used to diagnose pregnancy because of teratogenic effects).

Calculation of Estimated Date of Conception

To calculate the estimated date of conception (EDC), apply Naegele's rule: Add 7 days to the first day of the last menstrual period (LMP), then subtract 3 months from that date. Considerations in calculating the EDC include:

- Find out the first day of the LMP. Make sure the patient is sure of the date because the EDC is based on the LMP. Conception usually occurs around 2 weeks after the LMP in a 28-day cycle.
- Review the patient's menstrual history, including frequency of menses, length of flow, normalcy of the LMP, and contraceptive use.
- Ultrasound studies may also be used to estimate the gestational age.

Prenatal Laboratory Tests

Urine Tests

- Clean-catch midstream urine specimen, for glucose (to assess for diabetes), protein (to assess for PIH), and nitrites and leukocytes (to assess for infection).

Blood Tests

- Complete blood count (CBC), blood type and screen, Rh status, rubella titer, serological test for syphilis, hepatitis B surface antigen.
- Patients of African ancestry are also referred for a sickle cell anemia screen.
- Patients who are at high risk for human immunodeficiency virus (HIV) infection should be screened for this infection.
- Between 16 and 18 weeks' gestation, a multiple marker or "triple screen" for maternal serum level of alpha-fetoprotein (MSAFP), human chorionic gonadotropin (hCG), and unconjugated estriol (uE3) is usually obtained. High levels of alpha-fetoprotein are associated with neural tube defects; low triple screen values with Down syndrome and other chromosomal abnormalities.

Head-to-Toe Physical Assessment

APPROACH: Inspection, palpation, percussion, auscultation.

POSITION: Sitting, supine, lithotomy.

TOOLBOX: Stethoscope, light for pelvic examination, tape measure, fetoscope or fetal Doppler, equipment for pelvic exam (speculum, gloves, lubricant, glass slides, potassium hydroxide (KOH), normal saline, and cytology fixative).

Head-to-Toe Physical Assessment

SYSTEM/AREA, APPROACH, AND NORMAL FINDINGS	ABNORMAL FINDINGS
Integumentary: Inspection	
Linea nigra, striae gravidarum, chloasma, spider nevi, palmar erythema. Increased growth, softening, thinning of hair and nails.	*Pale skin:* Anemia. **Patient is anemic if hemoglobin drops below 10 g/dL.**

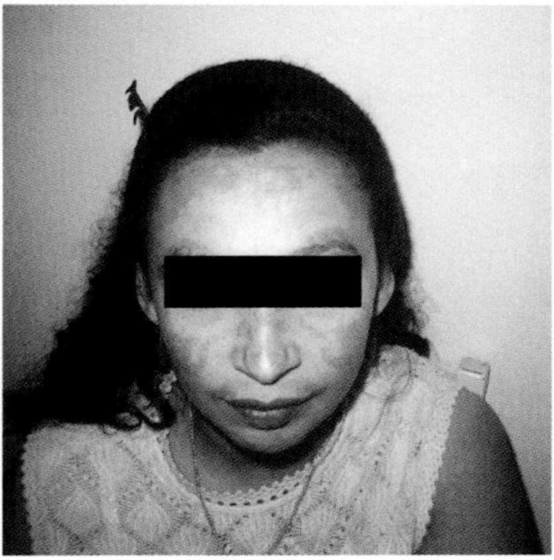

Chloasma

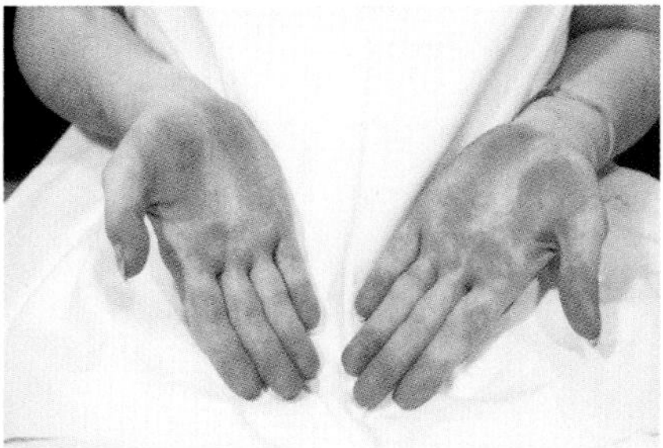

Palmar erythema

(box continued on page 388)

Head-to-Toe Physical Assessment (continued)

SYSTEM/AREA, APPROACH, AND NORMAL FINDINGS	ABNORMAL FINDINGS
HEENT	
Head and Neck: Palpation	
Palpable smooth, nontender, small cervical chain lymph nodes. Slight thyroid gland enlargement.	*Hard, tender, fixed or prominent cervical nodes:* Cancer. *Marked thyroid enlargement:* Hyperthyroidism.
Ears: Inspection	
Tympanic membranes clear, landmarks visible.	*Tympanic membranes red and bulging with pus:* Infection.
Nose: Inspection	
Mucosal swelling and redness, epistaxis (nosebleeds) common because of increased estrogen.	*Purulent discharge:* Upper respiratory infection.
Mouth/Throat: Inspection	
Gums: Gingival hypertrophy and epulis usually regress spontaneously after delivery.	*Bleeding gums:* Gingivitis. *Redness in throat:* Exudate present.

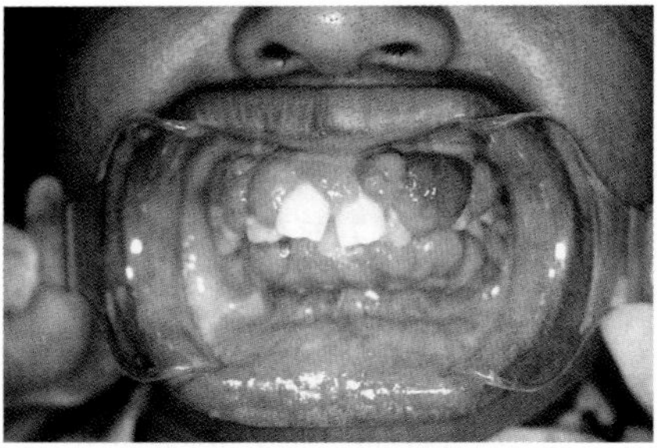

Gingival hypertrophy

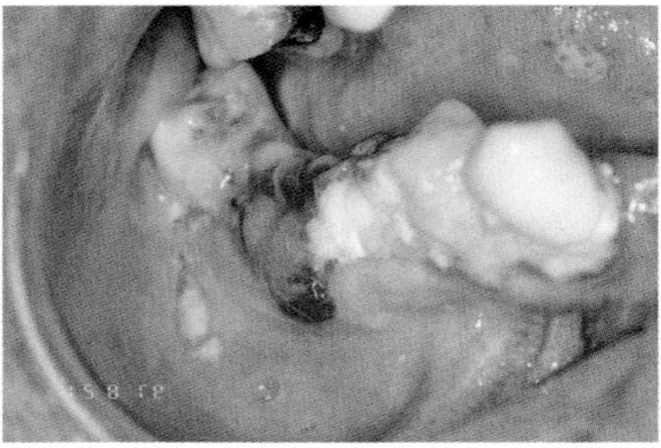

Epulis

SYSTEM/AREA, APPROACH, AND NORMAL FINDINGS	ABNORMAL FINDINGS
Throat: Pink, no redness or exudates.	*Enlarged tonsils:* Infection.
Respiratory: Inspection, Palpation, Percussion, Auscultation	
Increased anteroposterior chest diameter, thoracic breathing, slight hyperventilation, shortness of breath in late pregnancy, lung sounds clear bilaterally.	*Dyspnea, crackles, rhonchi, wheezes, rubs, absence of breath sounds, unequal breath sounds, respiratory distress:* Pulmonary complications, such as pulmonary edema or acute respiratory distress syndrome.
Cardiovascular: Palpation, Auscultation	
Point of maximal impulse (PMI) may be displaced upward and laterally in the latter stages of pregnancy.	*Enlarged PMI:* HTN.
Normal sinus rhythm.	*Irregular rhythm:* Cardiac disease.
Soft systolic murmur caused by increased blood volume.	*Dyspnea, palpitations, markedly decreased activity tolerance:* Cardiovascular disease. *Midsystolic click and late systolic murmur:* Mitral valve prolapse.
Breasts: Inspection, Palpation	
Venous congestion with prominence of Montgomery's tubercles.	**Nipple inversion may be problematic for breast-feeding women.**
Increased size and nodularity; increased sensitivity; colostrum secretion in the third trimester.	*Localized redness, pain, and warmth:* Mastitis.
Hyperpigmentation of nipples and areolar tissue.	*Bloody nipple discharge and skin retraction:* Cancer.
Abdomen: Inspection, Palpation, Auscultation	
Note cesarean scars and location; obtain previous pregnancy records to confirm type and location of uterine incision.	Note any scars that may indicate previous abdominal surgery and influence type of delivery.

(box continued on page 390)

Head-to-Toe Physical Assessment (continued)

SYSTEM/AREA, APPROACH, AND NORMAL FINDINGS	ABNORMAL FINDINGS
Abdomen: Inspection, Palpation, Auscultation *(cont'd)*	
Note striae, linea nigra.	

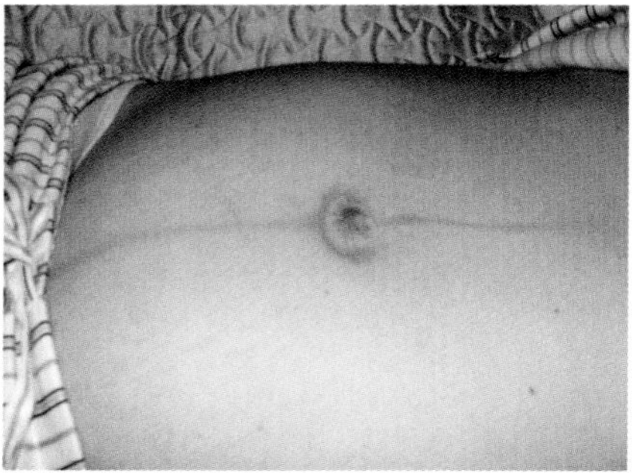

Linea nigra

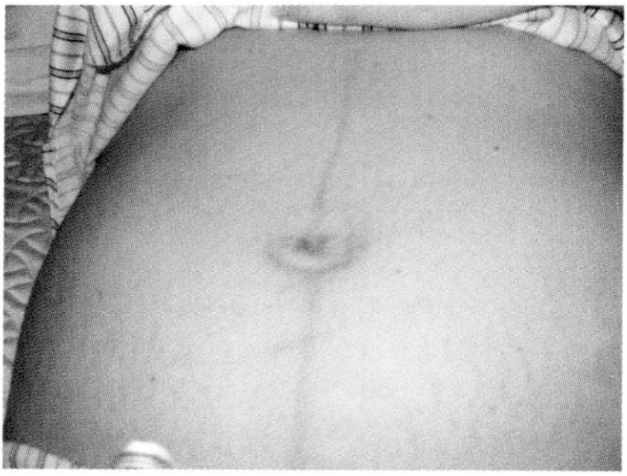

Linea nigra

SYSTEM/AREA, APPROACH, AND NORMAL FINDINGS	ABNORMAL FINDINGS
Enlargement caused by fetus; in later pregnancy, uterine shape may suggest fetal presentation and position. Palpable uterus at 10 to 12 weeks.	*Abnormal palpable masses:* Uterine fibroids or hepatosplenomegaly.
Fetal movement noticed by mother at 18 to 20 weeks (earlier for multipara).	*No fetal movement felt:* Wrong EDC or fetal demise.
Uterine contractions may be present; intensity is described as mild, moderate, or firm to palpation.	*Regular contractions before 37 completed weeks of gestation:* Preterm labor.
What is the duration of the patient's contractions? Time them from beginning to end of same	

SYSTEM/AREA, APPROACH, AND NORMAL FINDINGS	ABNORMAL FINDINGS
contraction. How frequent are they? Time them from beginning of one contraction to beginning of next.	
Fundal height measurement:	
Place zero point of tape measure on symphysis pubis and measure to top of fundus. Fundal measurement should approximately equal number of weeks of gestation; measurements may vary by 2 cm; measurements by different examiners should be approximately the same.	*Measurements greater than expected:* Multiple gestation, polyhydramnios, fetal anomalies, macrosomia. **Measurements > 4 cm from the estimated gestational age warrant further evaluation.** *Smaller than expected:* Fetal growth restriction.

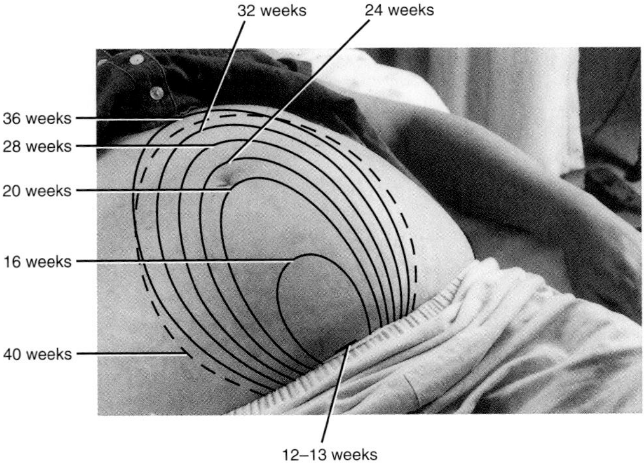

Fundal height assessment

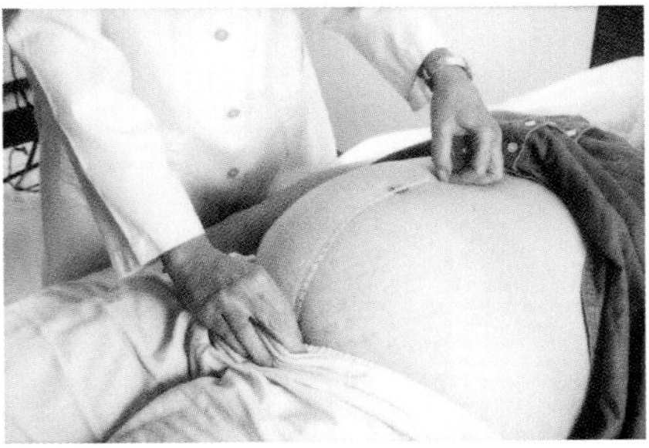

Fundal height measurement

(box continued on page 392)

Head-to-Toe Physical Assessment (continued)

SYSTEM/AREA, APPROACH, AND NORMAL FINDINGS	ABNORMAL FINDINGS
Abdomen: Inspection, Palpation, Auscultation *(cont'd)*	
Fetal heart tones (FHTs) are best auscultated through the back of the fetus. A fetal Doppler can be used after 10 to 12 weeks' gestation; a fetoscope may be used after 18 weeks' gestation.	*Inability to auscultate FHT with a fetal Doppler at 12 weeks:* Retroverted uterus, uncertain dates, fetal demise, false pregnancy.

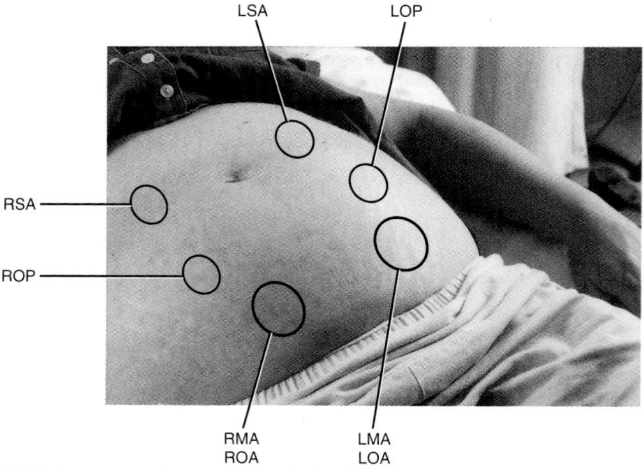

FHTs. Intensity varies according to fetal position.

- *RSA = right sacrum anterior*
- *LSA = left sacrum anterior*
- *ROP = right occipitoposterior*
- *LOP = left occipitoposterior*
- *RMA = right mentum anterior*
- *LMA = left mentum anterior*
- *ROA = right occipitoanterior*
- *LOA = left occipitoanterior*

Fetal heart rate (FHR) range: 120 to 160 beats per minute (BPM). In the third trimester, FHR accelerates with fetal movement.	*FHR decelerations:* Poor placental perfusion.
Fetal position: Use Leopold's maneuvers to palpate the fundus, lateral aspects of the abdomen, and lower pelvic area. Leopold's maneuvers assist in determining fetal lie, presentation, size,	*Oblique or transverse lie:* Breech presentation. If you hear fetal heart sounds above the umbilicus, it is a breech presentation; below the umbilicus, a vertex presentation.

SYSTEM/AREA, APPROACH, AND NORMAL FINDINGS	ABNORMAL FINDINGS
and position. A longitudinal lie is expected. Fetal presentation may be cephalic, breech, or shoulder. Fetal size is estimated by measuring fundal height and by palpation.	

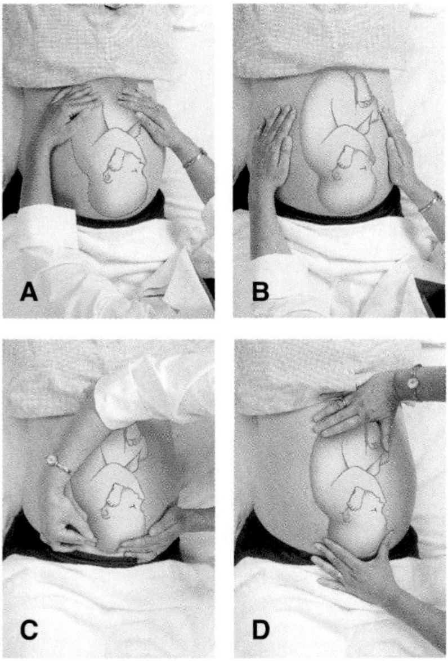

Fetal presentation/position

First maneuver: Face the patient's head and place your hands on the fundal area. You should palpate a soft, irregular mass in the upper quadrant of the mother's abdomen. The soft mass is the fetal buttocks; the round, hard part is the fetal head.

Second maneuver: Next, move your hands down to the lateral sides of the mother's abdomen. On one side you will palpate round, irregular nodules—the fists and feet of the fetus. Expect to feel kicking and movement. The other side of the

(box continued on page 394)

Head-to-Toe Physical Assessment (continued)

SYSTEM/AREA, APPROACH, AND NORMAL FINDINGS	ABNORMAL FINDINGS
Abdomen: Inspection, Palpation, Auscultation *(cont'd)*	
mother's abdomen feels smooth—this is the fetus's back.	
Third maneuver: Now move your hands down to the mother's lower pelvic area and palpate just above the symphysis pubis to determine the presenting part of the fetus. Grasp the presenting part with your thumb and third finger. If it is the fetus's head, it will be round, firm, and ballottable. If it is the fetus's buttocks, it will be soft and irregular.	
Fourth maneuver: Next, face your patient's feet, and place your hands on her abdomen, pointing your fingers toward her feet. Try to move your hands toward each other while applying downward pressure. If they move together easily, the fetus's head is not descended into the pelvic inlet. If they do not move together and stop because of resistance, the fetus's head is engaged into the pelvic inlet.	
Extremities: Inspection, Palpation	
In the third trimester, dependent edema is normal; varicose veins may also appear.	*Calf pain, presence of Homans' sign, generalized edema, diminished pedal pulses:* Deep venous thrombophlebitis (DVT).
Genitourinary: Inspection, Palpation	
External Genitalia	
Labial and clitoral enlargement, parous relaxation of introitus, scars from episiotomy or perineal lacerations (multiparous women).	*Labial varicosities:* Venous congestion.
Bartholin's and Skene's Glands	
No discomfort or discharge.	*Discharge and tenderness:* Infection.

SYSTEM/AREA, APPROACH, AND NORMAL FINDINGS	ABNORMAL FINDINGS
Vaginal Orifice	
Small amount of whitish discharge (leukorrhea).	*Thick, purulent vaginal discharge:* Gonorrheal infection. *Thick, white, cheesy discharge:* Yeast infection. *Gray-white discharge, sweet smell, positive clue cells:* Bacterial vaginosis infection.
Cervix	
Smooth, pink or bluish, long, thick, closed; 2.3 to 3 cm long. Softening of lower uterine segment (Hegar's sign) should be present. Bluish color (Chadwick's sign) indicates increased blood flow to pelvic area and is probable sign of pregnancy.	*Effaced, opened cervix:* Preterm labor or incompetent cervix if not a term gestation.

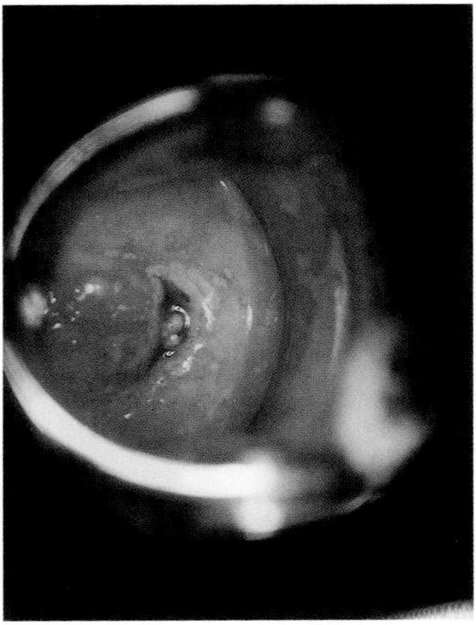

Chadwick's sign

(box continued on page 396)

Head-to-Toe Physical Assessment (continued)

SYSTEM/AREA, APPROACH, AND NORMAL FINDINGS	ABNORMAL FINDINGS

Abdomen: Inspection, Palpation, Auscultation *(cont'd)*

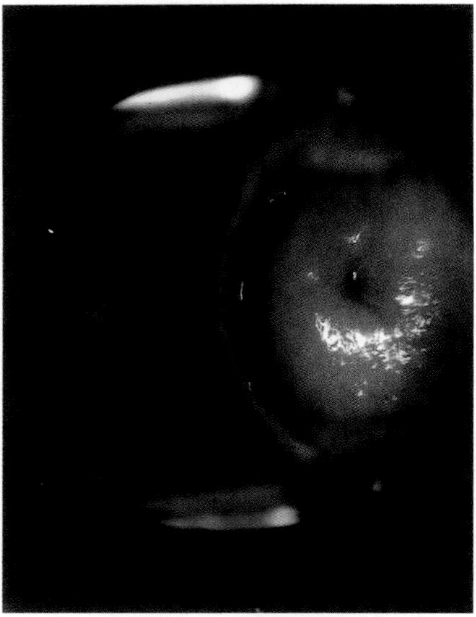

Circular cervical opening: nulliparous

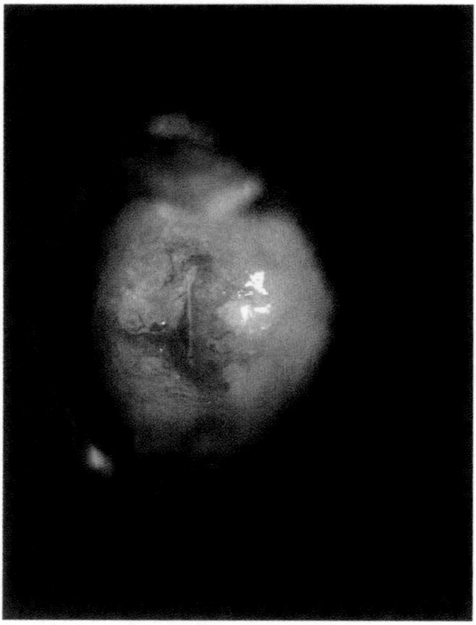

Slitlike cervical opening: multiparous

SYSTEM/AREA, APPROACH, AND NORMAL FINDINGS	ABNORMAL FINDINGS
Uterus	
Uterus is size of orange at 10 weeks; grapefruit at 12 weeks.	*Uterine size not consistent with dates:* Wrong dates, fibroids, multiple gestation.
No masses in left and right adnexa; some discomfort because of stretching of round ligaments.	*Palpable masses:* Ectopic pregnancy.
Musculoskeletal	
Accentuated lumbar curve (lordosis), wider base of support.	*Diastasis recti abdominis:* Separation of abdominal muscles from pregnancy.
Neurologic	
+ 1 to 2 deep tendon reflex.	*Hyperreflexia, clonus:* Preeclampsia, eclampsia.
Phalen's or Tinel's sign is absent.	*Presence of Phalen's or Tinel's sign:* Carpal tunnel syndrome.

HEENT = Head, eyes, ears, nose, and throat.

The Postpartal Assessment

The postpartal assessment includes a history and physical exam with focus on changes that occur after childbirth. In addition to reviewing your patient's prenatal records, ask the following questions:

- How many weeks' gestation? Were you full-term?
- How many times have you been pregnant? How many deliveries (children) do you have? Gravida (number of pregnancy)? Parity (number of pregnancies that reached viability)?
- What type of delivery? Vaginal or C-section?
- What type of anesthesia did you have?
- Do you have episiotomy? Tears? Hemorrhoids?
- When was the last time you went to the bathroom? Last void?
- How do you feel? Pain?
- Are you breast or bottle feeding?
- What is your blood type? Rh factor? Predelivery hemoglobin and hematocrit?

Postpartal Physical Exam

Postpartal Physical Assessment

AREA/NORMAL VARIATION	ABNORMAL VARIATION/RATIONALE
Vital Signs	
Temperature may increase to 38°C within first 24 hours due to dehydration.	*After 24 hours, elevated temperature:* May indicate puerperal sepsis, mastitis, endometritis, or urinary tract infection.
Pulse initially elevated few hours after delivery. Returns to prepregnancy rate within 8 to 10 weeks.	*Elevated pulse:* May be associated with hypovolemia secondary to hemorrhage.
Respirations return to prepregnancy rate within 6 to 8 weeks.	*Decreased respiratory rate:* Related to spinal block, pain medication. *Hypoventilation:* May occur with C-sections.
BP: Orthostatic hypotension for the first 48 hours due to splenchnic engorgement; slight transient rise in BP for 4 days after delivery.	*Hypotension:* May be associated with shock. *HTN:* May be associated with PIH.
HEENT: Neck	
Thyroid may be palpable during pregnancy, returns to prepregnant state after pregnancy.	Thyromegaly. *Palpable nodules:* Thyroiditis, hypothyroidism.
Respiratory	
Lungs: Clear.	Patient may hypoventilate after C-section, which would increase risk for atelectasis.
Cardiac	
PMI returns to normal as cardiac axis is restored. Systolic flow murmur usually disappears shortly after delivery.	*Tachycardia:* May signal shock. Murmur.
Breasts	
Lactating: Full, milk expressible.	Erythema, masses.
Nonlactating: Soft, without lymphadenopathy; bilateral galactorrhea (up to 3 months).	*Hard, masses, lymphadenopathy:* Mastitis.
Genitourinary	
Bladder: Nondistended. Voids within 8 hours postpartum. *Perenium:* Episeotomy, hemorrhoids usually regress after birth. Sutures intact. Perenium tender and edematous.	Overdistended bladder prevents involution, which can lead to hemorrhage. Inability to void secondary to birth-induced trauma and anesthesia, pain, episiotomy.

AREA/NORMAL VARIATION	ABNORMAL VARIATION/RATIONALE
	Increased risk for urinary tract infection. Severe perineal pain associated with a hematoma.

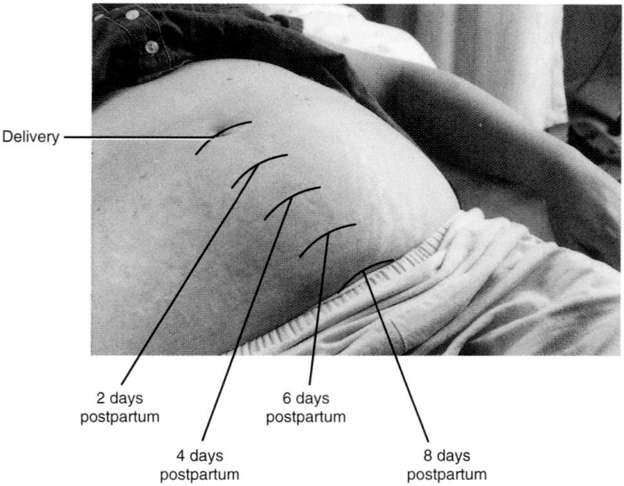

Fundal heights postpartum

AREA/NORMAL VARIATION	ABNORMAL VARIATION/RATIONALE
Lochia:	
Rubra (bloody) first few days postpartum. Rubra contains blood, decidual and thromboplastic debris. Serous (pink, brown) 3 or 4 to 10 days postpartum. Serous contains old blood, serum, leukocytes, and tissue debris. Alba (yellow, white) 10 days up to 6 weeks postpartum. Alba contains leukocytes, decidua, epithelial cells, mucus, serum, and bacteria.	Increase lochia rubra seen with hemorrhage, cervical or vaginal tears.
Vascular	
Extremities: Increased risk for thromboemboli due to hypercoagulable state. Negative Homans' sign. Varicosities usually regress after delivery. Edema usually decreases after delivery.	Positive Homans' may indicate phlebitis, DVT, varicosities.

(box continued on page 400)

Postpartal Physical Assessment (continued)

AREA/NORMAL VARIATION	ABNORMAL VARIATION/RATIONALE
Neurologic	
Carpal tunnel abates after delivery. Affect depends on outcome of delivery. Emotionally labile, postpartum blues common. Bonding well with baby.	Headaches may be caused by PIH, stress, or spinal fluid leaks secondary to spinal anesthesia. Can last 1 to 3 days to weeks dependent on cause. Postpartum depression or psychosis.
Musculoskeletal	
Joint stability returns within 6 to 8 weeks. Increase in shoe size is permanent.	

HEENT = Head, eyes, ears, nose, and throat.

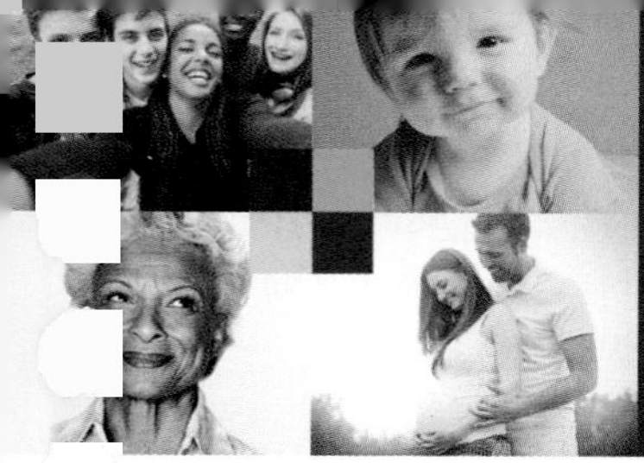

CHAPTER 15

Assessing the Newborn and Infant

During the first year of life, the infant experiences rapid growth and developmental changes. Many physical, gross motor, fine motor, primitive reflex, sensory, communication, and socialization changes are seen.

Developmental Considerations

- Psychosocial development focuses on establishing trust; infant establishes trust when his or her needs are met.
- Cognitive development during first year, also called the sensorimotor phase of development, involves three tasks:
  - Separation—realizing that self is separate from other objects.
  - Object permanence—realizing that objects are permanent even when not in sight.
  - Mental representation—recognizing symbols of objects without actually experiencing the object.
- Infant develops body image by exploring and playing with different parts of her or his body.
- Social development includes developing attachment to parents or caregivers and experiencing separation anxiety and fear of strangers.
- Communication and language development also occur.
- Denver Developmental Screening Test-II (DDST-II) and growth charts are frequently used to assess and track growth and development during well-baby check-ups.

- As you assess the infant, be sure to note if his or her physical development is appropriate for his or her age and whether he or she is performing appropriate developmental tasks for the age. Because growth and development are so rapid during the first year of life, even the slightest developmental delay may signal an underlying problem and warrant further investigation.
- Key physical changes:
  - Birth weight doubles by 6 months, triples by 12 months.
  - Height increases by 1 inch per month for first 6 months.
  - Fontanels are closing.
  - Lumbar curve develops with a lordosis once infant begins to walk.
  - Drooling and teething occur.
  - Primitive reflexes disappear as neurologic system matures.
- Gross motor changes:
  - Rolls, crawls.
  - Pulls to sit.
  - Begins to walk.
  - Achieves head control.
- Fine motor changes:
  - Grasps objects.
  - Puts objects in mouth.
  - Holds bottle.
  - Plays with toes.
  - Develops pincer grasp.
- Sensory changes:
  - Develops better vision.
  - Follows objects.
  - Responds to sounds.
- Communication changes:
  - Initially cries to convey needs.
  - Babbles.
  - Laughs.
  - Says three to five words by 12 months.
  - Begins to comprehend simple directions.
  - Imitates sounds.
- Socialization changes:
  - Identifies parents.
  - Develops social smile.

- Is aware of strange situations.
- Has increasing difficulty separating from parents.
- Becomes more fearful of strangers.
- Begins to develop memory.
- Shows emotions.

Cultural Considerations

Cultural or ethnic influences may affect your assessment findings. You need to be aware of these normal variations so that you do not mistake them for abnormal findings. Cultural or ethnic influences may also affect the relationship between child and parent and define the roles of both parent and child within the family. They may also affect the infant's health and wellness.

Cultural and Ethnic Variations in Infants*

African American

- Mongolian spots and other birthmarks more prevalent than in other ethnic groups.

Amish

- Babies seen as gifts from God. Have high birth rates, large families.

Appalachian

- Newborns wear bands around abdomen to prevent umbilical hernias and asafetida bags around neck to prevent contagious diseases.

Arab American

- Children "dearly loved."
- Male circumcision is a religious requirement.

Chinese American

- Children highly valued because of one-child rule in China.
- Mongolian spots occur in about 80 percent of infants.
- Bilirubin levels higher in Chinese newborns than in others, with highest levels seen on day 5 or 6.

*Adapted from Purnell, L.D., and Paulanka, B.J. (2012): *Transcultural Healthcare: A Culturally Competent Approach,* 4th ed. Philadelphia, F.A. Davis.

Cuban American

- Childbirth is a celebration. Family takes care of both mother and infant for the first 4 weeks.
- Tend to bottle-feed rather than breast-feed. If breast-fed, child is weaned early, around 3 months. If bottle-fed, weaned late, around 4 years.

Egyptian American

- Children very important.
- Mother and infant cared for by family for the first 50 days.

Filipino American

- Eyes almond shaped, low to flat nose bridge with mildly flared nostrils. Mongolian spots common.

French Canadian

- Five mutations account for 90 percent of phenylketonuria (PKU) in French Canadians. High incidence of cystic fibrosis and muscular dystrophy.

Greek American

- High incidence of two genetic conditions: thalassemia and glucose-6-phosphate dehydrogenase (G-6-PD).

Iranian American

- Believe in hot and cold influences, with baby boys "hotter" than baby girls. Infant may be confined to home for first 40 days. Ritual bath between 10th and 40th day.

Jewish American

- Children seen as valued treasure.
- High incidence of Tay-Sachs disease.
- Male circumcision is a religious ritual.

Mexican American

- Wears stomach belt *(ombliguero)* to prevent umbilicus from popping out when infant cries.
- Believe that cutting nails in the first 3 months after birth causes blindness and deafness.

Navajo Native American

- Infants kept on cradle boards until they can walk.
- Mongolian spots common.

Vietnamese American

- Mongolian spots common.

Assessment of Newborns

Apgar Scoring of Newborns

Heart rate	0 = Absent	1 = <100 BPM	2 = >100 BPM
Respirations	0 = Absent	1 = <30, irregular	2 = Strong cry, regular
Muscle tone	0 = Flaccid	1 = Some flexion in arms and legs	2 = Full flexion, active movement
Reflex irritability	0 = No response	1 = Grimace, weak cry	2 = Vigorous cry
Color	0 = Pale, blue	1 = Body pink, extremities blue	2 = Totally pink

Newborn Health History

MATERNAL HEALTH HISTORY	SIGNIFICANCE
General health, prenatal diseases or conditions, prenatal care, number of pregnancies	Maternal health problems (e.g., gestational diabetes, cardiac, or kidney disease) may cause potential risk factors in newborn.
Use of prescribed or over-the-counter (OTC) medications, tobacco, alcohol, illegal drugs	Medications and other agents may affect physiological systems (e.g., smoking during pregnancy related to low birth weights, alcohol use related to fetal alcohol syndrome).
Duration of pregnancy and labor, type of anesthesia, type of delivery, complications	Details of labor and delivery alert nurse to observe for potential newborn problems.

Physical Assessment of Newborns

APPROACH: Inspection, palpation, percussion, auscultation. Perform techniques that may evoke crying (e.g., otoscopic exam) at the end of the assessment. Be sure to keep the room and the baby warm.

TOOLBOX: Tape measure, stethoscope, thermometer, blood pressure (BP) cuff, penlight, otoscope, ophthalmoscope, baby scale.

(text continues on page 428)

Physical Assessment of Newborns

AREA/SYSTEM AND NORMAL VARIATIONS	ABNORMAL FINDINGS
General Survey/Anthropometric Measurements/Vital Signs: Inspection, Auscultation, Measurement	
Posture	
Head and extremities flexed.	*Limp posture with extension of extremities:* Birth injuries, anesthesia, acidosis, hypoglycemia, hypothermia, or congenital problems.
Head Circumference	
Measure head circumference from occiput to forehead.	
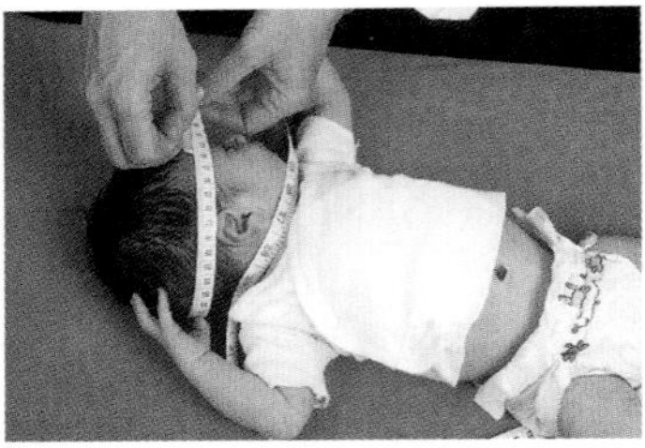 *Measuring head circumference*	
33 to 35 cm. Molding can affect measurement.	*Head circumference < 10 percent of normal:* Microcephaly related to congenital malformation or infection. *Head circumference > 90 percent of normal:* Macrocephaly related to hydrocephalus.
Chest Circumference	
Measure chest at nipple line.	
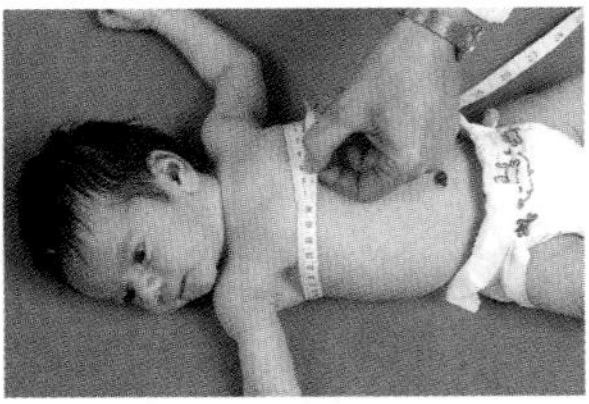 *Measuring chest circumference*	
30.5 to 33 cm (2 to 3 cm less than head). Breast engorgement can affect measurement.	

AREA/SYSTEM AND NORMAL VARIATIONS	ABNORMAL FINDINGS
Abdominal Circumference	
Measure abdomen above the umbilicus.	
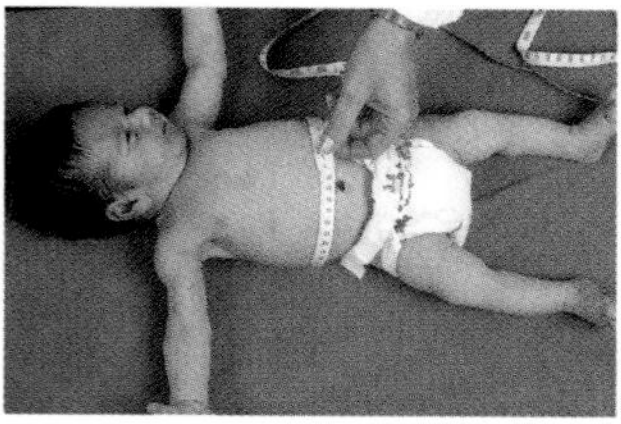 *Measuring abdominal circumference*	
Similar to chest measurement. Should not be distended.	
Length	
Crown to rump: 31 to 35 cm (about equal to head circumference). Head to heel: 45 to 55 cm (18 to 22 inches) at birth.	
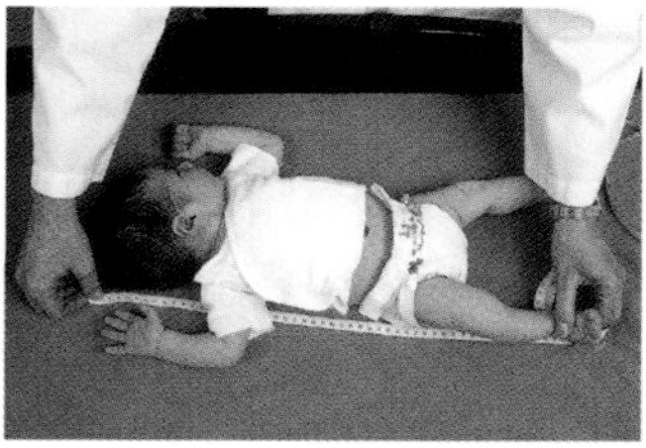 *Measuring length*	
Molding can affect measurement.	
Weight	
Newborn weight is usually between 2500 and 4000 g (5 lb, 8 oz and 8 lb, 13 oz).	Birth weights < 10 or > 90 percent are abnormal. *Low birth weight (small for gestational age):* Associated with prematurity. *Macrosomic infant (large for gestational age):* Associated with gestational diabetes in mother.
Temperature	
Axillary: 36.5°C to 37.2°C.	Hypothermia leads to cold stress. Sepsis, environmental extremes, and neurologic problems can cause hypothermia or hyperthermia.

(box continued on page 408)

Physical Assessment of Newborns (continued)

AREA/SYSTEM AND NORMAL VARIATIONS	ABNORMAL FINDINGS
General Survey/Anthropometric Measurements/Vital Signs: Inspection, Auscultation, Measurement *(cont'd)*	
Pulse	
Apical rate 120 to 160 beats per minute (BPM).	Irregular rhythms, such as bradycardia (<100 BPM) and tachycardia (>160 BPM).
Rate increases with crying and decreases with sleep.	Most murmurs are not pathological and disappear by age 6 months.
Respirations	
30 to 60 breaths/min; irregular.	Respirations < 30 or > 60 breaths/min.
Anesthesia during labor and delivery can affect respirations.	Periods of apnea > 15 seconds.
Blood Pressure	
Systolic: 50 to 75 mm Hg. *Diastolic:* 30 to 45 mm Hg.	*Low BP:* Hypovolemia.
Crying and moving increase systolic pressure.	Late clamping of umbilical cord can increase BP because of expanded blood volume from the "placental transfusion."
Integumentary: Inspection	
Skin	
Skin may be red, smooth, edematous, mottled (cutis marmorata).	*Persistent acrocyanosis:* Thermoregulation problem or hypoglycemia.
Hands and feet may be cyanotic (acrocyanosis).	*Extensive desquamation:* Post-term baby.
Physiological jaundice occurs after 24 hours.	Pathological jaundice occurs within first 24 hours.
Color may change with position (Harlequin sign).	*Plethora:* Polycythemia.
Cheesy substance (vernix caseosa) decreases as baby's gestational age increases to term.	*Pallor:* Anemia, hypothermia, shock, or sepsis.
Desquamation, ecchymosis, and petechiae may occur from trauma during delivery.	*Persistent ecchymosis or petechiae:* Thrombocytopenia, sepsis, or congenital infection.

AREA/SYSTEM AND NORMAL VARIATIONS	ABNORMAL FINDINGS
Milia (white papules) may occur on face. 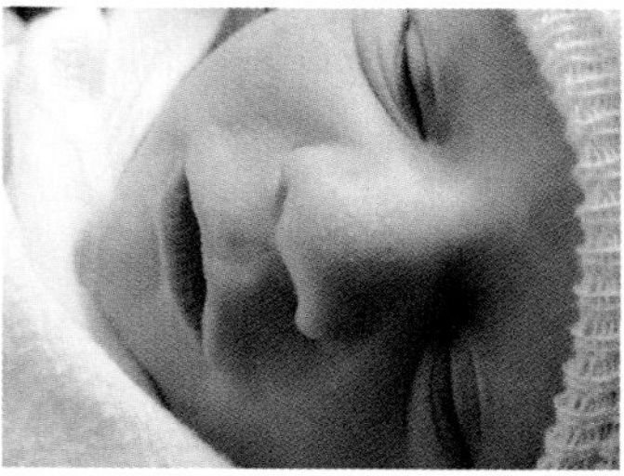 *Milia*	*Poor turgor:* Intrauterine growth retardation or hypoglycemia.
Miliaria or audamina (papules or vesicles on face) are caused by blocked sweat ducts.	*Café-au-lait spots:* >6 or larger than 4 x 6 cm may indicate neurofibromatosis; can become precancerous with age.
Mongolian spots (bluish discoloration in sacral area) are commonly seen in African, Asian, Latin, and Native American newborns.	*Nevus flammeus (port-wine stain):* Disfigures face; may be associated with cerebral vascular malformation.
Telangiectatic nevi.	Giant hemangiomas and nevus vasculosus ("strawberry marks") tend to trap platelets and lower circulating platelet counts. They usually disappear by age 5.
Flat hemangiomas ("stork bites") may be present at nape of neck. 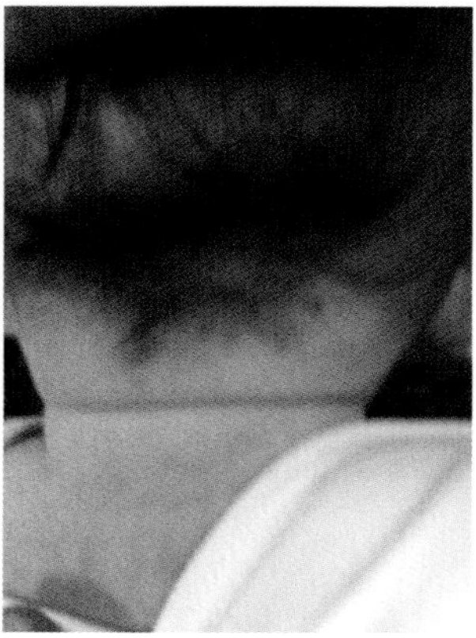 *Stork bite*	Reddish-blue round mass of blood vessels (cavernous hemangioma) must be monitored. If size increases, surgery may be necessary. Erythema toxicum, a common newborn rash of red macules and papules, usually disappears in 1 week. *Bullae or pustules:* Infections such as syphilis or staphylococcus. Thin, translucent skin and vernix caseosa are signs of prematurity. Genetic disorders may cause extra skin folds.

(box continued on page 410)

Physical Assessment of Newborns (continued)

AREA/SYSTEM AND NORMAL VARIATIONS	ABNORMAL FINDINGS
Integumentary: Inspection *(cont'd)*	
Hair	
Some fine hair (lanugo) is normal.	*Abundant lanugo:* Prematurity. Genetic disorders may cause abnormal hair distribution unrelated to gestational age.
Nails	Long nails seen in post-term babies.
HEENT	
Head/Face: Inspection, Palpation	
Palpate and transilluminate fontanels.	Fused sutures.

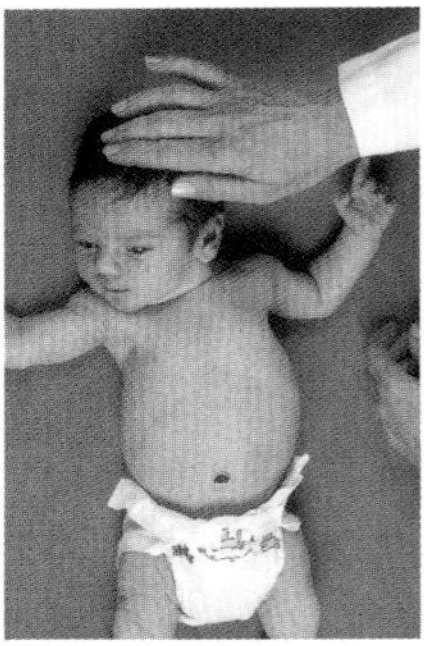

Palpating fontanel

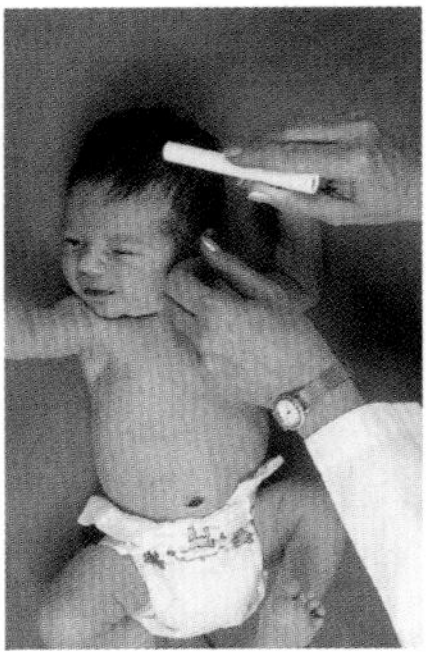

Transilluminating fontanel

AREA/SYSTEM AND NORMAL VARIATIONS	ABNORMAL FINDINGS
Molding in birth canal may cause asymmetry of face and skull and should resolve within 1 week.	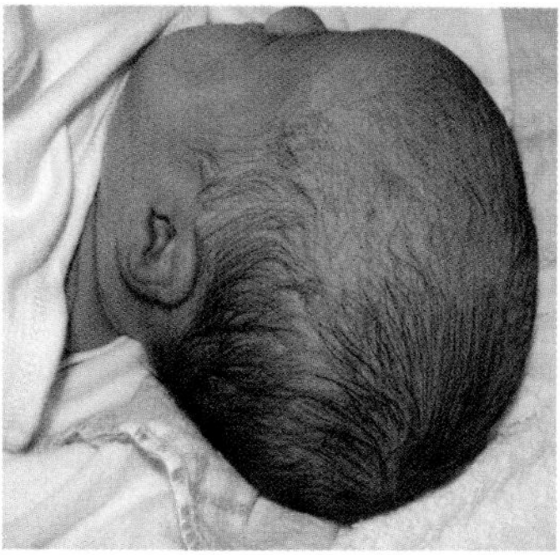 *Molding*
Anterior fontanel: Diamond shaped, 2.5 to 4 cm.	*Large fontanels:* Hydrocephaly, osteogenesis imperfecta, congenital hypothyroidism.
Posterior fontanel: Triangle shaped, 0.5 to 1 cm.	*Small fontanels:* Microcephaly.
Soft and flat.	*Bulging fontanels:* Increased intracranial pressure. *Depressed fontanels:* Dehydration. Craniosynostosis (premature closure of sutures). *Cephalohematoma (hematoma between periosteum and skull with unilateral swelling):* Most uncomplicated cephalohematomas totally resolve within 2 weeks to 3 months. Caput succedaneum (edema of soft scalp tissue from birth trauma) decreases gradually in several days.
Symmetrical facial movements.	*Asymmetrical facial movements:* Damage to facial nerve during forceps delivery.
Neck: Inspection, Palpation	
Positive tonic reflex.	*Absent tonic reflex:* Erb's palsy if unilateral or dislocation of cervical spine or fractured clavicle.
Short neck.	
Able to hold head up with "pull-to-sit" test.	*Head lag with "pull-to-sit" test:* Muscle weakness. Torticollis (wry neck).

(box continued on page 412)

Physical Assessment of Newborns (continued)

AREA/SYSTEM AND NORMAL VARIATIONS	ABNORMAL FINDINGS
HEENT *(cont'd)* *Eyes: Inspection*	
Avoid bright light because it will cause the newborn to avoid opening her or his eyes and make assessment difficult.	*Subconjunctival hemorrhage:* Trauma during delivery.
Eyes may be edematous after vaginal delivery.	*Brushfield spots, epicanthal fold, and Mongolian slant:* Down syndrome. *Absent red light reflex:* Congenital cataract.
Eyes equal and symmetrical. 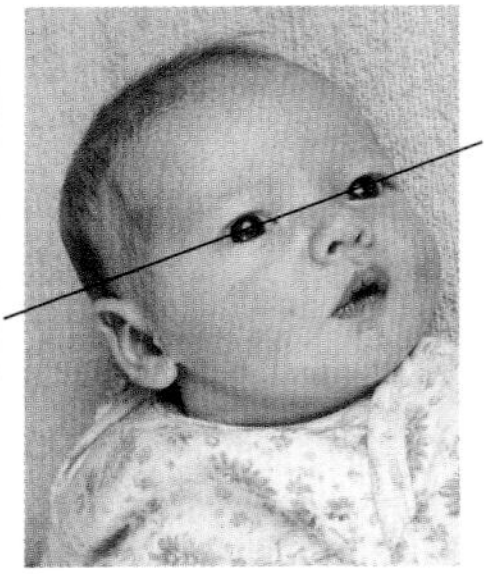 *Normal eye line*	*Ptosis:* Neuromuscular weakness. *Sun-setting (crescent of sclera over iris from retraction of upper lid):* Hydrocephalus.
Blue/gray or brown iris; white or bluish-white sclera. Antimongolian slant; Mongolian slant seen in Asian infants.	*Yellow sclera:* Jaundice. *Blue sclera:* Osteogenesis imperfecta.
Positive red light reflex. Positive blink reflex. Positive corneal reflex.	*Persistent nystagmus, absent blink reflex, inability to follow objects:* Vision problem, such as blindness.
No tears (tear production begins by 2 months).	*Dilated or fixed pupil:* Anoxia or neurologic damage.
Positive fixation on close objects. Positive pupillary reaction to light. Strabismus and searching nystagmus caused by immature muscular control.	Chemical conjunctivitis from eye prophylaxis may occur during first 24 hours.
Ears: Inspection, Palpation, Hearing Testing	
Pinna flexible, without deformity, aligns with external canthus of eyes. Presence of the startle reflex.	*Low-set ears:* Down syndrome. **The ears and kidneys develop at the same time in**

AREA/SYSTEM AND NORMAL VARIATIONS	ABNORMAL FINDINGS
American Academy of Pediatrics recommends hearing screening by auditory brainstem response or evoked otoacoustic emissions on newborns before discharge.	**utero, so malformed ears may be accompanied by renal problems.** *Absent startle reflex:* Possible hearing problem.
Nose: Inspection	
Nares patent. Small amount of thin white mucus.	Because infants are obligatory nose breathers, large amounts of mucus drainage may obstruct nostrils and result in respiratory difficulty.
May be flattened and bruised from birth.	***Nasal flaring:* Sign of distress.**
Mouth/Throat: Inspection	
Mucous membranes pink and moist.	*Cyanotic mucous membranes:* Hypoxia. Tongue-tied (ankyloglossia) 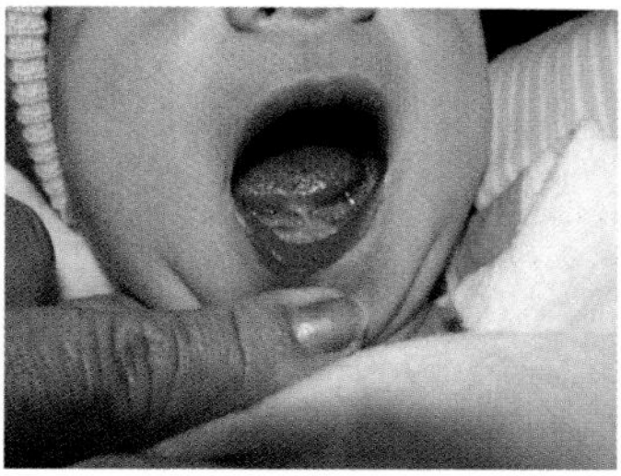 *Tongue tied*
Frenulum of tongue and lip intact. Palate intact, uvula midline.	Candida albicans *(thrush):* Contracted during vaginal delivery. 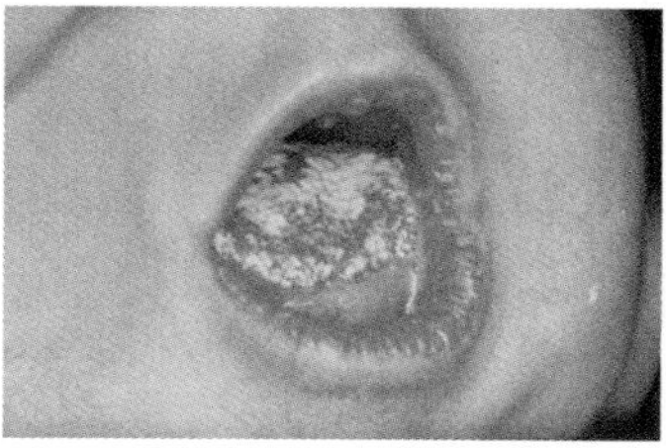 *Thrust*

(box continued on page 414)

Physical Assessment of Newborns (continued)

AREA/SYSTEM AND NORMAL VARIATIONS	ABNORMAL FINDINGS
HEENT *Mouth/Throat: Inspection (cont'd)*	
Strong sucking reflex; positive rooting, gag, extrusion, and swallowing reflexes.	*Weak sucking, swallowing reflex:* Maternal anesthesia or perinatal asphyxia.
Minimal saliva.	
Strong cry. Natal teeth may be benign or associated with congenital defects.	*Opening in palate or lips:* Cleft palate or lip. Any opening is abnormal. A series of surgical interventions will be necessary.
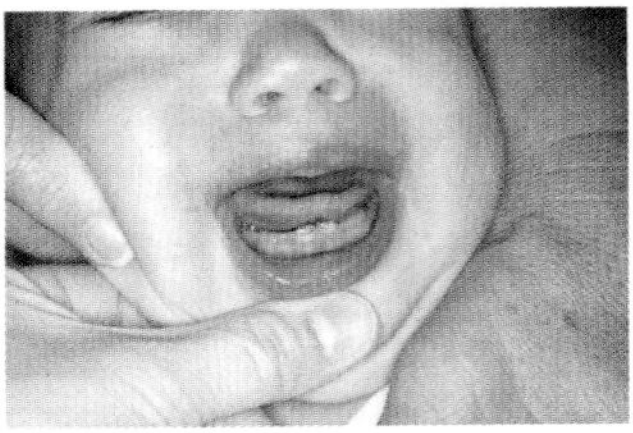 *Natal teeth*	
Natal teeth must be removed by a specialist because they usually fall out and can cause choking.	**Cleft lip or palate will cause newborn to have difficulty with feeding.**
Small white, pearl-like epithelial cysts on the palate (Epstein's pearls) disappear within a few weeks.	*Weak cry:* Neuromuscular problem, hypotonia, and prematurity.
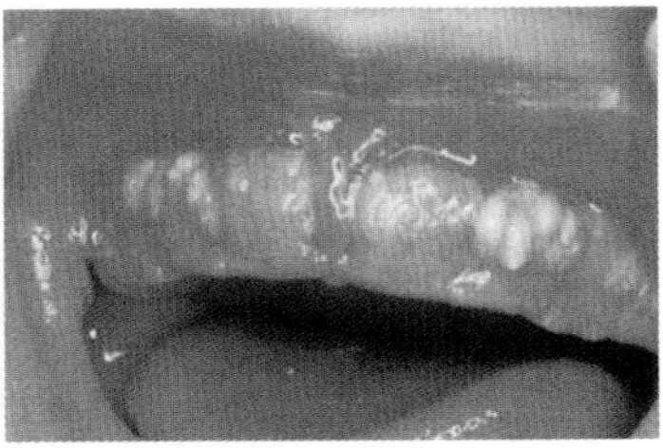 *Epstein's pearls*	
Chest: Inspection, Auscultation	
Anteroposterior:lateral (1:1).	*Funnel chest (pectus excavatum):* Congenital anomaly.
Equal chest excursion.	*Pigeon chest (pectus carinatum):* Obstructed respiration in infancy.

AREA/SYSTEM AND NORMAL VARIATIONS	ABNORMAL FINDINGS
Breast engorgement. 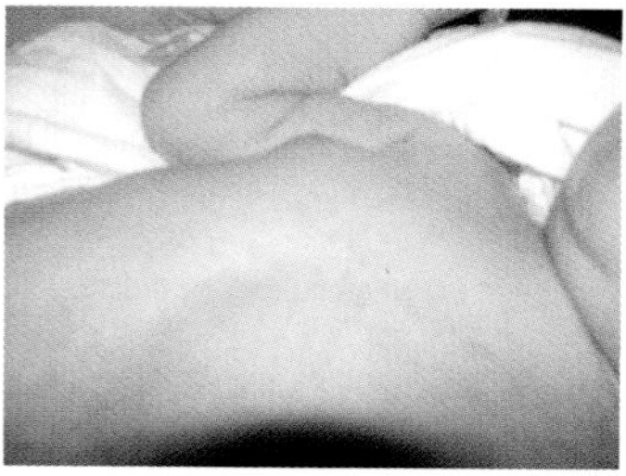 *Breast engorgement*	*Asymmetrical excursion, retraction:* Respiratory distress.
Clear or milky liquid from nipples ("witch's milk") develops from maternal hormones in utero.	
Supernumerary nipples.	Red, firm nipples.
Respiratory: Auscultation	
Lungs clear, bronchial breath sounds audible. Cough reflex absent at birth, but present 1 to 2 days later. Scattered crackles a few hours after birth.	Persistent crackles, wheezes, stridor, grunting, paradoxical breathing, decreased breath sounds, prolonged periods of apnea (>15–20 sec) are signs of respiratory problems.
Cardiovascular: Auscultation	
S_1, S_2, normal rhythm with respiratory variations.	Dextrocardia (heart on right side).
Point of maximal impulse (PMI): fourth left intercostal space midcostal line.	*Cardiomegaly:* Displaced PMI.
Quiet but clearly audible murmurs occur in 30 percent of newborns but should disappear in 2 days.	Murmurs often heard at base or along left sternal border and are usually benign, but need to be evaluated to rule out cardiac disorder. Thrills.
Abdomen: Inspection, Palpation	
Abdomen round. Positive bowel sounds. Liver edge palpable 2 to 3 cm. Tip of spleen, kidneys palpable.	*Abdominal distension, ascites, distended veins:* Portal hypertension.

(box continued on page 416)

Physical Assessment of Newborns (continued)

AREA/SYSTEM AND NORMAL VARIATIONS	ABNORMAL FINDINGS
Abdomen: Inspection, Palpation *(cont'd)*	
Cord bluish-white with two arteries and one vein.	*Green umbilical cord:* Infection.
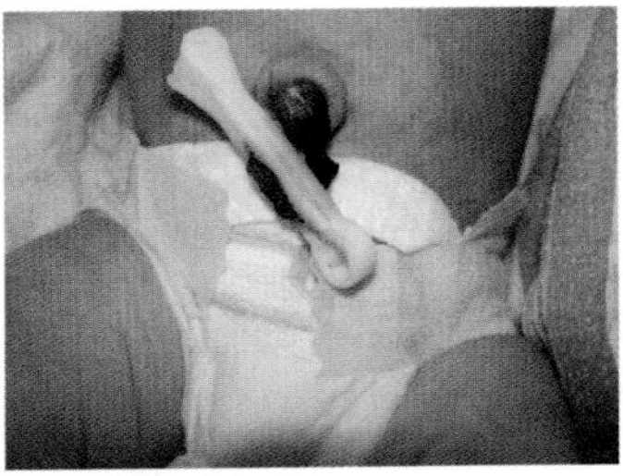 *Umbilical cord*	
Positive femoral pulses. Umbilical hernias and diastasis recti more common in African Americans; often resolves within a year.	*Absence of umbilical vessels:* Associated with heart and kidney malformations.
Rectum: Inspection	
Anus patent.	Anal fissures or fistulas.
Passage of meconium stool within 48 hours.	*No stools:* Malformation in gastrointestinal (GI) tract.
Positive anal reflex ("anal wink").	**Imperforate anus (absent anus) requires immediate surgical repair.**
Female Genitourinary: Inspection, Palpation	
Urination within 24 hours.	Inability to urinate within 24 hours.
Urinary meatus midline and uninterrupted stream noted on voiding.	Fused labia or absent vaginal opening.
Labia majora and minora may be edematous. Place thumbs on either side of labia and gently separate tissues to visualize perineum.	Ambiguous genitalia. Meconium from vaginal opening.
Blood-tinged vaginal fluid may be noted (pseudomenstruation).	
Note presence of clitoris, vagina, and hymen.	A newborn clitoris > 0.5 cm is abnormal.

AREA/SYSTEM AND NORMAL VARIATIONS	ABNORMAL FINDINGS

Male Genitourinary: Inspection, Palpation

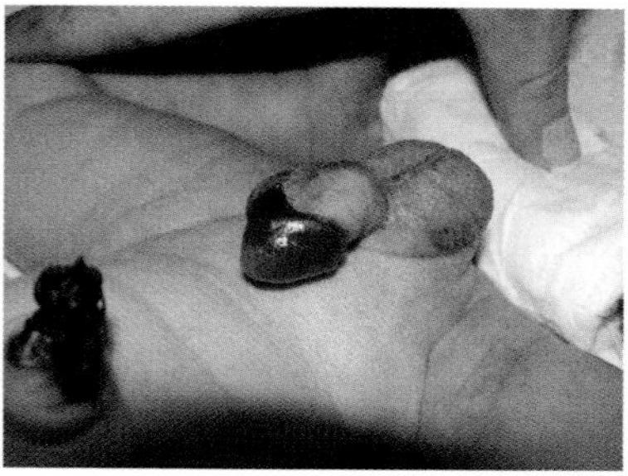

Circumcision

Urination within 24 hours.
Foreskin retracts.
Urethral opening at tip of penis.
Scrotum edematous.

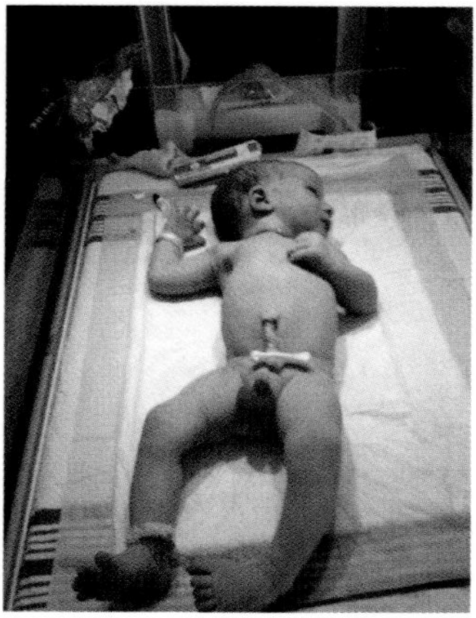

Scrotal edema

Inability to urinate within 24 hours.
Inability to retract foreskin.
Hypospadias.
Epispadias.
Chordee.
Hydrocele.
Undescended testicles.
Inguinal hernia.
Ambiguous genitalia.
Meconium from scrotum.

(box continued on page 418)

Physical Assessment of Newborns (continued)

AREA/SYSTEM AND NORMAL VARIATIONS	ABNORMAL FINDINGS
Male Genitourinary: Inspection, Palpation *(cont'd)* Smegma. Palpable testes.	

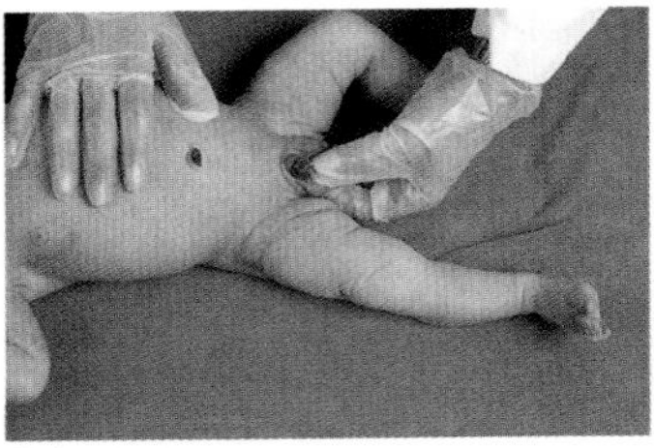

Palpating scrotum

Musculoskeletal: Inspection, Palpation	
10 fingers and 10 toes.	*Polydactyly:* Extra digits.
Full range of movement (ROM).	*Syndactyly:* Webbed digits.
No clicks in joints.	*Phocomelia:* Hands and feet attached close to chest.
Equal gluteal folds.	*Hemimelia:* Absence of distal part of extremity.

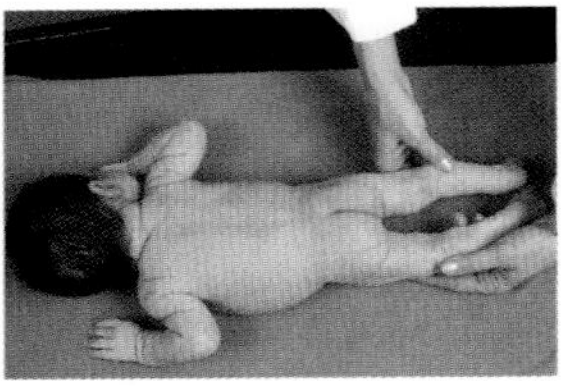

Checking gluteal folds

C curve of spine, no dimpling.	*Talipes (club foot):* Foot is permanently twisted out of shape.

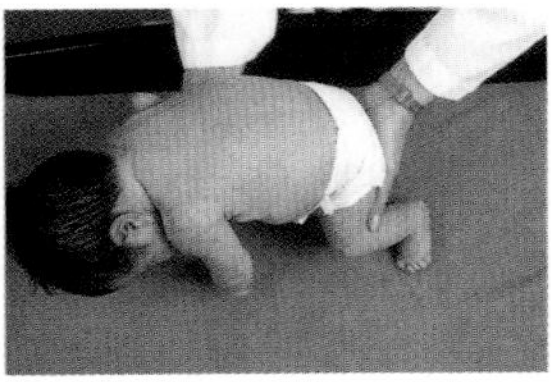

Checking for C curve

AREA/SYSTEM AND NORMAL VARIATIONS	ABNORMAL FINDINGS
When arms and legs are extended, muscles symmetrical with equal muscle tone, and arms and legs symmetrical in size and movement.	Severe bowing of legs is abnormal.
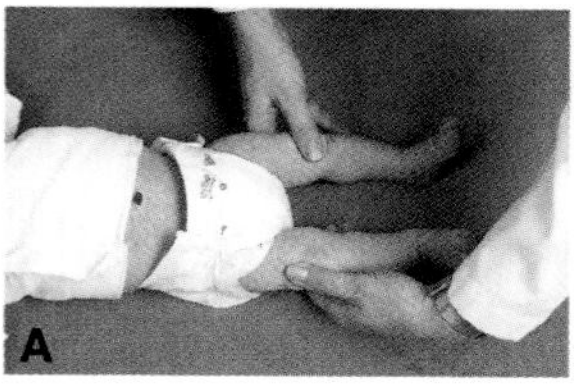 *A. Barlow-Ortolani maneuver #1*	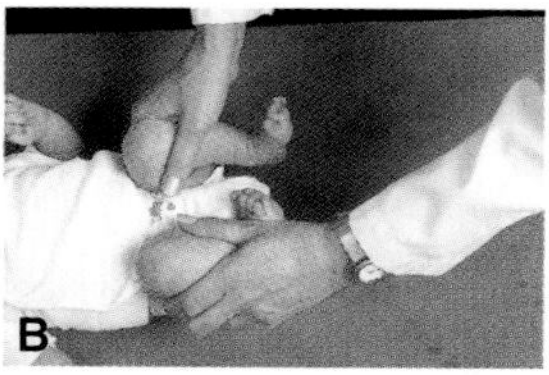 *B. Barlow-Ortolani maneuver #2*
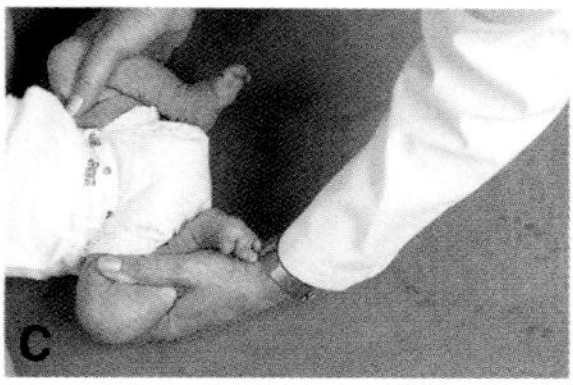 *C. Barlow-Ortolani maneuver #3*	*Unequal gluteal folds and positive Barlow-Ortolani:* Associated with congenial hip dislocation. Requires immediate referral.
Hands held as fists until after 1 month, when grasp becomes strong and equal.	
Position in utero may affect appearance.	Decreased ROM and muscle tone. *Swelling, crepitus, neck tenderness:* Possible broken clavicle. *Simian (transverse palmar) creases:* Down syndrome.
Neurologic: Inspection, Palpation, Percussion	
Positive newborn reflexes (Table 15.1).	*Hypotonia:* Floppy, limp extremities.
Positive knee reflex.	Paralysis. Marked head lag. Tremors. Asymmetrical posture. *Hypertonia:* Tightly flexed arms and stiffly extended legs with quivering. *Opisthotonic posture:* Arched back. *Dimpling of spine, tuft of hair:* Spina bifida or pilonidal cyst.

HEENT = Head, eyes, ears, nose, and throat.

TABLE 15.1 Newborn/Infant Reflexes

REFLEX AND TECHNIQUE	NORMAL RESPONSE	ABNORMAL RESPONSE
Moro		
Present at birth and lasts 1 to 4 months.	Quickly abducts and extends arms and legs symmetrically.	Premature or ill infants may have sluggish response.
Technique: Startle infant by suddenly jarring bassinet, or with infant in semi-sitting position, let head drop back slightly.	Makes "C" with index finger and thumbs. Legs flex up against trunk.	Positive response beyond 6 months indicates neurologic problem. Asymmetrical response may be caused by injury to clavicle, humerus, or brachial plexus during delivery.

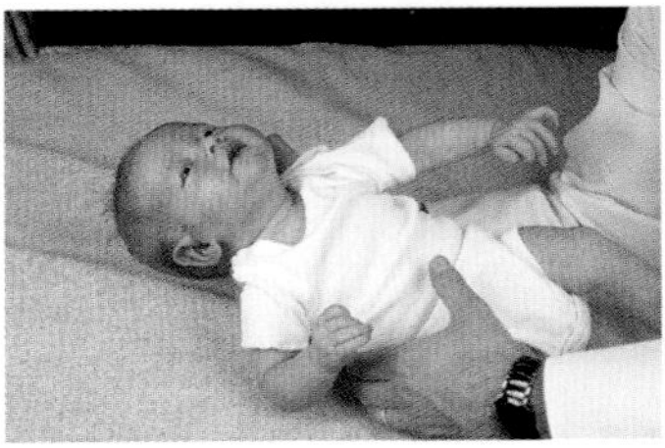

Moro reflex

REFLEX AND TECHNIQUE	NORMAL RESPONSE	ABNORMAL RESPONSE
Startle		
Present at birth and lasts 4 months. *Technique:* Startle infant by making loud noise.	Hands clenched, arms abducted, flexion at elbow.	Same as Moro.

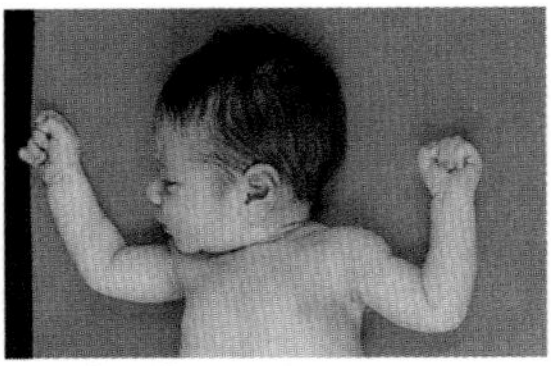

Startle reflex

REFLEX AND TECHNIQUE	NORMAL RESPONSE	ABNORMAL RESPONSE
Tonic Neck		
Present between birth and 6 weeks; disappears at 4 to 6 months.	Infant assumes "fencing position," with arm and leg extended in direction where head was turned.	Response after 6 months may indicate cerebral palsy.

REFLEX AND TECHNIQUE	NORMAL RESPONSE	ABNORMAL RESPONSE
Technique: With infant supine, rotate head to one side so that chin is over shoulder.		

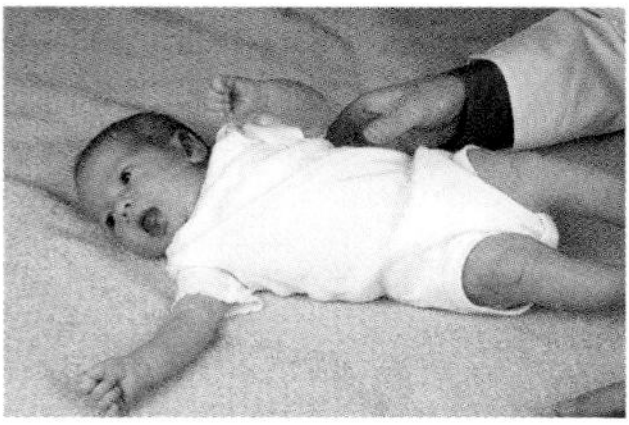

Tonic neck reflex

REFLEX AND TECHNIQUE	NORMAL RESPONSE	ABNORMAL RESPONSE
Palmar Grasp Present at birth; disappears at 3 to 4 months. *Technique:* Place object or finger in palm of infant's hand.	Infant grasps object tightly. If she or he grasps your fingers with both hands, she or he can be pulled to a sitting position.	Negative grasp seen with hypotonia or perinatal asphyxia.

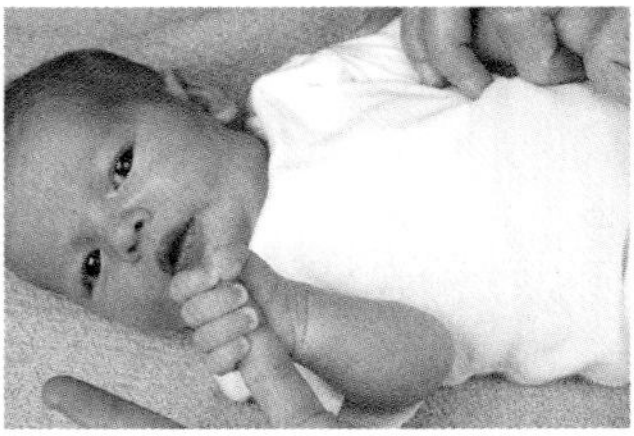

Palmar grasp reflex

REFLEX AND TECHNIQUE	NORMAL RESPONSE	ABNORMAL RESPONSE
Plantar Grasp Present at birth; disappears at 3 to 4 months. *Technique:* Place thumb firmly against ball of infant's foot.	Toes flex tightly downward in a grasping motion.	Negative grasp seen with hypotonia or spinal cord injury.

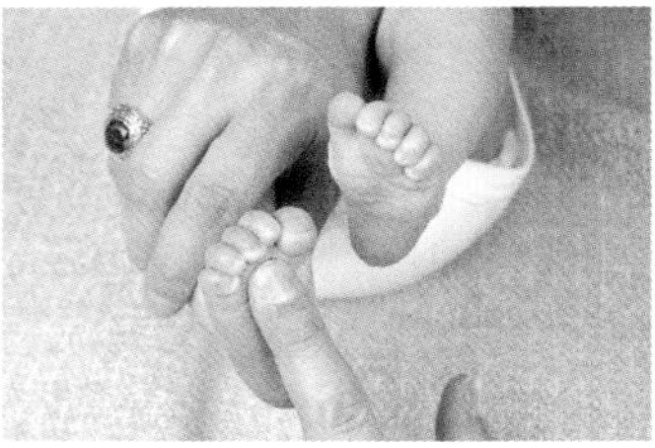

Plantar grasp reflex

(continued)

TABLE 15.1 Newborn/Infant Reflexes (continued)

REFLEX AND TECHNIQUE	NORMAL RESPONSE	ABNORMAL RESPONSE
Babinski Present at birth; disappears at 1 year. *Technique:* Stroke lateral surface of sole of infant's foot.	Toes should fan.	Diminished response associated with neurologic problem.
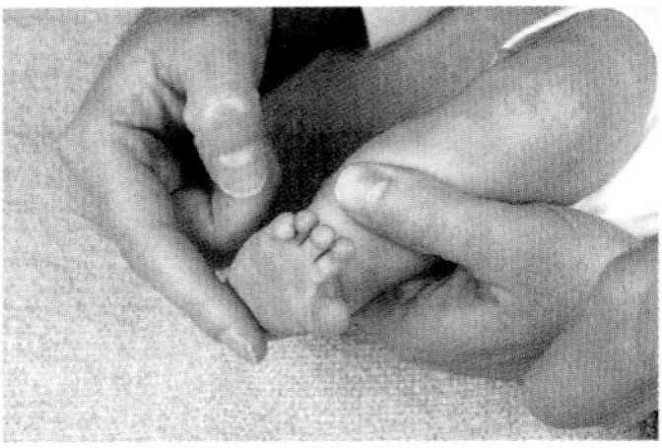 *Babinski reflex*		
Stepping or Dancing Present at birth; disappears at 3 to 4 weeks. *Technique:* Hold infant upright with feet touching a flat surface.	Infant steps up and down in place.	Poor response caused by hypotonia.
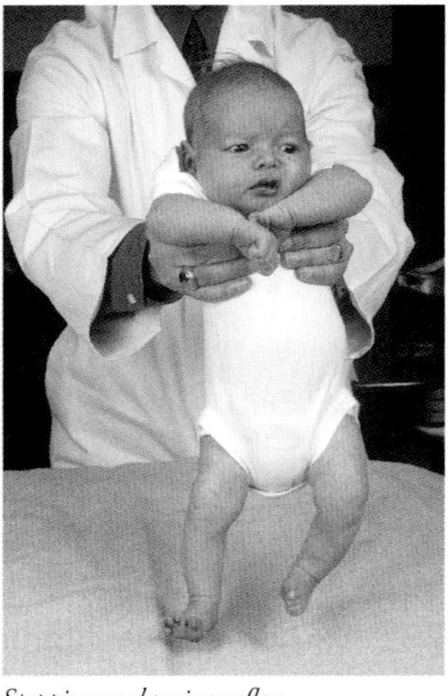 *Stepping or dancing reflex*		

REFLEX AND TECHNIQUE	NORMAL RESPONSE	ABNORMAL RESPONSE
Rooting Present at birth; disappears at 3 to 6 months. *Technique:* Brush cheek near corner of mouth.	Infant turns head in direction of stimulus and opens mouth.	Prematurity or neurologic problem may cause weak or absent response.
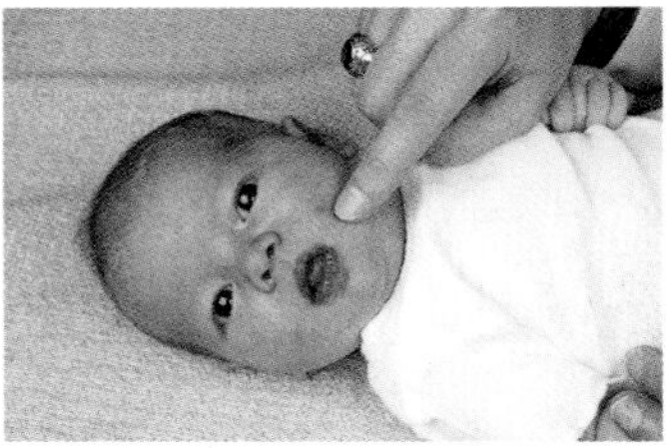 *Rooting reflex*		
Sucking Present at birth; disappears at 10 to 12 months. *Technique:* Touch lips.	Sucking motion occurs.	Weak or absent response associated with prematurity or neurologic defect.
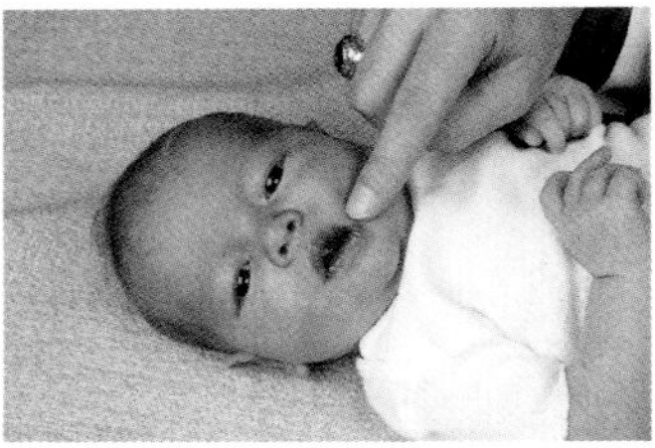 *Sucking reflex*		
Don't check for rooting or sucking responses immediately after a feeding—they will be difficult to elicit.		
Swallowing Present at birth and lasts throughout life. *Technique:* Automatically follows sucking response during feeding.	Sucking and swallowing should occur without coughing, gagging, or vomiting.	Weak or absent response associated with prematurity or neurologic problem.

(continued)

TABLE 15.1 Newborn/Infant Reflexes (continued)

REFLEX AND TECHNIQUE	NORMAL RESPONSE	ABNORMAL RESPONSE
Extrusion Present at birth to 4 months. *Technique:* Touch tip of tongue. 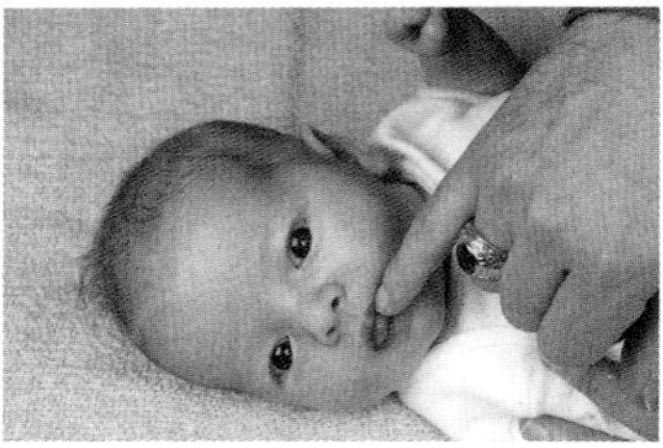 *Extrusion reflex*	Tongue protrudes outward.	Absence may indicate neurologic problem. Continued extrusion of large tongue associated with Down syndrome.
Glabellar Present at birth. *Technique:* Tap on forehead. 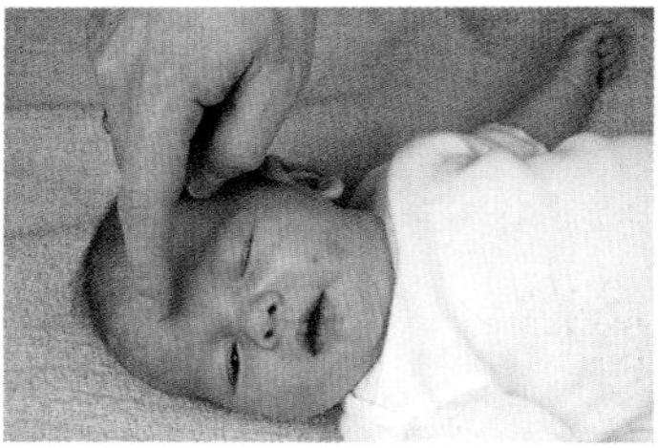 *Glabellar reflex*	Newborn blinks for first few taps.	Persistent blinking with repeated taps indicates extrapyramidal problem.
Crawling Present at birth; disappears at 6 weeks. *Technique:* Place infant on abdomen. 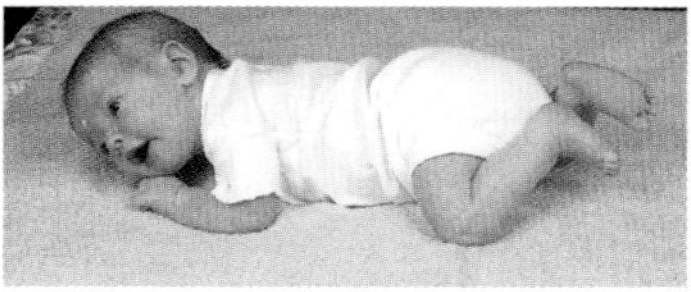 *Crawling reflex*	Newborn attempts to crawl.	

REFLEX AND TECHNIQUE	NORMAL RESPONSE	ABNORMAL RESPONSE
Crossed Extension Present at birth; disappears at 2 months. *Technique:* Infant supine with leg extended. Stimulate foot.	Flexion, adduction, then extension of opposite leg.	Peripheral nerve damage causes weak response. Spinal cord lesion causes absent response.

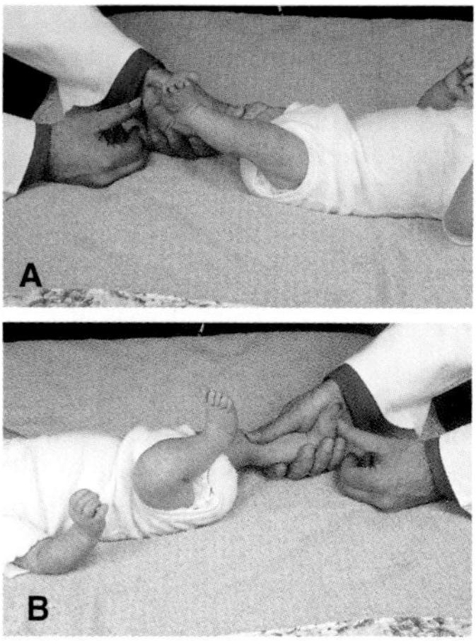

A. Crossed extension;
B. Stimulate foot

REFLEX AND TECHNIQUE	NORMAL RESPONSE	ABNORMAL RESPONSE
Pull-to-Sit Present at birth. *Technique:* Pull infant to sitting position.	Head lags as infant is pulled to sitting position, but then infant is able to hold up head temporarily.	Inability to hold up head suggests prematurity or hypotonia.

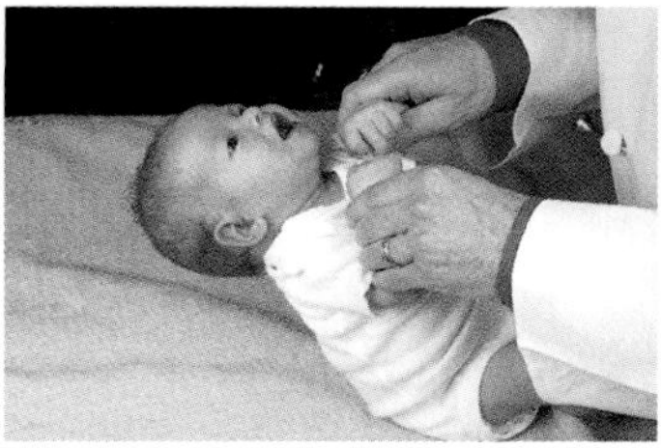

Pull-to-sit reflex

(continued)

TABLE 15.1 Newborn/Infant Reflexes (continued)

REFLEX AND TECHNIQUE	NORMAL RESPONSE	ABNORMAL RESPONSE
Trunk Incurvation Present at birth; disappears in a few days to 4 weeks. *Technique:* With infant prone, run finger down either side of spine. 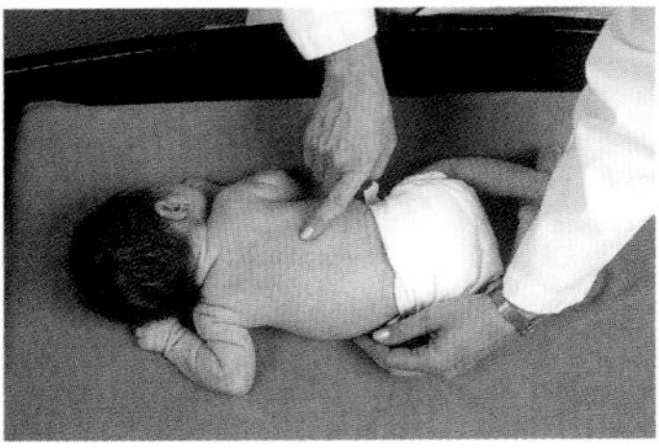 *Trunk incurvation reflex*	Flexion of trunk with hip moving toward stimulated side.	Absent response indicates neurologic or spinal cord problem.
Magnet Present at birth. *Technique:* With infant supine, flex leg and apply pressure to soles of feet. 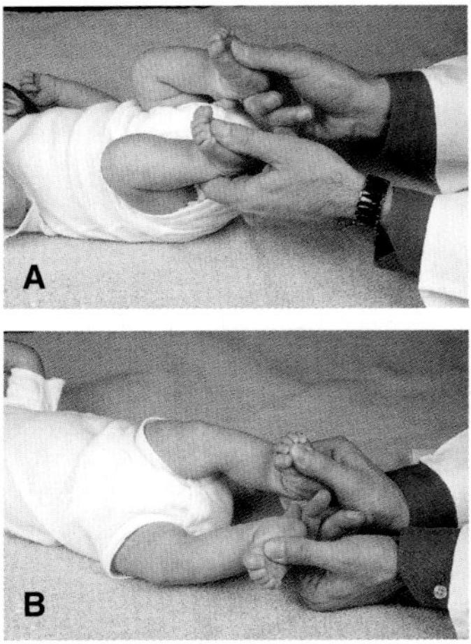 *A. Flex legs; B. Apply pressure to soles of feet*	Extends legs against pressure.	Breech birth may diminish reflex. Absent response caused by spinal cord problem.

Diagnostic/Screening Tests for Newborns

TEST	SIGNIFICANCE
PKU: Measures amount of phenylalanine amino acids in blood.	Test is collected after several days of feedings. High phenylalanine levels can cause brain damage.
Galactosemia: Transferase deficiency.	Elevated galactose and low fluorescence may result in mental retardation, blindness, or death from dehydration and sepsis.
Maple syrup urine disease	Elevated leucine can result in acidosis, seizures, mental retardation, and death.
Homocystinuria	Elevated methionine can lead to mental retardation, seizures, and behavioral disorders.
Congenital adrenal hyperplasia	Elevated 17-hydroxyprogesterone can lead to hyponatremia, hypokalemia, hypoglycemia, and ambiguous female genitalia.
Biotinidase deficiency	Decreased activity of biotinidase on colorimetric assay causes mental retardation, skin changes, hearing and vision problems, even death.
Thyroxine	Thyroxine is a thyroid hormone necessary for growth, development, and metabolism. Low values are associated with brain defects.
Blood type	Rh and ABO incompatibility can cause hemolysis and subsequent jaundice. If mother is Rh– and newborn is RH+, mother must be treated promptly to avoid sensitization to future Rh+ fetuses.
Sickle cell anemia	Detects presence of hemoglobin S. Electrophoresis identifies whether infant has the trait or disease.
Audiometric testing	Identifies hearing disorders early.
Human immunodeficiency virus (HIV): Newborns of mothers with HIV are tested for virus.	Early virus detection can permit start of early treatment that may enhance survival.
Gestational age: Normal gestational age is 38 to 42 weeks. Newborn less than 38 weeks is premature. A screening test, such as Ballard test, estimates fetal gestation.	Accurate estimate of gestational age influences care management and special monitoring needs. Full-term infant should have creases over entire sole of foot, full breast areolas, firm ear cartilage. Boys should have pendulous testes and deep scrotal rugae. In girls, the labia majora should cover clitoris and labia minora.

Assessment of Infants

Infant Health History

A complete health history can be obtained from the newborn's chart and from a parent or guardian. Review the chart, paying special attention to prenatal care, gestational or family health problems, and supports. The infant health history also addresses developmental milestones, home safety, and immunizations, which are critical for primary prevention of childhood diseases. Table 15.2 reviews the immunizations recommended for infants. For the most recent information about vaccines, visit the National Immunization Program Home Page at *http://www.cdc.gov/nip/,* or call the National Immunization Hotline at 800-232-2522 (English) or 800-232-0233 (Spanish).

AREAS AND QUESTIONS TO ASK	SIGNIFICANCE
General Health Status	
How is your infant doing now?	Determining the parents' view of their infant's general well-being provides a baseline for you to begin your assessment.
Body Weight	
Has infant been gaining weight?	Weight gain within normal parameters is an indicator of nutritional status.
Integumentary	
Does the infant have good skin turgor?	Skin tenting denotes dehydration.
Does skin appear healthy?	Scaly skin may be caused by an underlying medical condition or dryness from soaps or lotions.
Do hair and nails appear healthy or brittle?	Brittle hair and nails may be caused by poor protein intake.
Head and Neck	
Is head shape symmetrical?	Symmetry is normal.
Can infant hold head upright while sitting and move head from side to side?	Head control is a necessary motor development milestone.
Eyes, Ears, Nose, and Throat	
Can infant recognize toys you give him or her? Do eyes focus symmetrically?	Refer infants with signs of visual difficulties to specialist.

AREAS AND QUESTIONS TO ASK	SIGNIFICANCE
Is there eye exudate?	Infants are highly susceptible to eye infections and may require medications.
Does infant turn head when her or his name is called? Can he or she vocalize?	Ability to hear and speak is critical for development. If you notice signs of hearing or speaking problems, refer infant to specialist.
Is there exudate from the nose?	Nose exudate may signal infection or allergies or may be normal mucus production.
Respiratory	
Is breathing labored?	Monitor abnormal breathing patterns carefully.
Cardiovascular	
Is infant active?	Infants should be active and lively when awake.
Is skin ever blue-tinged?	Lethargy may be related to cardiac difficulties, of which cyanosis is a warning sign.
Gastrointestinal	
How is the infant's appetite?	Appetite denotes good health.
What does she or he usually eat and drink each day?	Adequate daily nutrient intake is necessary for growth.
How many bowel movements a day does he or she have?	Regular bowel movements suggest normal GI activity.
Genitourinary	
Is urination pattern consistent with fluid intake?	Adequate urination pattern denotes normal kidney function.
How many diaper changes a day?	Usually about eight diapers a day is normal, depending on fluid intake.
Musculoskeletal	
Does infant roll over, sit unsupported, transfer toy from one hand to the other? Can she or he creep forward or backward on tummy?	Body movements should be within developmental norms.
Neurologic	
Have you noticed any unusual movements such as tremors?	Tremors or other unusual movements may indicate seizures.
Problems with sucking, swallowing?	Diminished sucking or swallowing reflexes may indicate an underlying neurologic problem.
Infections	
Has infant had any colds, fevers, infections?	Usual infant infections may not be preventable. However, teach parents infection-control methods.

(continued)

AREAS AND QUESTIONS TO ASK	SIGNIFICANCE
Development	
Does infant prefer to play with people rather than toys? Does he or she search for an object that is out of sight? Is he or she afraid of strangers?	Deviations from these developmental milestones may impair social activities.
Relationships	
How do you feel about the new baby and about being a mother or father?	Mother may cry, feel irritable, and have loss of appetite and sleeplessness for first 10 days or so after delivery. If these problems persist for more than 2 weeks, it may signal postpartum depression and warrants referral.

TABLE 15.2 Recommended Immunizations for Infants

IMMUNIZATION	SCHEDULE
Hepatitis B	First dose within 2 months of age, second dose 1 month after first dose, and third dose 6 months after second dose.
Diphtheria, pertussis, tetanus toxoid (DPT)	Doses at 2 months, 4 months, and between 6 and 18 months.
Haemophilus influenzae type B (Hib)	Doses at 2 months, 4 months, and 6 months (check with manufacturer if third dose at 6 months is required).
Inactivated polio vaccine	Doses at 2 months, 4 months, and between 6 and 18 months.
Pneumococcal conjugate (PCV)	Doses at 2 months, 4 months, and between 6 and 18 months.

Physical Assessment of Infants

Physical Assessment of Infants

AREA/PA SKILL	NORMAL FINDINGS	ABNORMAL FINDINGS
Anthropometric Measurements *Head and Chest*		
Apply tape measure around widest part of head, just above eyebrows.	Head circumference increases by 1.5 cm each month for first 6 months and by 0.5 cm per month until age 12 months.	*Greater than normal head circumference:* Hydrocephalus.

AREA/PA SKILL	NORMAL FINDINGS	ABNORMAL FINDINGS
Measure chest at nipple line.	Chest circumference equals head circumference by 12 months.	*Smaller than normal head circumference:* Microcephaly.
Height and Weight		
Measure length from head to heels. Weigh without clothing or diaper.	Height should increase 50 percent by age 12 months. Birth weight should double by 6 months and triple by 12 months.	*Anthropometric measurements deviating from normal:* Underlying disease or inadequate eating or nutritional pattern.
Integumentary *Skin*		
Inspect skin appearance, folds, turgor.	Skin pigmentation varies. Newborns of dark-skinned parents may appear light skinned at birth. True skin color develops by 3 months of age. Good skin turgor in newborns and infants is a sign of adequate hydration.	Persistent cyanosis in the warm infant is never normal and requires immediate referral. *Red, excoriated skin:* Diaper rash (diaper dermatitis). Secondary yeast infection *(Candida)* causes bright, round scaling patches. *Dry, itchy patches on face and skin folds in infants with allergies:* Eczema (atopic dermatitis). *Flat, greasy scales on scalp:* "Cradle cap" (seborrheic dermatitis); may be caused by infrequent shampooing. *Depressed fontanels and skin tenting:* Signs of severe dehydration.
Note axillary temperature.	Axillary temperature range for newborns and infants is 35.9°C to 36.7°C (96.6°F to 98.0°F).	*Low temperature:* Hypothermia.
Never use a mercury thermometer on a newborn or infant. Mercury is highly toxic.		High temperatures can cause seizures in newborns and infants.

(box continued on page 432)

Physical Assessment of Infants (continued)

AREA/PA SKILL	NORMAL FINDINGS	ABNORMAL FINDINGS
Integumentary *(cont'd)* *Hair and Nails*		
Inspect amount and characteristics of hair.	As baby grows, amount of hair varies.	*Dry, brittle hair:* Malnutrition or malabsorption.
Check for presence of nails.	Nails present.	
HEENT *Head, Face, and Neck*		
Inspect and palpate infant's head, face, and neck.	Face and skull symmetrical.	
Some cultures fear touching fontanel area.	Fontanels flat and soft. At birth, anterior fontanel is 2.5 to 4 cm across; it closes between 12 and 18 months of age. Posterior fontanel is initially 2 cm and closes by 3 months. Neck is short and should rotate left to right.	*Sunken fontanel:* Dehydration. *Bulging fontanel:* Increased intracranial pressure.
Eyes		
Inspect and palpate external eye, eyelids, lacrimal ducts, conjunctiva, and sclera.	Bilateral blinking. Corneal reflex positive. Transient strabismus common.	Continued strabismus after 6 months is abnormal.
Test visual acuity using the DDST II. Check visual acuity.	No tearing in 1st month. Sclera may be blue tinged. Pupils constrict with light and are round and equal in size. Infants have full binocular vision.	*Lack of tears after 2 months:* Clogged lacrimal ducts; requires medical attention. *Fixed or dilated pupils:* Neurologic problem.
Ears		
Inspect and palpate external and internal ear. Check hearing.	Infant should respond to noise.	*Lack of response to noise:* Hearing problem.
To perform otoscopic exam, place infant flat and restrain arms above head. Pull auricle down and back to observe tympanic membrane.	Pinna flexible.	

AREA/PA SKILL	NORMAL FINDINGS	ABNORMAL FINDINGS
Nose		
Inspect nose.	Infants are nose breathers.	*Flaring of nares:* Sign of respiratory distress.
Check patency by closing one nostril, then the other.	Thin white mucus discharge and sneezing are normal.	Bloody discharge or large amount of nasal secretions may obstruct nares.
Mouth/Throat		
Inspect oral cavity: Palate, tongue, gums, tonsils.	White nodules (Epstein's pearls) may be found on hard palate and usually disappear by 3 months.	*Protruding tongue:* Associated with congenital disorders, such as Down syndrome or hypothyroidism.
Use light and tongue blade.	Tongue should not protrude from mouth. No coating in mouth. Suck should be strong. First primary teeth usually appear at 6 to 8 months.	
Chest/Back/Shoulders		
Inspect spinal curvature.	Convex spinal curvature (C-curve). By 12 to 18 months, lumbar curve develops and lordosis is present as walking begins.	Limited ROM may result from injury. Dimpling in spine may be associated with neural tube defects.
Note blemishes or skin openings.	No blemishes or skin openings.	
Respiratory		
Inspect chest.	Respiratory rate 25 to 50 breaths/min.	! **Apnea > 15 seconds accompanied by decreased heart rate is abnormal.**
Percuss chest lightly. Use direct percussion.	Apnea less common than in newborns.	! **Stressful breathing with flaring nares and sighing with each breath are signs of respiratory distress and require immediate attention.**

(box continued on page 434)

Physical Assessment of Infants (continued)

AREA/PA SKILL	NORMAL FINDINGS	ABNORMAL FINDINGS
Respiratory *(cont'd)*		
	Normal breath sounds more bronchial.	Inspiratory stridor, expiratory grunts, retractions, paradoxical (seesaw) breathing, asymmetrical or decreased breath sounds, wheezing, and crackles are abnormal.
Palpate back with two fingers while newborn is crying.	Infants are abdominal breathers.	Depressed sternum may affect normal respiration.
	Anteroposterior: lateral diameter is equal.	
Auscultate lungs.	Lungs clear, bronchovesicular breath sounds.	
Cardiovascular		
Auscultate heart and peripheral pulses.	Apical pulse felt in fourth or fifth intercostal space just medial to midclavicular line.	
Use a stethoscope with a small diaphragm and perform exam when infant is quiet.	Heart rate range 80 to 160 BPM. Capillary refill < 1 second.	Abnormal heart rate range requires attention. *Murmurs accompanied by cyanosis:* Congenital heart defects.
	Peripheral pulses present.	*Capillary refill times > 2 seconds:* Dehydration or hypovolemic shock. Evaluate newly discovered murmurs. Infant who eats poorly may have cardiovascular problem.
Gastrointestinal		
Inspect, palpate, percuss, and auscultate abdomen.	Bowel sounds present. Bowel soft. Tympany may be heard because of air swallowing.	

AREA/PA SKILL	NORMAL FINDINGS	ABNORMAL FINDINGS
	Umbilicus flat.	Umbilical hernias > 2 cm wide may require further evaluation. Abdominal pain may indicate childhood illnesses.
	Liver edge 1 to 2 cm below right rib cage (costal margin).	Enlarged liver or palpable spleen may indicate disease.
Extremities		
Inspect hands, arms, feet, legs, and hips.	Feet flat.	Inadequate ROM may indicate congenital malformation or birth injury or may result from pulling or lifting infant.
Test ROM.	Legs equal in length. Transfers objects from one hand to other by 7 months. Crawls and sits unsupported by 7 months. Pulls to standing position and holds on to furniture by 11 months.	Inability to meet developmental milestones may indicate neurologic or environmental deficits.
Genitourinary		
	Note infant's sex.	Ambiguous genitalia abnormal.
Boys		
Inspect and palpate penis and urethra.	In uncircumcised infant, foreskin may not be fully retractable until 1 year of age. Urethra midline.	Phimosis (tight foreskin) can constrict penis. Instruct parents on gentle retraction of foreskin to prevent phimosis.
	Urine flow straight and strong.	*Weak urine stream or dribbling:* Stricture at urinary meatus.
	No palpable masses in testes. Two testes should be palpated in scrotum or brought down from inguinal ring.	Solid scrotal masses are abnormal. Hernias present as scrotal masses. *Testes not palpable:* Undescended testicles.

(box continued on page 436)

Physical Assessment of Infants (continued)

AREA/PA SKILL	NORMAL FINDINGS	ABNORMAL FINDINGS
Genitourinary *Boys (cont'd)*		If scrotum swollen, transilluminate to determine if fluid (hydrocele) present.
Girls Inspect external genitalia.	External genitalia pink and moist.	Blood-tinged fluid from vagina abnormal after 1 week. Vaginal discharge or labial redness or itching may be caused by diaper or soap irritation or sexual abuse.
Anus and Rectum		
Inspect anus and rectum.	Bowel movements may occur with each feeding. By 1 year, they occur once or twice a day. Breast-fed babies have stools that are mustard colored and soft. Formula-fed babies have stools that are yellow-green and more formed.	*Watery stools and explosive diarrhea:* Infection. *Constipation or hard stools:* Inadequate hydration or nutrition.
Neurologic		
Inspect and test muscle strength, sensory function, and reflex movements. (See Table 15.1 for newborn/ infant reflexes.)	Infant's body stays erect when you support him or her with both hands under axilla. Motor control develops from head to toe. Infant opens eyes to noise and responds to touch.	*Delays in motor or sensory activity:* Brain damage, mental retardation, illness, malnutrition, or neglect. Asymmetrical posture or spastic movements need further evaluation.
	Presence of infantile reflexes denotes healthy neurologic system.	Maintenance of infant reflexes past usual age is abnormal.

PA = Physical assessment.

Diagnostic/Screening Tests for Infants

TEST	SIGNIFICANCE
Developmental Testing	
Should occur regularly throughout childhood. DDST II assesses skills in areas of personal/social, fine motor, language, and gross motor.	If delays are noted, refer child to specialist for further testing. Medications, malnutrition, neurologic, and emotional conditions affect test results.
Urine Screening	
Dipstick screening test is usually sufficient.	Any abnormalities require full urinalysis.
Hemoglobin or hematocrit.	Hemoglobin below 10 g/dL is low and infant is considered anemic. Hematocrit below 29 percent is low.
Lead Screening	
Only if environmental exposure is suspected.	Elevated blood lead levels can cause neurologic damage.

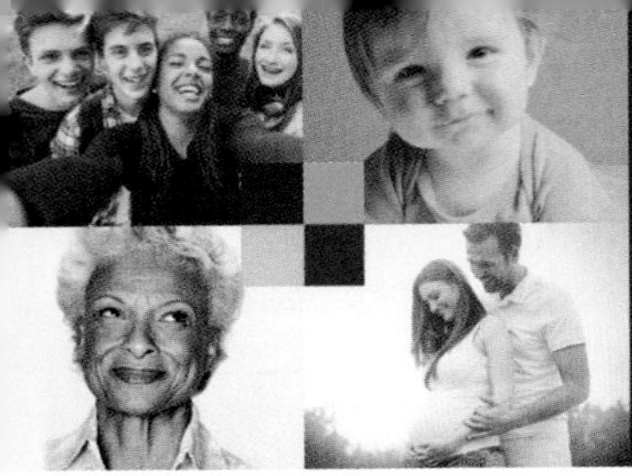

CHAPTER 16

Assessing the Toddler and Preschooler

The toddler years extend from 12 to 36 months and the preschool years from 3 to 5 years. The toddler years are often referred to as the "terrible 2s" as the child struggles to gain control; in the preschool years, the child is preparing for school.

Psychosocial and Emotional Changes

- Toddlers are struggling to develop a sense of autonomy.
- Toddlers work to gain control over bodily functions, tolerate separation from parents, differentiate self from others, develop socially acceptable behavior, develop verbal communication skills, become less egocentric, and tolerate delay in gratifying needs.
- Failure in developing autonomy results in doubt and shame.
- The negativism associated with this period often explains the term "the terrible 2s," when "No" seems to be the only word in the child's vocabulary.
- The child also looks for consistency in "ritualism," or sameness within his or her environment. This sameness provides a sense of safety and comfort.
- Sex role imitation, such as dressing-up, is common during toddler and preschooler years.
- The next developmental stage, initiative versus guilt, is a time of playing and learning. If the child goes beyond set limits, guilt results.
- Ability to tolerate a delay in satisfying needs reflects ego development in the child.
- Superego development is in its early stages.
- Behavior is seen as good or bad based on the outcome, either reward or punishment.

- Rapid cognitive development occurs during this time.
- The child begins to see causal and spatial relationships and develops object permanence.
- Language skills continue to develop during the preschool years.
- Play is an important means of expression and of learning.
- Preschoolers' perceptions of God are concrete and based on parental influence.

Health Promotion and Risk Factors for the Toddler and Preschooler

Common health issues seen with the toddler and preschooler include toilet training, sibling rivalry, temper tantrums, negativism and regression, fears, stress, and aggression. Health problems seen with toddlers and preschoolers include communicable diseases, accidents (such as poisonings), and injuries. Abuse or neglect can occur at any age, but younger children are more dependent on the parents for all needs, physical and psychological, and therefore, they are more vulnerable to neglect or abuse.

Assessment of the Toddler and Preschooler

Health History

Current Health Status

Ask about the health status of the child. Has the child been healthy, or is there an acute problem?

Current Medications

Ask about all prescription and over-the-counter (OTC) medications.

Past Health History

Include questions that relate to the pregnancy and the delivery of the child.

Immunizations

Additional immunizations recommended by or during the preschool years include:

- Polio dose 3 by 18 months,
- Diphtheria, tetanus, and pertussis (DTP) dose 4 between 15 and 18 months,

- Measles, mumps, and rubella (MMR) first dose between 12 and 15 months,
- Chickenpox (VZV) first dose between 12 and 15 months
- *Haemophilus influenzae* between 12 and 15 months,
- Hepatitis B (HBV) dose 3 between 6 and 18 months,

Significant Family Medical History

Ask about heart disease, strokes, cancer, and other serious health conditions within the family that present later in life.

Review of Systems

SYSTEM AND QUESTIONS TO ASK	SIGNIFICANCE
General Health Status	
How has the child been feeling?	Screen for any obvious problems.
How much does the child weigh? Changes in behavior are good indicators of how a child is feeling.	Changes in weight are closely monitored to evaluate normal growth and development.
Integumentary	
Any skin rashes, lesions, excessive itching?	Tinea capitis, ringworm, or contagious disorders can occur in toddlers and preschoolers, especially if the child is in day care. Eczema is often associated with allergies and has a familial tendency. Diaper rashes occur from prolonged exposure to an irritant, such as urine or feces. Head lice can occur in preschoolers in day care or preschool. Playing dressup or sharing hats can increase transmission.
Sun exposure? Use of sunblock?	Excessive exposure to sun (ultraviolet [UV] rays) without sunblock increases the risk for skin cancer later in life.
HEENT	
Eyes	
Does the child have vision problems? Crossed eyes?	Normal visual acuity is 20/40 for a toddler.
When was the child's last eye exam?	Depth perception is developing. Vision should be tested routinely during physical exams.
Ears	
Does the child have any hearing problems?	Hearing should be tested routinely during physical exams.

SYSTEM AND QUESTIONS TO ASK	SIGNIFICANCE
Does the child respond to sounds?	
Is the child talking, making sounds? When was the child's last hearing exam? Does the child have frequent ear infections? Does he or she exhibit irritability, poor appetite, poor sleeping?	Toddlers and preschoolers have a high incidence of otitis media, with the highest incidence between 6 months and 2 years.
Teeth	
How many teeth does the child have?	All 20 primary teeth should be complete by 2½ years.
Has the child had the first dental exam?	The first dental exam should occur shortly after onset of eruption of primary teeth. The child should have at least annual dental exam.
Does the child brush teeth?	Review tooth-brushing technique with child and parent.
Is your water fluoridated?	Fluoride decreases tooth decay. **Fluoride is toxic if ingested. Advise parents not to allow child to eat toothpaste.**
Does the child go to bed with a bottle?	Bedtime bottles, nocturnal breast-feeding, or coating pacifiers with sweet substance can cause baby-bottle caries; occurs most frequently between 18 months and 3 years.
Respiratory	
Does the child have a cough, sneezing, runny nose, or fever?	Upper respiratory infections (URIs) are common in toddlers and preschoolers. Respiratory syncytial virus (RSV) causes one-half of all bronchiolitis, usually occurring in children younger than age 2.
Does the child ever wheeze or have trouble breathing?	Asthma is the most common disease among children. Onset usually occurs between ages 3 and 8.
Is the child exposed to air pollutants (e.g., smoke or second-hand smoke)?	Exposure to second-hand smoke increases risk for respiratory and ear infections and asthma attacks.

(continued)

Review of Systems (continued)

SYSTEM AND QUESTIONS TO ASK	SIGNIFICANCE
Cardiovascular	
Were you ever told that the child had a heart murmur?	Although cardiovascular disease is not common in children, murmurs are a common finding. Most murmurs are innocent, functional murmurs, but follow-up is indicated to rule out pathology.
Has the child ever turned blue?	Change in skin color may indicate a cardiopulmonary problem.
Gastrointestinal	
Is the child potty trained? What is the child's bowel pattern?	Bowel control usually achieved before age 3. Bowel control usually precedes bladder control.
Genitourinary	
Does the child have bladder control?	Bladder control usually achieved by age 3.
Musculoskeletal	
Is the child walking?	The child should be able to walk without difficulty. **Even though the child is able to walk, the child still does not have refined coordination and full depth perception and, therefore, is still at risk for falls.**
Neurologic	
Is the child speaking? Using complete sentences?	Cognitive skills continue to develop. The child should be speaking. Speech development usually occurs between ages 2 and 4.
Does the child have any fears?	Fears, real and imaginary, are common (e.g., fear of dark).
Does the child have temper tantrums or aggressive behavior?	*Acting-out, aggressive behavior, temper tantrums:* May need to provide education to parents regarding effective ways to deal with the child's behavior.
Lymphatic/Hematological	
Have you noticed any lumps in the child's neck, groin, or underarms?	Enlarged nodes may indicate an infection.

Psychosocial History

Health Practices

When was the child's last health exam? Recommend health exams every year.

Typical Day

Can you tell me what your child's day is like? Does the child go to day care or preschool?

Nutrition

Screen diet by asking for a 24-hour recall. Is the child still nursing or bottle feeding? If yes, how often? Because breast milk contains immunoglobulin A (IgA) and breast-feeding minimizes reflux of milk into the eustachian tube, breast-feeding decreases the risk of otitis media and respiratory viruses and allergies. Ask about eating patterns: "How often do you eat breakfast?"; "What is a usual lunch for you?"; "What are your favorite snacks?" For the toddler, protein and caloric requirements are still high for growth, and calcium, iron, and phosphorus are needed for bone growth. After 18 months, the toddler's appetite decreases (physiological anorexia) in response to decreased nutritional needs. For the preschooler, an average of 1800 calories, with reduced fat, is needed per day. Calcium and minerals are still needed for bone growth. During the toddler and preschool years, the child develops taste preferences and may become a picky eater.

Activity/Exercise

Toddlers and preschoolers are usually very active. With this increased activity, close supervision is needed.

Sleep/Rest

Ask about sleep patterns and naps, bedtime rituals, sleep problems (nightmares, night or sleep terrors, somnambulism, enuresis). The toddler and preschooler usually sleep about 12 hours per day. The toddler usually requires a nap; the preschooler does not.

Personal Habits/Behaviors

Investigate personal habits of parents or caregivers, such as smoking or alcohol or drug use. Exposure to these substances (such as through second-hand smoke) places the child at risk for health problems. If drug or alcohol abuse is an issue, both the caregiver's ability and the home environment need to be assessed to ensure the child's safety. Referrals may be warranted.

Recreation/Hobbies

Safety is a major concern for the toddler and preschooler. If recreational activities or hobbies increase the risk for injury, ask if protective measures, such as bike helmets, are used. Also question the parent's hobbies; for example, ask about the presence of weapons in the home, and gun and hunting safety.

Play for the toddler is parallel; play for the preschooler is associative, group play. There is more social interaction in the play of preschoolers. With both age groups, safety is paramount, supervision is needed, and toys must be age appropriate.

Roles and Relationships

If there are siblings, ask the parent about the relationship. Sibling rivalry is not uncommon.

Sexuality/Reproductive

Toddlers and preschool children are curious by nature and exhibit sex-role imitation. They are also curious about their own bodies, and it is not uncommon for them to masturbate. How this behavior is addressed is important because it can have lasting effects.

Coping and Stress Tolerance

Does the child have aggressive behavior or temper tantrums? If the child's behavior is destructive to self or others, she or he needs to learn effective coping strategies.

Value/Belief Pattern

The toddler's and preschooler's perception of God is rather concrete and based on the beliefs and practices of the parents or caregivers. Prayer can be a source of comfort for a child; for example, prayers are often part of bedtime rituals.

Physical Assessment

SYSTEM/ ASSESSMENT	NORMAL VARIATIONS/ ABNORMAL FINDINGS
Anthropometric Measurements and Vital Signs	
Weigh the child and take measurements of height and head and chest circumference.	Toddler usually gains 4 to 6 lb a year and 3 inches a year in height. Head and chest circumferences are usually equal by age 2. The preschooler gains 5 lb a year and $2\frac{1}{2}$ to 3 inches a year in height.
Check child's vital signs.	Changes in vital signs include a gradual and slight increase in blood pressure and a slight decrease in temperature, pulse, and respirations.
General Health Survey	
Inspect overall appearance, noting appropriate growth and development for the child's age.	Toddler's general appearance: "Pot belly" and wide base of support are normal. Preschooler loses pot belly and becomes taller and leaner. Detect any delays or premature maturation. Note any obvious weight problems.
Integumentary	
Inspect skin for lesions.	Lesions, such as tinea capitis or ringworm, need treatment.
Inspect hair and scalp for lice.	Pediculosis common among preschoolers. **Suspect abuse if you find unexplained bruising or injury.**
HEENT	
Head and Face	
Inspect head and face.	Head size growth slows to 1 inch a year by end of age 2, then $\frac{1}{2}$ inch a year until age 5.
Palpate anterior fontanel.	Anterior fontanel closes by 18 months.
Eyes	
Test visual acuity.	Visual acuity is 20/40 during toddler years. Vision screening should begin between 3 and 4 years. Visual deficits warrant follow-up.
Test for "lazy eye" (strabismus) with corneal light reflex or cover-uncover test.	Referral needed for strabismus to prevent amblyopia (reduction or dimness in vision).
Ears	
Test hearing with pure tone audiometer.	Hearing deficits warrant follow-up.

(continued)

Physical Assessment (continued)

SYSTEM/ ASSESSMENT	NORMAL VARIATIONS/ ABNORMAL FINDINGS
HEENT	
Ears *(cont'd)*	
Inspect external ear canal and tympanic membrane.	Hearing should be tested by age 3 to 4 years.
You may want to leave the otoscopic exam until the end of the physical assessment.	Toddlers and preschoolers have a high incidence of otitis media.
Nose	
Inspect the nasal septum and mucosa.	Chronic rhinorrhea can result from allergic rhinitis. Boggy, bluish-purple, or gray turbinates are consistent with allergic rhinitis.
	When inspecting the nares or the external ear canal, always be alert for the presence of foreign objects.
Mouth	
Inspect oral mucosa and pharynx.	Generally, the tonsils are large.
Inspect number and condition of teeth.	Primary teeth eruption usually complete by $2\frac{1}{2}$ years. Note any nursing/baby-bottle caries. Review dental hygiene with parent and child.
Neck	
Palpate the neck for lymph nodes.	Enlarged lymph nodes may be associated with an infection or lymphoma.
Respiratory	
Inspect and measure size and shape of chest.	Anteroposterior:lateral diameter 1:2 by end of 2nd year.
Auscultate lungs.	Toddlers and preschoolers have a high incidence of respiratory infections.
Cardiovascular	
Auscultate heart; note rate and rhythm.	Children often have a sinus arrhythmia and a split second heart sound. Both the arrhythmia and the split second sound change with respiration. This is a normal variation. Systolic innocent murmurs and venous hum are common findings.
	If murmur is detected, refer for follow-up to rule out pathology.
Gastrointestinal	
Inspect, auscultate, and palpate abdomen.	A pot belly is normal for a toddler; the condition disappears as the abdominal muscles strengthen.

SYSTEM/ ASSESSMENT	NORMAL VARIATIONS/ ABNORMAL FINDINGS
Genitourinary	
Inspect external genitalia.	If child is still in diapers, inspect for diaper dermatitis.
Musculoskeletal	
Inspect gait.	Toddlers usually can walk alone by 12 to 13 months. Balance is unsteady with wide base of support. Genu valgus or varus may be present. Preschooler's gait more balanced, smaller base of support; walks, jumps, climbs by 3 years.
Test muscle strength.	Strength increases during preschool years.
Neurologic	
Test balance, coordination, and accuracy of movements.	During toddler and preschool years, the child's balance and coordination improve, with refinement of fine motor skills.

HEENT = Head, eyes, ears, nose, and throat.

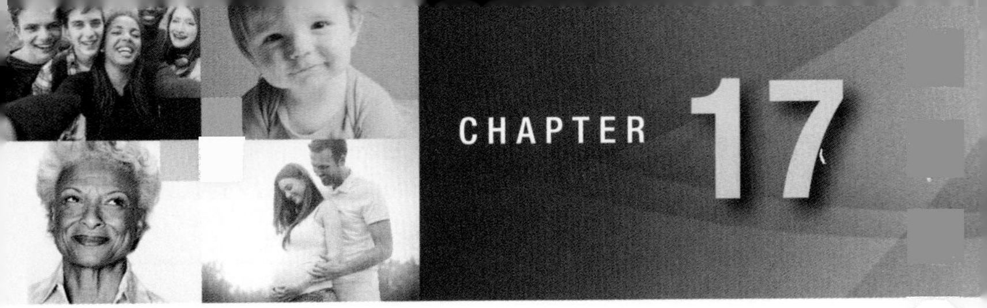

Assessing the School-Age Child and Adolescent

THE SCHOOL-AGE CHILD

The school-age child is the child between the ages of 6 and 12 years. This period is known as the "latency period." During this time, growth and development occur at a slower, steadier pace.

Growth and Developmental Changes

The changes that take place during the school-age years are subtle as the toddler and preschooler transforms into a child approaching preadolescence.

Physical Growth

- Measurements become more proportional as baby fat disappears.
- The child becomes more agile and coordinated.

Psychosocial and Emotional Changes

- Task of this stage is industry versus inferiority.
- The child becomes more independent, developing skills and competencies.
- Social skills also develop during this time as the child becomes more involved in school and community activities.
- Peer acceptance is very important: The child needs a sense of belonging, of fitting in.
- Peer pressure often has a greater influence on the child than parents do.

- Sex roles are established through peer relationships.
- The child chooses same-sex best friends.
- School provides the child with the opportunity to see different perspectives, argue, negotiate, resolve conflicts, work together, and develop friendships.
- Belonging to clubs, teams, and peer groups is important.
- Parents still have a major role in the child's development. The child will test parents, and limits and restrictions are needed to give the child a sense of security.
- Play involves team play, either active (such as sports) or quiet games.
- Sports, art, reading, collections, cooking, sewing, and the like are also important activities and often carry through adolescence and into adulthood.
- The child needs to feel special for a positive self-concept to develop.
- The child moves from preconceptual thinking to conceptual thinking, mastering the tasks of conservation and classifications.
- Reading is the most important skill that the child develops during this stage.
- The child becomes less egocentric and begins to develop a conscience. Initially, the child's views are black and white, right or wrong, based upon parents' moral values.
- God is seen in concrete terms. The child may see illness or injury as a punishment.

Health Promotion and Risk Factors

Common health problems seen with the school-age child include injuries related to accidents; drug, alcohol, and nicotine abuse; eating disorders; learning disorders; and emotional problems.

Cultural Considerations

CULTURE	PERSPECTIVE ON CHILDREN
African American	Good behavior, respectfulness, obedience, and conformity to rules are stressed. In violent communities, mothers try to protect children and keep them off the streets.
Amish	Children are seen as gift from God. Parents very directive of child throughout school.
Appalachian	Subscribe to physical punishment, which may be perceived as abuse. Having children associated with sense of importance.
Arab American	Child's character and success dependent on parental influence. Taught conformity and cooperation. A "good" child is an obedient child; behavior that would bring dishonor is avoided. Subscribe to physical punishment.
Chinese American	Boys and girls play together when young but separate when older. Pressure on children to succeed. Boys are more valued than girls. Help parents at home.
Cuban American	Children are expected to study and to respect parents.
Egyptian American	Children are expected to be studious and goal oriented; respectful and loyal to family.
Filipino American	Children are expected to honor and respect parents.
French Canadian	Children are well educated and a source of pride for family.
Greek American	Children are center of family. Children are disciplined through "teasing."
Iranian American	Culture is child oriented. Children expected to be respectful.
Irish American	Boys are expected to be more aggressive than girls. Children are expected to show self-restraint, discipline, respect, and obedience.
Jewish American	Children are seen as a valued treasure. Children are expected to respect and honor parents.

CULTURE	PERSPECTIVE ON CHILDREN
Mexican American	Children are highly valued. Children must respect parents.
Navajo Native American	Children are allowed to make decisions that might seem irresponsible, such as taking medicine.
Vietnamese American	Children are prized and valued. Children are expected to be obedient and devoted.

Adapted from Purnell, L.D., and Paulanka, B.J. (2012): *Transcultural Healthcare: A Culturally Competent Approach*, 4th ed. Philadelphia, F.A. Davis.

Assessment

Health History

Current Health Status

This is addressed in essentially the same way as with an adult.

Current Medications

Ask about all prescription and over-the-counter (OTC) medications.

Past Health History

Check with the parents or guardians for specifics of past health history questions.

Immunizations

Additional immunizations recommended by or during the school-age years include:

- Polio dose 4 by 6 years of age.
- Tetanus-diphtheria (TD) between 11 and 16 years.
- Measles, mumps, and rubella (MMR) between 11 and 12 years, if second MMR shot not given between 4 and 6 years.
- Chickenpox (VZV) between 1 and 12 years.
- HPV vaccine, 3 dose series between 11 or 12 years.

Significant Family Medical History

Ask about heart disease, strokes, cancer, and other serious health conditions within the family. It is also important to ask if anyone died at an early age (younger than age 35 years) from a sudden heart attack. This may be a risk factor for sports participation and may require additional investigation if present.

Review of Systems

SYSTEM AND QUESTIONS TO ASK	SIGNIFICANCE
General Health Status	
How have you been feeling?	Screen for any obvious problems.
Any recent weight changes?	Changes in weight, especially gains, may indicate poor eating habits.
Integumentary	
Any skin rashes, lesions, excessive itching?	Tinea capitis, (ringworm), verruca (warts); contact dermatitis; and poison ivy, oak, and sumac frequently seen in school-age children. Pediculosis capitis (head lice) common in school-age children.
Sun exposure? Use of sunblock?	Excessive exposure to sun (ultraviolet [UV] rays) without sunblock increases the risk for skin cancer later in life.
HEENT	
Eyes Any visual problems? Do you wear glasses or contact lenses?	Visual acuity reaches 20/20 by school age.
If yes, ask if child wears glasses consistently, especially while at school.	Many times children may not consistently wear glasses for fear of being teased by other children. May identify teaching need about care of contact lenses.
When was last eye exam?	Eyes should be tested routinely during physical exams.
Ears	
Do you have any hearing problems? Do you listen to loud music?	Cochlear damage can result from excessive exposure to loud noise, such as CD players and rock concerts. May identify teaching need about noise pollution's effect on hearing.
When was last hearing exam?	Hearing should be tested routinely during physical exams.
Teeth	
When was your last visit to the dentist? Orthodontist?	Should have at least annual dental exam.
How many second teeth do you have?	Primary teeth are lost during school-age years and replaced by secondary teeth. This stage is called "age of loose tooth" or "ugly duckling stage" because secondary teeth initially are too big for face. Common dental problems during school-age years include dental caries, periodontal disease, malocclusion, and dental injury.

SYSTEM AND QUESTIONS TO ASK	SIGNIFICANCE
	! In secondary tooth evulsion, tooth should be replanted as soon as possible. If replanted within 30 minutes, 70 percent successful.
Respiratory	
Do you have asthma?	Allergies and asthma are likely to become apparent during school-age years. Asthma is the most common disease among children.
Do you ever have trouble breathing or wheeze when exercising or running? Are you exposed to air pollutants, smoke, or second-hand smoke?	Exercise-induced bronchospasm is acute, reversible, self-terminating airway obstruction that occurs after vigorous exercise, peaks 5 to 10 minutes once activity stops, and then ceases within 30 minutes.
Cardiovascular	
Do you have any chest pain? Does your heart ever skip a beat?	Although cardiovascular disease is not common in children and adolescents, it can occur. Prolonged QT syndrome can cause sudden cardiac death in a seemingly healthy child. Include baseline ECG as part of sports physical.
Gastrointestinal	
Any stomach problems?	Recurrent abdominal pain is common during childhood and is often psychosomatic. Child usually has poor self-image. School can precipitate attacks. **! If child presents with recurrent abdominal pain, first rule out physiological causes.**
What is your bowel pattern?	Encopresis (fecal incontinence and voluntary or involuntary loss of bowel control) is more common in boys, usually secondary to constipation.
Genitourinary	
Do you have bladder control? Bedwetting?	Nocturnal bedwetting, often self-limiting, ends by age 6 to 8. More common in boys.
Musculoskeletal	
Do you have any back problems? Have you ever been told you had a spinal problem?	Heavy backpacks have been associated with low back problems in children. Scoliosis occurs more frequently in girls than in boys. Screening usually occurs in middle and high school. If present, determine if scoliosis is structural or postural (see Chapter 12). Physical maturity varies and does not always correlate with emotional or social maturity.

(continued)

Review of Systems (continued)

SYSTEM AND QUESTIONS TO ASK	SIGNIFICANCE
Neurologic	
How would you describe your mood?	Stress, anxiety, and fears can be seen in children. Depression, conversion reactions, and even schizophrenia can occur during childhood and be difficult to detect.
Lymphatic/Hematological	
Have you been tired?	
Any lumps in neck, underarms, or groin?	Non-Hodgkin's lymphomas occur most frequently in children before age 15.

Psychosocial History

Health Practices

When did you have your last health exam? (Recommend health exams every 2 years.)

Typical Day

Can you tell me what your day is like? How are you doing in school? This allows you to see the child through his or her eyes. You may be able to identify stresses confronting the child in everyday life. A change in academic performance or a sudden disinterest in school may reflect a more serious problem. Ask children what subjects they like, which ones they dislike. If they are having problems with a particular subject, have they sought help for this? How many days of school do they miss in a term? Attention deficit hyperactivity disorder (ADHD) and learning disabilities (LD) may become more apparent once the child starts school, and appropriate referrals should be made as indicated. School phobias are common at age 10, with the child trying to avoid school with somatic complaints such as nausea, headache, or abdominal pain. Characteristically, these complaints quickly subside once the child is assured that he or she does not have to go to school. If the child is a "latchkey child," one who is left without adult supervision after school, identify what the child does with his or her time until the parent or guardian returns home. Safety is an issue for children who are left home alone, which places them at higher risk for injury or delinquent behavior.

Nutrition

Screen diet by asking for a 24-hour recall. Ask about eating patterns: "How often do you eat breakfast?" "What is a usual lunch for you?" "What are your favorite snacks?" Junk and fast food amount to empty calories and contribute to the high incidence of obesity among children. Also, if suspected, screen for eating disorders.

Activity and Exercise (Such as Sports, if Applicable)

Ask about what children enjoy doing outside of the home. What sports do they play, if any? What do they like to do with their friends? How often do they watch TV during the week? How much time do they spend on the computer? You may identify a need for health education regarding the importance of routine exercise. If a child does participate in sports, does she or he use protective equipment? Is it a contact sport? Contact sports may increase the risk for injury.

If a child plays sports, he or she should engage in sports appropriate for his or her age.

Sleep and Rest

Ask about when the child usually goes to bed and when she or he awakens. The school-age child, age 8 to 11, may resist going to bed. Does she or he have a bedtime routine? Remember that enuresis can continue into adolescence.

Personal Habits and Behaviors

Substance abuse is occurring at younger and younger ages, so it is not uncommon for the school-age child to have tried smoking or alcohol. Experimentation is common for this age group, and peer pressure can be great. So you need to ask about substance use (drugs, alcohol, and nicotine). Ask, "If you smoke cigarettes, how many do you smoke in an average day?" "If you use alcohol, how much do you usually drink during the week?" "If you use drugs, what type and what method (smoking, snorting, huffing, ingesting, injecting)?" Asking questions in this way is less threatening to the child, and he or she is more likely to give an honest response.

Recreation and Hobbies

Ask, "What do you do for fun? Do you have any hobbies?" If recreational activities or hobbies increase the risk for injury, ask if protective measures (e.g., bike helmets) are used. Ask about presence of weapons in the home and gun and hunting safety courses, if appropriate.

Self-Perception and Self-Concept

Ask the child to describe herself or himself—"Tell me about yourself." A child's self-image and body image are often influenced by her or his perception of how she or he is seen by others, peers, and family. Anything out of the norm may become an easy target for teasing, and such teasing can have lasting effects on a child. If suspected, ask about bullying.

Role and Relationship

Ask the child to tell you about the family—"Who lives at home with you?" If there are siblings, ask about the relationship. Ask, "Is there an adult in your life whom you feel comfortable talking with?" Teachers can have a major influence on a child's development, either positive or negative. Ask about peer relationships. Ask if the child has a special friend and what things he or she enjoys doing with that friend. It is during the school-age years that a child develops close friendships with same-sex peers.

Sexuality and Reproductive Issues

The school-age child is curious by nature, and it is not unusual for school-age children to include some form of sexuality into play. This is the best time to begin sex education, and as a nurse you are in an ideal position to educate both children and parents.

Coping and Stress Tolerance

Ask questions such as "What do you do when you get angry?" and "What makes you angry?" Also ask questions such as "What do you do when you want to relax or have fun?" You need to identify whether the child has healthy coping strategies to deal with feelings and stresses in life. Violence is ever present in our society: in the home, at school, and within the community. If your patient uses violence as a coping mechanism, you may need to make referrals to help her or him develop more effective coping strategies.

Value and Belief Pattern

The school-age child's values and beliefs are often guided by those of the parents. God has to be depicted in concrete terms. Illness may be perceived as a punishment. Prayer can be a source of comfort for a child; for example, prayers are often part of bedtime rituals.

Physical Assessment of the School-Age Child

SYSTEM/ ASSESSMENT	NORMAL VARIATIONS/ ABNORMAL FINDINGS
Anthropometric Measurements and Vital Signs	
Obtain height and weight and vital signs. Plot height and weight on growth charts to note growth and development of child.	During school-age years, child will grow about 5 cm a year and gain about $4^1/_2$ to $6^1/_2$ lb a year. Boys and girls are relatively equal in size until they reach preadolescence, when girls tend to pass boys in both height and weight. Boys catch up during adolescence, but until then, this situation can be distressing for both boys and girls.
General Health Survey	
Inspect overall appearance, noting appropriate growth and development for child's age.	General appearance more slender, loss of baby fat. Detect any delays or premature maturation. Note any obvious weight problems.
Integumentary	
Inspect skin for lesions.	Lesions, such as tinea capitis or ringworm, need treatment.
Inspect hair and scalp for lice.	Pediculosis common among school-age children.
HEENT	
Head and Face	
Inspect head and face.	Head size becomes more proportionate to body.
Eyes	
Test visual acuity.	Visual acuity 20/20 by age 6. Visual deficits warrant follow-up.
Ears	
Test hearing with pure tone audiometer.	Hearing deficits warrant follow-up. Use opportunity to teach hazards of listening to loud music.
Nose	
Inspect nasal septum and mucosa.	Chronic rhinorrhea can result from allergic rhinitis. Boggy, bluish-purple, or gray turbinates are consistent with allergic rhinitis.
Mouth and Throat	
Inspect oral mucosa and pharynx.	Generally, the tonsils are large.
Inspect occlusion.	If malocclusion is present, refer to orthodontist.

(continued)

Physical Assessment of the School-Age Child (continued)

SYSTEM/ ASSESSMENT	NORMAL VARIATIONS/ ABNORMAL FINDINGS
HEENT	
Mouth and Throat ***(cont'd)***	
Inspect number of teeth.	Child loses first teeth during school age. Secondary teeth begin to erupt around age 6 years (with the 6-year molars): Most secondary teeth have grown in by the time 12-year molars erupt. Also assess for orthodontic devices and brushing technique around them.
Neck	
Palpate the neck for lymph nodes.	Enlarged lymph nodes may be associated with an infection or lymphoma.
Respiratory	
Auscultate lungs.	Children with exercise-induced asthma require bronchodilators before activity. Usually, albuterol administered through a metered-dose inhaler is given 20 to 30 minutes before exercise.
Cardiovascular	
Auscultate heart; note rate and rhythm.	Children often have a sinus arrhythmia and a split second heart sound. Both the arrhythmia and the split second sound change with respiration. This is a normal variation.
Gastrointestinal	
Inspect, auscultate, and palpate abdomen.	Appendicitis is the most common illness during childhood that requires surgery.
Genitourinary	
Inspect external genitalia.	Precocious puberty—sexual development before age 8 in girls and age 9 in boys—warrants follow-up evaluation.
Musculoskeletal	
Inspect and palpate spinal curves. Test for spinal deformities. (See Chapter 12.)	Scoliosis is the major variation within the musculoskeletal system. Screening for scoliosis should be done in the preadolescent period, generally during the fifth and sixth grade. Any significant curvature should be referred for evaluation and follow-up.
Test muscle strength.	Strength doubles during school-age years.
Neurologic	
Test balance, coordination, and accuracy of movements.	During school-age years, the child's balance and coordination greatly improve with refinement of fine motor skills.

Abuse

Abuse can occur at any age and comes in many different forms: neglect, physical injury, sexual abuse, or psychological abuse. You must be constantly alert for the following signs or symptoms of abuse or neglect in all children:

- Obvious physical signs of abuse or neglect.
- Repeated emergency room visits.
- Siblings blamed for injury.
- Inconsistent accounts of how injury occurred.
- Report of abuse by child.
- Inappropriate response by child or parent to injury.
- Inconsistency between physical findings and cause of accident.
- Inconsistency between injury and child's developmental level.
- Previous history of abuse.

A sudden change in a child's behavior may reflect an underlying problem that warrants further investigation.

THE ADOLESCENT

Stages of Adolescence

- Early adolescence begins at puberty (as early as 8 or 9 years but more typically 11 to 14 years for girls and 12 to 16 years for boys). This is a period of rapid physical growth and corresponds with the onset of menstruation in girls and sperm production in boys.
- Middle adolescence typically ranges from ages 14 to 16 in girls and 16 to 18 in boys. Girls have generally achieved adult height, but boys may continue their linear growth.
- Late adolescence typically starts around age 17 and can continue into the early 20s.
- Prepubescence is the 2-year period before puberty in which preliminary physical changes are occurring.
- Puberty is the time when sexual maturity occurs, reproductive organs begin to function, and secondary sexual characteristics develop.
- Postpubescence occurs 1 to 2 years after puberty, when skeletal growth is completed and reproductive function is regular.

Growth and Developmental Changes

Physical Growth

- There is a rapid period of growth in height, weight, and muscle mass.
- Sexual maturation occurs during this period and can be tracked by using the Tanner scale.
- For girls, the first sign of sexual maturation is breast development, and menstruation generally begins within 2 years of the onset of breast development.
- For boys, sperm production (spermatogenesis) corresponds with increased testicular size and penile enlargement. Nocturnal emissions ("wet dreams") typically start about 1 year after the penis begins to enlarge in size.
- The achievement of Tanner stage 5 for both girls and boys corresponds with adult sexual maturity.
- The rapid physical growth is responsible for much of the clumsiness and awkwardness associated with the adolescent period.

Psychosocial and Emotional Changes

- Adolescence is also a period of tremendous psychosocial and emotional changes.
- The developmental task of adolescence is "identity versus identity diffusion."
- Adolescents become preoccupied with "what others think about them" in an attempt to be accepted. The focus of influence shifts from the family to the peer group, and it is with this group that the adolescent begins to form a sense of identity.
- Ideally, the adolescent moves through this stage developing an internal set of personal values and a sense of self-competency while beginning to plan for a future career.
- Cognitive development is termed the "formal operational stage." The adolescent now begins a process of more logical thought.
- Conflicts begin to occur between adolescents and their parents. Traditional values of the adolescent's family may be challenged by the exposure to new ideas and values from peers.
- The adolescent struggles to develop his or her own set of moral principles, questioning established moral codes.

- Peers often have more influence on the adolescent than do her or his parents, but often pre-established values and morals persist.
- The adolescent questions his or her spiritual beliefs, often turning away from formal religion, and eventually resolving the questions and identifying his or her own sense of spirituality.
- Adolescence is also a time of increased risk-taking behavior. This is a result of several factors, including the desire to separate from parental influence, peer pressure and the need to "belong," and a thought process in which the adolescent does not see herself or himself as vulnerable ("It can't happen to me").
- A number of undesirable behaviors—such as unprotected sexual activity, substance use, and unsafe driving—are examples of risky behavior that is often exhibited by teens.

Health Promotion and Risk Factors

Common health problems seen with this age group include eating disorders, obesity, pregnancy, sexually transmitted diseases (STDs), emotional disorders, substance abuse, and violence.

Cultural Considerations

Cultural influences may affect adolescent behaviors by establishing expectations.

CULTURE	PERSPECTIVES ON ADOLESCENTS
African American	Adolescents are often expected to assume some responsibility for household chores and are encouraged to get jobs. Premarital teen pregnancy is not condoned, but it is accepted once child is born.
Amish	Adolescent may want to break away from cultural norms (e.g., dress), but it is expected that this is experimental and teen will return and assume adult role, adhering to prescribed norms.

(continued)

CULTURE	PERSPECTIVES ON ADOLESCENTS
Appalachian	Formal education is not stressed; adolescent expected to get job and support family. Adolescents marry young, 15 years and even as young as 13. Having children associated with sense of importance. Underage alcohol abuse common.
Arab American	Chastity and decency expected.
Chinese American	Expected to score well in national tests by age 18. Must make career choice during adolescent years. Teenage pregnancy not common. Expected to respect elders.
Cuban American	At age 15, girls have "rite of passage" (quince party) and are ready for courting. Unmarried couples may have chaperones.
Egyptian American	Loss of virginity affects marriageability, so parents very restrictive.
Filipino American	Short courtships.
Greek American	Girls have less freedom in dating than boys. Dating is often prohibited until upper grades of high school.
Iranian American	Girls are expected to maintain virginity.
Irish American	Expected to remain loyal to family.
Jewish American	Rite of passage at age 13 for boys and age 12 for girls.
Navajo Native American	Menarche for a teenage girl seen as passage to adulthood. Older children taught to be stoic and not complain.
Vietnamese American	Teens are expected to respect elders.

Adapted from Purnell, L.D., and Paulanka, B.J. (2012): *Transcultural Healthcare: A Culturally Competent Approach*, 4th ed. Philadelphia, F.A. Davis.

Assessment

Health History

Current Health Status

This is addressed in essentially the same way as with an adult.

Current Medications

Ask about all prescription and OTC medications. Many teens (especially those involved in athletics) take vitamin or protein supplements, and it is important to assess for these. Ask girls if they take oral contraceptives, get monthly "shots" (Depo-Provera), or have a contraceptive implant (Norplant). Also, ask all female patients about Accutane (an acne medication) because the risk of serious birth defects with this medication necessitates counseling about pregnancy prevention.

Past Health History

The questions are the same as for the adult, although the adolescent may not be aware of all his or her past health history.

Immunizations

Additional immunizations recommended by or during adolescence include:

- Tdap between 11 and 12 years.
- MMR between 11 and 12 years, if second MMR shot not given between 4 and 6 years.
- VAR, varicella, 2nd dose 4 to 6 years.
- Meningitis vaccine (Menomonee) administered before start of college.
- HPV2 vaccine for girls between 11 and 12 years, or HPV4 males and females.

Significant Family Medical History

If the teen is being interviewed alone, she or he may have limited knowledge in this area. Most, however, will be aware of heart disease, strokes, cancer, and other serious health conditions within the family. It is also important to ask if anyone died at an early age (younger than age 35) from a sudden heart attack. This may be a risk factor for sports participation and may require additional investigation, if present.

Review of Systems

SYSTEM AND QUESTIONS TO ASK	SIGNIFICANCE
General Health Status	
How have you been feeling?	Screen for any obvious problems.
Any recent weight changes?	Changes in weight, either loss or gain, may indicate an eating disorder.
Integumentary	
Any skin problems, such as acne?	Adolescents are very self-conscious about appearance and acne may affect self-image.

(continued)

Review of Systems (continued)

SYSTEM AND QUESTIONS TO ASK	SIGNIFICANCE
Changes in body hair growth?	Secondary sexual changes include increased growth of body hair (i.e., pubic hair, axillae, legs, and facial hair for boys).
Piercing or tattoos?	Body piercing and tattooing can increase risk for human immunodeficiency virus (HIV) or hepatitis B.
Sun tanning? Use of sunblock? Tanning salons?	Excessive exposure to sun (UV rays) without sunblock increases the risk for skin cancer later in life.
HEENT	
Eyes	
Any visual problems?	Visual refractive problems peak during adolescence.
Do you wear glasses or contact lenses?	May identify teaching need about care of contact lenses.
When was your last eye exam?	Eyes should be tested routinely during physical exams.
Ears	
Do you have any hearing problems? Do you listen to loud music?	Cochlear damage can result from excessive exposure to loud noise, such as CD players and rock concerts. May identify teaching need about noise pollution's effect on hearing.
When was your last hearing exam?	Hearing should be tested routinely during physical exams.
Teeth	
When was your last visit to the dentist? Orthodontist?	Should have at least an annual dental exam. The need for orthodontic work usually becomes apparent during adolescence and can make the teenager even more self-conscious about appearance.
Respiratory	
Do you have asthma?	Asthma is the most common disease among children and adolescents.
Do you ever have trouble breathing or wheeze when exercising or running? Are you exposed to air pollutants, smoke, or second-hand smoke?	Exercise-induced bronchospasm is acute, reversible, self-terminating airway obstruction that occurs after vigorous exercise, peaks in 5 to 10 minutes once activity stops, and then ceases within 30 minutes.
Cardiovascular	
Do you have any chest pain? Does your heart ever skip a beat?	Although cardiovascular disease is not common in children and adolescents, it can occur. Prolonged QT syndrome can cause sudden cardiac death in a seemingly healthy child.

SYSTEM AND QUESTIONS TO ASK	SIGNIFICANCE
Breasts	
Girls	
Do you have any tenderness of the breasts? Have they increased in size? Are they growing equally?	Need to determine if normal breast development is occurring. May identify areas for health teaching. Initially, breast development may be asymmetrical, but it will even out.
Boys	
Have your breasts enlarged?	During early puberty, boys may experience temporary gynecomastia, which usually disappears within 2 years. Because appearance is of great concern, gynecomastia can be very alarming for boys and make them very self-conscious.
Gastrointestinal	
Any stomach problems? What is your bowel pattern?	Identify underlying eating disorder.
Do you use laxatives?	Excessive use of laxatives associated with eating disorders.
Genitourinary	
Girls	
Did your periods start? When? Frequency? Description of flow?	Need to identify menarche and determine if cycle is normal.
Do you use pads or tampons?	Use of tampons has been associated with risk for toxic shock syndrome.
Do you have burning when you go to the bathroom? Urinary tract infections (UTIs)?	A history of frequent UTIs in girls can be the result of sexual activity and a clue to follow up more thoroughly in this area.
Are you sexually active? Have you had sex? Are you practicing safe sex?	May identify teaching need about STDs and safe sex practices. *Pubertal delay for girls:* No breast development by age 13 or no menarche within 4 years of initial breast changes.
Boys	
Are you sexually active? Have you had sex? Are you practicing safe sex?	May identify teaching need about STDs and safe sex practices. *Pubertal delay for boys:* No changes in testes or scrotum by age $13^1/_2$ to 14, incomplete genital growth within 4 years of initial change.

(continued)

Review of Systems (continued)

SYSTEM AND QUESTIONS TO ASK	SIGNIFICANCE
Musculoskeletal	
Do you have any back problems? Have you ever been told you had a spinal problem?	Heavy backpacks have been associated with low back problems in children and adolescents. Scoliosis occurs more frequently in girls than in boys. Screening usually occurs in middle and high school. If scoliosis is present, determine if it is structural or postural (see Chapter 12).
Neurologic	
How would you describe your mood? Do you feel sad a lot?	Adolescence is a time of change, and emotional response to these changes varies. Depression and suicidal ideations need to be identified and treated.
Endocrine	
Any swelling in neck? Difficulty swallowing? Hoarseness?	Thyroid is more active during puberty. Enlarged thyroid may indicate hypothyroid or hyperthyroid disease. Lymphocytic thyroiditis (Hashimoto's disease or juvenile autoimmune thyroiditis) peaks in adolescence. Graves' disease occurs between ages 12 and 14. If sexual maturation is not progressing, endocrine problems should be considered.
Lymphatic/Hematological	
Have you been tired?	Rapid growth and poor dietary habits increase the risk of iron deficiency anemia during adolescence.
Have you any lumps in neck, underarms, or groin?	Hodgkin's lymphoma is prevalent between ages 15 and 19. Non-Hodgkin's lymphomas occur more frequently before age 15.

HEENT = Head, eyes, ears, nose, and throat.

Psychosocial History

Health Practices

When did you have your last health exam? (Recommend health exams every 2 years.)

Typical Day

Can you tell me what your day is like? How are you doing in school? This allows you to see the teen through his or her eyes.

You may be able to identify stresses confronting the teen in everyday life. A change in academic performance or a sudden disinterest in school may reflect a more serious problem. Ask teens what subjects they like, which ones they dislike. If they are having problems with a particular subject, have they sought help for this? How many days of school do they miss in a term? High absenteeism (except for serious illness) correlates with other risky behaviors.

Nutrition

Screen diet by asking for a 24-hour recall. Ask questions about realistic body image, such as, "How much do you think you should weigh?" Further explore this issue if the response is unrealistic. Ask about eating patterns: "How often do you eat breakfast?" "What is a usual lunch for you?" "What are your favorite snacks?" These open-ended questions will provide a much clearer picture of the adolescent's nutritional status and potential risks. Dietary needs are greater for calcium, iron, and zinc. Calcium is needed for bone growth and the bone mass that develops during adolescence. It also influences the development of osteoporosis later in life. You need to assess for both overeating and undereating problems. Ask about dieting. Girls tend to be more concerned about losing weight, whereas boys may want to "bulk-up" and improve strength.

Activity and Exercise (Such as Sports, if Applicable)

Ask about what teens enjoy doing outside of the home. What sports do they play, if any? What do they like to do with their friends? How often do they watch TV during the week? How much time do they spend on the computer? You may identify a need for health education regarding the importance of routine exercise. If a teen does participate in sports, does she or he use protective equipment? Is it a contact sport? Contact sports may increase the risk for injury.

Sleep and Rest

Ask about when they usually go to bed and when they awaken. Do they feel refreshed in the morning or are they still tired? How does this pattern change on weekends? Even though sleep needs increase during growth spurts, teens often get less than ideal amounts of sleep during the week and sleep late into the day on weekends. Also ask about bedwetting, which is not entirely uncommon in teens, especially boys. Asking, "Many young people find they sometimes wet themselves during their sleep—Does this ever happen to you?" is a less threatening and less embarrassing way to assess for this.

Personal Habits and Behaviors

Ask about substance use (drugs, alcohol, and nicotine). Ask, "If you smoke cigarettes, how many do you smoke in an average day?" "If you use alcohol, how much do you usually drink during the week?" "If you use drugs, what type and what method (smoking, snorting, huffing, ingesting, injecting)?" Asking questions in this way is less threatening to the teen, and he or she is much more likely to give an honest response.

If the teen drives, did she or he attend a driver's education program? Does she or he wear seat belts? Is she or he aware of the hazards of driving under the influence of drugs or alcohol? If drug or alcohol use is identified, make appropriate referrals as indicated.

Recreation and Hobbies

Ask, "What do you do for fun? Do you have any hobbies?" If recreational activities or hobbies increase the risk for injury, ask if protective measures (e.g., bike helmets) are used. Ask about presence of weapons in the home and gun/hunting safety courses if appropriate.

Self-Perception and Self-Concept

Ask the teen to describe himself or herself—"Tell me about yourself: What do you like best about yourself, and what would you like to change?"

Role and Relationship

Ask the teen to tell you about her or his family—"Who lives at home with you?" If there are siblings, ask about the relationship. Ask, "Is there an adult in your life whom you feel comfortable talking with?" Ask about peer relationships. Ask if the teen has a special friend and what things she or he enjoys doing with that friend. Ask about dating or other significant relationships.

Sexuality and Reproductive Issues

For girls, ask about menarche and if they have any questions or concerns about menstrual issues. For boys, ask about physical changes and if they have questions about this. For example, one could ask a young man, "Many young men have questions about some of the changes in their bodies; do you have any questions I could answer for you?" Ask about sexual activity: "If you are sexually active, how do you protect yourself against STDs and unwanted pregnancy?" Sex role identity becomes established during adolescence. Sexual preferences—heterosexual, homosexual, or bisexual—become apparent during adolescence.

Coping and Stress Tolerance

Ask questions such as "What do you do when you get angry?" and "What makes you angry?" Also ask questions such as "What do you do when you want to relax?" You need to identify whether the teen has healthy coping strategies to deal with feelings and stresses in life.

Value and Belief Pattern

Ask about what is important to them—Do they have specific beliefs about God or a "higher power?"

Physical Assessment

The physical assessment of the adolescent does not differ greatly from the adult assessment, but there are specific variations that are unique to this developmental period.

It is important that weight measurements be done in private. Often, particularly in school settings, this is not done, and it is the source of much anxiety for adolescents, especially those who are overweight or who think they are.

Physical Assessment of the Adolescent

SYSTEM/ ASSESSMENT	NORMAL VARIATIONS/ ABNORMAL FINDINGS
General Health Survey	
Inspect overall appearance, noting appropriate growth and development for patient's age.	Detect any delays or premature sexual maturation. Note any obvious weight problems.
Integumentary	
Inspect skin for lesions. Note piercings and tattoos.	Acne is a common problem and a major concern for adolescents. This condition should be treated and not dismissed as insignificant. Severe acne can result in permanent scarring. Many effective treatments are now available for all types of acne.
Note body hair distribution.	Absence of or excessive body hair may relate to a problem with sexual maturation.

(continued)

Physical Assessment of the Adolescent (continued)

SYSTEM/ ASSESSMENT	NORMAL VARIATIONS/ ABNORMAL FINDINGS
HEENT	
Eyes	
Test visual acuity.	Many adolescents are reluctant to wear prescribed eyeglasses, yet many have some degree of myopia.
Ears	
Test hearing with pure tone audiometer.	Adolescents often listen to very loud music (often in very close ear contact using earphones); this can result in early hearing loss. Use opportunity to teach hazards of listening to loud music.
Nose	
Inspect nasal septum and mucosa.	Chronic rhinorrhea can result from allergic rhinitis. Boggy, bluish-purple turbinates are consistent with allergic rhinitis. Also assess for cocaine-induced rhinorrhea or mucosal damage.
Mouth	
Inspect oral mucosa and pharynx.	Hypertrophied tonsils of early childhood have usually shrunk to more normal proportions.
Inspect occlusion.	If malocclusion is present, refer to orthodontist.
Inspect number of teeth and presence of wisdom teeth.	Adolescents should have 28 permanent teeth, and third molars ("wisdom teeth") may erupt during this period. Referral may be needed if wisdom teeth are impacted. Also assess for orthodontic devices and brushing technique around them.
Neck	
Palpate the thyroid.	A tender, enlarged thyroid gland can signal acute thyroiditis.
Respiratory	
Auscultate lungs.	Adolescents with exercise-induced asthma will require bronchodilators before activity. Usually, albuterol administered through a metered-dose inhaler is given 20 to 30 minutes before exercise.
Cardiovascular	
Auscultate heart and note rate and rhythm.	Adolescents often have a sinus arrhythmia and a split second heart sound. Both the arrhythmia and the split second sound change with respiration. This is a normal variation.

SYSTEM/ ASSESSMENT	NORMAL VARIATIONS/ ABNORMAL FINDINGS
Breasts	
Inspect and palpate breasts.	Breast exams should begin during adolescence, along with instruction in breast self-exam. Gynecomastia occurs in about one-third of boys.
Gastrointestinal	
Inspect, auscultate, and palpate abdomen.	No specific variations occur with the abdomen during adolescence, except for pregnancy. It is not unusual to detect pregnancy during a routine exam of the abdomen in an adolescent who is denying this possibility. By 20 weeks' gestation, the fundus is at the level of the umbilicus.
Genitourinary	
Inspect external genitalia.	Sexually active teens should be examined for STDs.
For girls: Perform pelvic examination with Pap smear at age 21 or 3 years after onset of sexual activity.	Sexually active girls should have annual gynecological examinations.
For boys: Perform testicular exam.	Instruction in testicular self-exam should be provided to all adolescent boys. Tanner staging should be noted for both boys and girls.
Musculoskeletal	
Inspect and palpate spinal curves. Test for spinal deformities. (See Chapter 12.)	Scoliosis is the major variation within the musculoskeletal system. Screening for scoliosis should be done in the preadolescent period, generally during the fifth and sixth grade. Any significant curvature should be referred for evaluation and follow-up.
Neurologic	
Focus on affect and cognitive functioning.	Depression and suicidal ideations warrant immediate intervention.

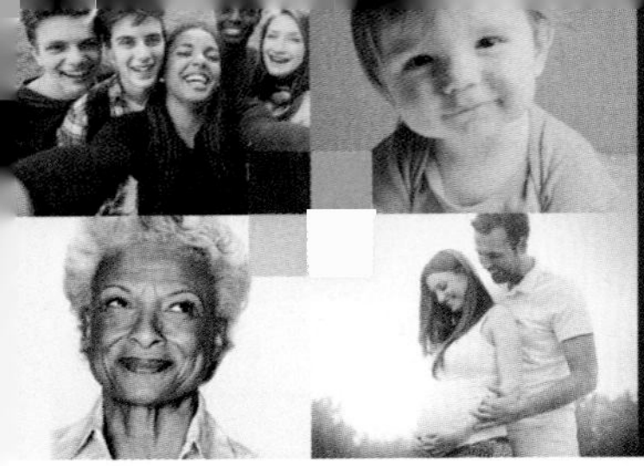

CHAPTER 18

Assessing the Older Adult

Developmental Considerations

- Erikson identifies the final stage of development as ego integrity versus despair, and this stage of life correlates well with Maslow's Theory of Human Needs self-actualization need, in which self-fulfillment of one's potential is actualized.
- Ideally, adults older than age 65 will be able to do a life review with a sense of satisfaction and accomplishment and will be able to accept their own mortality.

Cultural Considerations

CULTURE	PERSPECTIVE ON AGING
African American	Elders are valued and treated with respect. Grandmother has central role, often offers economic and child care support. Grandchildren often raised by grandmother.
Amish	Elders are respected members of the community. Grandparents turn over farming responsibilities to their children, live close to them, and assist with child care. Elder care usually within the family setting, and Amish prefer to die at home.
Appalachian	Elders respected and honored. Live close to children and participate in childcare.
Brazilian American	Elders live with children and are included in all activities.
Chinese American	Elders are highly valued, respected, and considered very wise. Children are expected to care for parents.
Cuban American	Elders live with children. Multigenerational households are common.

CULTURE	PERSPECTIVE ON AGING
Egyptian American	Elders are respected and are thought to become wiser with age. Family expected to take care of elders. Women gain status with age and childbearing; however, older women are expected to care for older men.
European American	Value is on youth and beauty, so elders are seen as less important and little attention is paid to their problems.
Filipino American	Multigenerational households are common. Grandparents act as surrogate parents while parents work.
Greek American	Elders well respected. Children are expected to care for parents, who actively participate in family activities.
Iranian American	Believe that with age come experience, worldliness, and knowledge; so elders seen with respect. Caring for them is children's obligation.
Irish American	Elders are well respected, and their opinions are valued. Elders are cared for in home.
Jewish American	Elders respected and seen as having wisdom. Honoring and caring for parents is important. Old age is a state of mind.
Korean American	60 is considered old age, and one is expected to retire then.
Mexican American	Elders live with children. Large extended family.
Navajo Native American	Elders with many children seen with respect. They have important role in teaching and keeping rituals to children and grandchildren.
Vietnamese American	Elders are honored, have key role in family activities, and are consulted on major family decisions.

Adapted from Purnell, L.D., and Paulanka, B.J. (2012): *Transcultural Healthcare: A Culturally Competent Approach,* 4th ed. Philadelphia: F.A. Davis.

Assessment

Health History

Remember that older adults may not present in the same way as younger people when ill.

- Older adults may minimize or ignore symptoms.
- They often have several concurrent medical problems.
- They often present with atypical signs and symptoms of disease.

Key points to remember when obtaining a history from an older adult:

- Realize that age differences between you and your patient may influence his or her response.
- Be aware of your own views and values associated with aging.
- Explain what you are doing and why.
- Allow more time than with younger patients.
- Realize that you may need to obtain the history over several visits.
- Ask the patient if she or he can hear you.
- Sit at same level in front of patient without invading his or her personal space.
- Maintain eye contact.
- Speak slowly and clearly, the lower the pitch the better.
- Set time limits for your interview.
- Redirect the interview as needed, but respect the patient's need to reminisce.
- Allow the patient to respond to each question before asking another.
- Listen to what your patient is saying, being alert for any signs of fatigue or discomfort.
- Use lay terminology that is culturally relevant to elicit more comprehensive information (e.g., "sugar" rather than "glucose" in diabetes).

The history and physical assessment are essentially the same as with other adults, but keep in mind:

- Symptom reporting may differ because the older patient may be either a health pessimist or a health optimist.
- Cost of health-care is a concern.
- The older patient may delay treatment.
- The older patient may have multiple pathologies.
- Disease presentation may differ in older adults.
- Polypharmacy may account for many of your patient's symptoms.
- Common surgeries for older adults include cataracts, joint replacement, and skin lesion removal.
- History should include functional assessment, and family history should include history of Alzheimer's disease and dementia.
- The patient needs to be asked about advance directives.
- History taking should begin with questions that focus on orientation and past information, as a way of establishing the patient's cognitive status.

Review of Systems

Review of Systems

SYSTEM AND QUESTIONS TO ASK	SIGNIFICANCE
General Health Status	
How would you describe your usual state of health? Are you able to do what you usually do?	Helps to identify current heath status and activity tolerance.
Have you noticed any changes in your height or weight? Do you notice any difference in how your clothes fit?	Loss of height (normally 1 cm every 10 years after age 40 with a total 1-3 inches as you age) occurs with aging. Changes in weight distribution occur with age; a decrease of subcutaneous fat is seen on the face and extremities with an increase on the abdomen and hips. Differences in the way clothes fit may signal subtle changes in weight that warrant further investigation.
Integumentary	
Skin	
Have you noticed any changes in your skin; for example, dryness, itching, rashes, blisters?	There are many age-related changes in the skin, some of which are also caused by the environment. They result in uncomfortable symptoms such as pruritus and xerosis (dry skin), which occur frequently in older adults during the winter.
How often do you bathe? What type of soap do you use? Do you use lotions, sunscreens? Have you been in the sun a great deal? What type of work did you do?	Skin care practices, sun exposure, and occupational history may influence current skin condition.
Have you noticed any skin changes such as changes in size of growths or open, sore, cracked, itchy, bleeding areas that won't heal?	The incidence of skin cancer increases with age.
Have you noticed any new rough areas of your skin that do not seem to go away?	**Remember that visual changes that occur with aging may make early recognition of skin changes more difficult.**

(continued)

Review of Systems (continued)

SYSTEM AND QUESTIONS TO ASK	SIGNIFICANCE
Integumentary *(cont'd)* **Hair**	
Any hair loss, increased hair growth, graying, dry scalp, or other hair changes? What are your usual patterns of hair care? Have you undergone hair replacement treatments?	Changes in hair growth and distribution are commonly associated with aging. Dry scalp is a normal and common complaint. Hair loss may be distressing for both men and women. Women may also be concerned about increased facial hair. You need to differentiate normal changes from possible disease.
Nails	
How do you care for your nails? Do you cut them yourself? Do you see a podiatrist?	Nails thicken with age and may be more difficult to trim. Fungal nail infections are common. A podiatry consult may be indicated, especially if the patient has a history of diabetes or vascular disease.
HEENT **Head, Face, and Neck**	
Do you have facial pain?	Increased incidence of temporal arteritis in older adults may explain pain over temporal artery.
Can you move your head easily?	ROM in the head and neck may be limited because of musculoskeletal changes or osteoarthritis.
Eyes	
Have you noticed any changes in your vision? Can you read normal-sized print or large-print materials? Do you have problems going from light to dark areas? Do you drive at night?	Common problems (e.g., cataracts, macular degeneration, and glaucoma) can affect vision. Normal age changes include increased sensitivity to glare and decreases in visual acuity, lens elasticity, peripheral vision, color intensity (specifically blue, green, and purple), night vision, accommodation to changes in lighting, tear production and viscosity, depth perception; and presbyopia. Dry eyes are very common. They may be caused by decreased tear production or blocked tear ducts, so further investigation is warranted.
Do your eyes feel dry? Do you have floaters? Do you see flashes of light? Does it look like a shade is being pulled over your eye?	There are several eye complaints that require immediate attention, such as a sudden onset of floaters or flashes of light peripherally, with decreased visual acuity. The patient may describe

SYSTEM AND QUESTIONS TO ASK	SIGNIFICANCE
	this as like a curtain coming down over the field of vision (amaurosis fugax). These symptoms indicate retinal detachment or TIA or stroke. A complaint of a sudden onset of painless unilateral loss of vision also requires immediate attention because this may be caused by retinal vein occlusion.
Ears	
Do you have any problems with your hearing?	Problems with pitch discrimination are common, especially with high-pitched sounds (s, t, f, and g). Presbycusis is common in older adults.
Do you have balance problems?	Balance problems may be caused by a problem in the inner ear or a more serious neurologic problem.
Nose	
Have you noticed any changes in your sense of smell?	Anosmia—a decreased ability to identify and discriminate odors—occurs with aging.
Do you have a runny nose? Do you sneeze frequently? Do you have postnasal drip?	Atrophic changes associated with aging may cause vasomotor rhinitis.
Mouth and Throat	
Do you have difficulty chewing, swallowing, tasting, smelling, or enjoying food?	Age-related changes on the surface of the tongue and atrophy of taste buds affect the ability to eat and enjoy food. In particular, there is a decrease in the ability to taste sweets and salt. Gums become thinner and recede, resulting in loose teeth and exposure of the roots.
Do you wear dentures? Do they fit properly? Do you have any sores in your mouth? When was the last time you saw your dentist?	Poorly fitted dentures may lead to poor nutrition and mouth sores. May identify need for referral.
When you are eating, do you ever cough or choke? Does this occur with liquids and/or solids? Do you have problems swallowing?	Dysphagia may be related to a variety of underlying problems and is not a normal part of aging. It warrants further investigation.
Does your mouth always feel dry with a bad taste? Do you have difficulty swallowing dry food or speaking for long periods?	Dry mouth (xerostomia) is a very common problem in older adults, caused by medication, decreased production of saliva, inadequate fluid intake, atrophy of the oral mucosa, vitamin deficiencies, poor

(continued)

Review of Systems (continued)

SYSTEM AND QUESTIONS TO ASK	SIGNIFICANCE
Integumentary	
Mouth and Throat *(cont'd)*	nutrition, and poor oral hygiene. Burning mouth syndrome is also common in the older adult. It causes dry mouth, altered taste, thirst, difficulty swallowing, swelling in the face and cheeks, and altered sense of smell.
Respiratory	
Do you have any difficulty breathing? If yes, when does it occur and with how much exertion? Has it affected your ability to perform usual activities?	Respiratory disorders are common in older adults. Patients may describe themselves as having breathing difficulties or trouble getting a deep breath or sufficient air. With chronic obstructive pulmonary disease (COPD), dyspnea is usually insidious in onset and progressive.
Do you have a cough?	Lung cancer most frequently occurs between ages 55 and 74 years. There has been a recent increase in tuberculosis among older adults. If there is a new-onset cough, determine if the patient has been exposed to a change in environment or has taken any new medications, such as angiotensin-converting enzyme (ACE) inhibitors.
Cardiovascular	
Do you get short of breath when walking or making the bed? Do you have swelling in the feet, hands, face, or abdomen; weight gain; or shoes or clothing that no longer fit? Does the swelling get worse as the day goes on and disappear in the morning?	Cardiovascular disease is not a normal change associated with aging, but it is the most common problem. Unfortunately, it often does not exhibit the typical signs and symptoms found in younger people. For example, an older adult may present with atrial fibrillation but have no symptoms at all or complain vaguely of just not feeling right. If the patient reports swelling, explore if this is related to his or her activity level or to a change in medication or diet.
Do you get dizzy? When? Does the dizziness get worse when going from lying to standing, or is it worse with exertion? Are there any changes in your energy level?	Orthostatic (postural) hypotension can cause dizziness.

SYSTEM AND QUESTIONS TO ASK	SIGNIFICANCE
Do you have a cough? Is it worse at night? Do you get more short of breath when lying flat? Do you need to sleep with several pillows?	Cough may be related to congestive heart failure or a cardiac medication. Vascular disease increases with age.
Do you have headaches?	Headaches may be associated with hypertension (HTN), stroke, or temporal artery disease.
Do you have leg pain when walking? Skin changes, swelling, ulcers, or varicose veins in your legs?	Intermittent claudication (pain in legs when walking) and skin changes (thin, shiny, and hairless) suggest arterial vascular disease. High incidence of venous disease in older adults.
Gastrointestinal	
What is your typical diet for a day? Any change? Any food intolerance?	Food intolerance is a common complaint and may be associated with hiatal hernia and esophageal reflux.
What are your usual bowel patterns? Diet and fluid intake? Medications, prescribed and over-the-counter (OTC)?	Constipation is one of the most common digestive complaints in the older adult, and accounts for 2.5 million physician visits annually. The prevalence of constipation increases with age, is more common in women than in men, in nonwhites than in whites, and in those with lower family income and education. Constipation may have dangerous complications in older adults, including acute changes in cognition, urinary retention, urinary incontinence, and fecal impaction. Fecal impaction can result in intestinal obstruction, ulceration, and urinary problems. Chronic straining to defecate can have adverse effects on cerebral, coronary, and peripheral-vascular circulation. Constipation can be categorized as functional (slow transit of stool) or rectosigmoid outlet delay (anorectal dysfunction, 10 minutes or more needed to defecate). Bowel changes associated with bleeding and weight loss suggest a malignancy.

(continued)

Review of Systems (continued)

SYSTEM AND QUESTIONS TO ASK	SIGNIFICANCE
Genitourinary **Urinary** Do you have trouble getting to the bathroom on time? Do you need to wear a pad? If so, how many times a day do you have to change it? Does the incontinence occur with coughing or sneezing, on the way to the bathroom, or at night? Does it interfere with your ability (or desire) to do daily activities or engage in social activities?	Urinary incontinence is not a normal aspect of aging, but it is a common problem. Approximately 10 million Americans suffer from urinary incontinence. Report of new-onset incontinence, loss of appetite, vomiting, falls, nocturia, difficulty urinating, or behavioral and cognitive changes should alert you to a possible urinary tract infection. Prostate enlargement can cause incontinence. See Table 18.1 for types of incontinence.
Ask men about frequent urination, hesitancy, weak or intermittent stream, a sensation of incomplete emptying of the bladder, dribbling after voiding, and nocturia.	
Female Reproductive Do you have any vaginal discharge? If so, what is the type, color, odor, and consistency of the discharge?	Changes in vaginal secretions, amount, and pH increase the risk for vaginal infections.
Do you have vaginal pressure, or an uncomfortable, bearing-down sensation, in addition to symptoms of urinary incontinence?	Symptoms may be related to the presence of a uterine prolapse, cystocele, or rectocele.
Do you have any vaginal bleeding? Are you taking hormone replacement therapy? When did you go through menopause? When was your last Pap test?	Bleeding may be related to hormone replacement therapy. If patient is not on hormones, bleeding that occurs after 1 year postmenopause is abnormal and needs follow-up.
Do you do breast-self-exams? When was your last mammogram? Do you get them yearly?	Incidence of breast cancer increases with age. Yearly mammograms are recommended for women older than age 40. May identify teaching needs.
Are you satisfied with your sexual activity? Do you have pain during intercourse (dyspareunia) or vaginal dryness?	Older adults continue to be sexually active, unless they no longer have a sexual partner, have a disease, or are exposed to a treatment that decreases libido or makes intercourse uncomfortable. None of the age-related changes in either men or women precludes the

SYSTEM AND QUESTIONS TO ASK	SIGNIFICANCE
	continuation of a satisfying sexual life. Decreased vaginal secretions may result in dyspareunia. If it is present, an appropriate plan of care should be developed.
Have you ever had a sexually transmitted disease? Do you practice safe sex?	Because older women do not fear pregnancy, they are less likely to ask their partners to use condoms as a form of protection.
Male Reproductive	
When was the last time you had your prostate checked? Have you ever had a prostate specific antigen (PSA) test? Do you have any urinary changes or problems?	Increased incidence of prostate cancer in older men. Yearly prostate exams should begin at age 50. May identify need for health teaching.
Are you satisfied with your sexual activity? Have you been feeling more tired than usual?	Sexuality does not normally decrease with age. However, the physical act and response may require more time and be less intense. Be alert for vague complaints. Give men the opportunity to talk about impotence and associated feelings so that individualized plans can be developed.
Musculoskeletal	
Do you have pain, stiffness, joint enlargement, decreased ROM, and functional changes?	Osteoarthritis is the most common joint disease in the older adult and affects over 80 percent of those age 65 and older. Rheumatoid arthritis also increases with age. Gout is also common, exacerbated by use of diuretics or alcohol.
Do you have pain, stiffness, and decreased ROM in the neck, shoulders, or hips that persists for at least 1 month? Do you have severe headache, visual loss, scalp tenderness, and mouth pain?	Common problems in older adults include polymyalgia rheumatica, a syndrome that involves the musculoskeletal system; giant cell arteritis, a vasculitic disorder of the cranial arteries associated with polymyalgia rheumatica; and osteoporosis.
Have you had any fractures, bone pain, or loss of height? Do you take calcium and vitamin D? Do you exercise? If so, what type of activity do you do? Are you taking any additional bone-building medication?	Identifies participation in measures to prevent further bone loss and possible teaching needs.

(continued)

Review of Systems (continued)

SYSTEM AND QUESTIONS TO ASK	SIGNIFICANCE
Musculoskeletal *(cont'd)*	
Do you have balance problems or a history of falls?	Refer to Box 18.1 for the checklist *Evaluating the Risk Factors for Falls.* This can help determine whether the fall is caused by a gait or balance disorder or another underlying problem for which the patient needs to be evaluated and treated.
Do you have any foot problems? How do your shoes fit? Do you see a podiatrist? How do you care for your feet?	Foot problems are common in older adults and may result from poorly fitted shoes or poor foot care. Referrals may be warranted.
Neurological	
Do you have problems with balance, mobility, coordination, sensory interpretations, level of consciousness, intellectual performance, personality, communication, comprehension, emotional responses, and thoughts?	Changes in the neurological system may be normal or the result of disease. Stroke is the most common neurologic problem in older adults. Parkinson's disease is the most common extrapyramidal problem.
Do you have dizziness? Feel the room is spinning or you're spinning?	Vertigo is a common problem, and diagnosis is based mainly on clinical symptoms.
Do you have a known history of seizures? Do you have repetitive shaking or muscle contractions, brief lapses of consciousness, or any abnormal sensations?	Incidence of seizures significantly increases in people over age 65 because of an increase in strokes, tumors, subdural hematomas, metabolic disorders, dementia, and medications.
Endocrine	
Have you been feeling depressed? Experiencing weight loss/gain? Does your heart ever flutter, race, or skip beats?	Thyroid disease presents differently than in younger adults. Signs of hyperthyroidism include apathy, depression, and emaciation rather than hyperactivity. Atrial fibrillation also often occurs. Hypothyroidism is the most frequent thyroid disorder in older adults, but it is easy to miss because signs (dry skin and hair, hypotension, slow pulse, sluggishness, depressed muscular activity, goiter, weight gain) are often attributed to aging.
Do you have increased thirst, urination, and appetite?	The incidence of diabetes mellitus increases with age.

SYSTEM AND QUESTIONS TO ASK	SIGNIFICANCE
Immune/Hematological	
Have you been feeling more tired than usual?	When an older person becomes sick, symptoms may be vague because of changes in the immune system. Fatigue may be associated with anemia, a common problem in older adults, usually caused by iron deficiency.

HEENT = Head, eyes, ears, nose, and throat.

TABLE 18.1 Types of Incontinence

TYPE OF INCONTI-NENCE	DEFINITION	PATHO-PHYSIOLOGY	SIGNS AND SYMPTOMS
Stress	Involuntary loss of urine caused by urethral sphincter failure with increases in intra-abdominal pressure.	Usually caused by weakness and laxity of pelvic floor musculature or bladder outlet weakness. Also may be caused by urethral hypermobility.	Urine is lost during coughing, sneezing, laughing.
Urge	Leakage of urine because of inability to delay voiding after sensation of bladder fullness is perceived.	Associated with detrusor hyperactivity, central nervous system disorders, or local genitourinary conditions.	Urine is lost on the way to the bathroom or as soon as the urge to void is felt.
Overflow	Leakage of urine resulting from mechanical forces on an overdistended bladder.	Results from mechanical obstruction or an acontractile bladder.	Variety of symptoms including frequent or constant dribbling, increased incontinence at night, frequency, and urgency.
Functional	Urine leakage caused by inability to get to toilet because of cognitive or physical impairment.	Cognitive and physical functional impairment.	Patient is aware of the need to void, but urine is lost on the way to the bathroom.

Psychosocial History

A psychosocial history of the older adult patient should address subjects such as a description of the patient's typical day, nutritional history, physical activity and exercise, sleep/rest patterns (Box 18.2), personal habits, support systems, and possible environmental hazards.

BOX 18.1 Evaluating the Risk Factors for Falls

Patient's Name ______________________________

Age__________ Gender___________ Date___________

1. History of previous falls:
   - ☐ Yes ☐ No
2. Medications:
   - ☐ Four or more prescriptions
   - ☐ New prescription in the last 2 weeks
   - ☐ Use of any of the following medications: Tranquilizers, sleeping pills, antidepressants, cardiac medications, antidiabetic agents
3. Known gait problem or muscular weakness:
   - ☐ Yes ☐ No
4. Dizziness, vertigo, or loss of consciousness at time of fall:
   - ☐ Yes ☐ No
5. Visual changes:
   - ☐ Yes ☐ No
6. Environmental problems:
   - ☐ Clutter
   - ☐ Dim lighting
   - ☐ Uneven flooring
   - ☐ Inappropriate footwear/lack of footwear
   - ☐ Inappropriate assistive device
7. Major illnesses:
   - ☐ Neurologic: Parkinson's disease, stroke, dementia
   - ☐ Musculoskeletal: Arthritis, contracture, fracture
   - ☐ Cardiac: Hypotension, arrhythmia, acute infarct
   - ☐ New acute illness: Infection
   - ☐ Other
8. What was the patient doing at the time of the fall?

____

____

____

9. Were there any injuries associated with the fall?
   - ☐ Laceration ☐ Persistent pain
   - ☐ Sprain/strain ☐ Head trauma
   - ☐ Fracture ☐ Other

10. How has course been since the fall?
    - ☐ Associated fear of falling
    - ☐ Change in function
    - ☐ Change in cognition

    Is the patient able to carry on usual activities? If not, who is available to help her or him?

____

____

____

BOX 18.2 How Age Affects Sleep

- Longer time to fall asleep
- Increased time in stages 1 and 2 sleep
- Decreased time in deeper stages of sleep (stages 3 and 4)
- Decreased rapid eye movement (REM) sleep
- Increased and shorter repetition of sleep cycle
- Increased nighttime awakenings
- Altered circadian rhythm with a need to fall asleep earlier and awaken earlier

Functional Assessment

Exploring functional performance is a very important component of the history for older patients. The Katz Index (Box 18.3), the Barthel Index (Table 18.2), and the Instrumental Activities of

BOX 18.3 The Katz Index of Activities of Daily Living

Abbreviations: I = independent; A = assistance; D = dependent.

1. Bathing (sponge, shower, or tub)
   - I: Receives no assistance (gets in and out of the tub)
   - A: Receives assistance in bathing only one part of the body
   - D: Receives assistance in bathing more than one part of the body
2. Dressing
   - I: Gets clothes and gets completely dressed without assistance
   - A: Gets clothes and gets dressed without assistance except in tying shoes
   - D: Receives assistance in getting clothes or in getting dressed or stays partly or completely undressed
3. Toileting
   - I: Goes to bathroom, cleans self, and manages clothes without assistance (may use an assistive device)
   - A: Receives assistance in going to bathroom or in cleaning self, managing clothes, or emptying a bedpan
   - D: Doesn't go to bathroom for elimination

(box continued on page 486)

BOX 18.3 The Katz Index of Activities of Daily Living (continued)

4. Transfer
   I: Moves in and out of bed or chair without assistance (may use assistive device)
   A: Moves in and out of bed or chair with assistance
   D: Doesn't get out of bed
5. Continence
   I: Controls urination and bowel movements independently
   A: Has occasional accidents
   D: Urine or bowel control maintained with supervision; patient is incontinent or has catheter
6. Feeding
   I: Feeds self without assistance
   A: Feeds self except for cutting meat or buttering bread
   D: Receives assistance in feeding or is fed partly or completely by tubes or intravenous fluids

TABLE 18.2 The Barthel Index

LEVEL OF CARE	INTACT	LIMITED	HELPER	NULL
Self-Care				
Feed	10	5	3	3
Dress (upper extremities)	5	5	3	0
Dress (lower extremities)	5	5	2	0
Don brace	0	0	–2	0
Grooming	4	4	0	0
Cleanse	4	4	2	0
Perineum				
Sphincters	Completely voluntary	Urgency/ appliance	Some help needed	Frequent accidents
Bladder	10	10	5	0
Bowel	10	10	5	0
Mobility/Transfer				
	Easy/No Device	With Difficulty Or Uses Device	Some Help Needed	dependent
1. Chair	15	15	7	0
2. Toilet	6	5	3	0
3. Tub	1	1	0	0
4. Walk 50 yards	15	15	10	0
5. Stairs	10	10	5	0
6. Wheelchair 50 yards	15	5	0	0

Adapted from Mahoney, F., and Barthel, D. (1965). Functional evaluation: The Barthel Index. *Maryland State Medical Journal 14*(2):61–65.

Daily Living tool (Box 18.4) are examples of instruments that will help you obtain baseline information on your patient's ability to perform activities of daily living (ADLs) and make appropriate referrals for care.

BOX 18.4 Instrumental Activities of Daily Living (IADL)

Abbreviations: I = independent; A = assistance; D = dependent.

1. Telephone:
   - I: Able to look up numbers, dial, receive, and make calls without help
   - A: Able to answer phone or dial operator in an emergency, but needs special phone or help in getting number or dialing
   - D: Unable to use the telephone
2. Traveling:
   - I: Able to drive own car or travel alone on bus or taxi
   - A: Able to travel but not alone
   - D: Unable to travel
3. Shopping:
   - I: Able to take care of all shopping with transportation provided
   - A: Able to shop but not alone
   - D: Unable to shop
4. Preparing meals:
   - I: Able to plan and cook full meals
   - A: Able to prepare light foods, but unable to cook full meals alone
   - D: Unable to prepare any meals
5. Housework:
   - I: Able to do heavy housework (scrub floors)
   - A: Able to do light housework, but needs help with heavy tasks
   - D: Unable to do any housework
6. Medication:
   - I: Able to take medications in the right dose at the right time
   - A: Able to take medications, but needs reminding or someone to prepare it
   - D: Unable to take medications
7. Money:
   - I: Able to manage buying needs, write checks, pay bills
   - A: Able to manage daily buying needs, but needs help managing checkbook and paying bills
   - D: Unable to manage money

From Duke University Center for the Study of Aging and Human Development. *The Multidimensional Functional Assessment Questionnaire*, ed. 2., pp. 169–170, with permission.

Physical Assessment

Approach

When examining the older patient, make sure the environment is as safe and appropriate as possible. To ensure a senior-friendly environment, do the following:

- Keep examination rooms warm (between 70°F and 80°F).
- Use bright but nonglaring lights.
- Keep background noise to a minimum.
- Provide higher than standard seating with arm rests on all chairs. (Patient might have trouble getting up, and if patient has degenerative joint disease [DJD] or has had joint replacement, she or he should not flex joint more than 90 degrees.)
- Use examination tables that mechanically elevate the patient from lying to sitting and vice versa and a broad-based step stool to help patients get onto the table.
- Use a private exam room, if possible, or at least pull the privacy curtain if there is a roommate.
- Minimize position changes to keep the patient from getting tired.
- Uncover only the area being assessed, making sure that patient is warm and covered with blankets or drapes.
- Provide reading materials with large print.
- Allow more time than usual for the exam. The complete exam may need to be scheduled over several meetings.
- Make safety a priority. If your patient cannot tolerate or perform what is expected for the exam, adapt the exam to meet his or her needs.
- Take the time to explain to your patient everything you are doing.

Toolbox

To perform the physical exam, you will need all the tools of assessment.

Physical Assessment

SYSTEM/AREA, APPROACH, AND NORMAL FINDINGS	ABNORMAL FINDINGS
Integumentary: Inspection, Palpation *Skin*	
Skin color uneven in areas, increased creases, wrinkle lines, and skin lesions. Some common skin lesions include seborrheic keratosis, lentigines (liver spots), and acrochordons. Senile purpura commonly found on hands and forearms is caused by frail capillaries.	Areas of pressure or pressure sores from immobility or splints/appliances. Body folds may develop intertrigo (inflammatory, moist erythema and scaling lesions) or fungal infections. Table 18.3 describes common skin lesions associated with aging.

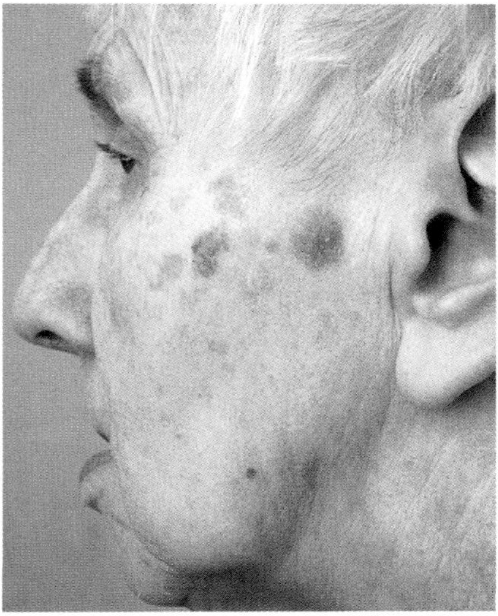

Seborrheic keratosis

(box continued on page 490)

Physical Assessment (continued)

SYSTEM/AREA, APPROACH, AND NORMAL FINDINGS	ABNORMAL FINDINGS

Integumentary: Inspection, Palpation
Skin (cont'd)

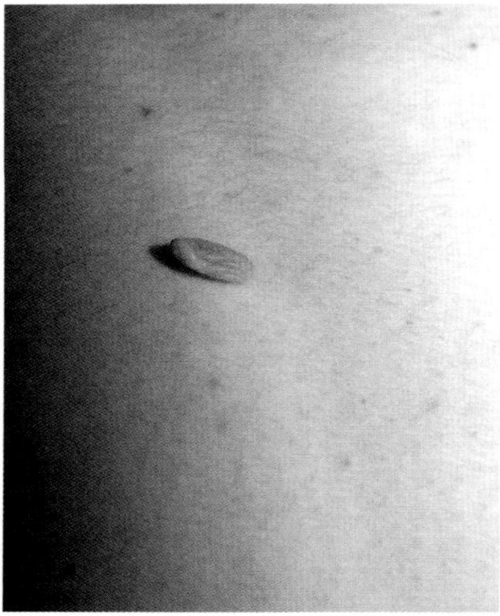

Acrochordon

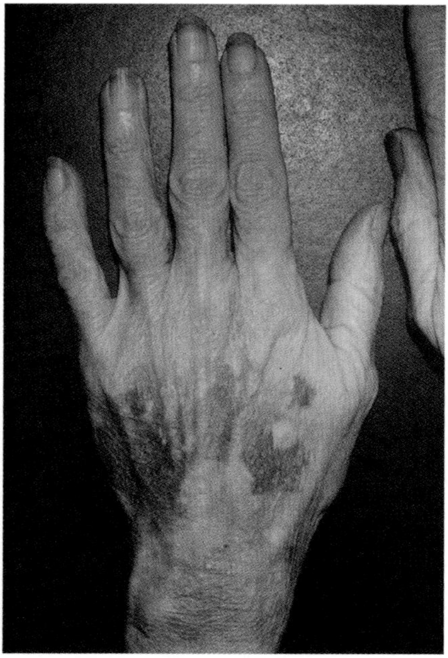

Senile purpura (normal)

SYSTEM/AREA, APPROACH, AND NORMAL FINDINGS	ABNORMAL FINDINGS
Temperature: Warm, but hands and feet may be cool.	Cool extremities may signal vascular disease. Unilateral cool temperature may indicate an occlusion and warrants medical attention.
Turgor: Normally decreased. Not a marker of hydration status.	Decreased turgor increases risk for injury and skin breakdown.
Hydration and texture: Dry, flaky, and thin.	Excessive dryness may indicate dehydration.
Hair and Scalp	
Hair color and distribution: Graying in both sexes; thinning and balding especially in men. Increased facial hair (hirsutism) in women. Coarse, dry hair and dry flaky scalp (senile xerosis).	Changes in hair may also relate to endocrine problems or may occur as a side effect of medications.
Nails	
Yellow, dry, brittle nails with longitudinal ridges.	Yellow, thick nails may also be caused by vascular disease or a fungal infection.
HEENT: Inspection, Palpation *Head/Neck*	
May have decreased range of motion (ROM) caused by musculoskeletal changes.	Decreased ROM of the neck may also be associated with DJD.
Lymph Nodes	
Lymph tissue decreases in size with aging and should be nonpalpable.	Palpable nodes warrant referral.
Thyroid	
Nonpalpable.	Palpable thyroid may signal thyroid disease (common in older patients) and warrants referral.
Temporal Artery	
Palpable and nontender.	Pain, nodularity, and presence of a pulse may indicate temporal arteritis.
Eyes	
Presbyopia may cause difficulty reading. Far vision may be intact.	Loss of peripheral vision, halos, and eye pain may indicate glaucoma and warrant referral. Loss of central vision may indicate macular degeneration.
Decreased peripheral vision.	Visual changes may also occur with cerebrovascular disease.

(box continued on page 492)

Physical Assessment (continued)

SYSTEM/AREA, APPROACH, AND NORMAL FINDINGS	ABNORMAL FINDINGS
HEENT: Inspection, Palpation *Eyes (cont'd)*	
Dry eyes.	
Enophthalmos (recession of eyeball into orbit).	Basal cell carcinoma frequently found on inner third of lower lid.
Arcus senilis (white to yellow deposit at outer edge of the iris), along with xanthelasma (yellowish, raised tumor on upper or lower lids).	Yellow or opaque lens associated with increased incidence of cataracts.
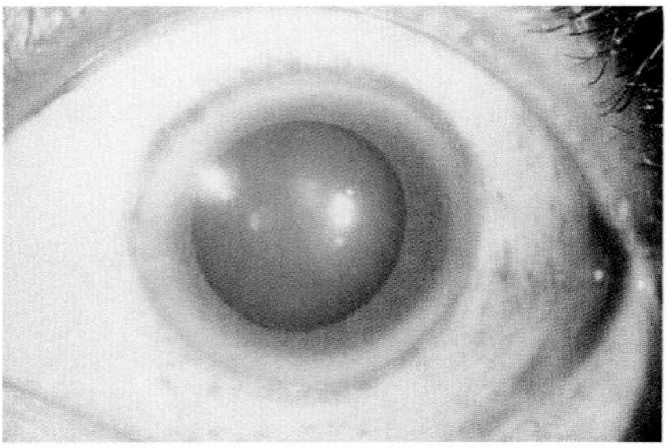 *Arcus senilis*	
Senile entropion (inversion of the lids and lashes).	Entropion increases the risk of corneal abrasions.
Senile ectropion (eversion of the lids and lashes).	Ectropion increases risk of dryness and conjunctivitis.
Xanthelasma (lipid deposits) on lids.	Macular degeneration.
Pale or yellow-tinted conjunctiva; pale iris; pingueculae (clear to yellow fleshy lesion on conjunctiva).	
Pterygium: Similar to pingueculae, but extends over cornea.	
Increased stimulation needed to elicit corneal reflex.	
Small pupils; reaction equal but may be less brisk.	
Funduscopic—Retina and optic disc paler.	Check for diabetic and hypertensive retinal changes; their incidence increases with age.
Ears *Internal*	
Gross hearing is intact but diminished with decreased pitch discrimination.	Balance problems and tinnitus may indicate a neurologic problem.
Potential conductive hearing loss (presbycusis).	
Increased difficulty hearing high-pitched sounds, especially, "s," "t," "f," and "g."	

SYSTEM/AREA, APPROACH, AND NORMAL FINDINGS	ABNORMAL FINDINGS
Difficulty understanding speech. Equilibrium-balance problems.	Balance problems increase risk for falls and injury.
External	
Lobes elongate. Increased external ear canal hair in men.	Dry ears with scratch marks related to senile pruritus.
Otoscopic	
Dry cerumen.	Cerumen impaction can decrease hearing acuity by 40 to 45 dB; removal of cerumen corrects the impairment.
Diminished cone of light.	Hearing aids can cause contact dermatitis.
Nose	
Elongated nose. Increased nasal hair. Decreased sense of smell (cranial nerve [CN] I).	Vasomotor rhinitis causes pale nasal mucosa and boggy turbinates.
Mouth and Throat	
"Purse-string" appearance of mouth. Teeth may show staining, chipping, or erosion.	Gum recession and bleeding (atrophic gingivitis).
Some teeth may be loose or missing. Buccal mucosa and gums thin and pale. Oral mucosa dry, causing halitosis.	Chewing and swallowing difficulty may be caused by poor dentition or poorly fitted dentures, or by more serious problem such as stroke.
Decreased sense of taste (CNs VII and IX). Decreased gag reflex (CNs IX and X). Decreased papillae on tongue. Varicose veins under tongue (caviar spots).	Leukoplakia (white precancerous lesion) in mouth, particularly under tongue.
Respiratory: Inspection, Palpation, Auscultation	
Senile kyphosis (increased anterior to posterior diameter) caused by musculoskeletal changes, barrel chest appearance. Decreased respiratory excursion. Cheyne-Stokes breathing may occur during sleep. Breath sounds may be decreased with few atelectatic crackles.	Respiratory changes increase risk for pulmonary problems, such as pneumonia.

(box continued on page 494)

Physical Assessment (continued)

SYSTEM/AREA, APPROACH, AND NORMAL FINDINGS	ABNORMAL FINDINGS
Cardiovascular: Inspection, Palpation, Auscultation	
Increase in premature beats and irregular pulse. Decreased pedal pulses.	Increased incidence of vascular disease. If present, carotid bruit and thrills may be detected.
Stiffer arteries.	Increased varicosities.
Slight increases in blood pressure and wider pulse pressure.	*Abnormal heart sounds:* Rate irregular with ectopic beats, S_4 common, systolic murmurs associated with aortic stenosis.
Orthostatic drops in blood pressure more common in older adults.	Differentiate arterial insufficiency from venous insufficiency.
Gastrointestinal: Inspection, Palpation, Percussion, Auscultation	
Bowel sounds may be slightly decreased.	Bruits may be heard over stenotic arteries or aneurysms with palpable enlarged aorta.
Abdomen very soft because of decreased musculature, so organs may be easier to palpate.	Dullness over bladder may signal urinary retention; dullness over bowel may signal stool retention. Do a follow up physical exam to determine that dullness is not caused by tumor.
Rectal examination: Stool negative for occult blood; no fecal impaction; prostate soft and smooth and not enlarged.	Palpable bladder with retention. Palpable intestines if filled with stool. A pulsatile mass in the abdomen may be an aneurysm. Incidence of abdominal aortic aneurysms increases with age. An aneurysm may have lateral as well as anteroposterior pulsation. Aneurysms are usually wider than 3 cm and often have an associated bruit. Surgical evaluation may be appropriate, particularly if aneurysm is greater than 5 cm.

SYSTEM/AREA, APPROACH, AND NORMAL FINDINGS	ABNORMAL FINDINGS
	Incidence of colorectal cancer peaks between ages 85 and 92 and accounts for 20 percent of all cancers found in people age 90 and above. Benign prostatic hypertrophy and prostatic cancer increase with age. If prostate feels abnormal, refer patient for urological evaluation.
Genitourinary: Inspection, Palpation *Urinary*	
Incontinence is a common problem. Evaluate urinary incontinence with the Pad test: With full bladder, have patient cough forcefully three times while standing. No leakage is normal.	Leakage of urine indicates stress incontinence. In urinary retention, bladder may be palpable above the symphysis pubis after voiding. You will also percuss dullness above the symphysis pubis after patient voids.
Female Reproductive	
Decreased elasticity, breast sag, cordlike feel to breasts. Decrease in and graying of pubic hair. External genitalia decrease in size, and skin becomes thin, inelastic, and shiny. Pelvic exam reveals pale vaginal walls, narrow, thick, glistening cervix as a result of decreased estrogen. Uterus and ovaries decrease in size. Ovaries should not be palpable.	Palpable ovaries, masses, rectocele, cystocele, or prolapsed uterus require referral.
Male Reproductive	
Gynecomastia may be seen. Decrease and graying of pubic hair. Scrotum and penis decrease in size. Testes hang lower and have fewer rugae.	Any mass requires referral.

(box continued on page 496)

Physical Assessment (continued)

SYSTEM/AREA, APPROACH, AND NORMAL FINDINGS	ABNORMAL FINDINGS
Musculoskeletal: Inspection, Palpation About half of people over 65 have decreased arm swing during gait; a wider base of support; a decline in step length, stride length, and ankle ROM; decreased vertical and increased horizontal head excursions; decrease in spinal rotation and arm swing; increased length of double support phase of walking, and a reduction in propulsive force generalized at the push-off phase. Decrease in sensory input, slowing of motor responses, and musculoskeletal limitations result in an increase in unsteadiness or postural sway under both static and dynamic conditions.	Musculoskeletal changes associated with aging increase the risk for falls and injury.

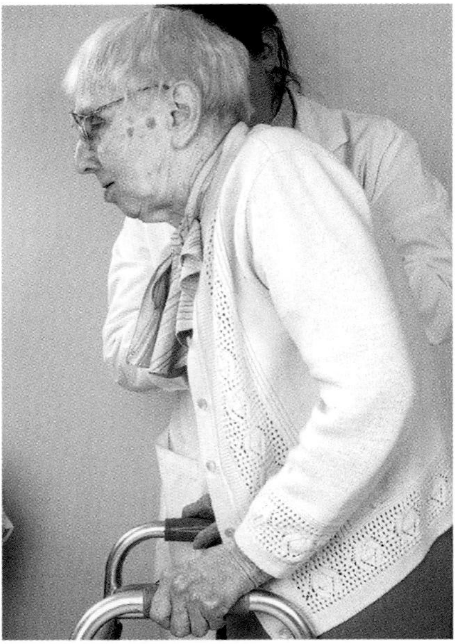

Thoracic curvature (senile kyphosis)

SYSTEM/AREA, APPROACH, AND NORMAL FINDINGS	ABNORMAL FINDINGS
ROM decreased.	Heberden's nodes, involving the distal interphalangeal joints, are commonly seen with osteoarthritis but are rarely inflamed.

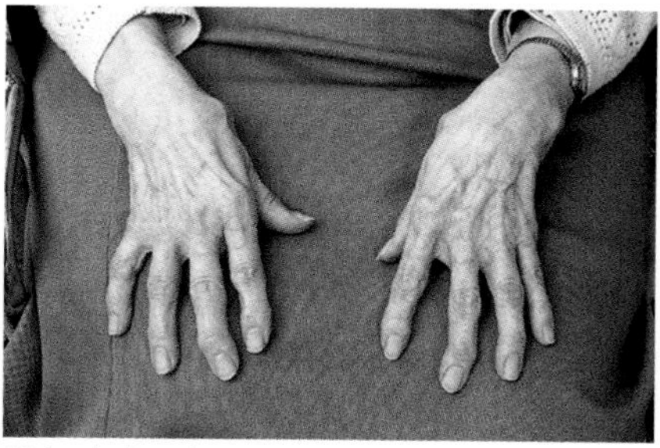

Heberden's nodes

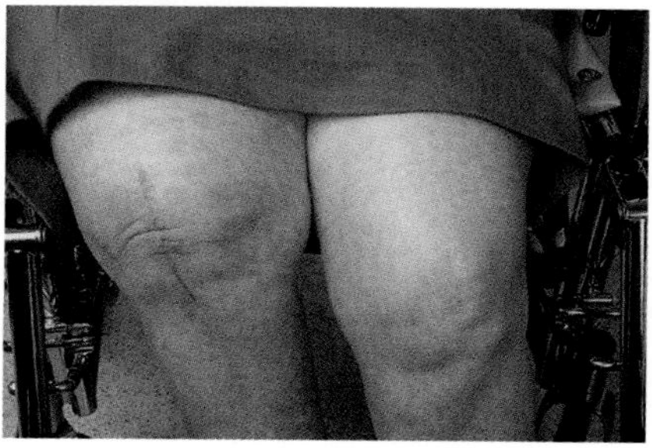

DJD (osteoarthritis)

SYSTEM/AREA, APPROACH, AND NORMAL FINDINGS	ABNORMAL FINDINGS
Crepitation, stiffness with ROM.	Asymmetrical decrease in strength and tone may be associated with transient ischemic attack (TIA) or stroke.

(box continued on page 498)

Physical Assessment (continued)

SYSTEM/AREA, APPROACH, AND NORMAL FINDINGS	ABNORMAL FINDINGS
Musculoskeletal: Inspection, Palpation *(cont'd)*	
Decreased muscle strength and tone. Muscle strength depends on muscle mass. Strong equal hand grip usually remains intact.	Diabetes-related ulcerations, fungal infections of the feet or toenails, calluses, bunions, hallux valgus, and other deformities are very common and can affect function.

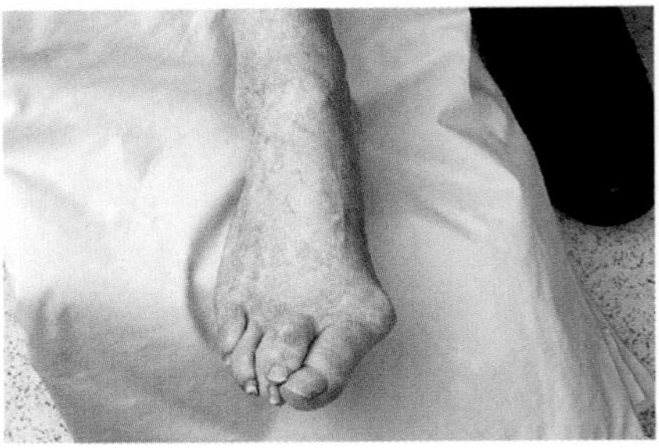

Hallux valgus and bunions

SYSTEM/AREA, APPROACH, AND NORMAL FINDINGS	ABNORMAL FINDINGS
Shoes fit well, wear evenly. No lesions, calluses, or deviations noted. Toenails well groomed.	
Neurologic: Inspection *Mental Status*	
Cognitive ability intact; benign forgetfulness; short-term memory and long-term memory for new information may decrease with age.	Confusion may be caused by delirium, an underlying dementia, or depression. These conditions may be difficult to differentiate and may occur independently or together. Patients with dementia will work hard to answer questions and confabulate answers. Delirium causes difficulty concentrating on the questions and attending to the task. Patients with depression are often unwilling to try to complete the task or answer the question. Detection of dementia, delirium, or depression warrants referral. Several bedside screening tools are available to differentiate between dementia, delirium, and depression and to evaluate cognitive function. See Box 18.5 for the Clock Scoring Test.

SYSTEM/AREA, APPROACH, AND NORMAL FINDINGS	ABNORMAL FINDINGS
Cranial Nerves	
Slower response time bilaterally. CN I Olfactory—Decreased. CN II Optic—Decreased visual acuity, presbyopia, funduscopic changes. CN III Oculomotor—Pupils smaller and reaction to light not as brisk. Extraocular movements should remain intact: • CN III Oculomotor. • CN IV Trochlear. • CN VI Abducens. CN V Trigeminal—Increased stimulation needed to elicit corneal reflex. CN VII Facial—Decreased taste. CN VIII Acoustic—Presbycusis, increased loss of high-pitched sounds progresses to loss of all frequencies. CN IX Glossopharyngeal—Decreased taste. CN X Vagus—Decreased gag reflex. CN XI Spinoaccessory—No change, but ROM and strength depend on musculoskeletal changes. CN XII Hypoglossal—No change.	Diminished response time on only one side warrants further investigation.
Neurological/Muscle Function Movements	
+Drifting with minimal weakness.	Tremors common in older patients.
No abnormal movements.	Types include: • Postural or physiological—Benign fine tremors. • Intention, essential, familial, and senile—Visible tremor associated with intentional movements, diminishes with rest. • Rest—Visible tremor at rest but absent/diminished with movement; "pill-rolling"; associated with Parkinson's disease. • Action—Large, irregular tremors of limbs, associated with cerebellar dysfunction (e.g., multiple sclerosis).

(box continued on page 500)

Physical Assessment (continued)

SYSTEM/AREA, APPROACH, AND NORMAL FINDINGS	ABNORMAL FINDINGS
Neurologic: Inspection *(cont'd)* *Cerebellar Function*	
Slight increase in swaying—Romberg's sign.	Loss of balance may be associated with Parkinson's disease.
Reflexes: Percussion	
Deep tendon reflex may be increased or decreased (+1 or +3).	Asymmetrical reflexes may indicate an underlying problem.
Achilles reflex more difficult to elicit. May need to use reinforcement techniques to elicit response. Superficial abdominal reflexes disappear with age.	
Older adults may demonstrate the release of some primitive reflexes, including the snout, glabellar, and palmomental.	Positive primitive reflexes may also indicate a severe neurologic assault.

HEENT = Head, eyes, ears, nose, and throat.

TABLE 18.3 Common Skin Lesions Associated With Aging

SKIN LESION	DESCRIPTION
Lentigines	Hyperpigmented macular lesions (liver spots)
Ichthyosis	Dry, scaly, fishlike skin
Acrochordons	Small, benign polyp-growths (skin tags)
Actinic keratosis	Rough precancerous skin macule or papule from sun exposure
Seborrheic keratosis	Benign pigmented lesions with a waxy surface on face and trunk
Senile purpura	Vascular lesion of ecchymoses and petechiae on arms and legs caused by the frail nature of capillaries and decreased collagen support
Venous lakes	Bluish-black papular vascular lesions
Senile ectasias	Red-purple macular or papular lesions (senile or cherry angiomas)
Basal cell carcinoma	Pearly, papular or plaquelike cancerous lesions that may be ulcerated in the center; associated with sun exposure
Squamous cell carcinoma	Erythematous, indurated areas that may be scaly or hyperkeratotic; associated with sun exposure, and tend to grow more rapidly than basal cell

BOX 18.5 Clock Scoring

Give the patient a paper and ask her or him to draw a circle. Instruct her or him to draw the face of a clock inside the circle, putting the numbers in the correct positions. Then ask her or him to draw the hands to indicate 10 minutes after 11 or 20 minutes after 8.

Scoring:

Assign 1 point for each of the following:

- Draws closed circle
- Places numbers in correct positions
- Includes all 12 numbers in correct positions
- Places clock hands in correct positions

There are no specific cutoff scores. If performance on clock drawing is impaired, consider a complete diagnostic evaluation for dementia.

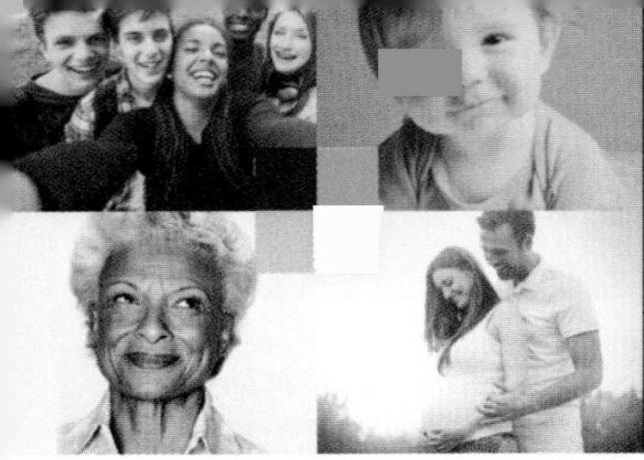

CHAPTER 19

Assessing the Homeless Person

The components of the health history and physical exam are the same as for other patients. However, when dealing with homeless patients, your approach and focus will differ.

Approach and Focus

- Provide unconditional positive regard for the homeless patient.
- Be accepting and nonjudgmental.
- Listen.
- Be sensitive to the reality of the homeless situation.
- Be direct in your communication with the patient.
- Ask permission to touch the patient. (Physical privacy may be one of the few prerogatives the patient has left.)
- Focus more on addressing an immediate problem than on getting a complete history and physical exam.
- Use event markers for time periods; days, months, and years may not be meaningful to the homeless person.
- Schedule healthcare appointments early in the day because shelter management requires a person to be present in the afternoon to secure a bed for the night. "Claiming a bed" may take priority over healthcare.
- Respond accurately and simply if the homeless person expresses concern about how his or her personal revelations are recorded and how the information will be used.
- Realize that the homeless person may be homeless by choice, be impatient, refuse to make eye contact, take a long time to respond, express minor complaints such as headache, not have a mailing address or contact person, and see healthcare needs and priorities differently from you.

Health History

AREA/TYPES OF QUESTIONS	SIGNIFICANCE
Biographical Data	
Ask where patient is staying.	Less threatening to ask than "What is your address?" Questions about family members, telephone numbers, or additional demographic data may not be appropriate and may be met with silence. May also be reluctant to identify government agencies.
Current Health Survey	
Ask about injuries first.	Patient may synthesize life and environmental factors to explain symptoms in ways that may not have occurred to you. Begin with questions about injuries; this may be a marker for time in an unstructured life.
Ask about symptoms of communicable diseases that may not have been reported.	Increased risk for communicable diseases as a result of crowded living quarters.
Ask about respiratory diseases, such as tuberculosis (TB).	Risk is high for those who sleep in close quarters in shelters or crowded spaces.
Ask about dermatological problems such as lesions, infestation.	No change of socks, no clean clothes, exposure to extremes, poor hygiene, living in close quarters increase risk.
Past Health History	
Ask about past injuries, infections, communicable diseases, hospitalizations, substance abuse, and psychiatric problems.	Determines compliance or completion of treatment and follow-up.
Family History	
	May not want to discuss family.
Review of Systems	
Ask about problems in the following systems that you may have missed in the current health survey.	Homeless patients are at increased risk for the problems identified by system below.

(continued)

AREA/TYPES OF QUESTIONS	SIGNIFICANCE
Integumentary	Skin problems: Scabies, lice.
HEENT	Ear and eye problems with children; dental problems with all ages.
Respiratory	Upper respiratory infection (URI), TB.
Cardiovascular	Hypertension (HTN).
Gastrointestinal	Poor nutrition complications **Alcohol abuse increases risk for gastrointestinal (GI) disorders and poor nutrition.**
Genitourinary	*Women:* Pregnancy, lack of prenatal care. Sexually transmitted diseases (STDs).
Musculoskeletal/ Neurologic	Neurologic and psychiatric disorders.
Hematological/ Immune/Endocrine	Anemia related to dietary deficiency, human immunodeficiency virus (HIV)/ acquired immunodeficiency syndrome (AIDS); diabetes.
Psychosocial Profile	
Health Practices and Beliefs	Give patient opportunity to present positive aspects of life. Acknowledging positive behaviors may help establish bond between you and patient. Barriers to healthcare and limited resources limit preventive behaviors. Patient's healthcare practices are often crisis or problem oriented and treated symptomatically. Follow-up is difficult.
Typical Day	May consist of being on feet all day, looking for food and a place to sleep.
Nutritional Patterns	Nutrition is a problem. Tell patient about available resources (e.g., food stamps, soup kitchens).

AREA/TYPES OF QUESTIONS	SIGNIFICANCE
Activity and Exercise Patterns	Center on survival and meeting basic needs.
Sleep/Rest Patterns	Finding a safe place to sleep is a problem.
Personal Habits	Substance abuse and associated health problems are common among homeless people, but do not assume this is the case with your patient. Ask, "Do you smoke, drink alcohol, or use drugs?" If the answer is yes, ask "How much?"
Occupational Health Patterns	Patient may be working, but income may not be sufficient to maintain housing.
Socioeconomic Status	Homelessness denotes low socioeconomic status, poverty. Ask if patient is a veteran. Identify available resources and make appropriate referrals.
Environmental Health Patterns	Thermoregulatory problems (hypothermia or hyperthermia) resulting from exposure. Alcohol increases risk for hypothermia. Using fire to keep warm increases risk for burns. Because the homeless person often wears everything he or she owns, risk for heat exhaustion, heat stroke, and dehydration increases in warm weather. Increased risk for being a victim of crime, robbery, assault, and rape.
Roles/Relationships/ Self-Concept	Low self-esteem, anxiety, and depression are common.
Cultural Influences	Can be seen in both legal and illegal immigrants. Many groups have high poverty rates (e.g., 30% of Hispanics live in poverty). In homeless, language barriers can also add to problem of accessing healthcare.

(continued)

AREA/TYPES OF QUESTIONS	SIGNIFICANCE
Religious Influences	Faith-based organizations are often major service providers for basic needs. Spiritual support may be integrated.
Sexuality Patterns	Homeless patient may still be sexually active and in a committed relationship. Ask, " Are you sexually active? With men, women, or both? Do you have genital itching, burning, or other symptoms?" Ask if patient is a victim of abuse—50 percent of homeless women with children have been victims of domestic abuse.

HEENT = Head, eyes, ears, nose, and throat.

Physical Assessment

Conduct the physical assessment using tools and techniques appropriate for the age and gender of the patient. Use gloves if risk for exposure to bodily fluids exists; otherwise, direct touch can convey trust. With the homeless patient, the customary head-to-toe approach may not be practical. Close, face-to-face contact at the beginning of the exam may be seen as invasive or threatening by the patient. Simply reverse the order, working from toe to head. This also minimizes the power position of the nurse standing over the patient, giving directions while performing the exam.

Pay special attention to the patient's feet. The homeless are at risk for foot problems because they are often on their feet most of the day, wearing poorly fitting shoes with no change of socks. Regardless of your findings, the act of touching and examining the feet demonstrates a thoroughness of approach and simple caring.

Also keep in mind that the homeless person may have all of her or his possessions on her or his person and may be reluctant to remove clothes. Assure the person that her or his clothing and belongings will be safe, and allow her or him to keep personal items.

The table below outlines a thorough physical assessment of a homeless patient. Instead of performing a total assessment, you will usually focus on a specific area identified as a problem from the history data. Be as thorough as necessary to meet your patient's health needs and as thorough as your patient permits.

AREA	SIGNIFICANCE
General Health Survey	
Inspect general appearance, signs of injury, dress and grooming.	May have signs of injury—Homeless people are more vulnerable to crime. Poor hygiene resulting from lack of resources may warrant referral.
Note any odors.	Body odors may be caused by poor hygiene or alcohol abuse.
Take vital signs: temperature, respirations, blood pressure (BP).	Hypothermia or hyperthermia from exposure often present. Upper respiratory problems common. HTN is chronic health problem.
Integumentary	
Inspect skin for lesions, color changes; inspect hair for infestation.	Lice or scabies caused by crowded living conditions.
Inspect feet for lesions and edema.	High incidence of hepatitis related to intravenous (IV) drug use. Cirrhosis related to alcohol abuse. Minor skin problems common. Poor wound healing because of poor nutrition. Being on feet most of day increases risk for peripheral-vascular disease (PVD). Diabetes is also a chronic problem.
Inspect mouth and throat.	Dental problems and URIs common among homeless.
Respiratory	
Auscultate lungs.	Respiratory problems and TB common.
Cardiovascular	
Palpate peripheral pulses.	PVD common.
Auscultate heart for normal and extra sounds.	HTN common.
Gastrointestinal	
Auscultate bowel sounds.	GI problems common.
Palpate abdomen.	Cirrhosis, pancreatitis associated with alcohol abuse common.

(continued)

AREA	SIGNIFICANCE
Genitourinary	
Inspect genitalia.	Homeless people, especially women, are susceptible to rape, increasing risk for STDs and pregnancy.
Musculoskeletal	
Inspect and palpate muscles.	Homeless people are susceptible to trauma from beatings.
Neurologic	
Assess mental status.	Head trauma may result from beatings. Substance abuse (drugs and alcohol) can affect neurologic status. Seizures can result from trauma and substance abuse. Psychiatric problems common, including depression, schizophrenia, and organic brain syndrome.

HEENT = Head, eyes, ears, nose, and throat.

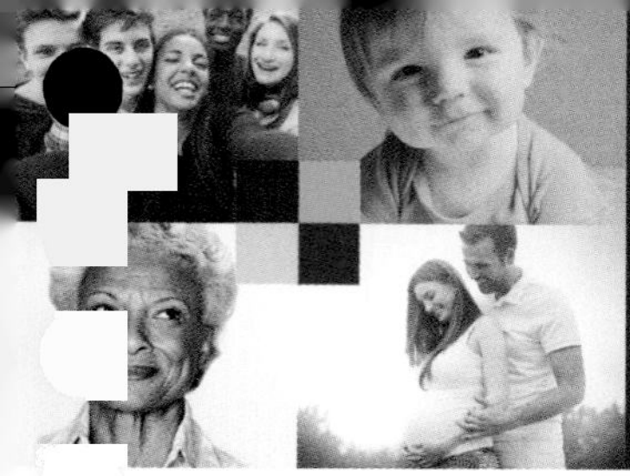

CHAPTER 20

Assessing Pain

Although pain is referred to as the fifth vital sign, it is a symptom. Subjective in nature, pain is "whatever the person says it is, whenever s/he says it does" (McCaffery, 1999). Types of pain are described in Table 20.1.

Mechanism of Pain

- **Transduction** is response to noxious stimuli.
- **Transmission** is activation of nociceptors; a nerve impulse is transmitted to the spinal cord and brain.
- **Perception** is awareness of pain. The pain threshold is the point where stimulus is perceived as pain. This is consistent from one person to next.
- **Pain tolerance** is the amount of pain one is able to endure. This differs from one person to the next.
- **Modulation** is the modulation of nerve transmissions, such as inhibition, (for example, gate control theory of pain modulation: After stubbing a toe, a person will automatically rub the toe. The rubbing sensation is transmitted through the fast delta fibers, while the impulse from stubbing the toe travels along the slow C-fibers and is blocked.
- **Sensitization** can be peripheral or central.
  - Peripheral sensitization occurs with prolonged exposure to noxious stimuli. This lowers the threshold of pain, leading to hyperalgesia (increased response to pain) and allodynia (painful response to non-painful stimuli).
  - Central sensitization occurs with prolonged exposure to noxious stimuli with spinal neuron hyper excitability, and results in hyperalgesia and allodynia.
  - Sensitization can be a protective mechanism during healing, but if it persists, it can lead to chronic pain.

TABLE 20.1 Types of Pain

TYPE	CAUSE	DURATION	EFFECTS	EXAMPLES
Acute	• Injury or pathology. • Nociception and or sensitized central neurons.	• Self-limiting, resolves with healing. • Continuous or intermittent.	• Activates autonomic nervous system, such as increased heart rate, respirations, BP, diaphoresis. • Dilated pupils. • Protective responses, such as rubbing or guarding area of pain.	• Trauma • Medical or surgical procedures. • Labor. • Acute disease.
Chronic	• May or may not be associated with pathology. • Weak connection between cause and extent of pain. • May be nociceptive, neuropathic, or both.	• Persists beyond expected healing time. • Remote from the original cause. • Continuous, intermittent with or without acute exacerbation.	• Parasympathetic response. • Normal vital signs. • Dry, warm skin. • Depressed and withdrawn. • No protective behaviors.	• Injury. • Malignant conditions. • Chronic non–life-threatening diseases such as arthritis.
Cancer/malignant	• Associated with underlying malignancy, diagnostic procedure, or disease treatment.	• May be acute or chronic. • Pain level strongly correlates with the degree of pathology.	• Variable depending on location and duration.	• Malignancy and associated diagnostic tests and treatments.

TYPE	CAUSE	DURATION	EFFECTS	EXAMPLES
Chronic noncancer pain	• Weak connection between cause and extent of pain. • Associated with chronic disease or no identifiable cause. • Pain becomes disease.	• Prolonged. • Possibly life-long.	• Pain, ranging from mild to excruciating and possibly affecting any system or region.	• Osteoarthritis. • Low back pain. • Myofascial pain. • Fibromyalgia. • Headaches. • Central pain. • Chronic abdominal pain. • Sickle cell disease. • Complete regional pain syndrome. • Phantom limb pain. • Peripheral neuropathy. • Neuralgias.
Chronic pain syndrome	Chronic pain that consumes and incapacitates patient.	• Prolonged. • Possibly life-long.	• Psychosocial dysfunction, such as anger, depression, anxiety, substance abuse. • May stress personal and work relationships. • Life centers on obtaining pain relief.	

Developmental Considerations

Infants

Since the infant cannot verbalize pain, physiological and behavior indicators are used to assess for pain in the infant.

A good rule of thumb to remember when assessing for pain in an infant who is nonverbal is "whatever is painful for you, would most likely be painful for the infant/child" (Wong, 2001).

Infant physiological changes associated with pain include:

- *Integumentary system:* Pallor or flushing, diaphoresis, palmar sweating.
- *Cardiovascular:* Increased heart rate, increased blood pressure (BP).
- *Respiratory:* Rapid, shallow respirations, decreased arterial oxygen saturation and transcutaneous oxygen saturation.
- *Musculoskeletal:* Increased muscle tone.
- *Neurologic:* Increased intracranial pressure, dilated pupils, decreased vagal nerve tone.
- *Endocrine (hormonal release):* Increased catecholamines, growth hormones, glucagon, cortisol, corticosteroids, and aldosterone.
- *Metabolism:* Increased plasma lactate, pyruvate, ketone bodies, and fatty acids.
- *Laboratory values:* Increased blood glucose (hyperglycemia) and corticosteroid levels and decreased pH.

Infant behavioral changes associated with pain include:

- *Vocalization:* Intense, sustained crying; whimpering; and groaning.
- *Facial expression:* Eye squeeze, brow bulge, open mouth, taut tongue, chin quivering, and grimaces.
- *Body movements:* Limb withdrawal, thrashing, rigidity or flaccidity, and fist clenching.
- *Sleep/wake cycle:* Increased wakefulness and irritability.
- *Feeding:* Loss of appetite, vomiting, loss of interest and/or energy in sucking.
- *Activity level:* Decreased activity level; fussiness, irritability, and listlessness (Wong, 2001).

Children

Depending on the age of the child, assessing pain in children can be a challenge. The mnemonic QUESTT is helpful in assessing pain in children (Wong, 2001).

- Q = Question the child.
- U = Use a pain rating scale.

- E = Evaluate behavioral and physiological changes.
- S = Secure parents' involvement.
- T = Take cause of pain into account.
- T = Take action and evaluate results.

Question the Child

Self-report is the most accurate means for assessing pain, so ask the child to describe the pain. Self-report is more accurate than the child's behavior.

When questioning a child, it's often helpful to use these techniques:

- Use language the child will understand, such as "boo-boo."
- Use toys to enable the child to identify painful area by asking the child to show you where it hurts on a doll or puppet, having the child draw a picture of pain, or identifying the painful area with crayon on a drawing of human figure.

Use a Pain Rating Scale

Various pain rating scales are available for assessing pain in children. Be sure to select one that is age appropriate for your patient.

Evaluate Behavioral and Physiological Changes

If the child is nonverbal, unable to describe pain, detecting behavioral and/or physiological changes is essential. Physiological changes that may be seen with acute pain include increased BP, increased or decreased heart rate, increased respirations, flushing, sweating, and dilated pupils. Behavioral changes for a young child include crying, screaming, vocalizing hurt, thrashing of arms and legs, pushing away, clinging to parents, and increasing restlessness and irritability. Behavioral changes for a school-age child include crying, muscle rigidity, clenched fists, white knuckles, clenched teeth, closed eyes, and stalling techniques when anticipating a painful procedure. Behavioral changes for an adolescent include verbalization of pain and muscle tension.

Secure Parents' Involvement

Parents know their child, so rely on their assessment. Parents are more in tuned to subtle changes in their child's behavior. And, parents usually know what will best comfort their child.

Ask the parent:

- What is the child's past experience with pain?
- What is child's response to pain?

- How do you know your child is having pain?
- What relieves child's pain?

Take the Cause of Pain Into Account

Consider the pathophysiology of the underlying problem when evaluating the child's pain.

Take Action and Evaluate Results

After assessing the pain, develop a plan to treat the pain. After treating pain, you need to assess the child to evaluate the effectiveness of the treatment and revise the plan as needed.

Older Adults

It is important to realize that the elderly do experience pain both acute and chronic. Untreated pain increases the risk for complications such as pneumonia, constipation, deep vein thrombosis, impaired immune function, sleep disturbances, weight loss, social isolation, and depression. Often, the older patient experiences chronic pain and does not exhibit the typical signs of pain. Questions about the patient's functional level and quality of life are good indicators of the effects of pain.

If the patient is cognitively impaired, assessing for pain becomes a greater challenge. The degree of impairment will determine the use of pain scales. Keep questions simple, specific, and in the here and now. If the patient is unable to verbally communicate, rely on physiological signs—such as increased BP, heart rate, and respirations; diaphoresis; and behavioral changes, such as agitation, restlessness, facial expression of pain, and vocal sounds (moaning and groaning) of pain—associated with pain.

Cultural Considerations

Although the physiological response to pain is consistent across cultures, your patient's cultural/ethnic background influences his or her psychological and behavioral responses to pain.

CULTURE	RESPONSE TO PAIN
African American	• Pain a sign of illness or disease. • Absence of pain may affect compliance with treatment, for example, may not take medication as prescribed unless pain present. • Pain is seen as inevitable and must be endured. • Spiritual and religious beliefs account for high tolerance to pain. • Persistent pain associated with little faith. • Prayer and laying on of hands used to treat pain.
Appalachian	• Pain is endured and stoically accepted. • Expects to be cared for when experiencing pain. • Believes use of objects can rid pain, for example, knife or ax under the bed to "cut out" pain.
Arab American	• Pain seen as unpleasant and something to be controlled. • Expression of pain more reserved with strangers while more expressive with family, sends conflicting perceptions of pain. • Confidence in Western medicine, expects immediate relief of pain.
Chinese American	• Description of pain more diverse in terms of body symptoms such as pain more dull and diffuse. • Explain pain from the traditional influences of imbalances in yin and yang. • Cope with pain using oils, massage, warmth, sleeping on affected area, relaxation, and aspirin.
Cuban American	• Pain sign of physical problem that warrants traditional or biomedical healer. • Response to pain very expressive, for example, crying, moaning, groaning, and seen as pain-relieving function.
Egyptian American	• Avoids pain and seeks prompt treatment. • Expression of pain more reserved with strangers while more expressive with family, sends conflicting perceptions of pain. • Description of pain more generalized. • Age and birth order correlate with individual responses and description of pain, for example, younger children and first-born more expressive about pain. • Helpful to have close family member present during pain episodes, preferably woman who is seen as more nurturing, caring, and capable of comforting patient in pain.

(continued)

CULTURE	RESPONSE TO PAIN
Filipino American	• Pain seen as part of living honorable life. • Pain seen as means to atone for past transgressions and achieve fuller spiritual life. • Response to pain stoic and tolerant of high degree of pain. • May need to encourage use of pain interventions. • May use prayer in pain management.
French Canadian	• Pain described as more intense and more affectively described.
Greek American	• Pain, "ponos," cardinal symptom of ill health. • Pain considered evil and needs to be eradicated. • Family relied on to find resources to relieve pain. • Physical pain expressed publicly, but emotional pain kept within privacy of family.
Iranian	• Expressive about their pain. • Men more stoic than women in expressing pain. • May justify pain in light of later rewards after death.
Irish American	• Stoic response to pain, may ignore or minimize pain. • Denial of pain may delay treatment.
Jewish American	• Preservation of life paramount, therefore, would seek immediate treatment for pain. • Verbalization of pain is acceptable and common. • Wants not only relief from pain but also to know cause.
Mexican American	• Good health associated with being pain free. • Pain seen and accepted as necessary part of life. • Obligated to endure pain in performance of duties. • Type and amount of pain divinely predetermined. • Pain and suffering seen as consequence for immoral behavior. • Methods used to relieve pain maintain balance within person and environment. • Perceptions of pain may delay seeking treatment.
Navajo Native American	• Pain viewed as something to be endured, leading to inadequate pain control. • May use herbal medications to treat pain.
Vietnamese American	• Pain is endured, seen as part of life. • Cultural restraints against showing weakness limits use of pain medication.

Source: Purnell, L.D., and Paulanka, B.J. (2012). *Transcultural Healthcare: A Culturally Competent Approach*, 4th ed. Philadelphia: F.A. Davis.

Assessment

History

When your patient presents with pain, perform a symptom analysis. The mnemonic PQRST provides a thorough description of pain. Ask:

- **P = Precipitating/palliative/provocative factors**
  - What were you doing when the pain started?
  - Does anything make it better, such as medication or a certain position?
  - Does anything make it worse, such as movement or breathing?
- **Q = Quality/quantity**
  - What does it feel like?
    - *Superficial somatic pain* is sharp, pricking, or burning.
    - *Deep somatic pain* is dull or aching.
    - *Visceral pain* is dull, aching, or cramping.
    - *Neuropathic pain* is burning, shocklike, lancing, jabbing, squeezing, or aching.
  - How often are you experiencing it?
  - To what degree is the pain affecting your ability to perform your usual daily activities?
- **R = Region/radiation/related symptoms**
  - Can you point to where it hurts?
  - Does the pain occur or spread anywhere else?
    - *Localized pain* is confined to the site of origin, such as cutaneous pain.
    - *Referred pain* is referred to a distant structure, such as shoulder pain with acute cholecystitis or jaw pain associated with angina.
    - *Projected (transmitted) pain* is transmitted along a nerve, such as with herpes zoster or trigeminal neuralgia.
    - *Dermatomal pattern* as with peripheral neuropathic pain.
    - *Nondermatomal pattern* as with central neuropathic pain, fibromyalgia.
    - No recognizable pattern as with complex regional pain syndrome.
  - Do you have any other symptoms (e.g. nausea, dizziness, shortness of breath)?
    - *Visceral pain–related symptoms* include sickening feeling, nausea, vomiting, and autonomic symptoms.

  - *Neuropathic pain–related symptoms* include hyperalgesia and allodynia.
  - *Complex regional pain syndrome–related symptoms* include hyperalgesia, hyperesthesia, allodynia, autonomic changes and skin, hair, and nail changes.
- **S = Severity**
  - Use appropriate pain scale. (See pain scales below.)
- **T = Timing**
  - When did the pain begin?
  - How long did it last?
    - *Brief flash*: Quick pain as with needle stick.
    - *Rhythmic pulsation*: Pulsating pain as with migraine or toothache.
    - *Long-duration rhythmic*: As with intestinal colic.
    - *Plateau pain*: Pain that rises then plateaus, such as angina.
    - *Paroxysmal:* Such as neuropathic pain.
  - How often does it occur?
    - *Continuous fluctuating pain:* As with musculoskeletal pain.
  - Do you have times when you are pain-free?

Another mnemonic used to assess pain is OLDCART.

- O = Onset
- L = Location
- D = Duration
- C = Characteristics
- A = Aggravating factors
- R = Radiation
- T = Treatment

Pain Scales for Adults

Unidimensional and multidimensional pain scales are available. The unidimensional scale assesses one dimension, usually intensity of pain, and is often used to assess acute pain. Multidimensional scales provide additional information about pain such as the pain's characteristics and the effects on the patient's daily life. A multidimensional scale is useful in assessing chronic pain.

Unidimensional Scales

These scales usually use numerical, verbal, or visual descriptors to quantify pain. Examples include the Numerical Rating Scale, Visual Analogue Scale, and categorical scales.

- *Numerical Rating Scale:* The Numerical Rating Scale rates pain on a scale of 0 (no pain) to either 5 or 10 (worst pain) by asking the patient to rate her or his current pain level.

- *Visual Analogue Scale:* The Visual Analogue Scale utilizes a vertical or horizontal 10-cm line with anchors. One end of the line is labeled "No pain" and the opposite end of the line is labeled "Worst pain." The patient marks his or her current pain level on the line (Fig. 20.1).

[____]

0 cm (no pain) — 10 cm (worst pain)

Visual Analogue Scale

- *Categorical Scales:* Categorical scales use verbal or visual descriptors to identify pain intensity. The patient selects the descriptor that she or he feels best represents the current pain level. Verbal descriptors include:
  - Mild, discomforting, distressing, horrible, excruciating.
  - No pain, mild pain, moderate pain, severe pain, very severe pain, worst possible pain.

Visual descriptors include the Faces Pain Scale for Adults and Children (FPS), which utilizes illustrated faces with facial expressions ranging from happy (no pain) to sad and crying (worst pain). The FPS scale has eight faces to select current pain level. The patient is asked to select the face that best represents his or her current pain level.

Multidimensional Pain Scales

These scales assess pain characteristics and effects on patient's activities of daily living.

- *Initial Pain Assessment Inventory (IPAI):* The IPAI is used for initial assessment of pain. It assesses characteristics of pain; effects of pain on the patient's life, such as daily activities, sleep, appetite, relationships, and emotions; and the patient's expression of pain. This assessment tool includes a diagram to note pain location, a scale to rate pain intensity, and space to document additional comments and the treatment plan.
- *Brief Pain Inventory (BPI):* The BPI is used to quantify pain intensity and associated disability. It assesses pain intensity, location, effects on life, type and effectiveness of treatment over the last 24 hours. Benefits of the BPI include that it's quick and easy to use and available in multiple languages.
- *McGill Pain Questionnaire (MPQ):* The MPQ uses descriptive words to assess pain on three levels: sensory, affective and

evaluative. It can be used with other tools, and is available in short and long form.

- *Neuropathic Pain Scale:* The Neuropathic Pain Scale assesses the type and degree of sensations associated with neuropathic pain. The patient rates eight common qualities of neuropathic pain (sharp, dull, hot, cold, sensitive, itchy, deep, or surface pain) on a scale of 0 (no pain) to 10 (worst pain). This scale is still in the development stages, but early testing holds diagnostic and therapeutic promise.

Pain Scales for Children

Color Tool

This assessment tool assesses pain for children as young as 4 years by having the child create a body outline using colored markers or crayons. The child selects four colors. The first color represents "most hurt," the second represents "little hurt," the third represents "least hurt," and the last represents "no hurt." Using all four colors, the child identifies areas and degree of hurt on the body outline (Eland and Banner, 1999).

FACES Pain Rating Scale

This scale assesses pain for children ages 3 years and up. The Wong-Baker has five faces from which the child can select her or his current pain level (Fig. 20-2).

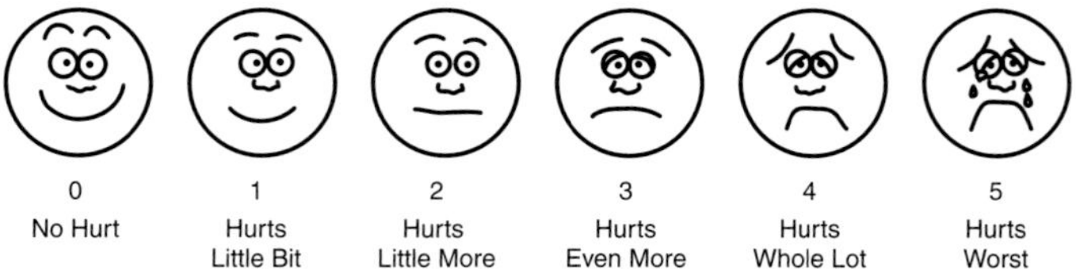

Wong-Baker Faces Scale

Numerical Scale

The Numerical Scale assesses pain for children ages 5 years and older (Fig. 20.4). It uses a horizontal linear scale with numbers from 0 to 5 or 10, with 0 being "no pain" and 5 or 10 being "worst pain." The child is asked to identify his or her current pain level on the scale. Although similar to a scale used for adults, this provides the child with a visual to help assess his or her pain.

No pain					Worst pain
[					]
0	1	2	3	4	5

Numerical scale

Oucher

This scale assesses pain for children ages 3 to 13 years with photos or a numerical scale. The photographic scale uses six photographs of children ranging from a child with "no hurt" to a child with a "lot of hurt." The photographs are arranged vertically from 0 to 5, with 0 (no hurt) on the bottom and 5 (lot of hurt) on the top. This scale also has photographs of African American and Hispanic children available.

The Numerical Scale vertically ranges from 0 to 100 with 0 being "no hurt" and 100 being "biggest hurt" (Beyer, Denyes, and Villaruel, 1992).

- 0 = No hurt.
- 1–29 = Little hurt.
- 30–69 = Middle hurt.
- 70–99 = Big hurt.
- 100 = Biggest hurt.

Poker Chip Tool

The Poker Chip Tool scale assesses pain in children 4 years of age and up. The nurse places red poker chips horizontally in front of the child, with the poker chips denoting "pieces of hurt." She then asks the child to select how many pieces of hurt he or she has (Hester et al., 1998).

Visual Analogue Scale

This scale, which assesses pain in children ages 4½ and older, is similar to that uses for adults. The child is asked to identify her or his pain level by marking the line in the area that represents her or his level of pain (Cline et al., 1992).

Word-Graphic Rating Scale

The Word-Graphic Rating scale assess pain in children ages 4 to 17 years (Fig. 20.3). It uses words on a horizontal linear scale to assess pain. The child is asked to identify her or his current pain level on the scale (Tesler et al., 1991).

[				]
No Pain	Little Pain	Medium Pain	Large Pain	Worst Pain

Word-Graphic Rating Scale

Physical Assessment

SYSTEM/ AREA	ABNORMAL FINDINGS/RATIONALE
General Appearance	Abnormal body posture, splinting, guarding.
Facial Expression	Grimacing, frowning, crying.
Gross Abnormalities	Weight loss, muscle atrophy, deformities. Change in vital signs, fever, increased heart and respiratory rate, shock due to altered release of multiple hormones (e.g., adrenocorticotropic hormone [ACTH], cortisol, catecholamines, insulin).
Integumentary	*Pallor, diaphoresis:* possible signs of shock.
HEENT	Pained facial expression. Clenched teeth. Abnormal sounds, such as moans and groans. Dilated pupils.
Respiratory	Increased respiratory rate. *Atelectasis and pneumonia:* Decreased air flow due to involuntary (reflex muscle spasm) and voluntary (splinting) mechanisms that limit respiratory effort.
Cardiovascular	Increased heart rate. Increased BP. *Unstable angina (chest pain) or myocardial infarction (heart attack):* Increased vascular resistance and increased myocardial oxygen demand. *Deep vein thrombosis (blood clot):* Hypercoagulation.
Gastrointestinal	*Hypoactive bowel sounds:* Delayed gastric emptying and peristalsis resulting in constipation, anorexia, ileus.
Genitourinary	*Decreased urine output:* Abnormal release of hormones that affect urine output, fluid volume, and electrolyte balance. Hypertension (fluid retention). Electrolyte disturbances.
Musculoskeletal	Limited mobility. Involuntary, reflexive movements. Muscle tensing/spasm. Muscle weakness and fatigue.
Neurologic	Altered affect, depression. Screening neurologic exam revealing sensory deficits, motor abnormalities, coordination problems, signs of sympathetic responses, and orientation and memory deficits.
Immune	*Infection:* Impaired immune function.
Other Regions	Findings dependent on site of pain.

HEENT = Head, eyes, ears, nose, and throat.

Pain scales have been developed to objectively assess pain by scoring behavioral and physiological responses to pain.

Pain Scales for Infants

Cries CRIES (C, crying; R, requiring increased oxygen; I, increased vital signs; E, expression; S, sleeplessness) assesses postoperative pain from 32 weeks' gestation to 20 weeks' post-term. Each of the five categories is scored from 0 to 2. A score of 10 equates to the "worst pain," and any score greater than 4 identifies significant pain.

	0	1	2
Crying	No	High pitched	Inconsolable
Requires Oxygen	No	<30%	> 30%
Increase in Vital Signs	Heart rate and BP less than or equal to preoperative state	Heart rate and BP increase <20% of preoperative state	Heart rate and BP increase >20% of preoperative state
Expression	None	Grimace	Grimace/grunt
Sleepless	No	Wakes at frequent intervals	Constantly awake

From Krechel, S., MD, and Bildner, J., RNC, CNS (1995) from University of Missouri-Columbia with permission.

Neonatal Infant Pain Scale (NIPS) This assessment tool is used to assess infants at an average gestational age of 33.5 weeks. It grades six categories: facial expression (0 to 1), cry (0 to 2), breathing pattern (0 to 1), arms (0 to 1), legs (0 to 1), and state of arousal (0 to 1). A final score of 0 identifies no pain while a score of 7 identifies worst pain (Lawrence, 1993).

Pain Assessment Tool (PAT) This assessment scale assesses pain from a gestational age of 27 weeks to full term. It grades 10 different categories: posture/tone (1 to 2), sleep pattern (0 to 2), expression (1 to 2), color (0 to 2), cry (0 to 2), respirations (1 to 2), heart rate (1 to 2), saturations (0 to 2), BP (0 to 2), and nurse's perception (0 to 2). A final score of 4 identifies no pain, while a score of 20 identifies worst pain (Hodgkinson, 1994).

Pain Rating Scale (PRS) This assessment tool assesses pain for infants ages 1 to 36 months. The infant is given a grade of 0 ("no pain") through 5 ("worst pain") based on the following guidelines. For a score of 0, the infant exhibits smiling, sleeping, and no change when moved or touched. Behaviors associated with a score of 1 include taking small amounts orally, restlessness, moving and crying. A score of 2 includes behaviors of not eating or drinking, short periods of crying but distracted with rocking or use of pacifier.

With a score of 3, a definite change in behavior is noted. The baby is irritable, with facial grimacing and arms and/or legs shake or have jerking movements. With a score of 4, the baby is inconsolable, flailing with a high-pitched wailing cry. A score of 5 is characterized by prolonged sleep periods interrupted by jerking movements, continuous crying, and shallow respirations (Joyce, 1994).

Postoperative Pain Score (POPS) This assessment tool assesses postoperative pain in infants ages 1 to 7 months. It scores each of its 10 categories (sleep, facial expression, quality of cry, spontaneous motor activity, spontaneous excitability, flexion of fingers and toes, tone, consolability, and sociability) on a scale of 0 to 2. A total score of 0 indicates worst pain, a score of 20, no pain (Attia, 1987).

Premature Infant Pain Profile (PIPP) This assessment tool assesses pain for gestational ages 28 to 40 weeks. It grades seven categories on a scale of 0 ("no pain") to 3 ("worst pain"). The categories are gestational age, behavioral stage, heart rate, oxygen saturation, brow bulge, eye squeeze, and nasolabial furrow. A final score of 0 identifies no pain, while a score of 21 identifies worst pain (Stevens, 1996).

Behavioral Pain Assessment Scales for Children

Behavioral Pain Score (BPS) This assessment tool assesses pain for children ages 3 to 36 months. It assesses three categories: facial expression (0 to 2), cry (0 to 3), and movements (0 to 3). A final score of 0 identifies no pain, while a score of 8 identifies worst pain (Robieux et al., 1991).

Children's Hospital of Eastern Ontario Pain Scale (CHEOPS) This assessment tool assesses pain for children ages 1 to 5 years. It assesses six categories: crying (1 to 3), facial (0 to 2), child verbal (0 to 2), torso (1 to 2), touch (1 to 2), and legs (1 to 2). A final score of 4 identifies no pain, while a score of 13 identifies worst pain (McGrath et al., 1985).

FLACC Postoperative Pain Tool This assessment tool assesses pain for children ages 2 months to 7 years. It assesses five categories using a scale of 0 ("no pain") to 2 ("worst pain"). A final score of 0 indicates no pain, while a score of 10 indicates worst pain.

Nurses Assessment of Pain Inventory (NAPI) This assessment tool assesses pain for infants and children from birth to age 16 years. It assesses three categories: body movement (0 to 2), facial (0 to 3), and touching (0 to 2). A final score of 0 identifies no pain, while a score of 10 identifies worst pain (Stevens, 1990).

Objective Pain Score (OPS) This assessment tool assess pain for infants and children from ages 4 months to 18 years. It assesses five categories, each on a scale of 0 ("no pain") to 2 ("worst pain"). The categories are BP, crying, moving, agitation, and verbal evaluation/body language. A final score of 0 identifies no pain, a score of 10 identifies worst pain (Hannallah et al., 1987).

Riley Infant Pain Scale (RIPS) This assessment tool assesses pain in children younger than 36 months and children with cerebral palsy. It assesses five categories on a scale of 0 ("no pain") to 3 ("worst pain") (Schade et al., 1996).

Riley Infant Pain Scale (Rips)

SCORE	FACIAL EXPRESSION	SLEEP	MOVEMENTS	CRY	TOUCH
0	Neutral. Smiling, calm.	Sleeping quietly.	Moves easily.	None.	–
1	Frowning Grimaces.	Restless.	Restless body movements.	Whimpering.	Winces with touch.
2	Clenched teeth.	Intermittent.	Moderate agitation.	Crying.	Cries with touch. Difficult to console.
3	Crying expression.	Prolonged with periods of jerking or no sleep.	Thrashing Flailing.	Screaming, high-pitched.	Screams when touched. Inconsolable.

FLACC Postoperative Pain Tool

SCORE	FACE	LEGS	ACTIVITY	CRY	CONSOLABILITY
0	Neutral or smile.	Relaxed, normal.	Moves easily.	None.	Content.
1	Grimace or frown, withdrawn.	Restless Tense.	Squirming.	Whimpers or moans, occasional complaint.	Reassured with touching, can be distracted.
2	Constant frown, clenched jaw, quivering chin.	Flexed Kicking.	Arched, rigid, jerking.	Crying, screams, verbal complaints.	Difficult to console.

Adapted from Wong, D., Hockenberry-Eaton, M., Wilson, D., Winkelstein, M., and Schwartz, P. (2001). *Wong's Essentials of Pediatric Nursing*, ed 6. Philadelphia: C.V.Mosby.

Behavioral Pain Scale for the Older Adult

Pain Assessment in Advanced Dementia Scale (PAINAD)

This assessment tool can be used to assess pain levels in patients with advanced dementia. It assesses five categories on a scale of 0 to 2. The higher the score, the greater the pain.

ITEM/POINT VALUE	0	1	2
Breathing, independent of vocalization	Normal.	Occasional labored breathing, short periods of hyperventilation.	Moisy, labored breathing; long period of hyperventilation; Cheyne-Stokes respirations.
Negative vocalization	None.	Occasional moan and groan; low-level speech with a negative or disapproving quality.	Repeated, troubled calling out; loud moaning and groaning; crying.
Facial expression	Smiling or inexpressive.	Sad, frightened, frowning.	Facial grimacing.
Body language	Relaxed.	Tense, distressed, pacing, fidgeting.	Rigid, fists clenched, knees pulled up, pulling or pushing away, striking out.
Consolability	No need to console.	Distracted or reassured by voice or touch.	Unable to be consoled, distracted, or reassured.

From Lane, P. (2004). Assessing pain in patients with advanced dementia. *Nursing 2004 34*(8):17.

Reassessment of Pain

Reassessment of pain is imperative to determine the effectiveness of treatment. Current recommendations for pain reassessment include:

- Within 30 minutes after parenteral administration of pain medication.
- Within 1 hour after oral administration of pain medication.
- After each and every report of new or changes in pain.

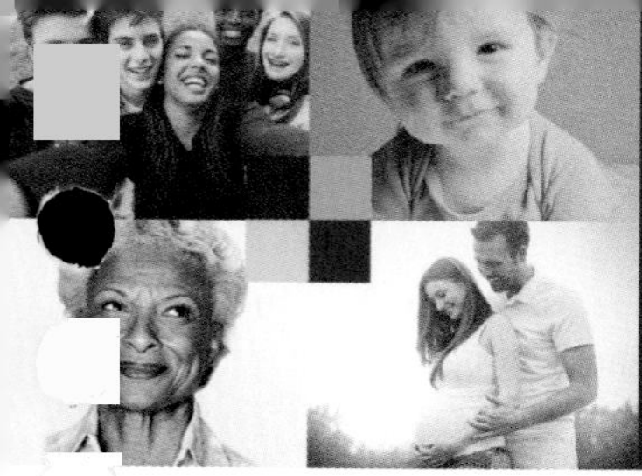

CHAPTER 21

Approach to the Mental Health Assessment

Mental health is a "state of successful performance of mental function, resulting in productive activities, fulfilling relationships with other people, and the ability to adapt to change and to cope with adversity" (Healthy People 2010). Mental health remains a leading health indicator (Healthy People 2020).

Developmental Considerations

Children

Various instruments are available to assess a variety of mental health disorders in children. Be sure to select the one best suited to meet the child's needs.

Children Rating Scales for Mental Health Disorders

INSTRUMENT	ASSESS FOR:
Behavior Assessment System for Children (BASC)	Behavior and emotions for children ages 2–18
Child Behavior Checklist (CBCL)	Psychopathology and competencies for children ages 4–16
Children's Depression Inventory (CDI)	Physical symptoms, harm avoidance, social anxiety and separation/panic disorders for children ages 7–17
Pediatric Anxiety Rating Scale (PARS)	Severity of anxiety for ages children 6–17
Yale-Brown Obsessive Compulsive Scale (YBOCS)	Obsessive compulsive disorder for children ages 6–17
Swanson, Nolan, and Pelham (SNAP)-IV	Inattention and overactivity (ADHD) and oppositional defiant disorders

Adapted from Boyd, M.A. (2005). *Psychiatric Nursing Contemporary Practice.* Philadelphia: Lippincott, Williams & Wilkins.

Risk Taking

Adolescents are known risk takers. Experimenting with drug and alcohol is common, and suicide is the second leading cause of death among adolescents (Box 21.1). Mental and substance abuse disorders or a combination of disorders are more times than not associated with suicide.

Another popular form of risk taking during childhood is the "choking game," which produces a high or a state of euphoria by cutting off the blood supply to the brain. If the blood supply is compromised for too long, the child will pass out and feel a "rush" as consciousness returns. Depriving the brain of oxygen may result in permanent and cumulative death to brain cells, stroke, seizures, retinal damage, or death. See Box 21.2 for the signs and symptoms of the choking game.

Pregnant Patients

Many mothers experience mild depression, also known as "baby blues," usually within 4 weeks following childbirth. If the "baby blues" persist for more than a few weeks, postpartum depression may have developed.

BOX 21.1 Risk Factors for Teen Suicide

- Depression
- Social isolation
- History of abuse
- Drug and alcohol abuse
- "Not fitting in with peers"
- School pressure

Source: Gorman, L. Raines, M., and Sultan, D. (2007). *Psychosocial Nursing for General Patient Care*, 3rd ed. Philadelphia: F.A. Davis.

BOX 21.2 Signs and Symptoms of the Choking Game

- Unexplained marks or bruises on neck
- Severe headaches
- Red eyes
- Belts, leashes, ropes, and shoelaces tied in strange knots or in unusual locations
- Disorientation after being alone
- Locked bedroom doors

Assessing for Postpartum Depression

Begin by identifying those at risk for developing postpartum depression. Risk factors include:

- History of mood disorders.
- Low self-esteem.
- Unwanted pregnancy.
- Unemployment of mother or head of household.
- Poor marital relationship.
- Father depressed.
- Poor support systems.
- External stressors.

Older Adult

Alzheimer's Disease is the 6th leading cause of death in adults, with 5.1 million Americans aged 65 years and older having Alzheimer's disease (Healthy People 2020). See Table 21.1 for the characteristics of dementia, delirium, and depression.

TABLE 21.1 Characteristics of Dementia, Delirium, and Depression

FEATURE	DEMENTIA	DELIRIUM	DEPRESSION
Onset	Gradual (months to years)	Abrupt (hours to a few weeks)	Either
Prognosis	Irreversible	Reversible	Variable
Course	Progressive	Worse in P.M.	Worse in A.M.
Attention	Normal	Impaired	Variable
Memory	Impaired recent and remote	Impaired recent and immediate	Selective impairment
Perception	Normal	Impaired	Normal
Psychomotor behavior	Normal/apraxia	Hypo/ hyperkinetic	Retardation/ agitation
Cause	Caused by many diseases, including alcoholism, acquired immunodeficiency syndrome (AIDS), cerebral anoxia, and brain infarcts	Caused by acute illness, fever, infection, dehydration, electrolyte imbalance, medications, and alcoholism	Usually coincides with life event, such as death in the family, loss of a friend or a pet, or a move

Delirium should be treated as an emergency since the acute onset may have an underlying life-threatening cause.

Depression

Depression is a major mental health problem for older adults, but can be easily missed. If left untreated, depression can lead to suicide or self-neglect. In the United States, the suicide rate is highest among older adults, with older men over age 80 at highest risk and guns the most frequent method (Gorman, Raines, and Sultan, 2002). But the suicide rate is probably higher, because older adults can easily commit passive suicide by not complying with medical regimens or failing to eat. See Boxes 21.3 to 21.5 for more information.

BOX 21.3 Signs and Symptoms of Depression in the Older Adult

TYPICAL

- Changes in appetite
- Decreased self-esteem
- Changes in sleep patterns
- Social withdrawal
- Feelings of helplessness
- Loss of motivation
- Constipation
- Hostility
- Pessimism
- Agitation
- Guilt
- Aggression

ATYPICAL

- Vague somatic complaints—such as constipation, joint pain, fatigue, and memory changes—that seem to be out of proportion to the actual problem.
- Client may become obsessed with the problems and feel that if the problems are relieved, he or she will be fine.

BOX 21.4 Geriatric Depression Scale

Are you basically satisfied with your life?	YES/**NO**
Have you dropped many of your activities and interests?	**YES**/NO
Do you feel that your life is empty?	**YES**/NO
Do you often get bored?	**YES**/NO
Are you in good spirits most of the time?	YES/**NO**
Are you afraid that something bad is going to happen to you?	**YES**/NO
Do you feel happy most of the time?	YES/**NO**
Do you often feel helpless?	**YES**/NO
Do you prefer to stay at home rather than going out and doing new things?	**YES**/NO
Do you feel you have more problems with memory than most?	**YES**/NO
Do you think it is wonderful to be alive now?	YES/**NO**
Do you feel pretty worthless the way you are now?	**YES**/NO
Do you feel full of energy?	YES/**NO**
Do you feel that your situation is hopeless?	**YES**/NO
Do you think that most people are better off than you are?	**YES**/NO

Bold answers = Depression

GDS Scoring:

12–15 Severe depression

8–11 Moderate depression

5–8 Mild depression

0–4 Normal

Source: Yesavage, J., Brink, T., Rose, T., Lum, O., Huang, V., Adey, M., and Leirer, O. (1983). Development and validation of a geriatric depression screening scale: A preliminary report. *Journal of Psychiatric Research 17*:37–49.

GDS website: http://www.stanford.edu/~yesavage/

BOX 21.5 Risk Factors for Suicide Among Older Adults

- Lives alone
- Widower
- Lack of financial resources
- Poor health
- Social isolation
- Drug and alcohol abuse

Source: Gorman, L. Raines, M., and Sultan, D. (2007). *Psychosocial Nursing for General Patient Care*, 3rd ed. Philadelphia: F.A. Davis.

Cultural Considerations

Cultural and ethnic variations often influence a patient's view of mental health.

CULTURE	PRACTICES/BELIEFS
Amish	Children with mental or physical differences are seen as "hard learners." The mentally ill are generally cared for at home.
Appalachian	Usually take care of own, so mentally deficient and handicapped are readily accepted. Mentally handicapped are not crazy, but rather have "bad nerves" or are "quite turned or bad turned." Behaviors that would warrant psychiatric treatment are seen as "lazy, mean, immoral criminal or psychic" and treated by punishment or tolerance.
Arab American	Mental illness seen as a social stigma; therefore, psychiatric symptoms may be denied, attributed to "bad nerves" or supernatural beings, or caused by a physical ailment or emotional trauma. Somatic orientation leads to patients' tolerance of emotional suffering, and relatives' tolerance of behavioral disorders. Patients with mental distress will somatize symptoms. Somatic treatment for psychiatric disorders preferred over psychotherapy.
Chinese American	Balance between yang and yin explains mental health/illness. Mental illness results from metabolic imbalance and organic problem. Stigma associated to mental illness so will seek folk healer first. Do not readily seek treatment for emotional or nervous disorders.
Cuban American	Emotional crises are treated by santero, a practitioner of santeria (a 300-year-old Afro-Cuban religion that combines Roman Catholic elements with ancient Yoruba tribal beliefs and practices). May act out emotional problems in a nonthreatening way, allowing person to maintain self-esteem.
Egyptian American	Mental illness considered a stigma. More tolerance for emotional problems. View mental health problems with a supernatural framework, including "curse" and "devil."

CULTURE	PRACTICES/BELIEFS
	Emotional problems of grief and losses due to wrongdoings of others or weakness and inability to control and snap out of distress. Mental and emotional issues expressed somatically so therefore treated with psychosomatic interventions. Seek family and friends for advice.
Filipino American	Stigma associated to mental illness. Mental illness caused by heredity. Take care of mentally ill family member rather than seek mental healthcare.
French Canadian	Federal Canadian laws protect the mentally disabled from discrimination.
Greek American	Stigma associated to mental illness. Mental illness seen as hereditarily linked, therefore, "polluting" the blood line, bringing shame to family. Families of mentally ill may experience loss of friends and social isolation. Mental illness often somatisized. Wide range of acceptable behavior leads to delay of seeking treatment. Folk model for "nerva" (nerves) is socially acceptable and treated with medication rather than psychotherapy.
Iranian	Stigma associated to mental illness. Mental illness is caused by a genetic problem, more likely to be labeled a "neurologic" problem. Avoids psychotherapeutic treatment. Symptoms somatasized and treated with psychopharmacology.
Irish American	High rate of mental illness. Difficulty expressing emotions and feelings. Family may take care of mentally ill family member. Some attribute mental illness to sin and guilt.
Jewish American	Mental health as important as physical health. Mental incapacity relinquishes one from all responsibilities.
Mexican American	Mental illness seen as God's will. Family prefers to care for patient at home.
Navajo Native American	Mental illness caused by witches; treated by healers. May wear turquoise to ward off evil. Some tribes view mentally ill as having special problems.

(continued)

CULTURE	PRACTICES/BELIEFS
Vietnamese American	Mental illness results from offending a deity. Brings disgrace to family and is therefore concealed, which delays treatment. Emotional disturbances caused by malicious spirits, bad luck of family inheritance. Buddhists see mental illness as bad karma from previous misdeeds. Sometimes nervous system seen as cause of mental problems.

Source: Purnell, L.D., and Paulanka, B.J. (2012). *Transcultural Healthcare: A Culturally Competent Approach*, 4th ed. Philadelphia: F.A. Davis.

Assessment

History

When obtaining a history, ask yourself, "What can the health history reveal about the mental health of the patient?" Identify factors that may affect mental health in either a positive or negative way.

Report any suspected abuse or any threat of child or elder abuse. Also report threats of suicide or homicide. Threats to self or others must always be taken seriously.

RISK FACTORS/ QUESTIONS TO ASK	RATIONALE/SIGNIFICANCE
Biographical	
Age How old are you?	• Response to stressors differs with age. • Identifies possible maturational crises related to developmental changes.
Gender Male/female?	• Increased incidence of depression greater in women than in men. • Men have greater incidence of psychosocial and substance abuse disorders. • Women have higher incidence of affective and anxiety disorders. • Later age of onset of schizophrenia in women than in men. • Men more likely to be aggressive and self-destructive than women.

RISK FACTORS/ QUESTIONS TO ASK	RATIONALE/SIGNIFICANCE
Socioeconomic and Educational Levels	
Level of education?	• The higher the socioeconomic and educational level, the lower the incidence of depression. • The higher the educational level, the more likely the individual to use mental health services if needed. • The lower the income, the higher incidence of psychological symptoms.
Ethnicity	
Cultural background?	• African Americans and Hispanics have twice the rate of being diagnosed with severe mental illness. • African Americans are diagnosed with most severe types of psychopathology and less affective disorders, and overdiagnosed with schizophrenia. • Ethnic groups have three times more hospitalizations for mental illness than the general population.
Marital Status	
Single/married/divorced?	• Married and partnered adults report less stress than single or divorced adults.
Religion	
Religious affiliation?	• Can affect mental health in either a positive or a negative way. • Influences perceptions of mental illness.
Contact Person	
Who is your contact person?	• Identifies supports.
Current Health Status	
	• Identifies any signs or symptoms that may reflect mental illness.
Past Health History	
Childhood Illnesses	
Any major health problems (physical or mental) while growing up?	• Identify any past mental health problems and treatments.
Past Hospitalizations	
Have you ever been hospitalized for mental health problems?	Previous psychiatric hospitalization.

(continued)

RISK FACTORS/ QUESTIONS TO ASK	RATIONALE/SIGNIFICANCE
Past Health History *(cont'd)*	
Family History Does anyone in your family have mental health problems?	• Identifies familial/genetically linked psychiatric disorders. • Familial/genetically linked disorders include: – Schizophrenia. – Depression. – Bipolar disorders. – Anxiety and panic disorders.
Medications Are you taking any medications, prescribed, over-the-counter [OTC], or herbal? If yes, what?	• Identify any psychiatric drugs. • Identify any possible drug interaction (Tables 21.2 and 21.3.) **OTC medications such as pseudoephedrine can cause anxiety symptoms.** **Herbal supplements such as St. John's wort, ephedra, ginseng, kava kava, and yohimbe can interact with psychotrophics or other medications, cause anxiety, drowsiness, or other adverse psychological effects (Pedersen, 2014).**
Military Service Are you or did you ever serve in the military? If yes, when and tour of duty?	• Identifies possible source of stressor related to post-traumatic stress syndrome.

TABLE 21.2 Drugs That May Adversely Affect Mental Health

DRUGS	EFFECT
Antihypertensives • Reserpine • Beta-blockers • Methyldopa Oral contraceptives Corticosteroids Benzodiazepine Cancer chemotherapeutic agents • Vincristine • Vinblastine • Interferon • Procarbazine	Depression

DRUGS	EFFECT
Psychoactive agents • Alcohol • Amphetamine or cocaine withdrawal • Opioids	
Corticosteroids Levodopa Amphetamines Tricyclic antidepressants (TCAs) Monoamine oxidase (MAO) inhibitors Methylphenidate Cocaine Thyroid hormone	Manic states
Amphetamines Antidepressants (particularly TCAs) Anticholinergics (atropine) Anticonvulsants (carbamazepine, valproic acid) Antiparkinsonians (levodopa) Antituberculars (isoniazid)	Psychotic reactions
Antivirals (acyclovir, amantadine) Antiarrhythmics (lidocaine) Alcohol Beta-blockers (propranalol) Corticosteroids H_2-receptor blockers (cimetidine) Cyclosporine Disulfiram (antabuie) Anesthetics (ketamine) Antibiotics (cephalosporins, ciprofloxacin, sulfonamides) Opioids (morphine, hydromorphone)	

Source: Gorman, L., Raines, M., and Sultan, D. (2007). *Psychosocial Nursing for General Patient Care,* 3rd ed. Philadelphia: F.A. Davis.

TABLE 21.3 Psychotropic Drugs and Some Related Side Effects

DRUG	SIDE EFFECTS
Lithium	Nausea, diarrhea, polyuria, acne, rashes, alopecia, tremors; weight gain, hypothyroidism, and can precipitate psoriasis and psoriatic arthritis.
Anticonvulsants	Sedation, hepatotoxicity, rash, and Stevens-Johnson syndrome (SJS), which is a life-threatening mucocutaneous reaction.

(continued)

TABLE 21.3 Psychotropic Drugs and Some Related Side Effects (continued)

DRUG	SIDE EFFECTS
Anticholinergics	Blurred vision, constipation, dry mouth.
TCAs	Sedation, blurred vision, dry mouth, constipation, life-threatening arrhythmias, and electrocardiogram (ECG) changes.
Selective serotonin reuptake inhibitors	Gastrointestinal (GI) symptoms, insomnia, and agitation.
Antipsychotics	Movement disorders (akathisia) and tardive dyskinesia (especially conventional antipsychotics [chlorpromazine]), dystonia, parkinsonism, gynecomastia and lactation, and possibly treatment-emergent diabetes. **Neuroleptic malignant syndrome (NMS) is a potentially fatal side effect from antipsychotic drugs characterized by fever, tachycardia, sweating, muscle rigidity, tremors, incontinence, stupor, leukocytosis, elevated creatine phosphokinase, renal failure.**

Adapted from Pedersen, D. (2014). *PsychNotes, 4th ed.* Philadelphia: F.A. Davis.

Review of Systems

As you proceed with the review of systems, note any problems that may affect your patient's mental health.

AREA/SYSTEM, QUESTIONS TO ASK	RATIONALE/ SIGNIFICANCE
General	
How have you been feeling?	• Fatigue may be associated with depression. • Restlessness may be associated with anxiety.
Integumentary	
Do you have any problems with your skin? If yes, describe.	• Sweating, itching associated with anxiety. • Cutting form of self-injury to deal with emotional pain
HEENT	
Do you have headaches? If yes, describe. Thyroid disease?	• Headaches associated with depression. • History of migraines and tension headaches affected by psychological factors.

AREA/SYSTEM, QUESTIONS TO ASK	RATIONALE/ SIGNIFICANCE
	• History of hyperthyroidism and diabetes can be affected by psychological factors, manifest with psychological signs or symptoms, or mimic psychological disorders.
Respiratory	
Do you have any breathing problems? If yes, describe.	• History of breathing problems, such as hyperventilation, associated with anxiety disorders. Sighing associated with depression.
Cardiovascular	
Do you have any cardiovascular problems? If yes, describe.	• Hypertension, angina affected by psychological factors. • Palpitations, racing heart associated with anxiety. **Use heterocyclic antidepressants with caution with cardiovascular disease.**
Gastrointestinal	
Do you have any GI problems? If yes, describe. Changes in weight? If yes, describes. Changes in appetite? If yes, describe.	• Changes in appetite associated with depression, anxiety, eating disorders, substance abuse. • History of peptic ulcer, irritable bowel syndrome, colitis affected by psychological factors. • GI complaints such as nausea, abdominal pain, diarrhea seen with anxiety. • Indigestion and constipation seen with depression. **Nausea is a common side effect of many psychotropic medications.**
Genitourinary	
Do you have any genitourinary problems? If yes, describe. For female, menstrual cycle? Do you have any concerns about you sexual performance? If yes, describe.	• History of sexual dysfunction, such as impotence, frigidity, and premenstrual syndrome (PMS), affected by psychological factors. • Menstrual irregularities associated with eating disorders. • Pressure and frequency of urination associated with anxiety. **Use TCAs (amitriptyline) cautiously with benign prostatic hyperplasia (BPH).**
Musculoskeletal	
Do you have any musculoskeletal problems? If yes, describe.	• History of rheumatoid arthritis and idiopathic low back pain affected by psychological factors. • Weakness associated with anxiety. • Osteoporosis associated with eating disorders.

(continued)

AREA/SYSTEM, QUESTIONS TO ASK	RATIONALE/ SIGNIFICANCE
Musculoskeletal *(cont'd)*	**Use of antipsychotics contraindicated with myasthenia gravis.**
Neurologic Do you have any neurologic disorders? Seizures, concentration or memory problems? Depression, anxiety? If yes, describe.	• Seizures associated with eating disorders. **Use TCAs cautiously with seizures; buproprion contraindicated with seizures.** • NMS and movement disorders are a side effect of antipsychotic medications. • Cognitive problems, difficulty focusing, and inability to concentrate associated with anxiety, depression, dementia, and schizophrenia.

HEENT = Head, eyes, ears, nose, and throat.

Psychosocial Profile

As you perform the psychosocial assessment, look for clues that would reflect your patient's mental health.

AREA	SIGNIFICANCE
Health Practices and Beliefs How would you describe your mental health? Do you or would you use mental health services?	• Identify perceptions of mental health, mental health practices, and use of mental health services.
Typical Day Can you tell me what your typical day is like?	• Identifies ability to maintain activities of daily living (ADLs). Mental health problems such as depression and schizophrenia, compulsive disorders may affect ability to perform ADLs.
Nutritional Patterns Can you tell me what you ate yesterday (24-hour recall)?	• Nutritional disorders associated with eating disorders, anxiety, depression.
Activity and Exercise Patterns Do you exercise regularly? If yes, describe.	• Excessive exercise associated with eating disorders. • Inactivity associated with depression.

AREA	SIGNIFICANCE
Recreation, Pets, Hobbies What do you do for fun? Pets? Hobbies?	• Inactivity associated with depression.
Sleep/Rest Patterns How many hours of sleep do you get a night? Do you have any problems falling asleep, staying asleep? Do you take or do anything to help you sleep?	• Problems with sleep and rest associated with many psychological disorders such as anxiety, depression, bipolar disorders, substance abuse.
Personal Habits Do you use alcohol, drugs, caffeine, nicotine? If, yes, how much?	• Identify history of substance abuse (use of alcohol, drugs, caffeine, nicotine).
Occupational Health Occupation? How do you feel about your work? Coworkers? Do you find your work stressful? If yes, how do you deal with it. Are there any health risks associated with your work? If yes, describe.	• Identify ability to maintain job. Work can be a source of stress. • Identify risk for head injury, such as construction work.
Environmental Where do you live? Are you exposed to any pollutants or toxins?	• Identify risk for exposure to toxic substances that can affect cognitive ability, such as lead, mercury, herbicides, solvents, cleaning agents, lawn chemicals.
Roles, Relationships, Self-Concept How do you see yourself? Identify various roles and relationships.	• Identify sense of worth and value, which may be affected by psychological factors such as low self-image associated with depression, eating disorders. • Roles and relationships may affect or be affected by psychological factors.
Cultural Influences What is your cultural background? What influence your perception of health?	• Identify culture's perception of mental health and illness.
Religious/Spiritual Influences What is your religious background? What influence does your religious beliefs have on your perception of health?	• Identify religious/spiritual influences on mental health and illness.

(continued)

AREA	SIGNIFICANCE
Family Roles and Relationships What is your role in your family? Relationships?	• Identify sources of support or stress on patient's mental health. • Mental illness smay affect patient's role and relationship in family.
Sexuality Patterns Do you have any concerns about sexual patterns? If yes, describe. Do you practice safe sex?	• Sexual problems often associated with mental illness such as depression. • Risk for unprotected sexual activity associated with substance abuse.
Stress and Coping Patterns How do you deal with stress? What do you do when you're upset?	• Identify current coping skills. • Determine effectiveness of coping skills.

Physical Assessment

AREA	SIGNIFICANCE
General Appearance, posture, grooming, dress and hygiene, eye contact, body size and type, speech	Poor grooming and personal hygiene seen with depression. Bright colors or unusual dress seen with mania. Poor eye contact seen with depression. Inability to maintain attention seen with schizophrenia, depression. Affect reflects mental health (labile affect associated with mania, flat incongruent associated with schizophrenia). Stooped posture seen with depression. Restlessness, tension seen with anxiety. Malnourished appearance may be seen with eating disorders. Slurred speech seen with drug and alcohol abuse. Pressured speech seen with mania. Disorganized speech seen with schizophrenia. Irritability associated with anxiety. Suspiciousness associated with paranoia.
Integumentary	Flushed or pallid skin color seen with anxiety. Excessive sweating seen with anxiety. Injury or scarring from self-injury or past suicide attempts or self-mutilation.

AREA	SIGNIFICANCE
HEENT	
	Dilated or constricted pupils seen with drug abuse. Poor eye contact seen with depression. Dental caries, parotid swelling seen with eating disorders. Erosion of nasal or oral mucosa secondary to drug use. In children, rope marks on the neck associated with "choking game."
Respiratory	
	Increased respiratory rate and hyperventilation seen with anxiety.
Cardiovascular	
	Increased pulse rate and BP seen with anxiety.
Abdominal	
	Increased bowel sounds seen with excessive use of laxatives in eating disorders. Abnormal liver size from substance abuse.
Musculoskeletal	
	Generalized weakness and tremors seen with anxiety. Abnormal muscle movement may be side effect of psychotropic drugs. Excessive body movements associated with anxiety, mania, or stimulant abuse. Minimal or no body movement associated with depression, catatonic states, or drug-induced stupor. Repeated movements associated with compulsive disorders. Repeated picking at clothes may be associated with hallucinations, delirium, or toxic conditions.
Neurologic	
	Cognitive changes, thought process disorders seen with schizophrenia. Loose association associated with schizophrenia. Flight of ideas associated with mania. Preservation associated with brain damage or psychotic disorders. Auditory hallucinations associated with schizophrenia. Visual hallucinations often organic in nature. Tactile hallucinations seen with organic problems, drug abuse, or DTs. Changes in mental status seen with mental illness such as schizophrenia, substance abuse, bipolar disorder. Increased reflexes seen with anxiety Movement disorders side effect associated with anti-psychotic medications.

Source: Stuart, G., and Laraia, M. (2001). *Principles and Practice of Psychiatric Nursing,* ed. 7. Philadelphia: Mosby.

Mental Status Examination

The components of the mental status assessment include:

- General appearance.
- Behavior/activity.
- Speech and language.
- Mood and affect.
- Thought process and content.
- Perceptual disturbances.
- Memory/cognitive.
- Judgment and insight.

AREA/ASSESS FOR:	NORMAL	ABNORMAL/ RATIONALE AND EXAMPLES
General Appearance		
Grooming/dress		
Dress appropriate for age, gender, season, situation? Dress neat and appropriate?	Dress neat and appropriate.	*Disheveled:* Associated with depression. *Bright colored:* Associated with mania.
Hygiene		
Are the patient and her or his clothing clean? Any unusual odors?	Clean, no unusual odors.	*Poor hygiene:* May be associated with depression.
Eye contact		
Does the patient maintain eye contact?	Maintains eye contact.	*Poor eye contact:* Associated with depression.
Posture		
Does the patient assume a specific position? Is posture erect?	Comfortably positioned, posture erect.	*Slumped posture:* Associated with depression. *Defensive posture:* Associated with paranoia.
Identifying marks/scars/ tattoos		
Are there any obvious marks or scars?	No obvious marks or scars.	Scars may indicate self-mutilation or past suicide attempts.
Appearance vs. stated age		
Does the patient appear stated age, or younger or older?	Appears stated age.	*Older than stated age:* May be associated with depression.
Behavior/Activity		
Do you notice any unusual activity? Is patient's behavior appropriate for the situation?	Calm, relaxed, no unusual havior or movements.	*Hyperactive:* Associated with anxiety, mania, or stimulant abuse.

AREA/ASSESS FOR:	NORMAL	ABNORMAL/ RATIONALE AND EXAMPLES
Behavior/ Activity *(cont'd)*		*Agitated:* May be seen with dementia or delirium. *Psychomotor retardation, slow movements:* May be associated with depression. *Tremors:* May indicate drug/alcohol withdrawal. *Tics:* May be a side effect of psychotropic medications. *Unusual movements such as jaw/lip smacking:* May be associated with tardive dyskinesia, a side effect from antipsychotic medications. *Catatonia:* May be seen with schizophrenia. *Akathisia (restlessness):* Seen with extrapyramidal side effect from antipsychotic medications. *Rigidity:* May be a sign of NMS.
Speech/Language What is the quality, tone, volume, fluency and pace of speech?	Quality and pace of speech normal with no exaggeration, fluent pleasant tone.	*Slow speech:* Associated with depression. *Rapid and pressured speech:* Associated with mania. *Mumbling:* Seen with Huntington's chorea. *Slurred speech:* Seen with alcohol intoxication. *Suspicious tone:* Associated with paranoia. *Volume:* Soft associated with depression. *Fluency (mute/hesitation/latency of response):* Less likely to talk with depression. Hesitancy seen with mistrust or paranoia.

(continued)

AREA/ASSESS FOR:	NORMAL	ABNORMAL/ RATIONALE AND EXAMPLES
Attitude		
What is the patient's attitude? Friendly? Hostile?	Cooperative	*Uncooperative:* Associated with paranoia. *Warm/friendly/distant:* Seen with personality disorders. *Suspicious/combative:* Seen with paranoia. *Guarded/aggressive:* Seen with psychosis. *Hostile/aloof:* Seen with psychosis. *Apathetic:* Seen with depression.
Mood		
Self-report of emotional state. How would you describe your mood?	Appropriate for situation.	*Sad:* Associated with depression. *Elated:* Associated with mania. *Irritable/anxious:* Associated with anxiety. *Fearful/guilty:* Seen with phobias. *Worried/angry:* Seen with personality disorder. *Hopeless:* Associated with depression. *Labile:* Associated with mania. *Mixed (anxious and depressed):* Seen with depression.
Affect		
Apparent emotional state.	Appropriate for situation.	*Flat affect:* Seen with schizophrenia. *Blunted or diminished affect:* Seen with psychosis.
What is your patient's affect?		*Inappropriate/Incongruent (sad and smiling or laughing):* Associated with schizophrenia.

AREA/ASSESS FOR:	NORMAL	ABNORMAL/ RATIONALE AND EXAMPLES
Thought Process What is the patient's level of consciousness? Does the patient respond appropriately?	Awake, alert, and oriented (AAO) x 3, thought process intact, responds appropriately.	Thought process disturbances often seen with psychosis or organic brain disorders. The following are examples of thought process disturbances. *Concrete thinking:* Unable to abstract, thinks in concrete terms. *Circumstantiality:* Excessive, irrelevant detail, but eventually gets to the point. *Tangentiality:* Digresses from topic to topic never getting to the point. *Loose association:* Loose connection between thoughts that are unrelated. *Echolalia:* Repetition of words spoken by another. *Flight of ideas:* Rapidly going from one topic to another. *Perseveration:* Involuntary, excessive repetition of a single response to different questions. *Clang association:* Association of words by sound. *Blocking:* Draws a blank. *Word salad:* Combination of words that have no meaning. *Derailment:* Off track.

(continued)

AREA/ASSESS FOR:	NORMAL	ABNORMAL/ RATIONALE AND EXAMPLES
Thought Content Does the patient's thought process and content seem reality based? Did you ever think about hurting yourself or someone else?	Thought content reality based.	*Delusions (grandiose/ persecution/reference/ somatic):* Associated with psychosis. *Suicidal/homicidal thoughts:* Associated with depression, anxiety or schizophrenia. **If homicidal thoughts, identify toward whom. Suicidal/ homicidal ideations require immediate attention.** *Obsessions:* Seen with obsessive-compulsive disorder (OCD). *Paranoia:* Seen with schizophrenia. *Phobias:* Seen with anxiety disorders. *Magical thinking:* Primitive form of thinking that thinking about something will make it happen. Poverty of speech.
Perceptual Disturbances Does the patient have perceptual disturbances? Auditory? Visual? Olfactory? Tactile?	No hallucination, illusions, or depersonalization.	*Visual hallucinations:* Often organic in nature. *Auditory hallucinations (commenting/ discussing/ commanding/loud/soft/ other):* Associated with schizophrenia. *Tactile hallucinations:* Seen with organic problems, drug abuse, or DTs. *Illusions:* Misperception of a real external stimuli; common with dementia of Alzheimer's and schizophrenia.

AREA/ASSESS FOR:	NORMAL	ABNORMAL/ RATIONALE AND EXAMPLES
		Depersonalization: Altered perception or experience that causes temporarily loss of self or personal identity; seen with OCD.
Memory/Cognitive		
Orientation		
Is the patient oriented to time, place, and person?	AAO x 3 (time/ place/person).	Orientation altered with organic disorders or schizophrenia; may be disoriented.
Memory		
Immediate: Can you repeat the following numbers...? Remote: Can you tell me what you had for breakfast? Or I'll name three objects and ask you to remember them later in the exam.	Immediate, recent, and remote intact. No confabulation.	*Memory problems and confabulation:* Seen with organic, dissociative, and conversion disorders. *Level of alertness:* Altered with substance abuse.
Insight and Judgment		
Insight (awareness of the nature of illness)		
Does patient have insight into his or her problem? Ask, Can you tell me what the problem is? Is judgment appropriate? Ask the patient to respond to a hypothetical situation, such as "If you were walking down the street and saw smoke coming from a window of a home, what would you do?"	Insight and judgment intact and appropriate.	*Poor insight:* With psychosis. *Poor judgment:* With psychosis. *Poor impulse control:* With OCD, psychosis, mania.

Additional Assessments

Depending of your assessment findings, additional mental health screenings may be indicated. Various mental health problems and assessment instruments are available to assess for a variety of mental health problems. Additional mental health assessments are presented below.

Crisis Assessment

FACTOR	QUESTIONS TO ASK
Perception of event	• Can you tell me what has happened? Please be specific. • What caused the crisis? • How has this affected you? • How did this make you feel?
Supports	• Is there anyone I can call? • Do you live alone? • Do you have family or friends who support you? • Are you active in any religious or community groups?
Coping mechanisms	• How have you handled stressful events in the past? • Can you talk the stressful event? • What do you do to relieve tension? Cry? Talk? Exercise? Use alcohol?

From Stuart, G., and Laraia, M. (2005). *Principles and Practices of Psychiatric Nursing*, ed. 8. Philadelphia: Mosby.

BATHE Technique

When you only have limited time to perform an assessment, it's important to keep the interview focused. The BATHE technique helps the patient identify problems and coping strategies and is supportive of the patient. The acronym is representative of the interview's components (Stuart and Lieberman, 1993):

- B = Background—What is going on? What brought you here?
- A = Affect—How does this make you feel?
- T = Trouble—What troubles you most in this situation?
- H = Handling—How are you able to handle this situation/problem?
- E = Empathy—Empathize with patient; shows an understanding of client's view of situation.

The BATHE technique is not intended for use with patients with severe problems, such as patients who are suicidal or those who have suffered severe abuse.

Assessing Depression

If you suspect that your patient is depressed, use the mnemonic SIGECAPS to easily recall and review the Diagnostic and Statistical Manual of Mental Disorders (*DSM)-IV* criteria for major depression:

- S = Sleep (increase/decrease).
- I = Interest (diminished).

- G = Guilty/low self-esteem.
- E = Energy (poor/low).
- C = Concentration (poor).
- A = Appetite (increase/decrease).
- P = Psychomotor (agitation/retardation).
- S = Suicidal ideation.

A depressed mood plus four or more SIGECAPS for 2 weeks or longer indicates a major depressive disorder. A depressed mood plus three SIGECAPS most days for 2 years or longer indicates dysthymia, which is a depressive neurosis with no loss of contact with reality (Brigham and Women's Hospital, 2001).

Symptoms of dysthymia are similar to those of a major depressive disorder, but milder.

Suicide Assessment

In the United States, suicide is a major public health problem. Suicide, the 11th leading cause of death in the United States, accounts for the deaths of approximately 30,000 Americans each year (Healthy People 2020). It is often the end result of mental illness. More women attempt suicide than men, but men are four and a half times more likely to succeed at suicide than women. If you suspect that your client is suicidal, perform a suicide assessment. It is important to identify those at risk for suicide and intervene promptly. (See Boxes 21.6 and 21.7 for more information.)

BOX 21.6 Risk Factors for Suicide

- Previous suicide attempts
- Past suicide of family member, close friend, or peer
- Impulsivity
- Mood disorders
- Substance abuse
- Recent loss of a spouse, partner, friend, or job
- Expressed hopelessness (patient sees no future)
- Social isolation (patient lives alone, has few friends or supports)
- Stressful life event
- Previous or current abuse (emotional, physical, sexual)
- Sexual identity crises/conflict
- Available lethal methods (guns)
- Legal issues/incarceration

From: U.S. Public Health Services (1999). *The Surgeon General's Call to Action to Prevent Suicide.* Washington, D.C.: USDHHS. http://www.surgeongeneral.gov/library/calltoaction.htm

BOX 21.7 Groups at Risk for Suicide

- Elderly persons who are isolated, widowed, or who have experienced multiple losses
- Males who are widowed and without close supports
- Adolescents and young adults
- Persons with serious or terminal illness who become depressed or hopeless
- Persons with mood disorders, depression, and bipolar
- Persons with schizophrenia, either those newly diagnosed or those experiencing auditory command hallucinations
- Persons who abuse drugs or alcohol, especially persons with a mental disorder
- Persons under stress (sometimes multiple stressors) with recent loss or losses

Suicide attempts are more likely to occur as the patient's symptoms improve because the patient now has the energy to commit suicide.

Performing a Suicide Assessment The following feelings and behaviors should be included in a suicide assessment.

ASSESSMENT AREA	QUESTIONS TO ASK
Feelings of hopelessness	• How are you feeling? • What are your plans for tomorrow, next week? What do you have planned for the rest of the year? **A key element in assessing for feelings of hopelessess is determining whether the patient is able to see a future with herself or himself in that future.**
Suicidal ideations	• Have you ever had thoughts about hurting youself?
Plan for suicide	• Do you have a plan to commit suicide?
Possessions	• Have you been putting affairs in order? • Have you been giving things away? • Have you been contacting old friends?
Auditory hallucinations	• Have you heard a voice telling you to hurt or kill yourself?
Lack of support network	• How often do you communicate with friends and family? • Have you found yourself withdrawing from friends and family? • Who are your supports?

ASSESSMENT AREA	QUESTIONS TO ASK
Alcohol or substance abuse	• Do you drink or do drugs while alone?
Precipitating event	• Have you recently experienced the death of a loved one or the loss of a job? • Have you recently had a tragedy or disaster in your life? **For many people, holidays can be a precipitating event to a suicidal episode.**
Media	• Take note if the local media has reported on the suicide of a famous person or local teenager.

Adapted from Pedersen, D. (2014). *PsychNotes*, 4th ed. Philadelphia: F.A. Davis.

Assessing Substance Abuse

If substance abuse is a concern with your client, it's important to ask the right questions and obtain an accurate history (Box 21.8). If there is no time to obtain a detailed assessment, a focused assessment tool such as the CAGE questionnaire can also identify a possible substance abuse problem (Box 21.9). See Table 21.4 for more information on the effects from use and withdrawal of certain drugs.

BOX 21.8 Substance Abuse History and Assessment Tool

1. When you were growing up, did anyone in your family use substances (alcohol or drugs)? If yes, how did the substance abuse affect the family?
2. When (how old) did you use your first substance (e.g., alcohol, cannabis) and what was it?
3. How long have you been using a substance(s) regularly? Weeks? Months? Years?
4. What is your pattern of abuse?
   a. When do you use substances?
   b. How much and how often do you use?
   c. Where are you when you use substances and with whom?
5. When did you last use, what was it and how much?
6. Has substance use caused you any problems with family, friends, job, school, the legal system, other? If yes, describe.
7. Have you ever had an injury or accident because of substance abuse? If yes, describe.

(box continued on page 556)

BOX 21.8 Substance Abuse History and Assessment Tool (continued)

8. Have you ever been arrested for driving under the influence (DUI) because of your drinking or other substance use?
9. Have you ever been arrested or placed in jail because of drugs or alcohol?
10. Have you ever experienced memory loss the morning after substance use (can't remember what you did the night before)? Describe the event and your feelings about the situation.
11. Have you ever tried to stop your substance use? If yes, why were you not able to stop? Did you have any physical symptoms such as shakiness, sweating, nausea, headaches, insomnia, or seizures?
12. Can you describe a typical day in your life?
13. Are there any changes you would like to make in your life? If so, what are they?
14. What plans or ideas do you have for making these changes?
15. History of withdrawal:

Other comments:

From Pedersen, D. (2014). *Psychnotes.* Philadelphia: F.A. Davis; and modified from Townsend, M.C. (2007). *Psychiatric Mental Health Nursing: Concepts of Care,* 3rd ed. Philadelphia: F.A. Davis.

BOX 21.9 CAGE Questionnaire

- Have you ever felt you should **Cut** down on your drinking/drug use?
- Have people **A**nnoyed you by criticizing your drinking/drug use?
- Have you ever felt bad or **G**uilty about your drinking/drug use?
- Have you ever had an **E**ye opener (use of alcohol or drugs first thing in the morning) to steady your nerves or get rid of a hangover?

A positive (yes) response to two or more questions suggests that there is an alcohol/substance problem.

Note: The need to "cut down" is related to tolerance (needing more substance for same effect) and the "eye opener" is related to withdrawal syndrome (reduction/cessation of substance).

From Ewing J.A. (1984). Detecting alcoholism: The CAGE questionnaire. *Journal of the American Medical Association 252*:1905–1907.

TABLE 21.4 Abused Substances: Effects From Use and Withdrawal

SUBSTANCE	INTOXICATION	OVERDOSE	WITHDRAWAL
Depressants			
Alcohol (booze, brew, juice, spirits)	Depressed cognitive functioning. Impaired psychomotor functioning. Increased reaction time. Decreased balance and coordination. Decreased rapid eye movement (REM) sleep.	Unconsciousness. Respiratory depression. Coma. Death.	Tremors. Diaphoresis. Anxiety. Hallucinations. Delusions. Increased pulse and blood pressure (BP). Delerium tremens (DTs). Sleep disturbances.
Sedatives, hypnotics, and anxiolytics, including barbiturates (barbs, beans, black beauties, blue angle, candy, downers, goof balls, BB, nebbies, reds, sleepers, yellow jackets, yellow) Benzodiazepine (downers)	Slurred speech. Labile mood. Inappropriate sexual behavior. Loss of inhibition. Drowsiness. Impaired memory.	Hypotension. Nystagmus. Stupor. Cardiorespiratory depression. Coma. Death.	Insomnia. Hand tremor. Agitation. Nausea and vomiting. Anxiety. Tinnitus (with benzodiazepines). Seizures. Cardiac arrest.

(continued)

TABLE 21.4 Abused Substances: Effects From Use and Withdrawal (continued)

SUBSTANCE	INTOXICATION	OVERDOSE	WITHDRAWAL
Stimulants			
Amphetamines (A, AMT, bam, bennies, crystal, diet pills, dolls, eye-openers, peppills, purple hearts, speed, uppers, wake-ups)	Euphoria. High energy. Impaired judgment. Anxiety. Aggressive behavior. Paranoia. Delusions.	Ataxia. High temperature. Seizures. Respiratory distress. Cardiovascular collapse. Coma. Death.	Depression. Agitation. Confusion. Vivid dreams followed by lethargy.
Cocaine (bernice, bernies, big C, blow, C, charlie, coke, dust, girl, heaven, jay, lady, nose candy, nose powder, snow, sugar, white lady) Crack (conan, freebase, rock, toke, white cloud, white tornado)	Euphoria. Grandiosity. Sexual excitement. Impaired judgment. Insomnia. Anorexia. Nasal perforation (inhaled route). Psychosis.	High temperature. Seizures. Transient vasospasms (may cause myocardial infarction, stroke, coma, death).	Fatigue. Depression. Anxiety. Suicidal behavior.
Marijuana			
Cannabis (marijuana, hashish, Acapulco gold, Aunt Mary, broccoli, dope, grass, weed, grunt, hay, hemp, J, joint, joy stick, killer weed, pot, ragweed, reefer, smoke, weed)	Euphoria. Intensified perceptions. Impaired judgment and motor ability. Increased appetite, weight gain. Sinusitis and bronchitis with chronic use. Anxiety, paranoia. Red conjunctiva.	Extreme paranoia. Psychosis.	None.

SUBSTANCE	INTOXICATION	OVERDOSE	WITHDRAWAL
Opiates			
Heroin (H, horse, harry, boy, scag, shit, smack, stuff, white junk, white stuff) Morphine Hydromorphone Meperidine Codeine Oxycodone Opium Methadone	Euphoria. Drowsiness. Impaired judgment. Constricted pupils.	Dilated pupils. Respiratory depression. Seizures. Cardiopulmonary arrest. Coma. Death.	Yawning. Insomnia. Anorexia. Irritability. Rhinorrhea. Muscle cramps. Chills. Nausea and vomiting. Feelings of panic and doom.
Hallucinogens			
Hallucinogens (lysergic acid diethylamide [LSD], dimethyltryptamine [DMT], Mescaline – acid, big D, blotter, blue heaven, cap, D, deeda, flash, L, mellow yellow, microdots, paper acid, sugar, ticket, yello)	Dilated pupils. Diaphoresis. Palpitations. Tremors. Enhanced perceptions of colors and sound. Depersonalization. Grandiosity.	Panic. Psychosis with hallucinations. Cerebral damage. Death.	None.

(continued)

TABLE 21.4 Abused Substances: Effects From Use and Withdrawal (continued)

SUBSTANCE	INTOXICATION	OVERDOSE	WITHDRAWAL
Hallucinogens *(cont'd)*			
Club Drug, methylenedioxymethamphetamine (MDMA [Ecstasy])	Euphoria. Muscle relaxation.	Confusion. Hallucinations. Severe anxiety. Hypertension. Seizures. High temperature.	Psychological dependence can cause depression, flashbacks.
Phencyclidine			
Phencyclidine (PCP, angel dust, DOA, dust, elephant, hog, peace pill, supergrass, tictac)	Impulsive behavior. Impaired judgment. Belligerent, violent behavior. Ataxia. Muscle rigidity. Nystagmus. Hypertension. Numbness or diminished response to pain.	Hallucinations. Psychosis. Seizures. Respiratory arrest. Death.	None.

SUBSTANCE	INTOXICATION	OVERDOSE	WITHDRAWAL
Inhalants			
Gasoline, glue, aerosol sprays, paint thinners (spray, rush, bolt, huffing, bagging, sniffing)	Euphoria. Impaired judgment. Blurred vision. Unsteady gait.	Psychosis with hallucinations. Cardiac arrhythmias. Central nervous system depression. Coma. Cerebral damage. Death.	None.
Nicotine (Cigarettes, cigars, bidis, kreteks, pipe tobacco, chewing tobacco, snuff, nicotine gum or patches)	Sense of anxiety reduction. Relief from depression. Satisfaction.	None.	Insomnia. Depression. Irritability. Anxiety. Poor concentration. Increased appetite.

Source: Gorman, L., Raines, M., and Sultan, D. (2007). *Psychosocial Nursing for General Patient Care*, ed. 3. Philadelphia: F.A. Davis.

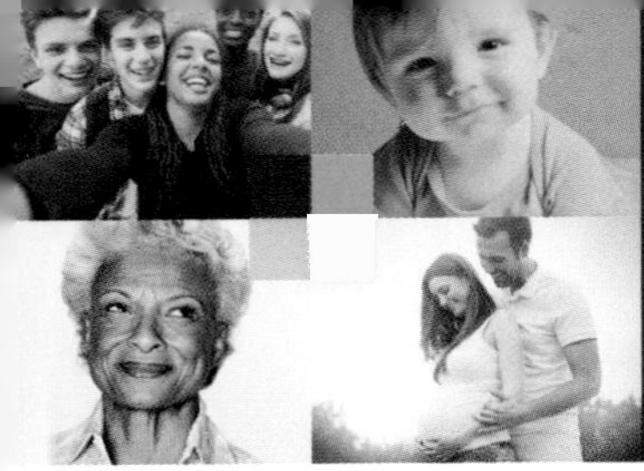

CHAPTER 22

Assessing Nutrition

Nutrition is the relative state of balance between nutrient intake and physiological requirements for growth and physical activity. Malnutrition can represent a nutrient deficit or excess. Assessing nutritional status achieves the following:

- Identifies actual nutritional deficiencies.
- Illuminates dietary patterns that may contribute to health problems.
- Provides a basis for planning for more optimal nutrition.
- Establishes baseline data for evaluation.

Performing the Nutritional Assessment

Nutritional assessment is recommended for people with any of the following nutritional risks:

- Weight less than 80 percent or more than 120 percent of ideal body weight.
- History of unintentional weight loss (>10 lb or 10 percent of usual weight).
- Serum albumin concentration < 3.5 g/dL.
- Total lymphocyte count < 1500 cells/mm^3.
- History of illness, surgery, trauma, or stress.
- Symptoms associated with nutritional deficiency or depletion.
- Factors associated with inadequate nutritional intake or absorption.

Health History

- Biographical: Note age of client to identify nutritional needs.
- Current health status: Any current health problems that may affect nutritional status.
- Past health history: History of GI disorders or nutritional disorders.
- Family history: Eating disorders, cancers, GI problems.

- Review of systems
  - Have you had unexplained weight loss, fatigue, activity intolerance, or inability to concentrate?
  - Have you noticed changes in skin texture, skin discolorations, poor wound healing, or bruising?
  - Do you have poor night vision or eye dryness?
  - Do you have nosebleeds or bleeding gums? Cavities or lost teeth?
  - Do you have chest pain or pressure?
  - Are you constipated?
  - Do you have diarrhea?
  - *Women:* Have you had frequent miscarriages or irregular menses? How much caffeine do you consume a day?
  - *Men:* Do you suffer from impotence?
  - Do you have muscle weakness?
  - Are you nervous or irritable? Do you have headaches, numbness or tingling, or muscle tics?
  - Do you have frequent infections? Allergies?
- Psychosocial profile
  - Who shops and prepares meals in your family?
  - Are you able to plan and cook meals yourself, or do you depend on others to do this?
  - When was your last dental exam?
  - Do you go for routine physical exams?
  - How do you usually spend your days? Do you go to restaurants frequently, and if so, where do you go and what types of foods do you eat? How much time do you spend shopping, preparing, and eating food?
  - What is your typical daily diet? How much water do you drink daily?
  - Do you actively try to maintain good nutrition and healthy weight? How?
  - Have your eating habits and appetite changed recently?
  - What is your usual activity and exercise level?
  - Do you feel that you have adequate energy? What activities do you not pursue because of lack of energy?
  - How many hours of sleep do you get a night? Do you wake up during the night? Are you taking more naps than usual? Do you feel rested? Do you use sleep aids? If so, what kinds?
  - Do you smoke?

- Do you drink alcohol? If so, how much per day? Do you drink coffee, tea, or soft drinks every day? If so, how much?
- Do you use over-the-counter (OTC) drugs?
- Do you use illegal drugs?
- What do you do for a living?
- How does your job affect daily meal routines?
- Is your income adequate to meet your food needs?
- Where do you buy your food? How do you store it? How do you prepare it?
- Do you have regular social interaction? Do you usually eat with other people or alone?
- Do you have any cultural influences that may affect your dietary practices? If so, what are they?
- Do you have any religious influences that may affect your dietary practices? If so, what are they?
- Are your social relationships satisfying or stressful? How much stress do you have in your life? How do you cope with it?

Focused Nutritional History

- Have you lost or gained weight unintentionally in the past 6 months?
- What is the most you have ever weighed?
- How much did you weigh 6 months ago, and how much do you weigh now?
- What do you normally eat every day? Has your diet changed significantly? If so, how?
- Do you have any stomach or bowel symptoms (e.g., nausea, vomiting, diarrhea, or anorexia) that have lasted more than 2 weeks?
- Has anything happened in your life that has affected your ability to obtain or prepare food? If so, what?

Comprehensive Nutritonal History

Two dietary analysis techniques are discussed below—24-hour recall and food intake records. You can use either technique as part of your comprehensive history.

24-Hour Recall

- Ask the patient to write down what he or she ate and drank during the previous 24 hours.
- Use the ChooseMyPlate.gov to sort and categorize the foods and determine the general quality of her or his diet.

- Ask the patient to record between-meal drinks and snacks, desserts, bedtime snacks, condiments, and food preparation items.
- Ask the patient to record water intake.
- Be sure to have the patient record the amount of each food or liquid he or she consumed, and translate these into standard servings according to MyPlate.

Food Intake Records

- Food intake records are typically done on people who are debilitated, have severe burns, or are on chemotherapy.
- A food intake record is a quantitative listing of all food and fluid consumed within a designated time frame—usually 3 to 5 days.
- To analyze the data, reduce the recorded food items into their constituent nutrients, using U.S. Department of Agriculture food composition tables.
- A less specific but more practical approach involves analyzing the patient's food intake record using food labels on packages.

Physical Assessment

APPROACH: You will mainly use the techniques of inspection and palpation. Evaluate the patient's hydration status simultaneously.

TOOLBOX: Weight scale, flexible measuring tape, calipers, stethoscope, growth charts, weight and height tables, anthropometric tables, laboratory values, a variety of containers.

Performing a Head-to-Toe Physical Assessment

- Look for changes in every system that might signal a nutritional problem.
- Anthropometry.
- Growth charts.
- Body mass index (BMI).
- Arm measurements
  - Triceps skin fatfold.
  - Midarm circumference.
  - Midarm muscle circumference.
  - Waist-to-hip ratio.

AREA/SYSTEM AND NORMAL FINDINGS	ABNORMAL FINDINGS
General Health Survey	
No unexplained weight changes.	*Weight changes in short time:* Fluid loss or gain.
Vital signs within normal limits for person's age.	*Elevated blood pressure (BP):* Fluid overload, high sodium intake, obesity. *Low BP:* Dehydration.
Integumentary *Skin*	
Skin intact, warm, and dry.	*Scaling:* Low or high vitamin A, low zinc, essential fatty acids.
Texture smooth, no lesions.	*Transparent, cellophane appearance:* Protein deficit.
Color consistent with ethnicity.	*Cracking (cracked-pavement appearance):* Protein deficit. *Follicular hyperkeratosis:* Vitamins A, C deficits. *Petechiae (especially perifollicular):* Vitamin C deficit. *Purpura:* Vitamins C, K deficits. *Pigmentation/desquamation of sun-exposed areas:* Niacin deficit. *Edema:* Protein and thiamin deficits. *Skin lesions, ulcers, nonhealing wounds:* Protein, vitamin C, zinc deficits. *Yellow pigmentation (except sclerae):* Excess carotene (benign). *Poor skin turgor:* Dehydration.
Integumentary *Hair*	
Even hair distribution, no alopecia.	*Transverse pigmentation of hair shaft; hair easy to pluck, breaks easily:* Protein deficit. *Sparse hair distribution:* Protein, biotin, zinc deficits; excess vitamin A. *Corkscrew hairs, unemerged hair coils:* Vitamin C deficit.
Nails	
Nails smooth and pink.	*Transverse ridges in nails:* Protein deficit. *Concave "spoon" nails:* Iron deficit.
HEENT *Eyes*	
Eyes clear and bright, vision intact.	*Papilledema:* Vitamin A excess. *Night blindness:* Vitamin A deficit. *Sunken eyeballs, dark circles, decreased tears:* Dehydration. *Sunken fontanels:* Dehydration.

AREA/SYSTEM AND NORMAL FINDINGS	ABNORMAL FINDINGS
Mouth and Throat	
Oral mucosa pink, moist, and intact without lesions.	*Angular stomatitis, cheilosis (dry, cracked, ulcerated lips):* Riboflavin, niacin, pyridoxine deficits.
Tonsils pink; gums pink and intact with no bleeding.	*Swollen, retracted, bleeding gums (if teeth present):* Vitamin C deficit. *Atrophic lingual papillae (coated tongue):* Riboflavin, niacin, folic acid, vitamin B_{12}, protein, iron deficits. *Glossitis (raw, red tongue):* Riboflavin, niacin, pyridoxine, folic acid, vitamin B_{12} deficits.
Parotid glands of normal size.	*Parotid gland enlargement:* Protein deficit (consider bulimia).
Taste sensation intact.	*Hypogeusia (blunting of sense of taste):* Zinc deficit.
Swallow and gag reflex intact. Full mobility of tongue.	Absent swallow and gag reflexes may impair eating. Impaired tongue mobility may cause dysphagia.
Nose	
Sense of smell intact.	*Hyposmia (defect in sense of smell):* Zinc deficit.
Nasal mucosa pink, moist, and intact without lesions.	Anosmia can affect taste. *Dry mucous membranes:* Dehydration.
Respiratory	
Lungs clear, respirations normal.	*Increased respiratory rate:* Iron deficiency anemia.
Cardiovascular	
Regular heart rate/rhythm. Point of maximal impulse (PMI) 1 cm at apex. No extra sounds.	*Heart failure, S_3:* Thiamin, phosphorus, iron deficits. *Sudden heart failure, death:* Vitamin C deficit. *Tachycardia and systolic murmur:* Iron deficiency anemia.
Gastrointestinal	
Abdomen soft, nontender; no organomegaly.	*Hepatomegaly, ascites:* Protein deficits, vitamin A excess. *Hyperactive bowel sounds:* Hyperperistalsis with absorption problem.
Musculoskeletal	
No deformities, tenderness, or swelling.	*Beading of ribs, epiphyseal swelling, bowlegs:* Vitamin D deficit. *Tenderness, superperiosteal bleeding:* Vitamin C deficit.

(box continued on page 568)

AREA/SYSTEM AND NORMAL FINDINGS	ABNORMAL FINDINGS
Neurologic	
No headache	*Headache:* Vitamin A excess.
Awake, alert, and oriented (AAO) x 3.	*Drowsiness, lethargy, vomiting:* Vitamins A, D excess.
Deep tendon reflex (DTR) +2/4	*Dementia:* Niacin, vitamin B_{12} deficit.
Senses intact.	*Confusion, irritability:* Dehydration. *Disorientation:* Thiamin (Korsakoff's psychosis) deficit. *Ophthalmoplegia:* Thiamin, phosphorus deficit. *Peripheral neuropathy (weakness, paresthesia, ataxia, decreased DTRs; diminished tactile, vibratory, and position sensation):* Niacin, pyridoxine, vitamin B_{12} deficits. *Tetany, increased DTRs:* Calcium, magnesium deficits.

HEENT = Head, eyes, ears, nose, and throat.

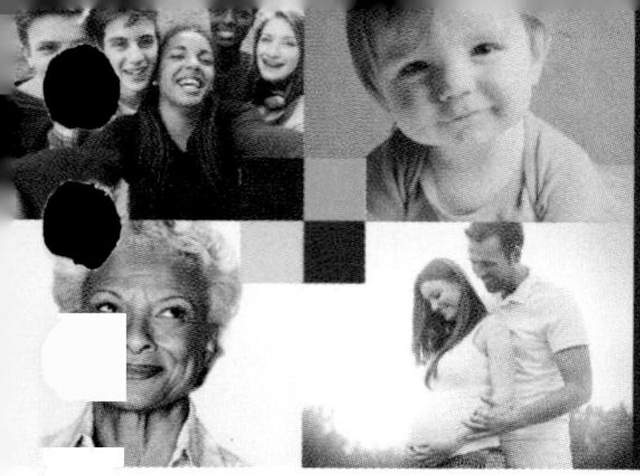

CHAPTER 23

Assessing Spirituality

Brief Review of Spiritual Health

- Does the patient identify with any organized religion? If so, what religion?
- If the patient does not identify with a particular religion, does he or she have a belief system that provides comfort and strength?
- Is the patient an agnostic or an atheist? If so, does any belief system give meaning to her or his life?
- Bear in mind what is the primary nature of the patient's religion.
- Are people of the patient's religion monotheistic or pantheistic?

Developmental Considerations

Infants

- What concerns do the parents have about their child's illness?
- How can you help support your patient's use of religious practices (e.g., by referral to the hospital chaplain or hospital meditation room)?
- Do parents ask why their child is ill?
- Do the parents see the infant's illness as a religious punishment?
- Are the parents practicing religious rituals?

Toddlers, Preschoolers, and School-Age Children

- How does the child feel about what is happening to him or her?
- To whom does the child talk when she or he is in trouble, sad, lonely, or scared?
- What makes the child feel better when he or she is scared, sad, or lonely?

- Does the child express concerns or show anxiety about illness and dying?
- Does she or he speak of being punished by a deity for "being bad?"
- Is he or she practicing religious rituals, such as saying bedtime prayers?

Adolescents and Young Adults

- How does the adolescent feel about what is happening to her or him?
- To whom does the adolescent usually go for support?
- What gives meaning to the adolescent's life? Has this changed since he or she got sick?
- Does the adolescent express concerns about dying or the seriousness of her or his illness?
- Does he or she practice any religious rituals?
- Does she or he verbalize her or his own beliefs and values?

Older Adults

- Ask the same questions as you would of an adolescent or young adult.
- Older patients often suffer many losses and, therefore, have fewer support systems, so you may need to make referrals to community services.

Cultural Considerations

- Familiarize yourself with your patient's cultural domain.
- Learn about the use of prayer, meditation, and other activities or symbols that help people of your patient's cultural or ethnic group reach fulfillment.
- Know what gives meaning to life for the patient's cultural group. Identify the patient's individual sources of strength.
- Become familiar with the way in which spiritual beliefs affect this cultural group's healthcare practices.

Health History

- Biographical data
  - Review the patient's admission sheet for basic religious information, and be sure to ask questions to clarify this information.

- Inquire about marital status and contact person.
- Ask the patient's age.
- Be aware that the absence of religious identification does not mean that the patient has no spiritual needs.

■ Current health status
- Your patient's current physical health and spiritual health are intertwined.
- Patients with chronic or terminal diseases are especially prone to spiritual distress.

■ Past health history
- Explore the connection between your patient's health and her or his spiritual needs.

■ Family history
- The family history is invaluable in identifying familial problems that pose a threat to your patient's health, which may affect his or her spiritual needs.

■ Psychosocial profile
- Examine your patient's typical day for activities that reflect spirituality.
- Determine whether dietary preferences may also be influenced by religious practices.

Spiritual Assessment

Assessing Behavior

Is the patient:

- Praying or meditating?
- Shutting others out?
- Constantly complaining?
- Having sleep difficulties?
- Pacing?
- Requesting frequent pain or sleep medication without apparent need?

Assessing Verbal Communication

Is the patient talking about:

- God or another deity?
- Church, temple, mosque, or other place of worship?
- Prayer, hope, faith, or the meaning of life?
- The effect of the diagnosis on her or his quality of life?

Assessing Relationships

Does the patient:

- Have many visitors? Who are his or her visitors (family, friends, clergy, or other spiritual support people)?
- Interact with them well?

Assessing Environment

Does the patient have:

- A Bible, Koran (Qur'an), or other religious reading material?
- Religious jewelry or symbols, such as a cross, Star of David, prayer cap or shawl, flowers from a church altar, or religious greeting cards?

Additional Questions for the Patient

- Who are your support people?
- What provides you with strength and hope?
- What gives your life meaning and purpose?
- How has your life changed since you became ill?
- What is important to you?
- How is your religion, deity, or faith important to you?
- Is prayer important?
- What accommodations can be made to assist you in continuing any spiritual practices (e.g., religious symbols and/or dietary needs)?

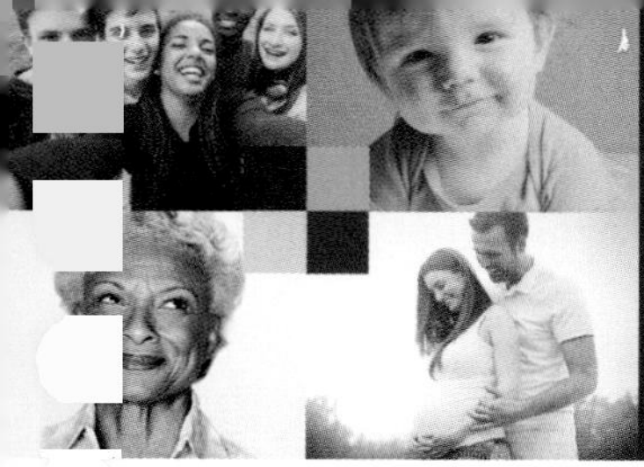

CHAPTER 24

Assessing Culture

Because cultural background encompasses every aspect of a person's life, you need to be aware of how it influences your patient's health and wellness. Consider the following areas—as adapted from Purnell, L.D., and Paulanka, B.J. (2012): *Transcultural Healthcare: A Culturally Competent Approach,* (ed. 4), Philadelphia: F.A. Davis—when determining the influence of culture on your patient's health.

Overview

- Inhabited localities and topography
  - In what part of the world does this person's cultural or ethnic group originate?
  - What are the climate and topography there?
- Heritage and residence
  - Where does this person's cultural or ethnic group reside now?
- Reason for migration and associated economic factors
  - What were the major factors that motivated this person's cultural or ethnic group to emigrate?
- Educational status and occupations
  - What value does the person's cultural group place on education?
  - What are the predominant occupations of the group's members?

Communication

- Dominant language and dialects
  - What is the dominant language of the group?
  - Does the person use that language or a dialect that may interfere with communication?

- Are there specific contextual speech patterns for this group? If so, what are they?
- What are the usual volume and tone of speech?

■ Cultural communication patterns
- Is the person willing to share thoughts, feelings, and ideas?
- What are the practice and meaning of touch in the person's society? With family, friends, strangers, same sex, opposite sex, and healthcare providers?
- What are the personal spatial and distancing characteristics when communicating one-to-one? With friends versus strangers?
- Does this group use eye contact? Does avoidance of eye contact have special meaning? Is eye contact influenced by socioeconomic status?
- Do various facial expressions have specific meanings? Are facial expressions used to express emotions?
- Are there acceptable ways of standing and greeting outsiders? If so, what are they?

■ Temporal relationships
- Are people primarily past, present, or future oriented? How do they see the context of past, present, and future?
- Are there differences in interpretation of social time versus clock time? If so, what are they?
- Are people expected to be punctual in terms of jobs, appointments, and social engagements?

■ Format and names
- What is the format for a person's name?
- How does the person expect to be greeted by strangers and healthcare practitioners?

Family Roles and Organization

■ Head of household and gender roles
- Who is the perceived head of household?
- How does this role change during different developmental aspects of life?
- What are the gender-related roles of men and women in the family system?

■ Prescriptive, restrictive, and taboo behaviors
- What are the prescriptive, restrictive, and taboo behaviors for children?

- What are the prescriptive, restrictive, and taboo behaviors for adults?

- Family roles and priorities
  - What family goals and priorities are emphasized by this culture?
  - What are the developmental tasks of this group?
  - What are the status and role of older people in the family?
  - What are the roles and importance of extended family members?
  - How does one gain social status in this cultural system? Is there a caste system?
  - How are alternative lifestyles and nontraditional families viewed by the society?

Workforce Issues

- Culture in the workplace
  - Are workforce issues, such as education, affected by immigration? If so, how?
  - What are the specific multicultural considerations when working with this culturally diverse person or group?
  - What factors influence patterns of acculturation in this cultural group?
  - How do the person's or group's healthcare practices influence the workforce?
- Issues related to autonomy
  - What are the cultural issues related to professional autonomy, superior or subordinate control, religion, and gender in the workforce?
  - Are there language barriers? For example, do people sometimes misunderstand English expressions by interpreting them concretely?

Biocultural Ecology

- Skin color and biological variations
  - Are there skin color and physical variations for this group? If so, what are they?
  - What special problems or concerns might the skin color pose for healthcare practitioners?
  - What are the biological variations in body habitus or structure?

- Diseases and health conditions
  - What are the risk factors for people related to topography or climate?
  - Are there any hereditary or genetic diseases or conditions that are common with this group? If so, what are they?
  - Are there any endemic diseases specific to this cultural or ethnic group? If so, what are they?
  - Are there any diseases or health conditions for which this group has increased susceptibility? If so, what are they?
  - Does this group have any specific variations in drug metabolism, drug interactions, and related side effects? If so, what are they?

High-Risk Behaviors

- Are any high-risk behaviors common in this group? If so, what are they?
- What are the patterns of use of alcohol, tobacco, recreational drugs, and other substances in this group?

Healthcare Practices

- What are typical health-seeking behaviors for this group?
- What is this group's usual level of physical activity?
- Do people in this group use safety measures, such as seat belts?

Nutrition

- What does food mean to this group?
- Common foods and food rituals
  - What specific foods, preparation practices, and major ingredients are commonly used by this group?
  - Are there any specific food rituals for this group? If so, what are they?
- Dietary practices for health promotion
  - Are enzyme deficiencies or food intolerances commonly experienced by this group? If so, what are they?
  - Are large-scale or significant nutritional deficiencies experienced by this group? If so, what are they?
  - Are there native food limitations in America that may cause special health difficulties? If so, what are they?

Pregnancy and Childbearing Practices

- Fertility practices and views regarding pregnancy
  - What are the cultural views and practices related to fertility control?
  - What are the cultural views and practices regarding pregnancy?
- Prescriptive, restrictive, and taboo practices in the childbearing family
  - What are the prescriptive, restrictive, and taboo practices related to pregnancy, such as food, exercise, intercourse, and avoidance of weather-related conditions?
  - What are the prescriptive, restrictive, and taboo practices related to the birthing process, such as reactions during labor, presence of men, position of mother for delivery, preferred types of health practitioners, or place of delivery?
  - What are the prescriptive, restrictive, and taboo practices related to the postpartum period, such as bathing, cord care, exercise, food, and roles of men?

Death Rituals

- Death rituals and expectations
  - Are there culturally specific death rituals and expectations? If so, what are they?
  - What is the purpose of the death rituals and mourning practices?
  - What specific practices (e.g., cremation) are used for disposal of the body?
- Responses to death and grief
  - How are people expected to show grief and respond to the death of a family member?
  - What is the meaning of death, dying, and afterlife?

Spirituality

- Religious practices and use of prayer
  - How does the dominant religion of this group influence healthcare practices?
  - Are there activities such as prayer, meditation, or symbols that help people reach fulfillment? If so, what are they?

- Meaning of life and individual sources of strength
  - What gives meaning to people's lives?
  - What is the person's source of strength?
  - What is the relationship between spiritual beliefs and healthcare practices?

Healthcare Practices

- Health-seeking beliefs and behaviors
  - What predominant beliefs influence healthcare practices?
  - What is the influence of health promotion and prevention practices?
- Responsibility for healthcare
  - Is the focus of acute-care practice curative or fatalistic?
  - Who assumes responsibility for healthcare in this culture?
  - What is the role of health insurance in this culture?
  - What are the behaviors associated with the use of over-the-counter medications?
  - How do magicoreligious beliefs, folklore, and traditional beliefs influence healthcare behaviors?
  - Are there barriers to healthcare, such as language, economics, and geography, for this group? If so, what are they?
- Cultural responses to health and illness
  - Are there cultural beliefs and responses to pain that influence interventions? If so, what are they?
  - Does pain have special meaning?
  - What are the beliefs and views about mental and physical illness in this culture?
  - Does this culture view mental handicaps differently from physical handicaps?
  - What are the cultural beliefs and practices related to chronicity and rehabilitation?
  - Are there any restrictions to the acceptance of blood transfusions, organ donation, and organ transplantation for this group? If so, what are they?

Healthcare Practitioners

- Traditional versus biomedical care
  - What are the roles of traditional, folklore, and magicoreligious practitioners, and how do they influence health practitioners?

  - How does this culture feel about healthcare practitioners providing care to patients of the opposite sex?
  - Does the age of the practitioner make a difference? If so, what?
- Status of healthcare providers
  - How does this culture feel about healthcare providers?
  - What is the status of healthcare providers in this culture?
  - How do different healthcare practitioners in this culture view each other?

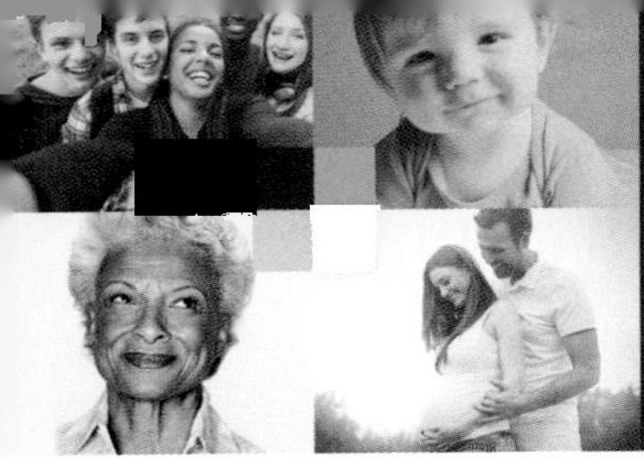

CHAPTER 25

Assessing the Patient's Environment

Shorter stays in acute-care settings have increased the need for nursing care at home. Home care nursing can occur at both the primary and the tertiary levels. At the primary-care level, you will make postpartum visits to new mothers and babies. At the tertiary level, you will make follow-up visits to patients discharged from the hospital.

Assessing the Home

In the home, your assessment is based on the health history and physical exam findings. You need to assess your patient's response to the treatment plan and also identify any risk factors in his or her environment that may affect his or her health and well-being. Remember, the treatment plan established in the hospital will be effective only if your patient is able to follow it at home.

Begin by determining if your patient is able to perform activities of daily living (ADLs); then assess basic needs and environmental safety hazards. Also assess support systems and self-esteem or self- actualization. Keep in mind that financial status and religious and cultural beliefs influence health beliefs and practices.

AREAS/QUESTIONS TO ASK	FACTORS IDENTIFIED BY QUESTIONS
Physical Needs	
Food	
What does the patient eat and drink?	Need for referrals for assistance, such as financial support, Meals on Wheels, home health aides.
Who prepares food? Who buys food? Is food being stored properly?	Self-care deficits. Teaching needs.
Is kitchen accessible? Clean? Are appliances in good operating condition?	Nutritional deficits or problems affecting nutritional status.
If you detect a nutritional deficit, does patient's illness have an effect on appetite? Is there an unexplained weight loss or gain? Does the patient drink alcohol? Does she or he have a dental problem? Are financial hardships limiting purchase of foods? Is the patient taking multiple medicines? Does he or she eat alone? Does she or he need assistance in eating?	
Elimination	
Is the bathroom accessible?	Need for assistive devices.
Does patient need a commode?	Self-care deficits.
Does he or she need a raised toilet seat? Grab bars?	Risk for falls. Risk for incontinence problems.
Bathing	
Does patient take baths, showers, or sponge baths?	Need for assistive devices. Self-care deficits.
Does she or he care for her or his hair and teeth?	Risk for falls.
Does he or she need assistance in bathing? Does he or she have a shower chair? Does the bathtub have grab bars? Rubber mats? Nonskid tiles?	
Dressing	
Does patient have clean clothes?	Self-care deficits.
Do clothes fit?	Risks for falls or skin breakdown.
Does she or he need assistance with dressing? Do shoes fit properly? Who does the laundry?	Need for home health aide.

(continued)

AREAS/QUESTIONS TO ASK	FACTORS IDENTIFIED BY QUESTIONS
Physical Needs *(cont'd)*	
Sleep	
Where does the patient sleep?	Risk for skin breakdown.
How much time does he or she spend in bed?	Need for special equipment. Safety issues.
Does the patient need a special mattress or bed? Are bedrails needed? How far is the bed from the bathroom? From other family members? Is there privacy for members in household?	
Medications	
Is patient able to take own medications as prescribed?	Compliance with medical treatment plan and reasons for noncompliance.
Is she or he taking any over-the-counter (OTC) medications, vitamins, or herbal supplements?	Problems associated with polypharmacy (e.g., side effects, drug interactions).
Does he or she need medications prepoured?	Safety issues surrounding medication preparation and administration.
Does she or he have any impairments that would prevent her or him from self-administering medications safely (e.g., cognitive or visual impairments)?	Need for assistive devices. Need for referral or visiting nurse. Teaching needs. Financial needs for obtaining prescriptions.
Are medications safely stored?	
Can patient open medication containers?	
If using syringes, how does patient dispose of them? Obtain supplies? What is the name of patient's pharmacy? His or her medication insurance plan? Does patient have the finances to pay for medications and treatment? Does patient understand what medications she or he is taking and their purpose?	
Shelter	
Is home maintained and clean?	Safety issues.
Who is responsible for managing and cleaning it? Are plumbing and sewage systems working properly?	Need for referrals. Need for assistance with home management and maintenance.

AREAS/QUESTIONS TO ASK	FACTORS IDENTIFIED BY QUESTIONS
What type of heating is there (gas, electric, oil, wood)? Central heating or space heating? Is heating system working properly? Is there air conditioning? Fans? Is ventilation adequate? Do windows open and close easily and completely? What type of insulation is there? Is home in need of repair (e.g., peeling paint or cracks in foundation or windows)? Is there evidence of insect or rodent infestation? Has home been tested for radon?	
Assessing Environmental Safety	
Mobility/Fall Prevention	
Is patient able to walk? Is her or his gait steady? Does patient use assistive devices correctly? Do devices fit through pathways and doorways? Is house one level or more? Are there elevators or stairs? Can patient enter and exit home without difficulty? Are pathways and stairs clear? Are there throw rugs? Are there sturdy handrails on the stairs? Are first and last steps clearly marked? Are floors slippery or uneven? Is there adequate lighting in hallways, stairs, and path to bathroom? Is there need for restraints? If yes, what type and when? Are carpets in good repair without tears? Can patient walk on carpet? Does he or she have to hold on to furniture to maintain balance? If yes, is furniture sturdy and stable enough to provide support? Are chairs sturdy and stable? Are there any cords or wires that may present a tripping hazard?	Risk for fall/injury. Need for assistive devices. Need for referrals. Need for teaching.

(continued)

AREAS/QUESTIONS TO ASK	FACTORS IDENTIFIED BY QUESTIONS
Assessing Environmental Safety *(cont'd)*	
Fire/Burn Prevention	
Are there working smoke detectors on each floor? Carbon monoxide detectors? Fire extinguisher? Is there an escape plan in case of fire? Are wires, plugs, and electrical equipment in good working condition? Is patient using a heating pad or portable heaters safely? Does she or he smoke? If yes, does she or he smoke safely? Are there signs of cigarette burns? Are there signs of burns in the kitchen? Is stove free of grease? Does patient use oxygen? If yes, is tank stored safely away from heat or flame?	Risk for injury. Safety issues. Teaching needs. Referrals (e.g., local fire company for free smoke detectors).
Crime/Injury	
Are there working locks on doors and windows? Is patient able to make emergency calls? Are emergency numbers readily available? Is phone readily accessible? Are there firearms in home? If yes, are they safely secured, with ammunition stored separately? Is there any evidence of criminal activity? Are poisonous or toxic substances properly stored?	Safety issues. Need for referral to local police. Teaching needs.
Assessing Support Systems, Self-Esteem, and Self-Actualization	
Roles	
What roles does person play because of illness? How has this affected other family members?	Source of stress, depression, and anxiety. Need for referrals.
Caregivers	
Is there a caregiver? Is caregiver competent, willing, and supportive? Does caregiver need support?	Supports. Need for referrals (e.g., caregiver may need support, respite care, or home health aide).

AREAS/QUESTIONS TO ASK	FACTORS IDENTIFIED BY QUESTIONS
Can caregiver hear patient? Is there a need for an intercom, "baby monitor," or bell?	Need for assistive devices. Teaching needs.
Communication	
Is phone in easy reach?	Emergency supports.
Can patient dial phone and see numbers? Does he or she need oversized numbers, audio enhancer, or memory feature?	Teaching needs. Need for assistive devices. Safety issues.
Is there a daily safety check system? Should there be an alert system like Lifeline?	
Are emergency numbers for police, fire, ambulance, nurse, doctor, relative, or neighbor clearly marked? How does patient get mail?	
Family/Friends/Pets	
Who visits patient? Family, friends, church members?	Supports. Need for referrals.
Who can drive patient to doctor appointments, church, and other places?	Ability to maintain follow-up care. Teaching needs.
Are there any pets? Is patient able to take care of them properly? Are pets well behaved?	
Self-Esteem and Self-Actualization	
What does patient like to do? Are there creative ways to enable her or him to do activities she or he enjoys?	Sources of meaning in patient's life. Need for referral to community resources (e.g., library, senior citizen groups).
Are there meaningful solitary activities patient can do, such as reading or listening to music? Interactive activities?	

Adapted with permission from Narayan, M. (1997). Environmental assessment. *Home Healthcare Nurse, 15*(11):798. Philadelphia, Lippincott-Raven.

Assessing the Community

Assessment involves assessing the people within the community, the environment of the community, and the interaction between the two to identify any actual or potential health problems.

QUESTIONS TO ASK YOURSELF	SIGNIFICANCE
Boundaries	
What is the geographic description of the community (e.g., a town) or the criteria for membership in the community (e.g., a school)?	Boundaries can be real, concrete or conceptual. Identifies who and what is included in the community.
What are the neighboring areas (e.g., a city if the community is a suburb)?	Allows you to focus assessment on the community.
Are boundaries open or closed?	Some boundaries may exclude certain groups (e.g., communities with only high-priced housing may exclude lower socioeconomic groups).
What is the purpose or goals of the community (e.g., a school's mission statement)?	Identifies purpose of community (e.g., goal of a Catholic school is to educate children in Christian values).
Physical Characteristics	
How old is the community?	Older, well-established community may have more resources available than new, developing community. Or, older community's resources may be outdated, not meeting current needs.
What are community's demographics (e.g., age, race, sex, ethnicity, housing, density of population)?	You can identify healthcare needs of community by identifying health problems associated with age, gender, or race.
What are community's physical features?	Physical features can influence community's behavior and health (e.g., exposure to toxic substances).
Psychosocial Characteristics	
What is the community's predominant religion, socioeconomic class, educational level, type of occupation, and marital status?	Religion influences what and how health issues are addressed (e.g., abortion/birth control contradicts Catholic beliefs). Socioeconomic class reflects affordability and accessibility of healthcare services. People in low socioeconomic areas may not

QUESTIONS TO ASK YOURSELF	SIGNIFICANCE
	have financial resources for healthcare or be able to practice preventive healthcare. Limited financial access to healthcare raises community's morbidity and mortality rates. Educational level identifies health teaching needs and approaches. The higher their educational level, the more likely people are to practice preventive health behaviors. Occupation can identify specific health issues for the group (e.g., blue collar workers may have a higher incidence of musculoskeletal problems; white collar workers may have a higher incidence of stress-related diseases). Marital status may identify stability and support sources within community.
External Influences	
Does the community receive any external funding?	Federal or state funding and grants may be available for health services.
Are there facilities outside community that are available to community members? Is there access or transportation to these facilities? Are adequate healthcare providers available to community?	Identifies healthcare facilities needed (e.g., rural areas may need to go outside community for health services).
Are volunteer groups available to the community?	Volunteer groups can be a valuable resource, especially if healthcare providers are limited.
How is health information communicated to community?	Determines if there is a need for further and better means of communication.
What laws affect the community?	Laws, such as zoning or pollution laws, can influence healthcare issues. Federal and state programs also can affect the health and well-being of some members of the community, such as senior citizens.
Are values of external influences consistent with those of community?	Inconsistent values can affect healthcare issues.

(continued)

QUESTIONS TO ASK YOURSELF	SIGNIFICANCE
Internal Functions **Human Services**	
What human services are available within community? Nurses, doctors, volunteers? Is access to services adequate?	Determines if services meet community's needs.
What is community's budget? How much is allocated for healthcare services?	Identifies value of healthcare services and need for external funding sources.
What and how many healthcare facilities (hospitals, nursing homes, daycare centers) are available in community? Are there enough to meet people's needs? Are they well equipped? Accessible?	Determines availability and accessibility of healthcare facilities.
Does facility have goods and supplies to produce its goods? What is the product? What is the facility's contribution to the community?	Identifies both positive and negative effects to community (e.g., if facility is drug treatment center, drug dealers and abusers, as a community in itself, exert a negative effect on community at large).
Is education appropriate, accessible, and adequate for community? What types of schools are there? How much money is budgeted for education?	Identifies adequacy and availability of schools.
Internal Functions **Politics**	
What is the organizational structure of the community? Elected vs. appointed positions? Terms? Formal vs. informal leaders?	Helps identify how decisions are made and who has power.
How are decisions made? Majority rule or consensus? Is community independent or dependent?	Identifies approaches needed to bring about change. Identifies role of nurse within community (e.g., if community is dependent, nurse may need to take more active role).
What are rules and laws of community? Formal and informal?	Identifies laws that regulate behaviors. Identifies expectations, peer pressures.
Communication	
Nonverbal: What is personality of community? How do people respond to outsiders?	Identifies approaches toward community.

QUESTIONS TO ASK YOURSELF	SIGNIFICANCE
Verbal: Who communicates with whom? What are means of communication? Is communication vertical or horizontal?	
Values	
What does the community value? What is important?	Identifies what is important to community.
Does the community have any traditions?	Can influence healthcare practices.
Are there subgroups within the community?	Can have own values and norms that affect community and influence healthcare practices.
What is the condition of the physical environment? Clean, dirty, in disrepair?	Condition of environment reflects value placed on it by community.
How is health defined by the community? How much does community value health? What type of healthcare facilities are there? How frequently are they used?	Identifies value community places on health.
Is the community homogeneous or heterogeneous?	Identifies approaches toward community.
Health Behavior/Health Status	
People	
What is the growth rate of the community? Relationship between birth and death rates? Relationship between immigration and emigration? Is population young or old? Is it mobile?	Identifies health status and needs of community (e.g., health needs for retirement community are different from those of a community with mostly young couples). Indirectly identifies teaching needs. Identifies factors within community that affect health.
What are morbidity and mortality rates? The prevalence and incidence of disease?	Identifies focus and direction of healthcare needed by community. Identifies health teaching needs for community.
What types of risky behavior occur in the community? Are there at-risk groups?	Identifies at-risk groups. Identifies need for intervention and teaching.
What is the incidence of presymptomatic illnesses, such as human immunodeficiency virus (HIV), hypertension (HTN), or high cholesterol?	Identifies need for screening programs. Determines effectiveness of existing screening programs. Identifies health teaching needs.

(continued)

QUESTIONS TO ASK YOURSELF	SIGNIFICANCE
Health Behavior/Health Status	
People *(cont'd)*	
What is the level of functioning of community (e.g., dependent vs. independent)?	Identifies type and direction of intervention needed to maintain and promote health.
Are there people with disabilities? How many people and what types of disabilities?	Identifies resources required to meet need of community members with disabilities.
Environment	
What is the quality of the air?	Identifies possible exposure to pollutants.
What is the quality of the food supply?	Identifies possible contamination causing gastrointestinal (GI) diseases.
What is the quality of the water supply? Is the water public or well? Is it fluoridated?	Identifies possible contamination causing GI problems.
What is the quality of the soil?	Identifies possible contamination with radioactive material, human or animal excreta, *Ascaris* worm.
Is there adequate housing?	Identifies possible crowding, radon and lead exposure.
What is the quality of home and work site?	Identifies possible occupational health risks.
What is the quality of solid waste disposal?	Identifies possible source of contamination.
What is the quality of hazardous waste disposal?	Identifies possible contamination from toxic substances.
Is there infestation by insects, rodents, and animals? Use of pesticides?	Identifies disease carriers. Pesticide use increases risk for exposure to toxic chemicals.
Are there natural disasters in the community? Incidences of violence or terrorism?	Identifies sources of stress.

Data from Smith, C., and Maurer, F. (2000). *Community Health Nursing Theory and Practice*, ed. 2. Philadelphia: W.B. Saunders.

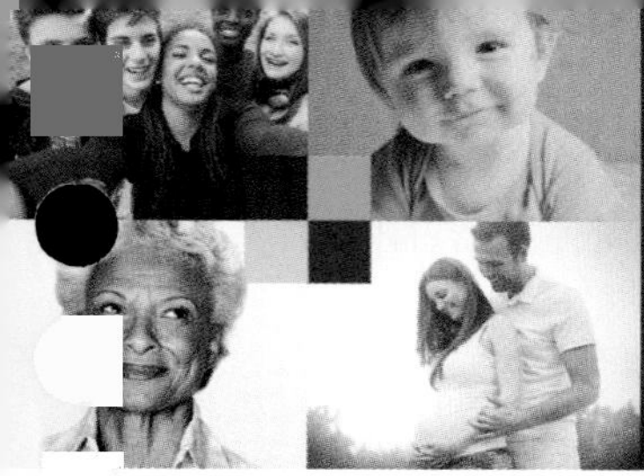

CHAPTER 26

Assessing Abuse

Abuse can take many forms, can affect any age group, and knows no socioeconomic boundaries. It can be physical, sexual, emotional, or a combination of two or all of these. It may also be directed at property. As a nurse, you need to be alert for signs and symptoms of abuse at all levels of healthcare for all of your patients. This chapter covers child abuse, spousal or partner (domestic) abuse, and elder abuse.

Types of Abuse

- *Physical abuse:* Physical contact with intent to harm, ranging from slapping, hitting, and biting to murder. Physical abuse includes neglect—depriving a person of basic needs such as food, water, or sleep.
- *Sexual abuse:* Sexually oriented behavior without the consent of the other person or persons involved, ranging from sexually degrading remarks to rape.
- *Psychological (emotional) abuse:* Verbal abuse or actions that can be considered degrading, belittling, or threatening, used for control, often by evoking fear in the victim. This type of abuse is difficult to assess.
- *Property abuse:* Deliberate destruction of a person's belongings.

Assessing Child Abuse

Child abuse and neglect are the leading cause of death in children younger than 3. More than 3 million cases are reported every year. Child abuse can take the following forms:

- *Physical abuse:* Includes actual physical trauma, such as bruising, breaking bones, intentional burns, and shaken-baby syndrome. It also includes Munchausen's syndrome by proxy (MSBP), in which the parent or caretaker intentionally causes a child to be ill to gain sympathy and recognition.

- *Neglect:* Failure to meet the child's basic needs.
- *Sexual abuse:* Includes actual intercourse with either vaginal or anal penetration, genital fondling and other inappropriate touching, or pornographic photography of the child.
- *Psychological abuse:* Includes emotional detachment from the child, constant belittling, fostering and enabling substance abuse and delinquency, and failing to provide adequate supervision.

Assessing for Physical Abuse

As you go through the assessment, ask yourself: Are the injuries inconsistent with the child's age or developmental stage (e.g., 1-month-old baby falling out of crib)? Is evidence of old fractures or trauma seen on current x-rays?

Taking the Health History

- Obtain separate statements from parents or caregivers. Be alert for inconsistencies (e.g., parent saying that hand-mark bruising on the child was inflicted by another child).
- Ask yourself: What is your perception of the child (e.g., difficult or quiet)?
- Ask the parent or caregiver:
  - Does the child have a history of past health problems? Where was the child treated? (Frequent emergency room [ER]) visits signal abuse. Parents may use different healthcare centers to avoid suspicion.)
  - What is the child's feeding history? (Compare the history given with the child's physical growth and development.)
  - Ask the child (if old enough): What types of stress do you have in your life? Who are your supports?
- Suspect MSBP if:
  - Child does not respond to usual treatment.
  - Laboratory results are inconsistent with history or physically impossible.
  - Parent seems very knowledgeable about medical treatment.
  - Signs and symptoms of illness do not occur when parent is not present.
  - Similar findings or unexplained deaths have occurred in siblings.
  - Parent craves adulation for his or her care of child.

Performing the Physical Exam

- Obtain growth measurements and compare them with previous measurements. Nutritional neglect can cause failure to thrive.
- Look for distended abdomen, a sign of malnutrition.
- Observe child's grooming, dress, and hygiene.
- Examine all body surfaces for bruises, burns, and skin lesions, looking especially for the following signs of physical abuse:
  - Bruises that form the outline of a hand (from parent grabbing child).
  - Linear bruises (from belts).
  - Bruises on head, face, ears, buttocks, and lower back (consistent with abuse).
  - Obviously nonaccidental burns (e.g., burns on both lower legs).
  - Burn outline of an entire object, such as multiple cigarette burns on various parts of body.
  - Detached retina and hemorrhages and subdural hematoma (shaken-baby syndrome).

Assessing for Sexual Abuse

Taking the Health History

Be nonjudgmental when questioning caregivers about possible sexual abuse. Obtain the following information from patients or their caregivers:

- Ask children over 2½ 2 years directly about being touched in "private parts." With older children, use an approach such as: "Sometimes people you know may touch or kiss you in a way that you feel is wrong. Has this ever happened to you?" With adolescents, use an approach such as: "Sometimes people touch you in ways you feel are wrong. This can be frightening, and it is wrong for people to do that to you. Has this ever happened to you?"
- Determine whether there has been a sudden onset of bedwetting in a child who was previously not a bedwetter.
- Determine whether the child masturbates or sexually acts out with other children.
- Determine whether the child has genitourinary symptoms, such as burning, itching, or vaginal discharge.
- Determine whether the child has a history of running away from home, especially to unsafe situations as opposed to a friend's home.

Performing the Physical Assessment

- Look for genital and anal irritation, discharge, swelling, redness, and bruising. In girls, carefully evaluate the vaginal introitus for evidence of penetration.
- During the exam, observe the child's behavior:
  - Is the child overly solicitous in a sexual manner?
  - Does she or he dress or act provocatively?
  - Is he or she overly fearful of the exam, especially the genital exam?

Assessing for Psychological Abuse

Taking the Health History

Ask the parent or caregiver the following questions:

- Was this child the result of a planned pregnancy? What were the birth and postpartum period like? Were there many stressors at home at the time of your child's birth?
- How would you describe your child now?
- How is this child compared with others in your family?
- Is there a history of physical or developmental problems? If so, what kinds of supports do you receive?
- Has the child had many illnesses? If so, what are they? How has this affected your life?
- What are your expectations of the child?
- What form of discipline works best for the child?

Performing the Psychological Assessment

During the exam, observe the following:

- Compare parental description of the child with what you actually observe.
- Observe child-parent interaction. Is it distant or engaging? How does the parent comfort the child?
- If other siblings are present, does the parent respond to them differently from the child in question?
- Does the parent openly and repeatedly belittle the child (e.g., saying: "You're so dumb")?
- Does the child have developmental delays, poor social skills, speech problems, or regression?

Assessing Spousal or Partner Abuse (Domestic Violence)

Domestic violence is the leading cause of injury to women. One in every four women has been abused by a spouse or partner at least one time during the relationship. Here are more facts about domestic violence:

- Fifty percent of homeless women and children have been victims of abuse.
- The battering cycle consists of the tension-building phase, the battering phase, and the apologetic phase.
- Abuse occurs in same-sex relationships as well as heterosexual relationships.
- Abusers are usually emotionally dependent and egocentric.
- The battered partner is usually unsure, economically and emotionally dependent, and exhibiting learned helplessness.
- Spousal or partner abuse can take the form of physical, sexual, or psychological abuse (or a combination of two or all of these), or property abuse.
- Emotional abuse is difficult to assess because the effects are not as visible as those of physical abuse.
- To gain power and control, the abuser may:
    - Use coercion and threats, such as threatening to leave the partner or commit suicide.
    - Use intimidation to evoke fear by destroying personal belongings or hurting pets.
    - Degrade and belittle, making the partner feel that it is her or his fault; make her or him feel guilty or blame abuse on her or him.
    - Isolate the partner by limiting contacts with family and friends.
    - Control or limit finances.
    - Put children in the middle of the situation or threaten to take them away.
    - If male, use male privilege by enforcing dominant role.

Assessing for Physical Abuse

Taking the Health History

Ask the patient:

- What is your chief complaint? Complaints are often vague and nonspecific; for example, headaches, gastrointestinal (GI) complaints, asthma, fatigue, and chronic vague pain.

- Do you have trouble sleeping? Do you have nightmares?
- Have you ever been hospitalized? Frequent ER visits are common, with injuries becoming progressively more severe. Current radiographs may reveal old fractures.
- How did the injury happen? Injury may not match the explanation (e.g., black eye from walking into door).
- Do you have a history of depression or attempted suicide? Abuse victim with a sense of hopelessness and powerlessness may be depressed and attempt suicide.
- Are you taking any prescribed or over-the-counter (OTC) medications? Do you drink alcohol? If so, how much? Substance abuse may be used as an attempt to deal with physical abuse.
- Have you had any weight or appetite changes? Anorexia and bulimia are not uncommon.
- Have you ever been sexually assaulted? Are you satisfied with your sexual relationship with spouse or partner? Domestic violence can take the form of sexual abuse.

Performing the Physical Exam

- Assess for injuries suggesting abuse, such as cigarette burns; black eyes; facial injuries; injuries to the chest, back, breast, or abdomen; bruising on genitalia; or bruises in the shape of a hand or belt.
- During the exam, observe for the following:
  - Patient's lethargic, passive behavior.
  - Patient's poor eye contact and anxious or fearful behavior.
  - Patient's visible fear when partner is in room; looking to partner before responding to questions.
  - Partner answering for patient and being overly condescending.

Assessing Elder Abuse and Neglect

An estimated 2.1 million older Americans are victims of some type of abuse annually. Elder abuse can be physical, sexual, or psychological. It can also take the form of neglect or financial or property abuse. During your assessment, be alert if the caregiver speaks for the patient, refuses to let the patient be examined alone, or underreacts when confronted with findings suggesting abuse.

Assessing for Physical Abuse

Taking the Health History

Ask the following questions of the patient and caregiver:

- How did the injury happen? Suspect abuse if injury does not match explanation (e.g., caregiver says injury is from fall, but patient has no difficulty with balance or walking).
- When did the injury occur? Lengthy interval between injury and treatment suggests abuse.
- Who is the primary healthcare provider? "Doctor shopping" (using different healthcare providers) suggests abuse.
- To patient: Do you feel safe in your home?
- To patient: Are there any situations in which you feel afraid?
- To patient or caregiver: Have you ever given/taken the wrong dose of medication? Repeated medication errors by caregiver (e.g., oversedating patient) suggest abuse.

Performing the Physical Exam

During the exam, observe for the following:

- Whiplash burns from rope or cord.
- Cigarette burns on palms and soles of feet.
- Injuries with a pattern, such as that of a belt buckle or electrical cord.
- Oral ecchymosis or injury from forced oral sex.
- Whiplash injuries from shaking.
- Hyphema, subconjunctival hemorrhage, detached retina, ruptured tympanic membrane.
- Bruises on trunk, breast, abdomen, genitalia, and buttocks (bathing suit zone).
- Bleeding or bruising of genitalia, poor sphincter tone, and bruises on inner thighs.
- Bruising on wrists and ankles from being bound or restrained.
- Immersion burns (may follow a stocking-glove pattern).
- Evidence of old injuries.
- Anxiety and depression.

Assessing for Neglect

The following are signs of neglect in a patient:

- Never changing clothes, or wearing clothes that are dirty or inappropriate for the weather.
- Poor hygiene or body odor.
- Ingrown nails.

- Decayed or missing teeth.
- Untreated sores or pressure sores.
- Matted hair.
- Hypo/hyperthermia.
- Untreated medical problems.
- Dehydration.
- Malnutrition, failure-to-thrive syndrome.
- Weight loss.
- Abnormal blood chemistry.
- If you are making a home visit: Clutter, disconnected utilities, neglected pets, animal or human excrement, spoiled food.

Assessing for Financial Abuse

The following are signs of financial abuse:

- Unusual activity in patient's bank account.
- Bank statements diverted from patient's home.
- Sudden disappearance of caregiver.
- Patient asked to sign documents such as power of attorney.
- Large withdrawals from patient's account.
- Family that is reluctant to spend money on patient.
- Disappearance of personal belongings.
- Isolation of patient by caregiver.
- Forged signatures on checks and documents.
- Caregiver who is evasive about sources of income.
- Lack of solid legal financial arrangements in place for older person.

Documentation

Physical, sexual, and financial abuse are crimes in all states. In most states, suspicion of abuse is grounds for reporting. Make sure that you document your findings clearly and objectively. Be specific and thorough because your assessment findings are crucial in early detection and prompt intervention.

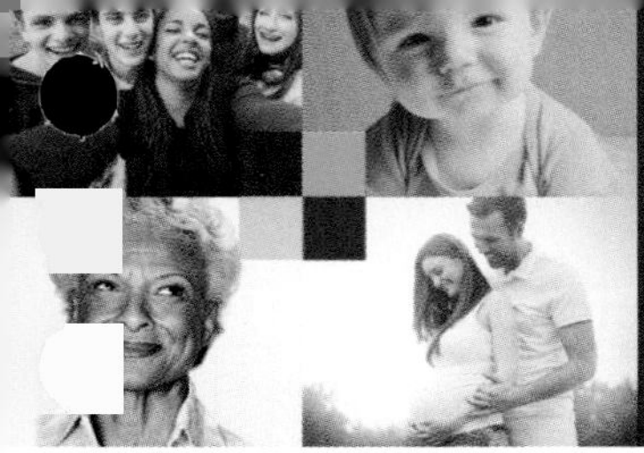

CHAPTER 27

Assessing the Dying Patient

Death is an immensely significant event in the life of the patient and the family. Care of the patient cannot be provided without caring also for the family who is equally suffering.

Cultural Considerations

Death is defined as permanent cessation of all vital bodily functions, and yet this simple definition is lacking in the societal and cultural definitions of death. Although death is a natural part of life, society, culture, and religion attach additional meanings to death. In some cultures, death can mean simply that the numbered days are up. In others, it could mean that a bad spell has been cast. In the United States, we tend to see death as a failure of the health care system as if death were a choice.

Death Rituals and Expectations

CULTURE	DEATH/DYING RITUALS
African American	Family oriented Important for family members to be at bedside May be reluctant to sign do-not-resuscitate (DNR) order or make funeral preparations. Less likely to donate organs or have autopsy. Response to loved one's death may result in "falling out," sudden collapse, paralysis or inability to see or speak, and severe emotional shock. Burial fifth to seventh day after death, viewings and religion are important.

(continued)

Death Rituals and Expectations (continued)

CULTURE	DEATH/DYING RITUALS
Amish	Expectation that family care for elderly and ill, prefer to die at home. Support derived from family and community. Funeral ceremony is simple.
Appalachian	Family and friends provide comfort and support to the immediate family. Friends and family remain with family after death to prevent loneliness. Funeral service and viewing are important and simple.
Arab	Muslims believe that life is preparation for death. Patient's bed is turned facing the holy city of Mecca. Readings from the Qur'an stress hope and acceptance. Immediately after death, the body is washed 3 times by a Muslim of the same sex, wrapped in white cloth, and buried same or next day.
Chinese	Death is feared. Hesitant to buy life insurance for fear of inviting death. Cremation is preferred. Death is viewed as a part of the natural cycle.
Cuban	Family is very important, at bedside of the dying person. May request Santero, performs death rites at bedside. Candles lit after death to light the path to the afterlife. Grief expressed openly.
European American	Death perceived as failure to cure an illness. May try to prolong death. Belief of self-determination and autonomy explains why Americans want to control end-of-life issues. Family remains with dying patient at the bedside. Usually buried or cremated within 3 days after death. Hospice may be used for end-of-life care for both patient and family.
Filipino	Roman Catholic religion influences views on death. May be seen as punishment. Fatalistic view, reluctant to prepare for death, or sign advanced directive. Family provides care. Wakes can last for a few days; funeral follows religious practice. One-year anniversary of death ends mourning period.
German	Death is seen as a part of life cycle; transition to God. Viewings allow friends and family time to pay condolence. Bereaving family limits social events for several months after death.

CULTURE	DEATH/DYING RITUALS
Haitian	Prefer to die at home with family at bedside. Open expression of grief. Family gathers after death to remember loved one, called veye. Seven consecutive days of prayer follow, dernie priye. Strong belief in resurrection, therefore cremation not acceptable.
Hindu	Prefer to die at home. Death rite, antyeshti, purifies body and supports family. Death is considered rebirth. Cremation within 24 hours. Ashes spread in Ganges River. There are 12 days of mourning. Women openly express grief.
Hmong	Death seen as continuation to next existence, reincarnation. Funeral unique, lasts few days, can include animal sacrifice.
Japanese	Paternalistic view to death, but becoming more Western oriented. Family at bedside. Mourning period is 49 days and ends with a family gathering and prayer service.
Jewish	Death seen as a part of life cycle. Family stays with patient. Funerals occur within 24 to 48 hours after death. No viewing. Family and friends visit deceased's relatives for 7 days after the burial, known as Shiva. This is a time of prayer and support for family.
Korean	Family assists in care of dying family member. Openly express grief. Cremation is acceptable. Rice wine sprinkled around grave.
Mexican	Death seen as a natural part of life. Death rituals are based on religion. Deceased buried within 24 hours. Family is the source of support.
Polish	Stoic acceptance of death. Family stay with dying patient. Wake and Mass are a part of funeral process.
Puerto Rican	Death is a crisis for family. Body respected and guarded. Death rituals are religion oriented, rosary and novenas. Openly express grief. Mourners may develop psychosomatic symptoms.
Russian	Family will stay with dying family member. Family reluctant to share bad news with patient. Family may resist with-holding treatment, and do everything possible to restore health. Death rituals are based on religion. Cremation not likely. Period of mourning is 1 year.

Source: Purnell L. *Transcultural Health Care: A Culturally Competent Approach.* 4th ed. Philadelphia, PA: F. A. Davis; 2013.

Timing of Death

Death can occur at any time throughout the life cycle. This discussion will focus on deaths that are expected from chronic, terminal conditions, which can occur at any age.

Stages of Grief

Kubler-Ross[1] has aptly identified the stages of grief that patients and families go through when diagnosed with terminal illness. Not all patients neatly follow the stages. More importantly, not all members of the family are in the same stage at the same time. It is easier on the caregivers and health care workers if the patient dies in the final grief stage. Kubler-Ross calls acceptance, but, in reality, some patients and/or families stay angry or in denial and the challenge to the nurse is to accept the patient and family at whatever stage they are and work with them accordingly. There are hospice agencies in all communities across the United States (and in most countries around the world) that can be called to help nurses in all settings to care for dying patients.

[1] Kubler-Ross E. On Death and Dying. New York, NY: Macmillan Publishing Company; 1969.

Coping Mechanisms Identified by Kubler-Ross

STAGE	MECHANISM	BEHAVIOR	SPEECH
I	Denial and isolation	Patient/family does not believe the diagnosis. Search for a second opinion.	I don't believe you That's not true
II	Anger	With the realization of the diagnosis, the patient/family can lash out at family members or health care providers. Frequently, this stage is accompanied by questions about spirituality and faith.	Why me? God has forsaken me!

STAGE	MECHANISM	BEHAVIOR	SPEECH
III	Bargaining	Once some of the anger is controlled, the patient begins to bargain—usually with God about the time of death.	"OK but can I live long enough to witness a wedding, christening, graduation, etc"
IV	Depression	When bargaining is over, the patient is overcome with a sense of loss—body image, independence, and so on. Sleeps a lot. Stays secluded.	What good have I done in my life? What's the use in living?
V	Acceptance	Patient speaks little. Sleeps a lot. May motion to visitors with a hand signal instead of speaking.	Very little verbal communication. Desires touch in the way of holding a hand rather than verbal communication.

Adapted from Kubler-Ross E. *On Death and Dying.* New York, NY: Macmillan Publishing Company; 1969.

Course of Events

- When patients are first told that they have a diagnosis that is not treatable, there may be outbursts of anger and denial from the patient or family member.
- As time progresses, increased sleeping and weakness is a common occurrence.
- As the dying patient gets weaker, he is usually confined to bed and may not be arousable even for meals.
- There are normal changes that occur to prepare the body for death. Knowledge of these will help the nurse care for the dying patient as well as help the nurse educate and provide anticipatory guidance for caregivers of dying patients.

Do-Not-Resuscitate Orders

Many times it is the nurse who initiates the discussion of do-not-resuscitate (DNR) paperwork and asks about funeral arrangements.

Although when the diagnosis is made, all parties involved know these issues need to be addressed, there is a fear that by talking about it, the death becomes more real and sometimes families feel this discussion will hasten the death. The nurse, as an impartial party, can discuss this with the patient and ask about preferences so as to free the family from making these difficult decisions at the time of the death when emotions are likely to run high. The more the nurse knows the patient as a person, the better able she is to make sure the patient's wishes are followed at the time of his death.

Complete History

DATA	SIGNIFICANCE/CONSIDERATIONS
Biographical Data	
Name, address, gender, religion, race, ethnicity	Issues of gender do come up in same sex relationships. Many religions and cultures have specific practices related to death and dying. It is important to clarify with the patient what his specific religious/cultural needs are at the time of death.
Does the patient have Advanced Directives? Are funeral plans in place?	These discussions are easier to have when the patient is feeling reasonably well than when the patient is in coma. It allows the patient to make choices and takes some of the burden from the family.
Marital status	
Are there any children? Where do they live? Who has the Medical Power of Attorney?	Identify the primary caregiver and availability of caregiver support systems. Need contact information for the medical power of attorney when the patient can no longer make decisions. If small children live in the home with the patient, their bereavement needs have to be also assessed.
Current Health History	
How long has the patient been ill? What is the patient's current functional ability? What was the patient's functional ability a week ago? A month ago?	Prolonged illness stresses the patient and the family. Caregiver needs to be assessed for caregiver burnout? Decline of function over time can indicate the speed with which the illness is progressing.

DATA	SIGNIFICANCE/CONSIDERATIONS
Are there any known medication allergies? If so, to what drug and what happens when the drug is taken?	If the patient reports an allergy to a drug, it is important to differentiate between a true allergy and a side effect. Nausea and vomiting when taking opioids are side effects and would not preclude use of these drugs for pain management if needed.
What is the list of current medications being taken?	Examine list and assess patient/family knowledge about the medication and administration
Past Medical History	
Past illnesses and surgeries	Other diagnosis may affect the course of the terminal disease Identify coping strategies with past events
Family History	Determine exposure of family members to death and dying. Identify if the patient/family dealt with this illness in other family members and may have a preconceived idea of how dying will occur.

Review of Systems

Review of systems

AREA/SYSTEM	SIGNIFICANCE
Skin	With immobility and impaired nutrition comes the risk of skin breakdown.
Head, Eyes, Ears, Nose, and Throat	
Any visual or auditory losses	Visual or auditory losses need to be considered when planning communication patterns with the patient.
Respiratory	Coughing or difficulty breathing may be indicative of fluid overload or dysphagia depending on when these symptoms are occurring.
Cardiovascular	Chest pain or changes in heart rate or blood pressure may signify decline or need to make adjustment to some medications.

(continued)

Review of systems (continued)

AREA/SYSTEM	SIGNIFICANCE
Genitourinary	Is the patient continent? Answer to this will alert the nurse to check for skin breakdown and identify need for additional supplies like diapers, blue pads, and so on.
Gastrointestinal	Decrease in appetite is normal in the dying process. Create opportunity to teach caregiver about nutrition and hydration at the end of life. Use of opioids for pain management frequently causes constipation.
Musculoskeletal	Assess ability of caregiver to assist with ambulation and other activities of daily living. Perform a safety assessment for falls. May need to provide assistive devices such as wheelchairs, walkers, and bedside commodes to help caregiver.
Neurologic	Decrease in level of consciousness, talking to deceased family members, and confusion are all part of the dying process. Behaviors described by family members will help to determine the stage of grief the patient is in.
Psychosocial **Nutrition** **Sleep/rest** **Supports**	While the patient is still conscious, attempt to meet requests. As death nears, peristalsis slows and then stops so that no bowel sounds will be heard. Feeding may cause more discomfort. Sleep and rest may be sporadic. Having family members, friends, pets may be a source of support for the patient. Also consider the needs of the supports.

Physical Assessment

It is important to note that death, like birth, is an individual experience. The time of death cannot be predicted with any accuracy although families ask that question regularly. Death is a process, and by understanding that process, the nurse can help families deal with the burden of caring for and ultimately losing a loved one.

General Health Survey

AREA/PHYSICAL ASSESSMENT SKILL	SIGNIFICANCE
Assess for general appearance, cleanliness, behavior, overview of immediate environment.	Evaluates the ability of caregiver to provide care and identify teaching needs for caregiver.
Assess patients comfort level.	McCaffery & Pasero[2] define pain as "whatever the person says it is, experienced whenever they say they are experiencing it." Pain is a subjective response and includes dimensions of psychologic, social, and spiritual distress in addition to physical pain. Patients with chronic pain do not demonstrate the same behaviors as those with acute pain, which is the model for pain we have in acute care settings. If the patient has had oral doses of opioids over the course of his illness and is now unable to take anything by mouth, it is imperative that opioids be continued in the sublingual or rectal route so as to prevent opioid withdrawal at a time that the body is preparing for death.
Vital signs	In the days preceding death, body temperature goes up, pulse rate frequently goes up, and blood pressure decreases, and respirations become faster and uneven.
Integumentary	
Inspect skin color.	As death approaches, the skin undergoes a phenomenon called Mottling, which is a bluish hue that usually appears first in the lower extremities (toes, feet, and knees) and progresses to other parts of the body.
Inspect pressure points for skin breakdown.	With fever, skin may be warm and moist.
Head, Eyes, Ears, Nose, and Throat	
Assess mouth for dryness or secretions.	Mouth breathing at the end stages of life cause lips and tongue to become dry.

(box continued on page 608)

[2] McCaffery M, Pasero C. *Pain: Clinical Manual.* 2nd ed. St. Louis, Mo: Mosby; 1999.

General Health Survey (continued)

AREA/PHYSICAL ASSESSMENT SKILL	SIGNIFICANCE
	Secretions at the back of the throat contribute to noisy respirations known as the "death rattle."
Respiratory	
Auscultate lungs	As death approaches, patient will have Cheyne-Stokes respirations with progressively longer periods of apnea. If the patient has continued to receive fluids by intravenous route or percutaneous endoscopic gastrostomy after his body systems have started shutting down, respirations will be labored with crackles throughout.
Cardiovascular	
Assess pulses	As blood pressure decreases, peripheral pulses will be harder to palpate. Pulse rate becomes rapid and thready as the heart tries to compensate for the drop in blood pressure.
Gastrointestinal	
Assess bowel sounds	Initially, the patient reports poor appetite and early satiety. As death approaches, peristalsis slows and then stops so that no bowel sounds will be heard. It is very important to teach the caregiver that any attempts at hydrating or feeding the patient at this point will lead to a more uncomfortable death. Once body systems begin to shut down, fluid infused accumulates ultimately in the lungs adding to the characteristic death rattle and contributing to discomfort at the time of death.

AREA/PHYSICAL ASSESSMENT SKILL	SIGNIFICANCE
Genitourinary	
Check output	There may not be any urine output for 2-3 days before the death as the kidneys begin to shut down. Urine present in a Foley bag will be concentrated and dark. Patients who have struggled with edema, either peripheral or ascites, will experience a reabsorption of some of those body fluids.
Musculoskeletal	
Assess muscle tone	Extremities that have been spastic become flaccid as death approaches.
Neurologic	
Assess level of consciousness	Not all patients are in coma for several days before death. Some (especially children) can be reasonably alert and mobile, and just die during sleep. Teach the family that death can occur in many ways and each is individual. It is common for the patient to see deceased family members in the room (usually on the ceiling) before the death. The patient may also experience a period of increased lucidity and alertness some time before the death giving the family some hope that the death may not be imminent. A symptom that is also common as death approaches is "terminal restlessness." The patient grows restless, trying to get out of bed, although confused and non-communicative.

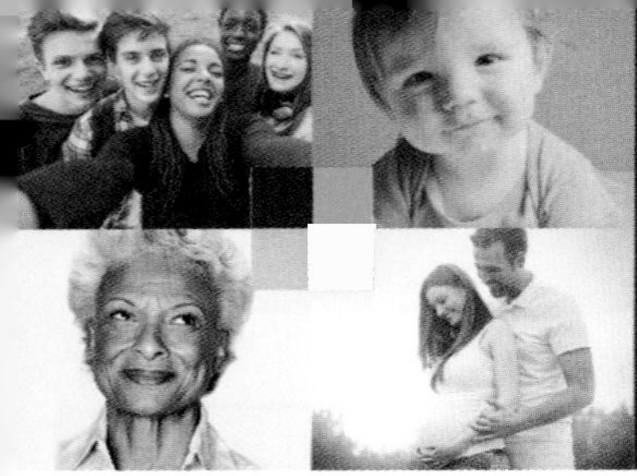

INDEX

Note: Page numbers followed by **b, f or t** refer to boxes, figures, or tables, respectively.

A

Abdomen, 245–274
anatomical landmarks of, 260f
collecting histories, 247, 248, 249–252
cultural considerations of, 246–247
developmental considerations, 245–246
drugs effecting gastrointestinal system, 252t–254t
four-quadrant method, 260b–261b, 260f
girth of, 234t
newborn's
inspecting and palpating, 415b–416b
measuring, 407b
nine regions of, 260f, 261b
older adults, 494b
pain
collecting history of, 247, 248, 249–252
rating intensity of, 248t
significance by quadrant, 247b
physical assessments
262b–274b
auscultation, 265b–266b
conducting, 26
during pregnancy, 389b–394b
fundal height measurements, 391b
inspections, 262b–264b
mental health, 545t
palpation for, 270b–274b
percussion for, 267b–269b
shapes, 262b
primary functions of, 245
relationship to
254t–259t
cardiovascular system, 257t
ears, 139t
endocrine system, 259t
eyes, 114b, 256t
general system, 254t–255t
genitourinary system, 257t–258t, 286t
HEENT, 256t
immunological/hematological systems, 259t
integumentary system, 255t–256t
musculoskeletal system, 258t–259t
neurologic system, 259t
PV/lymphatic systems, 212t, 215b–216b
respiratory system, 257t
tools for, 262
Abdominal reflex, 273b, 370b
Abdomino jugular reflux, 187b
Abducens nerve, 361b
Abnormal gaits, 342t–343t
Abstract reasoning, 358b
Abuse, 591–598
about, 591
of children
forms of, 591–592
preschoolers/toddlers, 439
school-age children, 459
contributing to suicide risk, 553–554, 553b, 554t–555t
documenting, 598
older adults, 596–598

reporting, 536
sexual, 591, 592, 593–594
spousal or partner, 595–596
substance
assessing, 555, 555b–556b
CAGE questionnaire, 555, 556b
effects of use and withdrawal, 557t–561t
suicide risks for, 554b
types of, 591
Accuracy of movements, 329b
Achilles reflex, 369b
ACL (Anterior cruciate ligament), 340b
Acoustic nerve, 362b
Acrochordon, 490b
Activity/exercise
adolescents, 467
homeless patients, 505t
mental health and, 542t
preschoolers/toddlers, 443
school-age children, 455
Acute pain, 510t
ADHD (attention deficit hyperactivity disorder), 454
Adolescents, 459–471
activity of, 467
boys
genitourinary system of, 297, 298t
maturation states in, 298t
cultural views of, 461t–462t
daily activities, 454, 466–467
depression, 466t, 530b
developmental considerations
changes in integumentary system, 30
growth and developmental changes, 460–461
skin disorders, 31t
girls
genitourinary system of, 275
maturation states in, 276t–277t
menarche for, 465t, 468t
pregnancies, 375
use of birth control pills, 282t, 462–463
health history
assessing, 462–463
current medications, 462–463
family medical history, 463
immunizations for, 463
neurologic system of, 345–346
physical assessments, 469t–471t
breasts, 471t
cardiovascular system, 470t
gastrointestinal system, 471t
general health survey, 469t
genitourinary system, 471t
HEENT, 470t
integumentary system, 30, 469t
musculoskeletal system, 471t
neurologic system, 471t
respiratory system, 470t
promoting health of, 461
psychosocial history of, 466–469
questions to ask, 463t–466t
breasts, 465t
endocrine system, 466t
gastrointestinal system, 465t
general health status, 463t
HEENT, 464t
integumentary system, 463t–464t
musculoskeletal system, 466t
neurologic system, 466t
pubertal delays, 465t
respiratory system, 464t
risks/risk taking of, 461, 530, 530b
spirituality of, 570
stages of, 459
suicides by, 530b
Adults. *See also* Older adults
Eustachian tube of, 135f
pain scales for, 518–520, 528
African Americans
childbirth practices, 377
death/dying for, 599t
mental health of, 537t
response to pain, 515t
views on
adolescents, 461t
infants, 403
older adults, 472t
school-age children, 450t

Age. *See also* Developmental considerations; *and specific age categories*
appearance vs. stated, 546t
developments of eyes by, 107–109
effect on vital signs, 23t
infant development appropriate for, 402
loss of height, 475t
mental health history, 536
skin disorders related to, 31t
AIDS
cultural considerations for, 205
maintaining weight with, 259t
men, assessing symptoms of, 302t, 304t
women
concerns about, 280
effects on genitourinary system, 287t
Alcohol use
effects of and withdrawal from, 557t
Allen's test, 108, 219b
around preschoolers/toddlers, 443–444
Allergies
food, 259t
tearing of eyes, 159t, 160t
Alpha-thalassemia, 377
Alzheimer's disease, 357b, 531, 550t
Amaurosis fugax, 477t
Amenorrhea, 280, 286t
Amish
childbirth practices, 377
death/dying for, 600t
views on
adolescents, 461t
infants, 403
mental health, 534t
older adults, 472t
school-age children, 450t
Amnesia, 357b
Amplitude scale for pulses, 219b
Anal assessments
infants, 436b
men, 312b–313b
women, 296b
Anal reflex, 370b
Anatomical landmarks
abdomen, 260f
breasts, 236f
cardiovascular system, 182f–183f
ears, 140, 141f
eyes, 115
head, neck, and face, 85f–86f
PV/lymphatic systems, 214f
respiratory system, 163f
synovial joints, 321t–322t
Anemia, 285t, 483t
Ankles
ankle-brachial index, 221b–223b
inspecting/palpating joints of, 341b
Anterior chamber of eyes, 125b–126b
Anterior cruciate ligament (ACL), 340b
Anterior thorax assessments, 25–26
Anthropometric measurements
about, 16
infants, 430b–431b
newborns, 406b–408b
in nutritional assessments, 565
older adults, 475t
preschoolers/toddlers, 445t
school-age children, 457t
Aorta, palpating, 270b
Aortic regurgitation, 200b
Aortic stenosis, 200b
Apgar score, 405t
Apley's test, 340b
Apnea, infant, 433b
Apneustic respiratory rate, 164b
Appalachians
childbirth practices, 378
death/dying for, 600t
response to pain, 515t
views on
adolescents, 462t
infants, 403
older adults, 472t
school-age children, 450t
Appearance
changes in grooming and, 351t
stated age vs., 546t
Appendicitis, 271b–272b
Appetite loss in women, 286

Arab Americans
childbirth practices, 378
death/dying for, 600t
mental health views, 534t
response to pain, 515t
views on
adolescents, 462t
infants, 403
school-age children, 450t
Arcus senilis, 125b, 492b
Arms. *See* Upper extremities
Arousal state, 372t–373t
Arteries and veins. *See also* Peripheral vascular system
assessing
carotid arteries/jugular veins, 184t, 184b–187b, 352t
in eye, 131b
insufficiencies of, 217b, 218b
auscultation during BP checks, 223b–225b
color change test for radial/ulnar arteries, 220b–221b
Homans' sign and, 219b, 222b
PV anatomical landmarks, 214f
Assessments. *See also* Physical assessments; *and specific system assessments*
approach to, 15
beginning/ending, 15–16
collecting histories, 32–33
complete health history, 17–21
complete physical, 21–28
data used for, 2
defined, 1
documentation methods for, 3–4
documenting, 16
doing process in, 2
feeling process in, 2
general surveys in, 16
head-to-toe approach, 16, 21, 22, 24–27
levels of preventative health care, 2
prioritizing data from, 3
thinking process for, 1
tools for, 12t–15t
types of physical, 4–11, 21–22
vital signs and anthropometric measurements, 16
Asterixis, 162t
Asthma, 170b
Atrial fibrillation, 198f, 352t, 482t
Attention deficit hyperactivity disorder (ADHD), 454
Auditory hallucinations, 550t, 554t
Auscultation. *See also* Murmurs
abdomen, 265b–266b
during pregnancy, 389b–394b
arteries and veins, 223b–225b
cardiovascular system
assessing, 179t, 320t
during BP checks, 223b–225b
extra heart sounds, 285t
heart rhythm, 352t
murmurs, 192b–193b, 194f–199f, 203t
neck vessels, 190b–191b
newborn, 415b
sites for, 184t
chest, 160t, 169b–171b
gastrointestinal system, 212t
head, neck, and face, 106b
infant lungs, 434b
liver, 266b
respiratory system
assessing, 169b–171b, 320t
distress related to female genitourinary system, 285t
newborn, 406b–419b
scrotum, 313b
using, 11f, 22
Awareness. *See* Levels of consciousness
Axilla of breast, 240b
Axillary temperature, 431b

B

Babinski's reflex, 371b, 422t
Balance
asking older adults about, 477t, 482t
inspecting, 326b–327b
neurologic conditions effecting, 353t
problems with, 137
Romberg test, 151b, 326b–327b, 500b
toddler/preschooler, 447t
Balance's sign, 273b
Ball and socket joints, 322t
Ballottement, 273b, 385t

Barlow-Ortolani maneuver, 419b
Barthel Index, 486t
Bartholin's glands, 294b, 394b
Beginning assessments, 15–16
Behavior. *See also* Substance abuse
assessing
for mental status, 546t–547t
pain from, 525b–528b
changes in
cardiovascular causes of, 181t
due to pain, 513
groups with high-risk, 576
personal habits and
adolescents, 468
preschoolers/toddlers, 443–444
school-age children, 455
related to patient's spirituality, 571
Behavioral Pain Score (BPS), 525
Beliefs. *See* Childbirth practices; Values
Bell's palsy, 362b
Benign prostatic hypertrophy, 495b
Beta-thalassemia, 377
Biflex reflex, 368b
Biocultural ecology, 575–576
Biographical data, 17
Biot's respiratory rate, 164b
Birth control pills
adolescents use of, 462–463
adverse reactions to, 181t, 235t
investigating history of, 282t
risk of stroke and, 353t
thrombophlebitis and, 285t
Birthing. *See* Childbirth practices
Bladder
effect of stroke on, 353t
percussion of, 269b
Bleeding
gums, 211t
menstruation and vaginal, 279
nosebleeds, 179t
risk of stroke and disorders in, 354t
Blindness
causes of, 109
color, 117b
Blink reflex
infant's, 107
newborn's, 412b
Blood. *See also* Immunological/hematological systems
in stool, 296b, 312b
tests estimating conception date, 386
Blood pressure (BP)
auscultating arteries/veins, 223b–225b
measuring ankle and brachial, 221b
newborn, 408b
older adults, 494b
Body piercing, 469t
Bones. *See* Musculoskeletal system
Bouchard's nodes, 337b
Boutonnière deformity, 337b
Bowel. *See also* Gastrointestinal system
adolescent eating disorders and, 465t
auscultation of, 265b
changes in
abdominal assessments and, 249–250
neurologic problems and, 352t–353t
function related to stroke, 353t
incontinence and cauda equina syndrome, 259t, 353t
infant bowel movements, 436b
sounds, 320t
auscultating, 265b
investigating, 212t
pregnant women, 246
Bowlegs, 314
Boys
breast enlargement in, 465t
genitourinary system of, 297, 298t
maturation states of, 298t
BP. *See* Blood pressure
BPI (Brief Pain Inventory), 519
BPS (Behavioral Pain Score), 525
Brachioradialis reflexes, 369b
Bradypnea respiratory rate, 165b
Brain
assessing side with problems, 356
cerebral functions, 356b–363b
abstract reasoning, 358b
communication skills, 359b–360b

general knowledge and vocabulary, 358b
judgment, 358b
levels of consciousness, 356b
mathematical and calculative ability, 357b
memory, 357b
thought process, 358b
Braxton Hicks contractions, 385t
Brazilian Americans, 472t
Breast cancer
palpations finding, 241b
symptoms of, 232
Breast feeding, 235t
Breasts, 226–244
adolescents, 465t, 471t
adverse reactions to drugs on, 232t–233t
anatomical landmarks of, 236f
collecting symptoms of, 229, 231–232
cultural considerations of, 228
developmental considerations of, 226–228, 227f, 228f
evaluating changes in, 286t
functions of, 226
newborn's, 415b
physical assessments
approach to, 236f
axilla, 240b
breast, 237b–239b
during pregnancy, 389b
general survey of, 22
nipple and areola, 239b–240b
palpations for, 240b–244b
postpartal assessment of, 398b
relationship to, 233t–235t
cardiovascular system, 234t
endocrine system, 235t
female genitourinary system, 286t
gastrointestinal systems, 234t
general system, 233t
genitourinary system, 234t–235t
HEENT, 234t
integumentary system, 234t
lymphatic/hematological system, 235t
male genitourinary system, 302t–304t
musculoskeletal system, 235t
respiratory system, 234t
self-examination of, 229b–230b
tools for examining, 237
Breathing. *See also* Respiratory system
abdomen's relationship to, 257t
assessing patterns of, 164b–165b
asthma, 170b
auscultation and patterns of, 169b–171b
cardiovascular health and, 179t, 478t–479t
COPD and, 158t, 159t, 160t, 161t, 170b, 285t, 352t
infant's, 429t, 433b
neurological factors in, 352t
older adults, 493b
symptoms of breathlessness, 153–154
Brief Pain Inventory (BPI), 519
Bronchial sounds, 170b
Brudzinski's sign, 372b
Brushfield spots, 412b
Buerger's disease, 352t
Bulbar conjunctiva, 123b
Bulbocavernosus reflex, 371b
Bulbourethral gland, 313b
Bullying, 456

C

Café-au-lait spots, 409b
CAGE questionnaire, 555, 556b
Cancer
breast
palpations finding, 241b
symptoms of, 232
cultural factors in incidence of, 228
pain associated with, 510t
prostatic, 495b
related symptoms in breast, 234t–235t
Candida albicans
newborns with, 413b
signs of vaginal, 293b
Cardiac rates and rhythms. *See also* Pulses
assessing abnormal, 186b
atrial fibrillation, 198f, 352t, 482t

auscultation of, 352t
cardiac rates and, 178t, 186b, 389b
dizzy spells and, 178t
during pregnancy, 398
preschoolers/toddlers, 446t
Cardiovascular system, 172–203. *See also* Cardiac rates and rhythms; Murmurs; Pulses
adverse drug reactions of, 174t–175t
anatomical landmarks of, 182f–183f
approach, position, tools for, 184
assessing CVD symptoms, 181t
auscultation, 190b–199b
during BP checks, 223b–225b
heart sounds, 199b–200b, 201f, 202t
murmurs, 192b–193b, 196f, 203t
of newborn, 415b
sites for cardiac, 184t
collecting histories of, 173–174
cultural considerations for, 173
developmental considerations, 172
evaluating in death process, 605t, 606, 608b
health history
homeless patients, 504t
older adults, 494b
physical assessments, 21–22 184b–193b
abnormal pulses, 199f
adolescents, 470t
auscultation of, 190b–193b
carotid arteries/jugular veins, 184t, 184b–187b, 352t
during pregnancy, 389b
homeless patients, 507t
mental health, 545t
nutrition, 567b
precordium, 185b, 187b–193b
preschoolers/toddlers, 446t
school-age children, 458t
valvular heart sounds, 199b–200b
postpartal assessment of, 398b–400b
primary functions, 172
questions to ask
adolescents, 464t
older adults, 478t–479t
preschoolers/toddlers, 442t
relationship to
abdomen, 257t
breasts, 234t
ears, 139t
endocrine system, 181t
eyes, 114b
gastrointestinal system, 180t, 257t
general system, 176t
genitourinary system, 180t–181t, 285t, 303t
head, neck, and face, 82t
HEENT, 178t–179t
integumentary system, 38t–39t, 176t–177t
lymphatic system, 182t, 212t
musculoskeletal system, 181t, 320t
neurologic system, 352t
PV system, 212t
respiratory system, 160t, 179t, 320t
Caregivers, 584t–585t
Carotid arteries
auscultation of, 190b–191b, 352t
palpations of, 185b–187b
Carpal tunnel syndrome, 336b, 337b
Cataracts, 125b
Catatonia, 547t
Categorical Scales, 519
Cauda equina syndrome, 259t, 353t
Cellulitis, 215f
Cerebellar function, 326b–327b, 500b
Cerebral functions, 356b–363b
abstract reasoning, 358b
communication skills, 359b–360b
general knowledge and vocabulary, 358b
judgment, 358b
levels of consciousness, 356b
mathematical and calculative ability, 357b
memory, 357b
thought process, 358b

Cerumen, 135–136, 145b
Cervical lymph nodes. *See also* Lymphatic system
  illustrated, 101f
  location of, 73
  physical assessments, 100b–101b, 106b
Cervical spine joints, 334b
Cervix
  assessing during pregnancy, 395b–396b
  inspecting, 288b, 290b–293b
  palpation of, 295b
Chadwick's sign, 277, 290b, 385t, 395b
Changes. *See also* Growth
  behavioral, children's pain and, 513
  developmental
    adolescent integumentary system, 30
    infant, 401–403
  to extremities, 174
  grooming and appearance, 351t
  immune system, 483t
  mental health, 347
  psychosocial and emotional
    preschoolers/toddlers, 438–439
    school-age children, 448–449
  senses
    hearing, 351t
    smell, 351t
    taste, 351t, 362b, 363b
    touch, 351t
    vision system 178t
  swallowing, 351t–352t
  weight, 249, 284t, 304t, 428b
CHEOPS (Children's Hospital of Eastern Ontario Pain Scale), 525
Chest
  anatomical landmarks for, 182f–183f
  assessing
    infant's spinal curvature, 433b
    newborn's, 414b–415b
    respiratory system, 164b
    shape of, 165b–166b, 179t
  auscultation of, 160t, 169b–171b
  measuring
    infant's, 430b–431b
    newborn's, 406b–408b
  pain
    cardiovascular history of, 173–174
    related to respiratory system, 154
  palpating, 167b, 168b
  PV/lymphatic systems and, 212t
Cheyne-Stokes respiratory rate, 165b, 179t, 493b
CHF. *See* Congestive heart failure
Chickenpox (VZV) vaccine, 440, 451
Childbirth practices, 377–384
  African American, 377
  Amish, 377
  Appalachian, 378
  Arab American, 378
  Chinese American, 379
  Cuban American, 379
  Egyptian American, 379–380
  Filipino American, 380
  French Canadian, 380
  Greek American, 381
  Iranian American, 381
  Irish American, 381–382
  Jewish American, 382
  Mexican American, 382–383
  Navajo Native American, 383
  Vietnamese American, 383
Children. *See also* Adolescents; Infants; Newborns; Preschoolers/toddlers; School-age children
  abdomen of, 245
  abuse, forms of, 591–592
  assessing mobility of TM, 146b
  cultural perspectives about, 450t–451t
  developmental considerations
    age-related skin disorders, 31t
    breasts, 226–228, 227f, 228f
    cardiovascular system of, 172
    ears, 134–135
    female genitourinary system of, 275
    male genitourinary system 297, 298t
    musculoskeletal system, 314
    pain, 512–513

ear infections in, 139t
eyes of, 108
head, face, and neck, 73–74
maturation states
boys, 298t
girls, 276t–277t
neurologic system of, 345–346
pain scales, 520–521, 525, 526t, 527t
PV and lymphatic systems of, 204
school-age, 448–459
Children's Hospital of Eastern Ontario Pain Scale (CHEOPS), 525
Chinese Americans
childbirth practices, 379
death/dying for, 600t
response to pain, 515t
views on
adolescents, 462t
infants, 403
mental health, 534t
older adults, 472t
school-age children, 450t
Chlamydia trachomatis, 285t, 290b, 303t
Chloasma, 387b
Choking game, 530b
Chronic obstructive pulmonary disease (COPD)
cardiovascular indicators of, 179t
respiratory indicators of, 158t, 159t, 160t, 161t, 170b, 285t, 352t
Chronic pain, 510t, 511t
Cincinnati Prehospital Stroke Scale, 354
Circumcision
female, 289b
male, 299, 306b, 417b
as religious ritual, 382, 403, 404
Circumference of arms and legs, 330b, 331b
Claudication in legs, 39t, 479t
Cleft palate/lip, 414b
Clitoris
enlargement during pregnancy, 394b
examining, 289b
presence of newborn, 416b
Clock scoring, 501b
Clonus testing, 368b
Closed-angle glaucoma, 118b
Club foot, 418b
Cocaine, 558t
Color
iris, 107
rating pain with, 520
skin, 56t–58t, 575
Color assessment tool, 520
Color blindness, 117b
Color changes
nails, 158t, 177t
test for
lower extremities, 222b
upper extremities, 220b–221b
Color vision, 117b
Coma response scale, 355b
Communications
changes in infant, 402
cultural influences on, 573–574
home-care patients and, 584t, 585t
related to patient's spirituality, 571
skills for nurses, 3
testing skills in, 359b–360b
Community
boundaries of, 586t
external influences on, 587t
health status and needs of, 589t–590t
human services within, 588t
physical characteristics of, 586t–587t
politics within, 588t
Complete health assessment, 17–28. *See also* Patient histories; Psychosocial histories
approach to physical assessments, 21–22
biographical data for, 17
current health status, 17
family medical history, 18f, 451
past health history, 17
psychosocial profile, 21
reviewing body systems, 19–21
Condyloid joints, 321t
Congestive heart failure (CHF)
awakening to urinate, 180t, 213t

inspecting men for, 303t
respiratory indicator, 157t, 158t, 161t
Conjunctiva
infections of, 285t, 303t
physical assessments, 123b–124b
Consciousness. *See* Levels of consciousness
Constipation, 479t
Constrictive pericarditis, 198f
Contact lenses, 119b–120b
Contraceptive history, 282t
Coombs' test, 209b
Coordination testing, 328b–329b, 447t
COPD. *See* Chronic obstructive pulmonary disease
Coping strategies
adolescents, 469
mental health and, 544t
preschoolers/toddlers, 444
school-age children, 456
stages of grief and, 602, 602t–603b
Cornea, 124b–125b
Corrigan's pulse, 199f
Coughs
assessing symptoms of, 153
dry, 179t
incontinence and, 480t
Crack, 558t
Cranial nerves 360b–363b
acoustic, 362b
facial, 362b
glossopharyngeal and vagus, 362b–363b
hypoglossal, 363b
oculomotor, trochlear, and abducens, 361b
olfactory, 360b–361b
optic, 361b
response times of older adults, 499b
spinoaccessory, 363b
trigeminal, 361b
Crawling reflex, 424t
Cremasteric reflex, 370b–371b
CRIES pain rating, 523
Critical thinking skills, 1
Crossed extension reflex, 425t
Cuban Americans
childbirth practices, 379
death/dying for, 600t
response to pain, 515t
views on
adolescents, 462t
infants, 404
older adults, 472t
school-age children, 450t
views, 534t
Cullen's sign, 263b
Cultural influences, 573–579. *See also specific cultural/ethnic groups*
abdomen, 246–247
about, 573
biocultural ecology, 575–576
breasts, 228
cardiovascular system, 173
on communications, 573–574
death rituals, 577, 599t–601t
effecting health practices, 576, 578–579
eyes, 109
family roles and organization, 544t, 574–575
fear of touching fontanel, 432b
female genitourinary system and, 278t
head, neck, and face, 74
high-risk behaviors of groups, 576
with homeless patients, 505t
integumentary system, 32
male genitourinary system, 299
musculoskeletal system, 315–316
nutrition and, 576
patient's spirituality, 570, 577–578
perceptions of pain, 514, 515t–516t
psychosocial history and, 543t
PV/lymphatic systems, 205
respiratory system, 153
variations in infants, 403–404
views on,
adolescents, 461t–462t
children, 450t–451t
mental health, 537t, 534t–536t
older adults, 472t–473t
pregnancy, 376–377, 577
workforce issues, 575

Current health status, 17
Cushing's syndrome, 263b
Cushing's triad, 351
Cutaneous hypersensitivity, 272b
CVD (cardiovascular disease). *See* Cardiovascular system
Cyanosis
  inspecting
    cardiovascular causes of, 176t
    nails for, 158t, 177t
  murmurs accompanying
    infant, 434b

D

Daily activities. *See also* Activity/exercise; Sexual activity
  adolescents, 467–469
  assessing performance of, 580
  for homeless patients, 504t
  older adults, 485b–487b
    Barthel Index, 486t
    Instrumental Activities of Daily Living, 487b
    Katz Index of Activities of Daily Living, 485b–486b
  school-age children, 454
  toddlers/preschoolers, 443
DAR mnemonics, 4
Data
  documentation methods for, 3–4
  prioritizing, 3
  types and sources of assessment, 2
Death, 599–609
  cultural rituals about, 577, 599t–601t
  defining, 599
  do-not-resuscitate orders, 603–604, 604t–605t
  review of systems before, 605t–606t
  stages of grief, 602, 602t–603t
  timing of, 602
Deep sensation testing, 364b
Deep tendon reflexes, 367b–368b, 500b
Deep vein thrombosis (DVT), 219b, 394b
Delirium, 531t, 532
Dementia
  clock scoring test for, 501b
  screening older adults for, 498b
Dental health, relationship of abdomen and teeth, 157b
Dentures, 477t
Denver Developmental Screening Test-II (DDST-II), 401, 432b
Depersonalization, 551t
Depressants, 557t
Depression
  adolescent, 466t, 530b
  appearance vs. stated age, 546t
  assessing, 552–553
  dementia and delirium vs., 531t
  older adults, 532, 532b–533b
  spousal abuse and, 596
  suicide risks and, 554b
  women's 286t–287t
    postpartum depression, 531
Developmental considerations
  abdomen, 245–246
  breasts, 226–228, 227f, 228f
  cardiovascular system, 172
  ears, 134–135
  female genitourinary system, 275, 277–278
  head, neck, and face, 73–74
  history of infant's, 430t
  integumentary system, 29–30
  male genitourinary system 297, 298t, 299
  maturation states
    boys, 298t
    girls, 276t–277t
  musculoskeletal system, 314–315
  neurologic system, 345–346
  older adults, 472
  pain
    children, 512–513
    infants, 512
    older adults, 514
  pubertal delays, 465t
  respiratory system, 152
  spirituality, 569–570
    children, 569–570
    infants, 569
    older adults, 570
  stages of adolescence, 459
Developmental testing for infants, 437t

Diabetes
diabetic retinopathy, 132b
foot ulcerations related to, 498b
neuropathies and, 354t
relationship to,
abdomen, 259t
cardiovascular system, 181t
female genitourinary system, 287t
HEENT, 178t
Diagnostic and Statistical Manual of Mental Disorders (DSM)-IV, 552–553
Diastolic murmurs, 196f
Diet. *See* Nutrition
Diphtheria, pertussis, tetanus (DPT) toxoid, 430t, 439
Discharge
in male genitourinary system, 300
penile, 258t
vaginal, 279
Discriminatory sensory functions, 365b–366b
Disorientation, 356b–357b
Dizziness
assessing patient history of, 347, 482t
orthostatic hypotension, 478t
relationship to abdomen, 255t, 257t
Do-not-resuscitate (DNR) orders, 603–604, 604t–605t
Documenting
abuse assessments, 598
assessment methods, 3–4
physical assessments, 27
quality of, 16
Doing process in assessment, 2, 15
Domestic violence, 595–596
Double vision, 110, 178t
Down syndrome, 412b, 433b
Drugs
adverse effects on
breasts, 232t–233t
cardiovascular system, 174t–175t
ears, 137t
eyes, 111t–112t
female reproductive system, 282t–283t
gastrointestinal system, 252t–254t
head, neck, and face, 76t–78t
integumentary system, 34t–36t
lymphatic system, 208t–210t
male genitourinary system, 301t
mental health, 538t–539t
musculoskeletal system, 318t
neurologic system, 348t–350t
respiratory system, 155t–156t
skin/hair/nails, 34t–36t
assessing current medications
adolescents, 462–463
effect on mental health, 538t–539t
preschoolers/toddlers, 439
birth control pills, 181t, 235t, 282t
exposure to
newborns, 405t
preschoolers/toddlers, 443–444
school-age children, 451
psychotropic, 539t–540t
Dry eyes, 476t, 492b
Dry macular degeneration, 133b
DVT (deep vein thrombosis), 219b, 394b
Dysarthria, 352t
Dysmenorrhea, 279
Dysphagia, 352t
Dyspnea
abdomen's relationship to, 257t
assessing symptoms of, 153–154
exertion and, 176t
PV/lymphatic systems and, 212t
Dysthymia, 553

E

Ears, 134–151. *See also* Nose; Throat
adolescents', 464t, 470t
anatomical landmarks, 140, 141f
developmental considerations of, 134–135
drugs adversely effecting, 137t
functions of, 134
helix of, 143b–144b
history of, 136–137
infant's, 429t
older adults, 492b–493b
physical assessments, 140–141, 141b–151b
about, 19, 24
angle of attachment, 140f, 141b–142b

approach, position, and tools, 141
during pregnancy, 388b
external ear canal, 145b–146b
hearing, 148b–151b
infant's, 432b
inspecting external ear, 141b–142b
newborn's, 412b–413b
otoscopic exam, 144b–145b
palpation of external ear, 143b–144b
preschoolers/toddlers, 445t–446t
school-age children, 457t
tools for, 115
tympanic membrane, 146b–148b
primary functions of, 134
questions for
older adults, 477t
preschoolers/toddlers, 440t–441t
relationship to
abdomen, 139t, 256t–257t
cardiovascular system, 139t, 179t
eyes, 113b
gastrointestinal system, 139t
general systems, 138t
genitourinary/reproductive system, 139t
head, face, and neck, 80t–81t
HEENT, 138t
integumentary system, 38t, 138t
musculoskeletal system, 140t
neurologic system, 140t
respiratory system, 139t, 159t
Echolalia, 549t
Ectropion/entropion, 108, 122b, 492b
Edema
assessing, 218b
cardiovascular causes of, 177t–178t
collecting histories of, 173
lower extremities, 216b
upper extremities, 215b
Egyptian Americans
childbirth practices, 379–380
response to pain, 515t
views on
adolescents, 462t
infants, 404
mental health, 534t–535t
older adults, 473t
school-age children, 450t
Elbows, 335b–336b
Elder abuse, 596–598
Embolic stroke, 352t
Emotions. *See also* Psychosocial histories
changes in
adolescents, 460–461
preschoolers/toddlers, 438–439
school-age children, 448–449
emotional state and mental health, 548t
identifying suicide risks, 553–554, 553b, 554t–555t
Ending assessments, 15–16
Endocrine system
assessment of, 21
homeless patients, 504t
questions to ask
adolescents, 466t
older adults, 482t
relationship to
abdomen, 259t
breasts, 235t
cardiovascular system, 181t
female genitourinary system, 287t
head, neck, and face, 79t, 84t–85t
integumentary system, 41t
male genitourinary system, 304t
neurologic system, 354t
respiratory system, 162t
Environment
assessing patient's home, 580, 581t–585t
communications, 584t, 585t
evaluating safety, 582t–584t
family, friends, and pets in, 585t
meeting physical needs, 581t–583t
nursing care in home, 580
overview, 580

patient's community, 586t–590t
sources of self-esteem, 585t
support systems and caregivers for, 584t–585t
of homeless patients, 505t
items related to spirituality in, 572
mental health and patient's, 543t
Epstein's pearls, 414b, 433b
Erb's point, 192b–193b
Erectile dysfunction, 301–302
Erythema toxicum, 409b
Estimated date of conception (EDC), 386
Ethical skills, 2
Ethnicity
influences on infant assessments, 403–404
pregnancy and childbirth, 377–384
Eupnea respiratory rate, 164b
European Americans
death/dying for, 600t
views on older adults, 473t
Eustachian tube, 134f, 135f
Examination approaches
assessments, 15
breast exams, 236f
cardiovascular system, 184
female genitourinary system, 287t
homeless patients, 502
musculoskeletal system, 323
older adults, 488
respiratory system, 164
Exercise. *See* Activity
External ear
canal of, 145b–146b
inspecting, 141b–142b
palpation of, 143b–144b
External genitalia
histories of lesions, 279–280
inspecting
female, 288b–290b, 394b
male, 27
Extinction, 366b
Extraocular movement (EOM), 361b
Extraocular muscles, 118b–119b
Extremities. *See also* Lower extremities; Upper extremities
Extrusion, 414b, 424t
Eyelashes, 121b–122b
Eyelids, 120b–121b
Eyes, 102–133
adolescents, 464t, 470t
adverse drug reactions to, 111t–112t
anatomical landmarks, 115
assessing infant's, 428t–429t
consensual reaction of pupils, 127b, 128b
cultural considerations of, 109
developmental considerations, 107–108, 412b, 432b
function of, 107
funduscopic features of, 129b
gonorrheal infections of, 285t, 303t
history of symptoms, 109–110
focused eye history, 110–111
for preschoolers/toddlers, 440t
inspecting
infant's, 432b
newborn's, 412b
older adults, 491b–492b
preschoolers/toddlers, 445t
nutritional assessments and, 566b
physical assessments, 19, 24
anterior chamber, 125b–126b
approach, position, tools for, 115
conjunctiva, 123b–124b
cornea, 118b, 124b–125b
extraocular muscles, 118b–119b
eyeball, 122b
eyelashes, 121b–122b
eyelids, 120b–121b
general appearance, 119b–120b
with Glasgow Coma Scale, 355t
inspecting visual acuity, 108, 117b–118b
iris, 126b
lacrimal ducts, puncta, 122b
macula and fovea centralis, 133b
ophthalmoscope apertures, 116b
ophthalmoscopy in, 129b
overview, 115
palpation of, 128b–133b

pupils, 126b–128b
red reflex, 108, 129b–131b
retinal vessels, 131b–132b
school-age children, 457t
sclera, 124b
questions to ask
older adults, 476t–477t
school-age children, 452t
relationship to
abdomen, 114b, 256t
cardiovascular system, 114b, 178t
ears, 113b
general system, 112b–113b
genitourinary/reproductive system, 114b, 285t
HEENT, 80t, 113b
integumentary system, 37t, 113b
musculoskeletal system, 114b–115b
neurologic system, 115b
respiratory system, 113b
Sjögren's syndrome, 319t
tearing of, 159t, 160t, 285t

F

Face. *See also* HEENT
anatomical landmarks for, 85f–86f
collecting histories, 74–76, 78
cultural considerations, 74
developmental considerations, 73–74
drugs adversely effecting, 76t–78t
expression of, 356b
facial droop, 354
infants, 73–74
inspecting preschoolers/toddlers, 445t
newborn, 411b
physical assessments, 86b–99b, 101b–102b
anatomical landmarks, 85–86
approach, position, tools for, 86
infant's, 428t
making, 19, 22, 24
older adults, 491b
primary functions of, 73
questions to ask, for older adults, 476t
relationship to, 78, 79t–85t
cardiovascular system, 82t
endocrine system, 79t, 84t–85t
eyes, 37t–38t, 80t, 113b
gastrointestinal system, 82t
genitourinary/reproductive systems, 82t–83t
immunological/hematological systems, 85t
integumentary system, 37t, 79bt–80t
musculoskeletal system, 83b
respiratory system, 81t
FACES pain rating scales, 248t, 519, 520
Facial nerve, 362b
Falling, 484b–485b
Family medical history
collecting, 18f, 451
from adolescents, 463
for infants, 428, 428t–430t
from school-age children, 451
genogram, 18f
mental health, 538t
Far vision, 117b
Fatigue
immune system changes and, 483t
relationship to
abdomen, 255t
cardiovascular system, 173, 176t
female genitourinary system, 284t
PV/lymphatic systems, 207
Feeling process, 2
Feet. *See also* Lower extremities
ankle-brachial index for, 221b–223b
examining toes and, 341b–342b
inspecting newborn's, 418b
problems of older adults, 482t, 498b
Female genitourinary system, 275–296. *See also* Pregnancy; Sexuality
collecting histories
reproductive/menstrual/sexuality history, 280, 281t–282t
symptoms, 279–280

cultural considerations and, 278t
developmental considerations, 275, 277–278
drugs adversely effecting, 282t–283t
female circumcision, 289b
functions of, 275
maturation states in girls, 276t–277t
physical assessments, 287, 288b–296b
approach, position, and toolbox for, 287
external genitalia, 288b–290b
female genitalia/rectal, 26, 290b, 296b
female reproductive system, 20
infant's, 436b
inspections during, 288b
newborns, 416b
older women, 495b
palpation during, 294b–296b
pelvic exams, 290b–293b
postpartal assessment of, 398b–400b
pregnancy assessments of, 394b
questions for older women, 480t–481t
relationship to, 284t–287t
breasts, 286t
cardiovascular system, 285t
endocrine system, 287t
eyes, mouth, and throat, 285t
gastrointestinal system, 286t
general system, 284t
HEENT, 284t–285t
integumentary system, 284t
lymphatic/hematological system, 287t
musculoskeletal, 286t
neurologic system, 286t–287t
respiratory system, 285t
Femoral hernia, 311b–312b
Fetus
assessments of, 375
causing abdominal enlargement, 390b–391b
complications with older mothers, 375, 376t
heart tones and rates of, 392b
measuring fundal height, 391b
movement of, 390b
position of, 273b, 392b–393b
positive signs of, 385t
Fibroadenoma, 240b
Fibrocystic breasts, 241b
Filipino Americans
childbirth practices, 380
death/dying for, 600t
response to pain, 516t
views on
adolescents, 462t
infants, 404
mental health, 535t
older adults, 473t
school-age children, 450t
Financial abuse of elders, 598
Fingers and thumbs
inspecting newborn's, 418b
inspecting/palpating, 337b–338b
FLACC Postoperative Pain Tool, 525, 527t
Fluid wave test, 216b, 272f
Focused physical assessments
breasts, 231
cardiovascular system, 174
collecting, abdomen, 251–252
ears, 137
eyes, 110–111
head, face, neck, 76, 78
integumentary system, 33
lymphatic, 208
musculoskeletal system, 317
neurologic system, 348
nutritional history, 564
peripheral-vascular, 208
respiratory system, 154
taking, 27–28
Fontanels
cultural fears of touching, 432b
newborn, 410b–411b
Food allergies, 259t
Foreskin
newborn's, 417b
physical assessment of, 306b
unable to retract, 307b, 310b
Forgetfulness, 357b
Four-quadrant method
abdominal inspections using, 264b
about, 260b–261b, 260f

FPS (Faces Pain Scale for Adults and Children), 519
French Canadians
  childbirth practices, 380
  response to pain, 516t
  views on
    infants, 404
    mental health, 535t
    school-age children, 450t
Friction rub
  abdominal, 266b
  illustration of cardiac, 197f
Functional assessments. *See* Daily activities
Functional incontinence, 483t
Fundal height measurements
    during pregnancy, 391b
    postpartum, 399b
Funduscopic features of eye, 129b
Funnel chest, 414b

G

Gag reflex
  testing, 362b
  testing oropharynx, 103b
Gait
  abnormal, 342b–343b
  inspecting, 325b–326b
  older adults, 496b
  toddler/preschooler, 447t
Gastroenteritis, 255t
Gastrointestinal system. *See also* Abdomen
  assessment of, 20
  auscultation of, 212t
  collecting histories of infant's, 429t
  drugs adversely effecting, 252t–254t
  evaluating in death process, 606, 606t, 608b
  health history for homeless patients, 504t
  physical assessments
    adolescents, 471t
    homeless patients, 507t
    infants, 434b–435b
    nutrition, 567b
    older adults, 494b–495b
    preschoolers/toddlers 446t
    school-age children, 458t
  questions to ask
    adolescents, 465t
    older adults, 479t
    preschoolers/toddlers, 442t
    school-age children, 453t
  relationship to
    breasts, 234t
    cardiovascular system, 180t, 257t
    ears, 139t
    female genitourinary system, 286t
    head, neck, and face, 82t
    integumentary system, 39t
    male genitourinary system, 303t–304t
    neurologic system, 352t
    PV/lymphatic systems, 212t
    respiratory system, 161t
General health survey
  adolescents, 463t, 469t
  details assessed in, 16
  evaluating in death process, 606, 607b–609b
  homeless patients, 503t, 507t
  mental health, 544t
  newborns, 406b–408b
  nutrition, 566b
  older adults, 475t
  preschoolers/toddlers, 440t, 445t
  school-age children, 452t, 457t
General system reviews
  abdomen, 254t–255t
  breasts, 233t
  cardiovascular system, 176t
  details of, 19–21
  ears, 138t
  eyes to, 112b–113b
  female genitourinary system, 284t
  head, face, neck, 79t
  integumentary system to, 36t–37t
  male genitourinary system, 302t
  mental health, 544t
  musculoskeletal system, 319t
  neurologic system, 351t
  PV/lymphatic systems 211f
  respiratory system, 157t
Genital herpes, 307b

Genitourinary system. *See also* External genitalia; Female genitourinary system; Male genitourinary system
assessment of, 20
bladder
effect of stroke, 353t
percussion of, 269b
collecting histories
homeless patients, 504t
for infants, 429t
older adults, 480t–481t
school-age children, 453t
evaluating in death process, 606, 606t, 608b
physical assessments, 508t
adolescents, 471t
during pregnancy, 394b–397b
female genitalia/rectal exams, 20, 26, 290b
infants, 435b–436b
male genitalia/rectal exams, 27, 309b, 312b–313b
older adults, 495b
preschoolers/toddlers, 447t
school-age children, 458t
postpartal assessment of, 398b–399b
questions for preschoolers/ toddlers, 442t
relationship to
abdomen, 257t–258t
ears, 139t
eyes, 114b
head, neck, and face, 82t–83t
integumentary system, 39t–40t
musculoskeletal system, 320t
neurologic system, 353t
PV/lymphatic systems, 213t
respiratory system, 161b
Geriatric depression scale, 533b
German Americans, death/dying for, 600t
Gingivae (gums)
assessing, 95b–96b
bleeding, 211t
during pregnancy, 388b
Girls. *See also* Birth control pills; Female genitourinary system; Menstruation
asking about menarche, 465t, 468t
maturation states, 276t–277t
pregnancies in, 375
use of birth control pills, 282t, 462–463
Glabellar reflex, 371b, 424t
Glands. *See also* Prostate; Thyroid
Bartholin's, 294b, 394b
bulbourethral, 313b
inspecting men's swollen, 303t
lacrimal apparatus, 128b
parotid and submandibular, 90b, 103b
Skene's, 294b, 394b
sublingual, 103b
Glasgow Coma Scale, 355t
Glaucoma
closed-angle, 118b
examining eyes for, 130b–131b
no palpation of eyeball in, 128b
Glossopharyngeal nerve, 362b–363b
Gluteal folds, newborn's, 418b
Goiter, 256t
Golf elbow, 336b
Gonorrhea
gonorrheal eye infections, 285t, 303t
physical assessments
men, 303t
women, 290b
Goodell's sign, 385t
Gouty arthritis, 338b
Graphesthesia, 365b
Grasping, 371b
Greek Americans
childbirth practices, 381
response to pain, 516t
views on
adolescents, 462t
infants, 404
mental health, 535t
older adults, 473t
school-age children, 450t
Grey-Turner's sign, 263b
Group suicide risks, 554b
Growth
adolescents and rapid periods of, 460
measuring
infants, 430b–431b
newborns, 406b–407b
school-age children, 448

Gums. *See* Gingivae
Gynecomastia, 465t, 471t

H

Haemophilus influenzae shots, 440
Hair
  adverse drug effects on, 34t–36t
  assessments of, 54b–56b, 101b
  infant's, 432b
  integumentary system and, 54b–56b
  loss of, 319t
  men's, 302t
  newborn's, 410b
  nutritional assessments and, 566b
  older adults, 476t, 491b
Haitian Americans, 601t
Hallucinations, 550t
Hallucinogens, 559t–560t
Hands, newborn's, 419b
Head. *See also* Headaches; HEENT
  anatomical landmarks for, 85f–86f
  collecting histories, 74–76, 78
  cultural considerations, 74
  developmental considerations, 73–74
  drugs adversely effecting, 76t–78t
  function of, 73
  infants, 73–74
  inspecting
    newborn fontanels, 410b–411b
    preschoolers/toddlers, 445t
  measuring
    infant's, 430b–436b
    newborn's, 406b
  physical assessments, 86b, 101b–103b
    anatomical landmarks, 85–86
    approach, position, tools for, 86
    conducting, 22, 24
    face and head, 19
    infants, 428t–429t
    neurologic symptoms, 347
    older adults, 491b
    school-age children, 457t
  questions for older adults, 476t
  relationship to, 78, 79t–85t
    cardiovascular system, 82t
    ears, 138t
    endocrine system, 79t, 84t–85t
    eyes, 113b
    gastrointestinal system, 82t
    general system, 79t
    genitourinary/reproductive systems, 82t–83t
    immunological/hematological systems, 85t
    integumentary system, 37t, 79t–80t
    musculoskeletal system, 83t
    neurologic system, 84t
    respiratory system, 81t
Head-to-toe assessments
  approach for, 16, 21
  performing, 22, 24–27
Headaches
  effect of cardiovascular disease on, 479t
  neurologic assessments of, 351t
  related to female genitourinary system, 284t
  vision changes and, 178t
Health histories. *See* Patient histories
Health practices. *See also* Childbirth practices
  cultural influences on, 576, 578–579
  of homeless patients, 504t
  mental health and, 542t
Hearing
  changes in sense of, 351t
  checking infant's, 432b
  exams assessing, 148b–151b
  loss of, 135–136
  in older adults, 492b–493b
  Rinne test for, 150b–151b
  testing verbal comprehension, 359b
  Weber test for, 149b–150b
Heart. *See also* Cardiac rates and rhythms; Cardiovascular system
  anatomical landmarks of, 182f–183f
  assessing auscultation of, 192b–193b, 194f–199f
  atrial fibrillation, 198f, 352t, 482t
  auscultation
    extra heart sounds, 285t
    infant heart and pulses, 434b
    for preschoolers/toddlers, 446t

fetal tones and rates of, 392b
sounds of, 199b–200b, 201b, 202t, 285t
Heberden's nodes, 337b, 497f
HEENT (head, ears, eyes, nose, and throat). *See also specific physical area*
collecting histories
homeless patients, 504t
infant, 428t–429t
physical assessments
adolescents, 470t
in death process, 605t, 606, 607b–608b
during pregnancy, 388b–389b
infants, 432b–433b
mental health, 545t
newborns, 410b–415b
nutrition, 566b–567b
older adults, 491b–493b
preschoolers/toddlers, 445t–447t
school-age children, 457t–458t
postpartal assessment of, 398b
questions to ask
adolescents, 464t
older adults, 476t
preschoolers/toddlers, 440t–442t
school-age children, 452t–453t
relationship to
abdomen, 256t
breasts, 234t
cardiovascular system, 178t–179t
ears, 138t
female genitourinary system, 284t–285t
male genitourinary system, 303t
musculoskeletal system, 319t–320t
neurologic system, 351t–352t
PV/lymphatic systems, 211t–212t
respiratory system, 159t–160t
Hegar's sign, 385t
Height
aging and loss of, 475t
fundal, 391b, 399b
of infants, 431b
Helix of ear, 143b–144b
Hemangiomas, 409b
Hematological system. *See* Immunological/hematological systems
Hemorrhoids
female, 296b
postpartal assessments of, 398b
Hepatitis B immunization, 430t, 440
Hernias
checking for abdominal, 263b
inguinal and femoral, 309b, 311b–312b
Herniated umbilicus, 263b, 416b
Herpes simplex virus, 307b
Hindu Americans, 601t
Hinge joints, 321t
Hips, 338b–339b
HIV. *See also* AIDS
about, 386, 304t
vaginal *Candida albicans* and, 293b
Hmong Americans, 601t
Homans' sign, 219b, 222b, 394b
Home care. *See* Environment
Homeless patients, 502–508
approach and focus with, 502
health history for
activity, 505t
cardiovascular, 504t
cultural influences, 505t
daily activities, 504t
environmental health patterns, 505t
gastrointestinal system, 504t
genitourinary system, 504t
health practices, 504t
HEENT, 504t
hematological/immune/endocrine systems, 504t
integumentary, 504t
musculoskeletal/neurologic system, 504t
nutritional patterns, 504t
occupational health patterns, 505t
overview, 503t
psychosocial profile, 504t
religious influences, 506t

roles/relationships/self-concept, 505t
sexuality patterns, 506t
sleep/rest patterns, 505t
socioeconomic status, 505t
values/beliefs, 504t
physical assessments, 506–507, 507t–508t
cardiovascular system, 507t
gastrointestinal system, 507t
genitourinary system, 508t
integumentary system, 507t
musculoskeletal system, 508t
neurologic system, 508t
respiratory system, 507t
Homicidal thoughts, 550t
Hormone replacement therapy (HRT), 181t, 235t, 320t
HPV2 (Human papillomavirus) vaccine, 463
HTN. *See* Hypertension
Human papillomavirus (HPV2) vaccine, 463
Human services within community, 588t
Hydration of skin, 491b
Hymen in newborn, 416b
Hypercapnia, 352t
Hypertension (HTN)
asking older adults about, 479t
cultural considerations, 205
symptoms
in ears, 38t
in eyes, 114b, 130b, 131b, 132b
nosebleeds, 179t
vison problems and, 212t
Hypertonia/hypotonia, 419b
Hyperventilation, 165b
Hypo-/hyperthyroidism, 105b, 285t
Hypoglossal nerve, 363b
Hypotension symptoms, 223b
Hypothermia, newborn, 407b
Hypoxia, 352t

I

IADL (Instrumental Activities of Daily Living), 487b
ICP (intracranial pressure), 361t
Ileocecal valve, 265b
Iliopsoas muscle test, 272b
Illusions, 550t
Immunizations
monthly contraceptive shots, 463
recommended
adolescents, 463
infants, 430t
preschoolers/toddlers, 439–440
school-age children, 451
resources on, 428
Immunological/hematological systems
fatigue and, 483t
homeless patients, 504t
physical assessments
adolescents, 466t
school-age children, 454t
questions for preschoolers/toddlers, 442t
relationship to
abdomen, 259t
breasts, 235t
female genitourinary system, 287t
head, face, neck, 85t
integumentary system, 41t
male genitourinary system, 304t
neurologic system, 354t
SCIDS, 205
Incontinence
bowel, 353t
urinary, 480t, 483t
Indigestion, 250
Infants, 401–437. *See also* Newborns
abdomen of, 245
breasts of, 226
breathing styles of, 166b
cardiovascular system of, 172
collecting histories of, 428, 428t–430t
cultural/ethnic influences on, 403–404
developmental considerations
male genitourinary system 297, 298t
musculoskeletal system, 314
pain, 512
spirituality, 569
summary of, 401–403
developmental testing for, 437t
ears of, 134–135

Eustachian tube of, 134f
eyes of, 107–108
female genitourinary system of, 275
head, face, and neck, 73–74
immunizations for, 430t
integumentary system of, 29–30
neurologic system of, 345
pain rating scales for, 523–524
physical assessments, 430b–436b
anus and rectum, 436b
cardiovascular system, 434b
extremities, 435b
gastrointestinal system, 434b–435b
genitourinary system, 435b–436b
HEENT, 432b–433b
integumentary system, 431b–432b
measuring, 430b–431b
neurologic systems, 436b
newborns, 405, 406b–419b
respiratory system, 433b–434b
PV and lymphatic systems of, 204
respiratory system of, 152
Infections
history of infant's, 429t
urinary tract, 465t
vaginal, 258t, 287t
Inguinal area
examining, 311b–312b
lymph nodes of, 274b, 309b, 312b
Inguinal hernia, 309b, 311b–312b
Inhalants, 561t
Initial Pain Assessment Inventory (IPAI), 519
Inspections, 4–5f
abdominal, 262b–264b, 389b–394b
breasts during pregnancy, 389b
cyanosis, 158t, 176t, 177t
external ear, 141b–142b
female genitourinary system, 288b
infant's eyes, 432b
joints, 333b–342b
nail assessments, 49b–54b
newborns
abdomen, 415b–416b
fontanels, 410b–411b
skin, 42b–49b
visual acuity, 117b–118b
Instrumental Activities of Daily Living (IADL), 487b
Integumentary system, 29–72. *See also* Hair; Nails; Skin
collecting histories, 32–33
cultural considerations, 32
developmental considerations of, 29–30
drugs adversely effecting, 34t–36t
physical assessments, 42, 42b–56b
adolescents, 469t
approach, position, and tools for, 42
during pregnancy, 387b
hair and scalp, 54b–56b
homeless patients, 504t, 507t
infants, 431b–432b
mental health, 544t
nails, 49b–54b
newborns, 408b–410b
nutrition, 566b
older adults, 489b–491b
preschoolers/toddlers, 445t
school-age children, 457t
skin, 42b–49b
primary functions of, 29
questions to ask
adolescents, 463t
for older adults, 475t–476t
school-age children, 452t
relationship to
abdomen, 255t–256t
breasts, 234t
cardiovascular system, 38t–39t, 176t–177t
ears, 138t
eyes, 113b
female genitourinary system, 284t
head/face/neck, 37t, 79t–80t
male genitourinary system, 302t
musculoskeletal system, 319t
neurologic system, 351t
other systems, 36t–41t

PV/lymphatic systems, 211t
respiratory system, 158t–159t
seasonal skin disorders, 33t–34t
skin color variations, 56t–58t
Interstitial fibrosis, 320t
Intracranial pressure (ICP), 361t
Introitus, 289b
IPAI (Initial Pain Assessment Inventory), 519
Iranian Americans
childbirth practices, 381
response to pain, 516t
views on
adolescents, 462t
infants, 404
mental health, 535t
older adults, 473t
school-age children, 450t
Iris, 107, 126b
Irish Americans
childbirth practices, 381–382
response to pain, 516t
views on
adolescents, 462t
infants, 404
mental health, 535t
older adults, 473t
school-age children, 450t
Irritable bowel disease, 265b

J

Japanese Americans, 601t
Jaundice
liver disease and, 255t, 262b
viewed in sclera, 114b
Jewish Americans
childbirth practices, 382
death/dying for, 601t
response to pain, 516t
views on
adolescents, 462t
infants, 404
mental health, 535t
older adults, 473t
school-age children, 450t
Jock itch, 307b
Joints
inspection/palpation 333b–342b
ankles, 341b
cervical spine, 334b
elbows, 335b–336b
feet and toes, 341b–342b
fingers and thumbs, 337b–338b
hips, 338b–339b
knees, 339b–340b
for newborn's, 418b
scapulae, 335b
shoulders, 335b
temporomandibular, 334b
thoracic and lumbar curve, 338b
wrists, 336b
types of synovial, 321t–322t
Judgment, 358b
Jugular vein
abnormal jugular venous waves, 198f
jugular waves correlated to cardiac cycle, 197f
palpations of, 185b–187b
pressure and pulsation of, 184b–185b
JVP (jugular venous pressure), 184b

K

Katz Index of Activities of Daily Living, 485b–486b
Kehr's sign, 273b
Kernig's sign, 372b
Kidneys
assessing newborn, 412b–413b
palpating, 270b, 271b
Kinesthetics, 364b–365b
Knees
inspecting/palpating, 339b–340b
physical assessments of, 323b
Knock knees, 314
Korean Americans
death/dying for, 601t
views on older adults, 473t
Korotkoff sounds, 224b–225b
Kübler-Ross, E., 602t–603t
Kussmaul's respiratory rate, 165b
Kyphosis, 324b, 493b

L

Labia
enlargement of, 394b
inspecting newborn, 416b
Lachman's test, 340b

Lacrimal ducts, 122b
Last menstrual period (LMP), 258t, 386
LD (learning disabilities), 454
Lead screening, 437t
Legs. *See also* Lower extremities
  circumferences of, 330b, 331b
  claudication in, 39t, 479t
  measuring lengths of, 330b–331b
Length of newborn, 407b
Lesions
  breast, 240b, 241b
  clinical description of, 66t–67t
  distribution of, 70t–72t
  external genitalia, 279
  in male genitourinary system, 299
  mouth, 211t, 285t
  of older adults, 500t
  oral, 285t, 303t
  pattern and configuration of, 68t–69t
  penile, 305b, 306b
  primary, 59t–61t
  related to
    female genitourinary system, 284t
    male sexual activity, 302t
  secondary, 61t–63t
  shingles, 255t, 263b
  vaginal, 293b
  vascular, 64t–65t
Levels of consciousness
  cerebral functions and, 356b
  terms used to describe, 373t
Lips
  cleft, 414b
  physical assessments, 90b–91b, 103b
Liver
  abdominal assessments of, 263b
  auscultating over, 266b
  diseases of, 303t–304t
    jaundice, 255t, 262b
    pruritus, 255t
  palpating, 270b–271b
  percussion of, 267b–268b
  scratch test for, 265b
Lochia, 399b
Lordosis, 325b
Lower extremities
  ankle-brachial index for feet, 221b–223b
  collecting histories of, 174, 205–208
  color change test, 222b
  coordination of, 329b
  exercise-induced pain of, 213t
  inspecting
    during pregnancy, 394b
    infant's, 435b
    joints of, 338b–342b
    newborn's, 419b
  intermittent claudication in legs, 39t, 479t
  measuring leg lengths, 330b–331b
  numbness of, 259t
  palpation of, 218b–219b
  physical assessments of, 26, 216b–217b
Lungs. *See also* Respiratory system
  anatomical landmarks of, 163f
  assessing with percussion, 168b
  auscultation of 169b–171b
    infant, 434b
  cultural considerations of, 153
Lyme disease, 319t
Lymph nodes. *See also* Cervical lymph nodes; Lymphatic system
  assessing
    enlarged, 319t
    in neck, 100b–101b, 159t
  inguinal, 274b, 309b, 312b
  physical assessments
    older adults, 491b
    palpating nipple and areola, 242b–244b
  swollen genitourinary
    men's, 300
    women's, 284t–285t
Lymphatic system, 204–225. *See also* Cervical lymph nodes; Immunological/hematological system; Peripheral-vascular system
  anatomical landmarks of, 214f
  collecting histories of, 205–208
  cultural considerations, 205

developmental considerations, 204–205
drugs adversely effecting, 208t–210t
homeless patients, 503t
physical assessments 214f, 215b–225b
adolescents, 466t
anatomical landmarks, 214f
assessing edema, 218b
auscultation during BP checks, 223b–225b
lower extremities, 216b–217b
palpation, 218b–221b
postpartal, 399b
school-age children, 454t
upper extremities, 215b–216b
primary functions, 204
questions to ask
adolescents, 466t
older adults, 483t
preschoolers/toddlers, 442t
school-age children, 454t
relationship to
breasts, 235t
cardiovascular system, 182t, 212t
female genitourinary system, 287t
gastrointestinal system, 212t
general system, 211f
genitourinary/reproductive systems, 213t
HEENT, 211t–212t
integumentary system, 211t
male genitourinary system, 304t
musculoskeletal system, 213t
neurologic system, 213t, 354t
respiratory system, 162t, 212t
vision, 212t
symptoms of STDs, 213t
tools for, 215
Lymphedema, 217f

M

Macula
assessing fovea centralis and, 133b
degeneration of, 133b
Magnet reflex, 426t
Male genitourinary system, 297–313. *See also* Prostate; Sexuality
assessing infant's, 435–436b
collecting histories, 299–302
erectile dysfunction, 301–302
sexual histories, 300–301
symptoms, 299–300
cultural considerations, 299
developmental considerations, 297, 298t, 299
drugs adversely effecting, 301t
physical assessments
anus and rectum, 27, 309b, 312b–313b
inguinal area, 309b, 311b–312b
male reproductive system, 20
newborns, 417b–418b
older men, 495b
palpations, 309b–313b
penis, 305b–307b, 309b–310b
prostate, 258t, 313b
scrotum, 308b
testes, 308b, 310b–311b, 418b
tools, 305
primary functions, 297
questions to ask older men about, 480t, 481t
relationship to, 302t–304t
breasts, 303t
cardiovascular system, 303t
endocrine system, 304t
gastrointestinal system, 303t–304t
general system, 302t
HEENT, 303t
integumentary system, 302t
lymphatic/hematological system, 304t
musculoskeletal system, 304t
respiratory system, 303t
Manual compressions tests, 222b
Marijuana, 558t
Mastoid palpation, 143b
Masturbation, preschooler/toddler, 444
Mathematical and calculative ability, 357b
Maturation states
boys, 298t
girls, 276t–277t

McBurney's point, 271b
McGill Pain Questionnaire (MPQ), 519–520
McMurray's test, 340b
Measles, mumps, and rubella (MMR) immunizations, 440, 451, 463
Measuring
arms and leg lengths, 330b–331b
infants, 430b–431b
newborns, 406b–407b
Memory
cardiovascular causes effecting, 181t
related to mental health, 551t
testing, 357b
Men. *See also* Male genitourinary system
breathing styles of, 166b
frequent or weak urination, 480t
incidents of breast cancer, 241b
prostate, 258t, 313b
sexual performance problems
cardiovascular-related, 180t
neurologic signs associated with, 353t
PV disease and, 213t
Menarche, 234t, 465t, 468t
Ménière's disease, 257t
Meningeal signs, 372b
Meningitis vaccine, 463
Meniscus tear, 340b
Menopausal women. *See also* Pre/postmenopausal women
genitourinary system of, 277–278
HRT and musculoskeletal system, 320t
integumentary system of, 30
Menstruation
amenorrhea, 280, 286t
asking about menarche, 465t, 468
dysmenorrhea, 279
hypercoagulable states in cycle, 353t
investigating history of, 281t
last period, 258t, 386
premenstrual syndrome, 281t
vaginal bleeding, 279
Mental health, 529–561. *See also* Psychosocial histories
assessing, 351t
with BATHE technique, 552
changes in, 347
crisis assessment, 552t
depression, 552–553
mental status, 546, 546t–551t
collecting history of, 536, 536t–538t
cultural views of, 534t–536t
daily activities and, 542t
developmental considerations 529–532, 529t, 530b, 531t, 532b, 533b
children, 529–530, 529t, 530b
older adults, 498b
pregnant women, 530–531
drugs adversely effecting, 538t–539t
physical assessments, 544t–545t
abdominal system, 545t
cardiovascular system, 545t
general system, 544t
HEENT system, 545t
integumentary system, 544t
musculoskeletal system, 545t
neurologic system, 545t
respiratory system, 545t
psychosocial history, 542t–544t
activity, 542t
cultural influences, 543t
daily activities, 542t
environment, 543t
family roles/relationships, 544t
health practices and beliefs, 542t
nutrition, 542t
occupational health, 543t
personal habits, 543t
recreation/hobbies, 543t
religious influence, 543t
roles/relationships/self-concept, 543t
sexuality patterns, 544t
sleep/rest, 543t
stress and coping patterns, 544t
suicide assessment, 553–554, 553b, 554b–555b

systems related to, 540t–542t
cardiovascular system, 541t
gastrointestinal system, 541t
general health, 540t
genitourinary system, 541t
HEENT, 540t–541t
integumentary system, 540t
musculoskeletal system, 541t–542t
neurologic system, 541t–542t
respiratory system, 541t
Mexican Americans
childbirth practices, 382–383
death/dying for, 601t
mental health of, 535t, 537t
response to pain, 516t
views on
infants, 404
older adults, 473t
school-age children, 451t
Migraines. *See* Headaches
Miliaria, 409b
Military service, 538t
Mitral regurgitation, 199b
Mitral stenosis, 200b
MMR (measles, mumps, and rubella) immunizations, 440, 451, 463
Mnemonics
BATHE technique, 552
CAGE questionnaire, 555, 556b
DAR, 4
OLDCART, 518
PIE, 4
PQRST, 517–518
SBAR, 3
SOAPIE, 4
Modulation of pain, 509
Mongolian spots, 409b
Moro reflex, 420t
Mothers-to-be. *See* Pregnancy
Motor responses. *See also* Musculoskeletal system
assessing, 355b
development in newborns and infants, 402
newborn facial movements, 411b
Mouth
adolescents, 470t
inspecting
infant's, 433b
newborn's, 413b–414b
older adult's, 493b
preschoolers/toddlers, 446t
lesions of, 211t, 285t
nutritional assessments and, 567b
physical assessments
during pregnancy, 388b–389b
pharynx and, 24
school-age children, 457t–458t
throat and mouth, 19
questions for older adults, 477t–478t
relationship to female genitourinary system, 285t
Movements
accuracy of, 329b
newborn facial, 411b
types of body, 333b
MPQ (McGill Pain Questionnaire), 519–520
Multidimensional pain scales, 519–520
Munchausen's syndrome by proxy (MSBP), 591, 592
Murmurs
accompanying infant cyanosis, 434b
continuous, 197f
developmental, 172
female anemia and, 285t
newborn, 415b
postpartal assessments of, 398b
pregnancy-related, 389b
sounds of, 192b–193b, 194f–199f, 203t
systolic and diastolic, 196f
Murphy's sign, 273b
Muscles
aging and decreasing strength of, 498b
cramps in, 181t
damage to spinoaccessory nerve, 363b
extraocular, 118b–119b
palpation of, 331b–332b
rating strength of, 344t

testing strength of, 332b, 436b
weakness of, 286t, 304t, 338b
Musculoskeletal system. 314–344. *See also* Posture
approach, position, and toolbox for, 323
assessment of, 20–21
newborn posture, 406b
collecting histories, 316–317
homeless patients, 504t
for infants, 429t
cultural considerations, 315–316
damage to spinoaccessory nerve, 353t
death process and, 606t, 609b
developmental considerations of, 314–315
drugs adversely effecting, 318t
physical assessments, 323b–342b
accuracy of movements, 329b
adolescents, 471t
cerebellar function, 326b–327b, 500b
during pregnancy, 397b
gaits, 325b–326b, 342t–343t
homeless patients, 508t
joint inspection/palpation, 333b–342b
mental health, 545t
motor responses, 355t
muscle palpation, 331b–332b
newborns, 418b–419b
nutrition, 567b
older adults, 496b–498b
posture and spinal curves, 323b–325b
preschoolers/toddlers, 447t
pronator drift, 330b, 354
school-age children, 458t
taking measurements, 330b–331b
testing coordination, 328b–329b, 447t
postpartal assessment of, 400b
primary function of, 314
questions to ask
adolescents, 466t
older adults about, 481t–482t
school-age children, 453t
rating muscle strength, 344t
relationship to, 319t–321t
abdomen, 258t–259t
breasts, 235t
cardiovascular system, 181t, 320t
ears, 140t
eyes, 114b–115b
female genitourinary system 286t
gastrointestinal system, 320t
general system, 319t
genitourinary/reproductive system, 320t
head, neck, and face, 83t
HEENT system, 319t–320t
integumentary system, 40t, 319t
male genitourinary system, 304t
neurologic system, 320t–321t
PV/lymphatic systems, 213t
respiratory system, 161t, 166b, 320t
tenderness of bones, 213t
types of synovial joints, 321t–322t

N

Naegele's rule, 386
Nails
color changes of, 158t, 177t
drug effects on, 34t–36t
infant's, 432b
inspecting, 49b–54b
newborn, 410b
nutritional assessments and, 566b
older adults, 476t, 491b
NAPI (Nurses Assessment of Pain Inventory), 525
Natal teeth, 414b
National Immunization Program, 428
National Institute of Health (NIH) Stroke Scale, 354–355
Nausea
associated with abdomen, 250–251
gastrointestinal causes of, 320t
neurologic problems and, 352t

Navajo Native Americans
childbirth practices, 383
influences on infants, 404
response to pain, 516t
views on
adolescents, 462t
mental health, 535t
older adults, 473t
school-age children, 451t
Near vision, 117b
Neck
adolescents, 470t
anatomical landmarks, 85f–86f
for cardiac assessments, 183f
collecting histories, 74–76
cultural considerations, 74
developmental considerations, 73–74
drugs adversely effecting, 76t–78t
goiter and, 256t
indicators of respiratory distress in, 160t
infants, 73–74
inspecting preschoolers/toddlers, 446t
newborn, 410b–411b, 420t–421t
physical assessments, 25, 100b, 103b–106b
anatomical landmarks, 85–86
approach, position, tools for, 86
carotid arteries and jugular veins, 184t, 184b–187b, 352t
conducting, 22, 25
during pregnancy, 388b
infant's neck, 428t
lymph nodes, 100b–101b, 159t
older adults, 491b
postpartal assessment, 398b
school-age children, 458t
primary functions of, 73
questions to ask, for older adults, 476t
relationship to, 78, 79t–85t
ears, 138t
endocrine system, 79t, 84t–85t
eyes, 113b
gastrointestinal system, 82t
genitourinary/reproductive systems, 82t–83t
integumentary system, 37t, 79t–80t
musculoskeletal system, 83b
neurologic system, 84t
PV/lymphatic systems, 211t
respiratory system, 81t
symptoms, 74–76
vein distension of, 159t, 160t
Neglect
children, 592
older adults, 597–598
preschoolers/toddlers, 439
Neonatal Infant Pain Scale (NIPS), 523
Neurologic system, 345–374
assessing arousal state, 372t–373t
Cincinnati Prehospital Stroke Scale, 354
collecting histories, 347–348
homeless patients, 504t
infant's, 429t
cultural considerations, 347
developmental considerations, 345–346
drugs adversely effecting, 348t–350t
evaluating at death, 606t, 609b
Glasgow Coma Scale, 355t
levels of consciousness
cerebral functions and, 356b
terms to describe, 373t
NIH Stroke Scale, 354–355
physical assessments, 21, 355–356, 356b–372b
adolescents, 471t
approach, position, tools for, 355
cerebral functions, 356b–363b
cranial nerves, 360b–363b
during pregnancy, 397b
homeless patients, 508t
infants, 436b
meningeal signs, 372b
mental health, 545t
newborns, 419b
nutrition, 568b
older adults, 498b–500b
postpartal, 400b

preschoolers/toddlers, 447t
school-age children, 458t
sensory functions, 363b–369b
superficial reflexes, 370b–371b
tools for, 164
primary functions, 345
questions to ask
adolescents, 466t
older adults, 482t
preschoolers/toddlers, 442t
school-age children, 454t
relationship to, 351t–354t
abdomen, 259t
breasts, 235t
cardiovascular system, 352t
ears, 140t
endocrine system, 354t
eyes, 115b
female genitourinary system, 286t–287t
gastrointestinal system, 352t
general system, 351t
genitourinary system, 353t
head, neck, and face, 84t
HEENT, 351t–352t
integumentary system, 40t–41t, 351t
lymphatic/hematological, 354t
musculoskeletal system, 320t–321t, 353t
PV/lymphatic systems, 213t
respiratory system, 162t, 352t
types of problems, 373t–374t
Neuropathic Pain Scale, 520
Neurosyphilis, 286t, 287t, 304t
Newborns, 401–437
Apgar scoring of, 405t
diagnostic/screening tests for, 427t
health history of, 405t
neurologic system of, 345
physical assessments 405, 406b–419b
abdomen, 415b–416b
chest, 414b–415b
female genitourinary, 416b
general observations, 406b–408b
HEENT, 410b–414b
integumentary system, 408b–410b
male genitourinary, 417b–418b
musculoskeletal system, 418b–419b
neurologic system, 419b
rectum, 416b
respiratory system, 415b
point of maximal impulse, 415b
reflexes 420t–426t
Babinski's, 371b, 422t
crawling, 424t
crossed extension, 425t
glabellar, 424t
inspecting, 414b
magnet, 426t
Moro, 420t
palmar grasp, 421t
plantar grasp, 421t
pull-to-sit, 425t
rooting reflex, 371b, 414b, 423t
startle, 412b, 420t
stepping, 422t
sucking, 371b, 414b, 423t
swallowing, 414b, 423t
tonic neck, 420t–421t
trunk incurvation, 426t
Nicotine, 561t
NIH (National Institute of Health) Stroke Scale, 354–355
Nipple and areola
collecting histories of, 231–232
illustrated, 236f
newborn's, 415b
palpating nodes associated with, 242b–244b
physical assessments of 239b–240b, 242b
NIPS (Neonatal Infant Pain Scale), 523
Nocturia symptoms, 161t
Nocturnal emissions, 460
Nose. *See also* Ears; Throat
assessments of, 19, 24, 88b–90b, 102b
adolescent's, 470t
infant's, 429b, 433b
newborn's, 413b
older adults, 493b
preschoolers/toddlers, 446t
school-age children, 457t

HTN and nosebleed, 179t
nutritional assessments and, 567b
questions to ask older adults, 477t
relationship to
abdomen, 256t–257t
cardiovascular system, 179t
ears, 138t
head, face, and neck, 80t–81t
integumentary system, 38t
Numerical Rating Scale, 248t, 518
Numerical Scale, 520–521
Nurses Assessment of Pain Inventory (NAPI), 525
Nursing
communications tips for, 3
doing assessments, 15
role of assessment in, 1
Nutrition, 562–568
about, 562
adolescents, 467
assessing, 562–564
food intake records, 565
health history, 562–564
24-hour recall, 564–565
cultural influences on, 576
diets of older adults, 479t
homeless patients, 504t
mental health and, 542t
physical assessments, 565, 566b–568b
cardiovascular, 567b
general health survey, 566b
HEENT, 566b–567b
integumentary, 566b
musculoskeletal, 567b
neurologic, 568b
respiratory, 567b
preschoolers/toddlers, 443
requests during death process, 606t
school-age children, 455

O

Objective Pain Score (OPS), 525
Obstetrics health history, 281t
Obturator muscle test, 271b
Occupational health
homeless patients and, 505t
mental health and, 543t
Oculocephalic reflex test, 361b
Oculomotor nerve, 361b
OLDCART mnemonic, 518
Older adults, 472–501. *See also* Cerebral functions
abuse and neglect of, 596–598
clock scoring for, 501b
collecting health history of, 473–474
common skin lesions of, 500t
cultural considerations, 472t–473t
depression of, 532, 532b–533b
developmental considerations
ears, 134–135
male genitourinary system, 299
musculoskeletal system, 315
pain, 514
pregnancy of older women, 375–376
psychological, 472
spirituality, 570
do-not-resuscitate orders for, 603–604, 604t–605t
eyes of, 108–109
falls by, 484b–485b
functional assessments 485b–487b
Barthel Index, 486t
Katz Index of Activities of Daily Living, 485b–486b
incontinence in, 480t, 483t
pain rating scales for, 528t
physical assessments, 488, 489b–500b
abdomen, 246
approach and tools for, 488
cardiovascular system, 172, 494b
female genitourinary system, 277–278
gastrointestinal system, 494b–495b
genitourinary system, 495b
head, face, and neck, 74
HEENT, 491b–493b
integumentary system, 30–31, 489b–491b
musculoskeletal system, 496b–498b
neurologic system, 346, 498b–500b
PV/lymphatic systems of, 205
respiratory system, 152, 493b
women's breasts, 228

questions to ask, 475t–483t
cardiovascular system, 478t–479t
endocrine system, 482t
gastrointestinal system, 479t
general health status, 475t
genitourinary system, 480t–481t
HEENT, 476t
immune/hematological system, 483t
integumentary system, 475t–476t
musculoskeletal system, 481t–482t
neurological system, 482t
respiratory system, 478t
skin disorders of, 31t
sleep patterns, 485b
testing knowledge and vocabulary, 358b
Olfactory nerve, 360b–361b
Ophthalmoscope apertures, 116b
Ophthalmoscopy of eyes, 129b
Opiates, 559t
Opisthotonic posture, 419b
OPS (Objective Pain Score), 525
Optic nerve, 131b–133b, 361b
Oral contraceptives. *See* Birth control pills
Oral mucosa
lesions of, 285t, 303t
physical assessments of, 91b–94b
Oropharynx, 99b–100b, 103b
Orthostatic hypotension, 478t
Orthostatic pitting, 218b
Ortolani's maneuver, 339b
Osteoporosis, 286t
Otalgia, 137
Otorrhea, 136
Otoscopic exam of ears, 144b–145b, 432b
Oucher pain rating scale, 521
Ovaries, 296b
Overflow incontinence, 483t

P

Paget's disease, 240b
Pain, 509–528. *See also* Pain rating scales
abdominal
abdominal aortic aneurysm, 257t
patient histories of, 247, 248–249
rating intensity of, 248t
significance of, 247b
about, 509
assessing during physical exams, 522t
breast, 229, 231
cultural considerations, 514, 515t–516t
developmental considerations, 512–514
children, 512–513
infants, 512
older adults, 514
dysmenorrhea, 279
exercise-induced, 213t
extremities, 205–206
indigestion, 250
mechanism of, 509
musculoskeletal system, 316
reassessment of, 528
symptoms
during woman's urination, 280
male genitourinary system, 299
PQRST analysis of, 517–518
testing sensation of, 363b–364b
types of, 510t–511t
wrist, 336b
Pain Assessment in Advanced Dementia Scale (PAINAD), 528
Pain Assessment Tool (PAT), 523–524
Pain Rating Scale (PRS) tool, 524
Pain rating scales
adults, 518–520, 528
behavioral assessment scales, 528
multidimensional, 519–520
unidimensional, 518–519
children, 520–521
behavioral assessment scales, 525, 526t, 527t
color tools, 520
Numerical Scale, 520–521
Oucher, 521
Poker Chip Tool, 521
visual analogue scale, 521
Wong-Baker FACES, 248t, 520
Word-Graphic Rating Scale, 521

infants, 523–524
selecting, 248t
using, 513
PAINAD (Pain Assessment in Advanced Dementia Scale), 528
Palmar erythema, 387b
Palmar grasp reflex, 421t
Palpation
abdomen,270b–274b
counterindications for, 216b
during pregnancy, 389b–394b
breasts
detecting cancer, 241b
during pregnancy, 389b
and lymph nodes, 240b–244b
carotid arteries and jugular veins, 185b–187b
cervix, 295b
external ear, 143b–144b
extremities, 218b–219b
eyes, 128b–133b, 432b
female genitourinary system, 294b–296b
head, neck, and face, 101b–106b
joints, 333b–342b
male genitourinary system, 309b–313b
mastoid, 143b
muscle, 331b–332b
newborns
abdomen, 415b–416b
eyes, 432b
fontanel, 410b
performing, 6f–7f, 21
precordium, 187b–189b
PV/lymphatic system, 218b–220b
sequences for respiratory, 167b, 168b
for ticklish patients, 274b
vagina, 294b–295b
Palpebral conjunctiva, 123b
Palpitations, 173
Paresthesia, 352t
Parkinson's disease, 353t
Parotid and submandibular glands, 90b, 103b
Paroxysmal nocturnal dyspnea (PND), 179t
Partner abuse, 595–596
Past health history, 17
PAT (Pain Assessment Tool), 523–524
Patellar reflex, 369b
Patient histories. *See also* Family medical history; Focused physical assessments; Psychosocial histories
collecting symptoms
abdomen, 247, 248, 249–252
breasts, 229, 231–232
cardiovascular system, 173–174
ears, 136–137
eyes, 109–111
female genitourinary system, 279–280
female sexual histories, 280, 281t–282t
head, neck, face, 74–76, 78
homeless patients, 503t
infant, 428, 428t–430t
integumentary system, 32–33
male genitourinary system, 299–302
pain symptoms, 517–521
pregnancy, 384
PV/lymphatic systems, 205–208
respiratory system, 153–154
general surveys of health, 16
including in do-not-resuscitate orders, 603–604, 604t–605t
information about spirituality, 569, 570–571
musculoskeletal system, 316–317
neurologic system, 347–348
nutritional assessments, 562–564
older adults, 473–474
past, 17
PQRST analysis of pain, 517–518
preschoolers/toddlers, 439–440, 443–444
signs of abuse
physical, 592–593
psychological, 594
sexual, 593–594
understanding nature of illness, 551t

PCL (posterior cruciate ligament), 340b
PCV (pneumococcal conjugate), 430t
Peers, 461, 468
Pelvic exams, 290b–293b
Penis
penile circumcision, 299, 306b, 417b
penile discharge, 258t
physical assessments of, 305b–307b, 309b–310b
Peptic ulcer disease, 255t–256t
Perceptions. *See also* Self-perceptions
of pain, 509, 524, 515t–516t
spatial, 353t, 356
temperature, 364b
Percussion
abdomen, 267b–269b
assessments using, 8f–10f, 22
bladder, 269b
chests of infants, 433b
during pregnancy, 389b
head, neck, and face, 106b
liver, 267b–268b
lungs, 168b
precordium, 190b
respiratory system, 168b
sounds produced by, 23t
spleen, 268b
Perimenopausal symptoms, 281t
Perineum, 398b
Peripheral-vascular (PV) system, 204–225. *See also* Blood pressure
collecting histories of, 205–208
cultural considerations, 205
developmental considerations, 204–205
effect on vision, 212t
physical assessments, 214f, 215b–225b
anatomical landmarks, 214f
assessing edema, 218b
auscultation during BP checks, 223b–225b
lower extremities, 216b–217b
palpation, 218b–221b
postpartal, 399b
upper extremities, 215b–216b
primary functions, 204
relationships to, 211t–213t
cardiovascular system, 212t
gastrointestinal system, 212t
general system, 211f
genitourinary/reproductive systems, 213t
HEENT, 211t–212t
integumentary system, 211t
musculoskeletal system, 213t
neurologic systems, 213t
respiratory system, 212t
tools for, 215
Peripheral vision, 118b, 491b
Peritonitis, 265b
Personal habits/behaviors
adolescents, 468
preschoolers/toddlers, 443–444
school-age children, 455
Petechiae, 351t
Phalen's test, 336b, 397b
Phencyclidine, 560t
Physical abuse
checking for, 592–593
of children, 591–592
Physical assessments, 4–11, 21–28. *See also* General health surveys
abdomen, 262b–274b
auscultation, 265b–266b
inspections, 262b–264b
newborns, 415b–416b
percussion for, 267b–269b
shapes, 262b
approach to, 21–22
assessing for physical abuse, 592–593
auscultation, 11, 22
breasts
adolescents, 471t
axilla, 240b
breast tissue, 237b–239b
nipple and areola, 239b–240b
cardiovascular system
abnormal pulses, 199f
adolescents, 464t, 470t
carotid arteries/jugular veins, 184t, 184b–187b, 352t
homeless patients, 507t
infants, 434b
older adults, 494b

preschoolers/toddlers, 446t
school-age children, 453t, 458t
documenting findings, 27
ears
angle of attachment, 140f, 141b–142b
ear canal, 145b–146b
external, 141b–142b, 143b–144b
hearing, 148b–151b
otoscopic exam, 144b–145b
tympanic membrane, 146b–148b
extremities of infants, 435b
eyes 115, 116b, 117b–133b
anterior chamber, 125b–126b
conjunctiva, 123b–124b
cornea, 118b, 124b–125b
extraocular muscles, 118b
eyeball, 122b
eyelashes, 121b–122b
eyelids, 120b–121b
general appearance of, 119b–120b
iris, 126b
lacrimal ducts, puncta, 122b
macula and fovea centralis, 133b
ophthalmoscopy in, 129b
palpation of, 128b–133b
pupils, 126b–128b
red reflex, 108, 129b–131b
retinal vessels, 131b–132b
sclera, 124b
female genitourinary system, 287, 288b–296b
approach, position, toolbox for, 287
genitalia/rectal, 26, 288b–291b, 296b
inspections during, 288b
palpation during, 294b–296b
pelvic exams, 290b–293b
reproductive system, 20
focused, 27–28
gastrointestinal system
adolescents, 465t, 471t
homeless patients, 507t
infants, 434b–435b
older adults, 494b–495b
preschoolers/toddlers 446t
school-age children, 453t, 458t
genitourinary system
adolescents, 471t
homeless patients, 508t
infants, 435b–436b
older adults, 495b
preschoolers/toddlers, 447t
school-age children, 453t, 458t
head, neck, and face, 85–86, 86b–106b
auscultation of, 106b
face, 87b–99b, 101b–102b
gingivae, 95b–96b
head, 86b, 101b
lips, 90b–91b, 103b
neck, thyroid, cervical lymph nodes, 100b–101b, 104b–106b
newborns, 410b–415b
nose, 88b–90b, 102b
oral mucosa, 91b–94b
oropharynx, soft palate, tonsils, uvula, 99b–100b, 103b
palpations of, 101b–106b
parotid and submandibular glands, 90b, 103b
percussion of, 106b
teeth, 96b–97b
tongue, 97b–99b, 103b
head-to-toe, 16, 21, 22, 24–27
HEENT
adolescents, 464t, 470t
infants, 432b–433b
older adults, 491b–500b
preschoolers/toddlers, 445t–447t
school-age children, 452t–453t, 457t–458t
homeless patients, 507t–508t
infants, 430b–436b
inspections, 4–5f
integumentary system, 41, 42b–56b
adolescents, 463t–464t, 469t
hair and scalp, 54b–56b
homeless patients, 507t
infants, 431b–432b
nails, 49b–54b
older adults, 489b–491b
preschoolers/toddlers, 445t

school-age children, 452t, 457t
skin, 42b–49b
lymphatic/hematological system
adolescents, 466t
school-age children, 454t
male genitourinary system
inguinal exams, 309b, 311b–312b
genitalia/rectal assessments, 27, 309b, 312b–313b
palpations, 309b–313b
penis, 305b–307b, 309b–310b
reproductive system, 20
scrotum, 308b
measurements and vital signs
preschoolers/toddlers, 445t
school-age children, 457t
mental health, 544t–545t
abdominal system, 545t
cardiovascular system, 545t
general system, 544t
HEENT system, 545t
integumentary system, 544t
musculoskeletal system, 545t
neurologic system, 545t
respiratory system, 545t
musculoskeletal system
accuracy of movements, 329b
adolescents, 466t, 471t
cerebellar function, 326b–327b, 500b
gaits, 325b–326b, 342b–343b
homeless patients, 508t
muscle palpation, 331b–332b
newborns, 418b–419b
older adults, 496b–498b
pronator drift, 330b, 354
school-age children, 453t
taking measurements, 330b–331b
testing coordination, 328b–329b, 447t
neurologic system, 355b–372b
about, 351t–354t
adolescents, 466t, 471t
cerebral functions, 356b–360b
cranial nerves, 360b–363b
homeless patients, 508t
infants, 436b
meningeal signs, 372b
older adults, 498b–500b
preschoolers/toddlers, 447t
school-age children, 454t, 458t
superficial reflexes, 370b–371b
newborns, 405, 406b–419b
Apgar scoring for, 405t
approach and tools for, 405
chest, 414b–415b
female genitourinary, 416b
integumentary, 408b–410b
male genitourinary, 417b–418b
neurologic system, 419b
rectum, 416b
respiratory system, 415b
nutrition, 565, 566b–568b
cardiovascular, 567b
general health survey, 566b
HEENT, 566b–567b
integumentary, 566b
musculoskeletal, 567b
neurologic, 568b
respiratory, 567b
older adults, 488, 489b–500b
palpations, 6f–7f, 21
percussion, 8f–10f, 22
PV/lymphatic systems, 214f, 215b–225b
respiratory system
adolescents, 464t, 470t
homeless patients, 507t
infants, 433b–434b
older adults, 493b
preschoolers/toddlers, 446t
school-age children, 453t, 458t
types of, 4–11, 21–22
Physical growth. *See* Growth
PIE mnemonic, 4
Pigeon chest, 414b
PMI (point of maximal impulse), 389b, 415b
PIPP (Premature Infant Pain Profile), 524
Piskacek's sign, 385t
Pivot joints, 321t
Plane/gliding joints, 322t
Plantar grasp reflex, 421t
Plantar reflex, 370b
Pleural effusion, 320t
PMS (premenstrual syndrome), 281t

Pneumococcal conjugate (PCV), 430t
Pneumonitis, 320t
Point localization, 366b
Point of maximal impulse (PIM), 389b, 415b
Poker Chip Tool, 521
Polio vaccine, inactivated, 430t, 439, 451
Polish Americans, 601t
Politics of community, 588t
POPS (Postoperative Pain Score), 524
Port-wine stain, 409b
Postconcussion syndrome, 357b
Posterior cruciate ligament (PCL), 340b
Posterior thorax/back assessments, 25
Postmenopausal women. *See* Pre/postmenopausal women
Postoperative Pain Score (POPS), 524
Postpartum exams
  depression, 400b, 531
  pregnancy assessments, 397, 398b–400b
Postpubescence, 459
Posture
  newborn's, 406b
  opisthotonic, 419b
  spinal curves and, 323b–325b
PQRST method. *See also* Patient histories
  pain analysis using, 517–518
Prayer, 444
Pre/postmenopausal women
  breasts of, 231, 235t, 240b
  cardiovascular risks of, 180t
Precordium
  assessments of, 185b
  auscultation of, 191b–193b
  palpations of, 187b–189b
  percussion of, 190b
Pregnancy, 375–400. *See also* Breasts; Childbirth practices; Fetus
  abdomen in, 245–246, 258t
  calculating conception date, 386
  cardiovascular system in, 172
  childbirth practices, 376–384
    African American, 377
    Amish, 377
    Appalachian, 378
    Arab American, 378
    Chinese American, 379
    Cuban American, 379
    Egyptian American, 379–380
    Filipino American, 380
    French Canadian, 380
    Greek American, 381
    how to assess, 577
    Iranian American, 381
    Irish American, 381–382
    Jewish American, 382
    Mexican American, 382–383
    Navajo Native American, 383
    Vietnamese American, 383–384
  collecting histories, 384, 405t
  developmental considerations
    adolescents, 375
    breasts, 227–228
    musculoskeletal system, 314–315
    older women, 375, 376
  diagnosing, 384, 385t
  fetal complications in, 375, 376t
  lordosis of, 325b
  mental health during, 530–531
  physical assessments 161t, 386–387, 387b–397b
    abdomen, 389b–394b
    approach, position, and tools, 386–387
    assessing fetal position, 273b, 392b–393b
    breasts, 389b
    cardiovascular system, 389b
    extremities, 394b
    female genitourinary system in, 275, 277–278
    genitourinary, 394b–395b
    head, face, and neck, 74
    HEENT, 388b–389b
    integumentary, 387b
    integumentary system in, 30
    musculoskeletal system, 397b
    neurologic system, 397b
    neurologic system in, 346

PV and lymphatic systems, 204–205
respiratory system, 152, 389b
postpartal assessments, 397, 398b–400b
prenatal lab tests, 386
teen, 375
Premature Infant Pain Profile (PIPP), 524
Premenstrual syndrome (PMS), 281t
Prepubescence, 459
Presbycusis, 135
Presbyopia, 108, 117b, 491b
Preschoolers/toddlers, 438–447
defined, 438
eyes of, 108
health history of, 439–440
physical assessments, 445t–447t
cardiovascular, 446t
gastrointestinal, 446t
general health survey, 445t
genitourinary system, 447t
HEENT, 445t–446t
integumentary system, 445t
measurements and vital signs, 445t
musculoskeletal system, 447t
neurologic system, 447t
respiratory, 446t
promoting health for, 439
psychosocial histories, 443–444
detecting emotional changes, 438–439
questions to ask, 440t–442t
cardiovascular system, 442t
gastrointestinal system, 442t
general health, 440t
genitourinary system, 442t
HEENT, 440t–441t
integumentary system, 440t
lymphatic/hematological system, 442t
neurologic system, 442t
respiratory system, 441t
spirituality of, 569–570
Pressure ulcers, 65t–66t
Preventative health care levels, 2
Priapism, 307b, 310b
Primary teeth, 452t
Primitive reflexes, 371b, 500b
Pronator drift, 330b, 354
Property abuse, 591
Propulsive gait, 342t
Prostate
abdomen and relationship to, 258t
benign prostatic hypertrophy, 495b
cancer of, 495b
palpating, 313b
questions to ask older men about, 481t
PRS (Pain Rating Scale) tool, 524
Pruritus and liver disease, 255t
Psychological abuse
checking for possible, 594
of children, 592
defined, 591
Psychosocial histories
adolescents, 460–461, 466–469
developing psychosocial profile, 21
evaluating in death process, 606, 606t
homeless patients, 504t
mental health, 542t–544t
activity, 542t
cultural influences, 543t
daily activities, 542t
environment, 543t
family roles/relationships, 544t
health practices and beliefs, 542t
nutrition, 542t
occupational health, 543t
personal habits, 543t
recreation/hobbies, 543t
religious influence, 543t
roles/relationships/self-concept, 543t
sexuality patterns, 544t
sleep/rest, 543t
stress and coping patterns, 544t
older adults, 484, 484b–485b
personal habits and, 543t
preschoolers/toddlers, 438–444
school-age children, 448–449, 454–456
Psychotropic drugs, 539t–540t
Pterygium, 492b
Pubertal delays, 465t

Puberty, 459
Puerto Rican Americans, 601t
Pull-to-Sit reflex, 425t
Pulses
  abnormal, 199f
  amplitude scale for, 219b
  auscultating during BP checks, 223b–225b
  checking in PV/lymphatic assessments, 219b–221b
  Corrigan's, 199b
  infant, 434b
  newborn, 408b
  palpating
    brachial, 223b
    neck vessels for, 186b–187b
  point of maximal impulse, 389b, 415b
  postpartal assessments of, 398b
Puncta, 122b
Pupils
  changes in reaction of, 113b
  consensual reaction of, 127b, 128b
  infant, 107
  physical assessments, 126b–128b
PV system. *See* Peripheral-vascular system

R

Radial and ulnar arteries, 220b–221b
Rashes
  meningitis and, 351t
  related to
    female genitourinary system, 284t
    musculoskeletal system, 319t
Rating scales
  children's mental health, 529t
  geriatric depression, 533b
  pain
    adults, 518–520, 528
    children, 520–521, 525, 526t, 527t
    infants, 523–524
  using, 513
Raynaud's disease, 352t
Rebound tenderness test, 272b
Recreation/hobbies
  adolescents, 468
  mental health and, 543t
  preschoolers/toddlers, 444
  school-age children, 455
Rectal exams
  female, 26, 290b, 296b
  infants, 436b
  male, 27, 309b, 312b–313b
  newborn, 416b
  older adults, 494b–495b
Red reflex of eyes, 108, 129b–131b
Reflexes
  abdominal, 273b, 370b
  Achilles, 369b
  assessing newborn's neurologic, 419b
  biflex, 368b
  brachioradialis, 369b
  corneal, 118b, 125b
  deep tendon, 367b–368b, 500b
  gag, 103b, 362b
  infant blink, 107–108
  newborn, 420t–426t
    Babinski's, 371b, 422t
    crawling, 424t
    crossed extension, 425t
    extrusion, 414b, 424t
    glabellar, 424t
    inspecting, 414b
    magnet, 426t
    Moro, 420t
    palmar grasp, 421t
    plantar grasp, 421t
    pull-to-sit, 425t
    rooting reflex, 371b, 414b, 423t
    startle, 412b, 420t
    stepping, 422t
    sucking, 371b, 414b, 423t
    swallowing, 414b, 423t
    tonic neck, 420t–421t
    trunk incurvation, 426t
  patellar, 369b
  primitive, 371b, 500b
  red, 108, 129b–131b
  superficial, 370b–372b
    anal, 370b
    bulbocavernosus, 371b
    cremasteric, 370b–371b
    plantar, 370b
  triceps, 368b–369b
Relationships. *See* Roles

Religious influences. *See also* Spirituality
  circumcision and, 382, 403, 404
  effect on mental health, 537t
  homeless patients, 506t
Replanting secondary teeth, 452t–453t
Reproductive system. *See also* Genitourinary system
  collecting histories, women, 280, 281t–282t
  physical assessments, 20
    adolescents, 469t–471t
    during pregnancy, 394b–397b
    female genitalia/rectal exams, 20, 26, 290b
    homeless patients, 508t
    infants, 435b–436b
    male genitalia/rectal exams, 27, 309b, 312b–313b
    older men, 495b
    pregnant women, 386–387, 387b–397b
    preschoolers/toddlers, 447t
    school-age children, 458t
  relationship to
    abdomen, 257t–258t
    ears, 139t
    eyes, 114b
    head, neck, and face, 82t–83t
    integumentary system, 39t–40t
    musculoskeletal system, 320t
    neurologic system, 353t
    PV/lymphatic systems, 213t
Respiration rates
  Cheyne-Stokes, 165b, 179t, 493b
  newborn, 408b
  types of, 164b–165b
Respiratory system, 152–171
  assessment of, 19
  auscultation of newborns, 415b
  collecting symptoms of, 153–154
  cultural considerations, 153
  developmental considerations, 152
  drugs adversely effecting, 155t–156t
  evaluating in death process, 605t, 608b
  infant's, 429t
  nutritional assessments and, 567b
  physical assessments
    adolescents, 470t
    anatomical landmarks, 163f
    approach, position, tools for, 164
    auscultation for, 169b–171b
    chest, 164b
    chest shapes, 165b–166b, 179t
    during pregnancy, 389b
    homeless patients, 507t
    infants, 433b–434b
    mental health, 545t
    muscles used, 166b
    nutrition, 567b
    older adults, 493b
    percussion for, 168b
    preschoolers/toddlers, 446t
    respiratory patterns, 164b–165b
    school-age children, 458t
    skin, 166b
    using palpation, 167b
  postpartal assessment of, 398b
  primary function, 152
  questions to ask
    adolescents, 464t
    older adults, 478t
    preschoolers/toddlers, 441t
    school-age children, 453t
  relationship to, 157t–162t
    abdomen, 257t
    breasts, 234t
    cardiovascular system, 160t, 179t, 320t
    ears, 139t
    endocrine system, 162t
    eyes, 113b
    female genitourinary system, 285t
    gastrointestinal system, 161t
    general system, 157t
    head, neck, and face, 81t
    HEENT, 159t–160t
    integumentary system, 158t–159t
    lymphatic/hematological system, 162t
    male genitourinary system, 303t
    musculoskeletal system, 161t, 320t

neurologic system, 162t, 352t
PV/lymphatic systems, 212t
Rest patterns. *See* Sleep
Restlessness, 547t
Retina
detachment of, 477t
retinal vessels, 131b–132b
Rheumatoid arthritis (RA)
effect on fingers and thumbs, 337b–338b
signs of, 319t, 320t, 321t
Ribs, 335b
Right ventricular hypertrophy, 198f
Riley Infant Pain Scale (RIPS), 525, 526t
Rinne test, 150b–151b
RIPS (Riley Infant Pain Scale), 525, 526t
Risks
adolescents, 461
risk taking, 530, 530b
suicide, 530b
found in patient's home, 582t–584t
high-risk behaviors of groups, 576
older adults
falls of, 484b–485b
suicide, 532, 533b
preschoolers/toddlers, 439
school-age children, 449, 454
suicide, 532, 533b, 553–554, 553b, 554b
Roles
families and cultural, 574–575
homeless patients, 505t
mental health and, 543t, 544t
with peers, 461, 468
preschool children, 444
related to patient's spirituality, 572
school-age children, 456
sex role identity, 469
Romberg test, 151b, 326b–327b, 500b
Rooting reflex, 371b, 414b, 423t
Rovsing's sign, 272b
Russian Americans, 601t

S

Saddle joints, 322t
Safety
patient's home, 582t–585t
preschoolers/toddlers, 444
SBAR mnemonic, 3
Scalp. *See* Hair
Scapulae, 335b
Schizophrenia, 547t, 550t–551t, 554b
School-age children, 448–459
abuse of, 459
changes
physical growth, 448
psychosocial/emotional, 448–449
cultural perspectives about, 450t–451t
defined, 448
eyes of, 108
immunizations for, 451
medications taken by, 451
physical assessments, 457t–458t
cardiovascular system, 458t
gastrointestinal system, 458t
general health, 457t
genitourinary system, 458t
HEENT system, 457t–458t
integumentary system, 457t
measurements and vital signs, 457t
musculoskeletal system, 458t
neurologic system, 458t
respiratory system, 458t
promoting health of, 449
psychosocial history of, 454–456
questions to ask, 451, 452t–454t, 463t–466t
cardiovascular system, 453t
gastrointestinal system, 453t
general health, 452t
genitourinary system, 453t
HEENT, 452t–453t
integumentary system, 452t
musculoskeletal system, 453t
neurologic system, 454t
respiratory system, 453t
spirituality of, 569–570
SCIDS (severe combined immunodeficiency syndrome), 205
Scissors gait, 343t
Sclera
infant's, 107
jaundice viewed in, 114b

newborn's, 412b
physical assessments, 120b, 124b
Scoliosis, 324b, 453t
Scratch test for liver, 265b
Scrotum
assessing, 308b
auscultation of, 313b
inspecting newborn, 417b
palpating, 310b
Seasonal skin disorders, 33t–34t
Seborrheic keratosis, 489b
Seizures, 482t
Self-perceptions
adolescents, 468
home-care patients, 585t
homeless patients, 505t
mental health and, 543t
school-age children, 456
Senile purpura, 490b
Sensitization to pain, 509
Sensory functions, 363b–369b. *See also* Neurologic system
biceps reflex, 368b
changes in, 347, 351t–353t, 361b–362b
deep sensations, 364b
deep tendon reflexes, 367b–368b, 500b
discriminatory, 365b–366b
kinesthetics, 364b–365b
touch, pain, and temperature tests, 363b–364b
Severe combined immunodeficiency syndrome (SCIDS), 205
Sexual abuse
checking for possible, 593–594
of children, 592
defined, 591
Sexual activity
changes related to
neurologic signs, 353t
respiratory signs, 161t
lesions related to male, 302t
UTIs and, 465t
Sexuality. *See also* Sexual activity; Sexually transmitted diseases
collecting histories
homeless patients, 506t
male genitourinary system, 300–301
from women, 281t–282t
developmental considerations
achieving sexual maturity, 460
adolescents, 444
older adults, 481t
preschoolers/toddlers, 444
school-age children, 456
men's performance problems, 180t, 213t, 353t
mental health and, 544t
musculoskeletal functioning and, 286t
sex role identity, 469
Sexually transmitted diseases (STDs)
abdominal indicators of, 257t–258t
adolescents' protection against, 468–469
effect on musculoskeletal system, 320t
eyes indicating, 114b
female concerns about, 280, 481t
men and, 304t
oropharynx and eyes as sites for, 285t, 303t
PV/lymphatic symptoms of, 213t
related neurologic signs of, 353t
Shingles, 255t
Shoulders, 335b, 433b
Sibling rivalry, 444
Sickle cell anemia, 259t, 304t, 310b, 376, 386
SIGECAPS mnemonic, 552–553
Sinuses
physical assessment of, 89b–90b, 102b, 106b
respiratory system effects on, 159t
Sjögren's syndrome, 319t
Skene's glands, 294b, 394b
Skills
communication, 359b–360b
critical thinking, 1
ethical, 2
nurse's communication, 3
writing, 360b
Skin
age-related disorders, 31t
assessments of, 42b–49b
conducting, 22
older adults, 489b–491b
color of, 56t–58t, 575
drugs adversely effecting, 34t–36t

homeless patients, 504t
lesions
clinical description of, 66t–67t
distribution of, 70t–72t
external genitalia, 279
older adults, 500t
oral mucosa, 285t, 303t
patterns of, 68t–69t
primary, 59t–61t
secondary, 61t–63t
vascular, 64t–65t
newborns, 408b–409b
nutrition and, 566b
older adults, 475t–476t
pressure ulcers, 65t–66t
relationship to
cardiovascular changes, 176t–177t
female genitourinary system, 284t
PV/lymphatic systems, 211t
seasonal disorders of, 33t–34t
SLE (systemic lupus erythematosus), 319t–321t
Sleep
adolescents, 467–468
during death process, 606t
homeless patients, 505t
mental health and, 543t
older adults, 485b
preschoolers/toddlers, 443
school-age children, 455
Slurred speech, 354
Smell
changes in sense of, 351t
checking olfactory nerve, 360b–361b
Smoking, second-hand, 443–444
Snellen E chart, 108
Snout reflex, 371b
SOAPIE mnemonic, 4
Socioeconomic status of homeless, 505t
Soft palate, 99b–100b
Sounds
assessing voice, 171b
bowel, 320t
auscultating, 265b
investigating, 212t
pregnant women, 246
breathing, 169b–170b
bronchial, 170b
cardiovascular
heart sounds, 199b–200b, 202t, 285t
murmurs, 192b–193b, 196f–197f, 203t
Korotkoff sounds, 224b–225b
produced by percussion, 23t
testing recognition of, 359b
Spastic gait, 343t
Spatial perception, 353t, 356
Speculum, 290b–294b
Speech
assessing
with Glasgow Coma Scale, 355t
for neurologic problems, 358b–359b
changes in, 351t
slurred, 354
Spinal bifida, 419b
Spinal stenosis, 353t
Spine
cauda equina syndrome, 259t, 353t
cervical spine joints, 334b
curvature of
infant's, 433b
posture and, 324b–325b
Spinoaccessory nerve, 363b
Spirituality, 569–572
assessing patient's, 569, 571–572
collecting in health histories, 570–571
cultural considerations about, 570, 577–578
developmental considerations, 569–570
adolescents, 570
children, 569–570
infants, 569
older adults, 570
prayers for preschoolers/toddlers, 444
questions to ask about, 572
Spleen
auscultating, 266b
palpating, 270b, 271b
percussion of, 268b
Spousal abuse, 595–596
Stages of grief, 602, 602t–603t

Staging criteria for pressure ulcers, 65t–66t
Startle reflex, 412b, 420t
STDs. *See* Sexually transmitted diseases
Stensen's ducts, 93b
Steppage gait, 343t
Stepping reflex, 422t
Stereognosis, 365b
Stiffness, musculoskeletal, 317, 497b
Stimulants, 558t
Stools
  breast-fed infants, 436b
  occult blood in, 296b, 312b
Strabismus, 108
Strawberry marks, 409b
Stress incontinence, 483t
Stress tolerance
  adolescents, 467, 469
  mental health and, 544t
  preschoolers/toddlers, 444
  school-age children, 456
Stroke. *See also* Neurologic system
  birth control pills and risk of, 353t
  bleeding disorders and risk of, 354t
  bowel and bladder function and, 35tb
  Cincinnati Prehospital Stroke Scale, 354
  increased risk of, 352t–353t
  indicators suggesting, 351t
  NIH Stroke Scale, 354–355
Sublingual glands, 103b
Submandibular glands. *See* Parotid and submandibular glands
Substance abuse
  assessing, 555, 555b–556b
  CAGE questionnaire, 555, 556b
  effects of use and withdrawal, 557t–561t
  spousal abuse and, 596
  suicide risks for, 554b
Sucking reflex, 371b, 414b, 423t
Suicide
  assessing risk of, 553–554, 553b, 554t–555t
  older adults, 532, 533b
  spousal abuse and, 596
  teen, 530b
  thoughts of, 550t
Superficial reflexes, 370b–372b
Support systems
  during death process, 606t
  for home care, 584t–585t
Swallowing
  aspiration risks and difficulty, 352t
  changes in, 351t–352t
  inspecting newborn's, 414b, 423t
  problems, 256t
  questions to ask older adults, 477t–478t
Swelling. *See also* Edema
  cardiovascular disease and, 478t–479t
  collecting patient histories for, 205–206
  in male genitourinary system, 300
Syncope
  assessing causes of, 178t
  assessing patient history of, 347
  cardiological causes of, 181t
  choking game and, 530b
  collecting histories of, 173
Synovial joints, 321t–322t
Syphilis
  assessing, 285t
  development of neurosyphilis, 287t
  effect on musculoskeletal system, 320t
  muscle strength and neurosyphilis, 286t, 304t
  newborn signs of, 409b
Systemic lupus erythematosus (SLE), 319t, 320t, 321t
Systolic murmurs, 196f

T

Tachypnea respiratory rate, 165b
Tactile fremitus, 167b
Tactile hallucinations, 550t
Tanner stages of breast development, 227f–228f, 460
Taste, 351t, 362b, 363b
Tattoos, 464t, 469t
Tay-Sachs disease, 377, 404
TD (tetanus–diphtheria) immunization, 451

Tdap immunization, 463
Teaching breast self-exams, 229b–230b
Tear glands and ducts
absence of tearing
in infants, 432b
in newborns, 412b
dry eyes, 476t
physical assessments of, 128b
tear production, 108, 109, 110
Teens. *See* Adolescents
Teeth. *See also* Gingivae
adolescents, 464t, 470t
natal, 414b
older adults, 493b
physical assessments, 96b–97b
questions to ask
preschoolers/toddlers, 441t
school-age children, 452t–453t
Temperature
extremities of older adults, 491b
infant's, 431b
newborn's, 407b
perceptions of, 364b
Temporal artery, 491b
Temporal bone, 144b
Temporomandibular joint, 334b
Tennis elbow, 335b
Testes, 308b, 310b–311b, 418b
Testing. *See also* Reflexes; *and specific tests*
accuracy of movements, 329b
Allen's, 108, 219b
for appendicitis, 271b–272b
arousal state, 372t–373t
clonus, 368b
color change tests, 220b–221b, 222b
communication skills, 359b–360b
Coombs', 209t
coordination, 328b–329b, 447t
corneal reflex, 118b, 125b
deep sensation, 364b
discriminatory functions, 365b–366b
ears
hearing tests, 148b–151b, 359b
Rinne test, 150b–151b
Weber test, 149b–150b
extraocular muscles, 118b–119b
fluid wave, 216b, 272f
gag reflex, 103b, 362b
infant developmental, 437t
kyphosis and scoliosis, 324b
memory, 357b
muscle strength, 332b, 436b
newborn diagnostic/screening, 427t
older adults' knowledge and vocabulary, 358b
peripheral vision, 118b
Phalen's or Tinel's, 336b, 397b
prenatal laboratory, 386
pupillary reactions to light, 127f
Romberg test, 151b, 326b–327b, 500b
scratch test for liver, 265b
speech, 358b, 359b
Thomas's, 339b
touch, pain, and temperature, 363b–364b
Trendelenburg test, 216b, 222b, 338b
urine tests, 386, 437t
verbal comprehension, 359b–360b
Tetanus-diphtheria (TD) immunization, 451
Thermometers, mercury, 431b
Thinking
assessing critical, 1
cerebral functions and process of, 358b
patient's mental state and, 549t–550t
Thomas's testing, 339b
Thoracic and lumbar curve, 338b
Thought process, 358b
Threats to self or others, 536
Throat. *See also* Ears; Nose
assessments of mouth and, 19
nutritional assessments and, 567b
physical assessments
during pregnancy, 388b–389b
infant's, 433b
newborn's, 413b–414b
older adults, 477t–478t, 493b
school-age children, 457t–458t
relationship to
abdomen, 256t–257t
cardiovascular system, 179t

ears, 138t
female genitourinary system, 285t
head, face, and neck, 80t–81t
integumentary system, 38t
PV/lymphatic systems, 212t
sore, 256t
Thrombophlebitis
oral contraceptives and, 285t
respiratory indicators of, 160t
symptoms of, 215b, 216b, 222b
Thumbs, 337b–338b, 418b
Thyroid
enlarged, 285t
hypo-/hyperthyroidism, 105b, 285t
neuropathies and disease of, 354t
physical assessments, 100b, 104b–105b
older adults, 482t, 491b
postpartal checkups, 398b
relationship to
abdomen, 256t, 259t
cardiovascular system, 181t
female genitourinary system, 287t
male genitourinary system, 304t
musculoskeletal system, 319t, 321t
neurologic system, 352t
respiratory system, 162t
TIA (transient ischemic attack), 351t
Time orientation, 356b–357b
Timing of death, 602
Tinea cruris (jock itch), 307b
Tinel's test, 336b, 397b
Tinnitus, 136, 139t, 179t
Toddlers. *See* Preschoolers/toddlers
Toe tapping, 329b
Toes. *See also* Lower extremities
inspecting newborn's, 418b
inspection/palpation of, 341b–342b
Tolerance of pain, 509
Tongue
hypoglossal nerve and, 363b
infant's protruding, 433b
physical assessments, 97b–99b, 103b
Tonic neck reflex, 420t–421t
Tonsils, 99b–100b
Tools for assessments
abdomen, 262
about, 12t–15t
breast examinations, 237
cardiovascular system, 184
color assessment, 520
ears, 141, 144b–145b
eyes and ears, 115
female genitourinary system, 287
head, face, and neck, 86
integumentary system, 42
male genitourinary system, 305
musculoskeletal system, 323
neurologic system, 355
newborns, 405
nutrition, 565
older adults, 488
PV/lymphatic systems, 215
respiratory system, 164
stethoscope for infants, 434b
used in pregnancy assessments, 387
Touch
changes in sense of, 351t
testing sense of, 363b–364b
Trachea, 167b
Tragus of ear, 143b
Transduction, 509
Transient ischemic attack (TIA), 351t
Transmission, 509
Trendelenburg test, 216b, 222b, 338
Triceps reflex, 368b
Trichomonas, 290b
Tricuspid regurgitation, 198f
Trigeminal nerve, 361b
Trochlear nerve, 361b
Trunk incurvation reflex, 426t
24-hour recall technique, 564–565
Two-point discrimination, 366b
Tympanic membrane (TM)
illustrated, 141f
physical assessments of, 146b–148b
position of, 140

U

Ulcers
pressure, 65t–66t
venous stasis, 217b

Umbilical hernias, 263b, 416b
Umbilicus, 263b
Unidimensional pain scales, 518–519
Upper extremities
assessing, 25, 215b–216b
color change test, 220b–221b
coordination of, 328b
exercise-induced pain of, 213t
inspecting
infant's, 435b
joints of, 334b–338b
newborn's, 419b
measuring arm lengths, 330b
numbness of, 259t
palpation of, 218b–219b
patient histories for, 174, 205–208
Urethra, 289b
Urge incontinence, 483t
Urinary meatus, 305b–307b
Urinary tract infections (UTI), 465t
Urination
CHF and nocturnal, 180t, 213t
newborn, 416b, 417b
symptoms
pain during female, 280
related to abdomen, 257t–258t
related to men's, 300
urinary incontinence, 480t
Urine tests
calculating fetal conception with, 386
infant urine screening, 437t
Uterus
assessing during pregnancy, 397b
palpating, 295b
uterine contractions, 390b–391b
Uvula, 99b–100b

V

Vagina
assessments during pregnancy, 395b
bleeding of, 279
discharge from, 279
infections of, 258t, 278, 290b
inspections of
cervix, 290b–293b
walls, 293b
palpation of, 294b–295b
presence of newborn, 416b
taking pool smear, 292b
Vagus nerve, 362b–363b
Values
adolescents, 469
community, 589t
homeless patients, 504t
preschoolers/toddlers, 444
school-age children, 456
Valvular heart sounds, 199b–200b
VAR immunization, 463
Varicosities, 216b, 222b
Vas deferens, 311b
Vascular disease, 114b
Vascular lesions, 64t–65t
Veins
auscultation of, 223b–225b
distension of neck, 159t, 160t
jugular
abnormal jugular venous waves, 198f
palpations of, 185b–187b
pressure and pulsation of, 184b–185b
waves correlated to cardiac cycle, 197f
thrombosis of deep, 219b, 394b
Venous hums, 190b–191b, 197f
Venous stasis ulcers, 217b
Vertigo
assessing patient history of, 347, 482t
symptoms of, 136, 139t
Vibratory sensations, 364b
Vietnamese Americans
childbirth practices, 382
response to pain, 516t
views on
adolescents, 462t
infants, 404
mental health, 536t
older adults, 473t
school-age children, 451t
Vision
assessing newborn's, 412b
changes in sense of, 351t, 352t
checking optic nerve, 361b
collecting history of, 109–111
double, 110, 178t

headaches/migraines and, 113b, 178t
hypertension and, 212t
inspecting visual acuity, 117b–118b
loss of, 109
PV/lymphatic systems effect on, 212t
testing visual recognition, 360b
Visual Analogue Scale, 519, 521
Visual hallucinations, 550t
Vital signs
anthropometric measurements of, 16
effect of age on, 23t
evaluating in death process, 606, 607b
postpartal assessment of, 398b
preschoolers/toddlers, 445t
school-age children, 457t
Voice
assessing sounds of, 171b
quality of, 362b
Vomiting, 251
VZV (chickenpox) vaccine, 440, 451

W

Waddling gait, 343t
Walking. *See* Gait
Weakness
assessing muscle, 332b, 340b, 353t–354t
of musculoskeletal system, 317, 320t
spinoaccessory nerve and muscle, 363b
Weber test, 149b–150b
Weight. *See also* Nutrition
cardiovascular symptoms and gain of, 176t
changes in
abdominal assessments and, 249
female genitourinary system and, 284t
infant, 428b
male genitourinary assessments and, 304t
distribution in older adults, 475t
edema of upper extremities and, 215b
weighing infants, 431b
Wet macular degeneration, 133b
Wharton's ducts, 93b
Women. *See also* Birth control pills; Female genitourinary system; Menstruation
abuse of, 595–596
birth control pills, 181t, 235t, 282t
breast self-examination for, 229b–230b
breathing styles of, 166b
development of breasts, 227f–228f, 460
HRT, 181t, 235t, 320t
last menstrual period for, 258t
mental health of pregnant, 530–531
pelvic exams, 290b–293b
pre/postmenopausal
breasts of, 231, 235t, 240b
cardiovascular risks of, 180t
reproductive/menstrual/sexuality history of, 281t–282t
vaginal infections, 258t, 278b
Wong-Baker FACES pain rating scales, 248t, 520
Word-Graphic Rating Scale, 521
Workforce issues, 575
Wounds, 177t
Wrists, 336b
Writing skills, 360b

X

Xanthelasma, 492b
Xerostomia, 477t–478t